GERIATRIC REHABILITATION MANUAL

EDITOR

TIMOTHY L. KAUFFMAN, Ph.D., P.T.

Kauffman-Gamber Physical Therapy
Lancaster, Pennsylvania

ASSOCIATE EDITORS

Osa Jackson, Ph.D., P.T.
Director
Physical Therapy Center
Rochester Hills, Michigan

Pamela Reynolds, M.S., P.T., G.C.S.
Assistant Professor
Chatham College
Pittsburgh, Pennsylania

John Barr, Ph.D., P.T.
Professor and Director
Physical Therapy Department
St. Ambrose University
Davenport, Iowa

Michael Moran, Sc.D., P.T.
Associate Professor
College Misericordia
Dallas, Pennsylvania

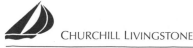
CHURCHILL LIVINGSTONE

A Division of Harcourt Brace & Company
New York, Edinburgh, London, Philadelphia, San Francisco

CHURCHILL LIVINGSTONE
A Division of Harcourt Brace & Company

The Curtis Center
Independence Square West
Philadelphia, Pennsylvania 19106

Library of Congress Cataloging-in-Publication Data

Geriatric rehabilitation manual/[edited by] Timothy L. Kauffman.—1st ed.

p.   cm.

ISBN 0–443–07651–0

1. Physical therapy for the aged Handbooks, manuals,
    etc.   2. Aged—Rehabilitation Handbooks, manuals, etc.   I. Kauffman,
    Timothy L.

[DNLM: 1. Rehabilitation—Aged.   WT 166 G3697 1999]

RC953.8.P58G48   1999

618.97—dc21

DNLM/DLC   99–19075

GERIATRIC REHABILITATION MANUAL   ISBN 0–443–07651–0

Copyright © 1999 by Churchill Livingstone.

Printed in the United States of America.

Last digit is the print number: 9   8   7   6   5   4   3   2   1

To my wife, Brenda
To my son, Ben
To my daughter, Emily
To my parents, Walter and Lillian
Bob and Lois

To the families
of all of the contributors

To all of our patients
who teach us so much

CONTRIBUTORS

Kristen D. Alexander, M.A., CCC/A

Audiologist, Crozer–Chester Medical Center, Upland, Pennsylvania

Louis R. Amundsen, Ph.D., P.T.

Professor and Chairman, Department of Physical Therapy, College of Pharmacy and Allied Health Professions, Wayne State University, Detroit, Michigan

E. Frederick Barrick, M.D.

Associate Clinical Professor, Department of Orthopaedic Surgery, Georgetown University School of Medicine, Washington, D.C.; Director of Orthopaedic Trauma, Inova Fairfax Hospital, Falls Church, Virginia

Margaret Basiliadis, D.O.

Independence Practice, Family Geriatrics, PLLC, Fort Worth, Texas

Randy Berger, M.D.

Clinical Instructor in Dermatology, Boston University School of Medicine; Assistant Dermatologist, Boston Medical Center, Boston, Massachusetts

Neil Binkley, M.D.

Assistant Professor of Medicine, University of Wisconsin, Madison, Wisconsin

Jennifer M. Bottomley, Ph.D., M.S., P.T.

Core Faculty, Harvard Division on Aging, Boston; Geriatric Rehabilitation Program Consultant, Wayland, Massachusetts

Mark A. Brimer, Ph.D., P.T.

Rehabilitative Services, Holmes Regional Medical Center, Inc., Melbourne, Florida

Mary M. Checovich, M.S.

Associate Researcher, Division of Orthopedic Surgery, Institute on Aging, University of Wisconsin, Madison, Wisconsin

Ronni Chernoff, Ph.D., R.D., FADA

Professor, Nutrition and Dietetics, University of Arkansas for Medical Sciences; Associate Director for Education and Evaluation, Geriatric Research Education and Clinical Center, Central Arkansas Healthcare System, Little Rock, Arkansas

Charles D. Ciccone, Ph.D., P.T.

Professor, Department of Physical Therapy, Ithaca College, Ithaca, New York

Joseph Cipriani, Ed.D., OTR/L

Associate Professor, Department of Occupational Therapy, College Misericordia, Dallas, Pennsylvania; Occupational Therapist, Penn State–Geisinger Wyoming Valley Medical Center, Wilkes-Barre, Pennsylvania

Meryl Cohen, M.S., P.T., C.C.S.

Adjunct Instructor, Division of Physical Therapy, Department of Orthopedics and Rehabilitation, University of Miami School of Medicine, Coral Gables, Florida; Adjunct Instructor, Massachusetts General Hospital Institute of Health Professions, Boston, Massachusetts

Deborah L. Cooke, Ph.D., P.T.

Associate Professor, Physical Therapy Education, Rockhurst College, Kansas City, Missouri

Paula Curliss, M.A., CCC/A

Audiologist, Crozer–Chester Medical Center, Upland, Pennslvania

Joanne Dalgleish, M.D.

Australia

Gordon M. Dickinson, M.D.

Professor of Medicine, University of Miami School of Medicine; Clinical Director, Special Immunology Section, Miami VA Medical Center, Miami, Florida

Joan E. Edelstein, M.A., P.T., F.I.S.P.O.

Associate Professor of Clinical Physical Therapy and Director, Program in Physical Therapy, Columbia University, New York, New York

Reenie Euhardy, M.S., P.T., G.C.S.

Faculty Associate, University of Wisconsin–Madison; Physical Therapist, Madison GRECC, VA Great Lakes Health Care System, Madison, Wisconsin

Walter R. Frontera, M.D., Ph.D.

Chairman and Associate Professor of Physical Medicine and Rehabilitation, Harvard Medical School; Chief, Physical Medicine and Rehabilitation, Spaulding Rehabilitation Hospital and Massachusetts General Hospital, Boston, Massachusetts

Barbara A. Gilchrest, M.D.

Professor and Chairman, Department of Dermatology, Boston University School of Medicine; Chief of Dermatology, Boston Medical Center, Boston, Massachusetts

Stephen A. Gudas, Ph.D., P.T.

Assistant Professor, Department of Anatomy, and Physical Therapist, Cancer Rehabilitation, Medical College of Virginia, Virginia Commonwealth University, Richmond, Virginia

Patricia A. Hageman, Ph.D., P.T.

Director and Associate Professor, Physical Therapy Education, University of Nebraska Medical Center, Omaha, Nebraska

June Hanks, M.S., P.T.

Assistant Professor, Physical Therapy Program, University of Tennessee at Chattanooga, Chattanooga, Tennessee

Osa Jackson, Ph.D., P.T.

Lecturer, Geriatric Special Interest Group, Norwegian Physical Therapy Association, Oslo, Norway; Director, Physical Therapy Center, Rochester Hills, Michigan

Jill Johnson, M.S., P.T.

Physical Therapist, Valley Regional Hospital, Claremont, New Hampshire

Joseph Kahn, Ph.D., P.T.

Clinical Assistant Professor Emeritus, Physical Therapy Program, State University of New York, Stony Brook; Private Practice, Syosset, New York

Robert R. Karpman, M.D.

Chief of Orthopedics, University of Arizona, College of Medicine, Phoenix, Arizona

Timothy L. Kauffman, Ph.D., P.T.

Kauffman-Gamber Physical Therapy, Lancaster, Pennsylvania

David E. Kelley, M.D.

University of Pittsburgh, Pittsburgh, Pennsylvania

Edmund M. Kosmahl, P.T., Ed.D.

Associate Professor, Department of Physical Therapy, University of Scranton, Scranton, Pennsylvania

Diane Krueger, B.S.

Research Program Manager, Institute on Aging, University of Wisconsin, Madison, Wisconsin

Gert Kwakkel, Ph.D., P.T.

Research Coordinator and Physical Therapist, Department of Physical Therapy, VU Hospital, Amsterdam, The Netherlands

Lars Larsson, M.D., Ph.D.

Marie Underhill Noll Professor, Noll Physiological Research Center, The Pennsylvania State University, University Park, Pennsylvania

David Levine, Ph.D., P.T.

UC Foundation Associate Professor of Physical Therapy, University of Tennessee at Chattanooga; Physical Therapist, Siskin Hospital for Physical Rehabilitation, Chattanooga, Tennessee

Rosanne W. Lewis, M.S., P.T., G.C.S.

Geriatric Clinical Specialist, Home Health Agency, Lodi Memorial Hospital, Lodi, California

Katie Lundon, Ph.D., P.T.

Assistant Professor, Department of Physical Therapy, Faculty of Medicine, University of Toronto, Toronto, Ontario, Canada

Michelle M. Lusardi, Ph.D., P.T.

Associate Professor, Physical Therapy, and Project Director of Elders 2000, College of Education and Health Professions, Sacred Heart University, Fairfield, Connecticut

Zoran Maric, M.D.

Chief, Orthopaedic Spine Service, Phoenix Orthopaedic Residency Program, Maricopa Medical Center and St. Luke's Medical Center, Phoenix, Arizona

Carolyn Marshall, M.P.H., Ph.D.

Associate Director, South Texas Geriatric Education Center, University of Texas Health Science Center, San Antonio, Texas

David C. Martin, M.D.

Clinical Professor of Medicine, Psychiatry, and Health Services Administration, University of Pittsburgh; Director, Geriatric Medicine Fellowship, UPMC Shadyside, Pittsburgh, Pennsylvania

Jeff A. Martin, M.D.

Formerly of Orthocare International, Phoenix, Arizona

Melen R. McBride, Ph.D.

Associate Director, Stanford Geriatric Education Center, Division of Family and Community Medicine, Stanford University, Palo Alto, California

Patrick McDonald, M.S.

Adjunct Professor, Sociology Department, Luzerne County Community College, Nanticoke; Director of Social Work and Coordinator of Bereavement Services, Hospice Preferred Choice, Clarks Summit, Pennsylvania

Wayne K. McKinley, P.T.

Clinical Manager, Nova Care, Inc., Outpatient Rehabilitation, Lebanon, Pennsylvania

Michael Moran, Sc.D., P.T.
Associate Professor, College Misericordia, Dallas, Pennsylvania

S. Scott Paist III, M.D.
Clinical Associate Professor, Temple University School of Medicine, Philadelphia; Director of Geriatrics, Department of Family and Community Medicine, Lancaster General Hospital, Lancaster, Pennsylvania

David Patrick, M.S., P.T., C.P.O.
Adjunct Instructor, College Misericordia, Dallas; President, Keystone Prosthetics and Orthotics, Inc., Clarks Summit, Pennsylvania

Lynn Phillippi, M.S., P.T.
Vice President, MJ Care, Racine, Wisconsin

Nancy M. Prickett, M.A., M.P.T.
Instructor, Thomas Jefferson University, Philadelphia, and Neumann College, Ashton, Pennsylvania; President/Owner, Aspen Physical Therapy, Mt. Holly, New Jersey

Carol Probst, M.S., P.T.
Instructor, Department of Physical Therapy, Duquesne University, Pittsburgh, Pennsylvania

Colleen Reynolds
Director, Speech Dysphagia Department, Crozer–Chester Medical Center, Upland, Pennsylvania

Pamela Reynolds, M.S., P.T., G.C.S.
Assistant Professor, Chatham College, Pittsburgh, Pennsylvania

James K. Richardson, M.D.
Assistant Professor, Department of Physical Medicine and Rehabilitation, University of Michigan Medical School, Ann Arbor, Michigan

Bruce P. Rosenthal, O.D., F.A.A.O.
Chief, Low Vision Programs, The Lighthouse International, New York, New York; Adjunct Distinguished Professor, State University of New York, State College of Optometry, and Adjunct Professor, Department of Ophthalmology, Mt. Sinai–NYU Hospital, New York, New York

Susan E. Rush, B.S., M.H.E., P.T., G.C.S.
Charlotte, North Carolina

John P. Sanko, Ed.D., P.T.
Associate Professor, University of Scranton, Scranton, Pennsylvania

Jane K. Schroeder, M.A., P.T.
Physical Therapy Staff, Queens Physical Therapy Associates, Forest Hills, New York

Ron Scott, J.D., L.L.M., M.S.B.A., M.S. (P.T.), O.C.S.
Director and Associate Professor, Physical Therapy Department, Lebanon Valley College, Annville, Pennsylvania

Shelley Slott
Senior Speech Pathologist, Crozer–Chester Medical Center, Upland, Pennsylvania

Everett L. Smith, Ph.D.
Associate Professor, Department of Preventive Medicine, University of Wisconsin, Madison, Wisconsin

Chris Stabler, M.D.
Family Practice Residency Program, Lancaster General Hospital, Lancaster, Pennsylvania

LaDora V. Thompson, Ph.D., P.T.
Assistant Professor, Program in Physical Therapy, Department of Physical Medicine and Rehabilitation, University of Minnesota, Minneapolis, Minnesota

Darcy Umphred, Ph.D., P.T.
Academic Vice-Chairman and Professor, Professional Masters Program in Physical Therapy; and Coordinator of Post-Professional Curriculum, University of the Pacific, Department of Physical Therapy, Stockton; International Lecturer, Consultant, and Clinician, Partners in Learning Clinic, Carmichael, California

Pamela G. Unger, P.T.
Clinical Director, Center for Advanced Wound Care, Wyomissing, Pennsylvania

Kristin von Nieda, M.Ed., P.T.
Assistant Professor, Department of Physical Therapy, Hahnemann University, Philadelphia, Pennsylvania

Robert C. Wagenaar, Ph.D.
Chairman of the Department of Physical Therapy and Associate Professor, Sargent College of Health and Rehabilitation Sciences, Boston University, Boston, Massachusetts

Chris L. Wells, M.S., P.T., A.T., C.
Research Assistant, Division of Cardiothoracic Surgery, Lung Transplant Program, University of Pittsburgh Medical Center, Pittsburgh, Pennsylvania

Mary Ann Wharton, M.S., P.T.
Associate Professor, Department of Physical Therapy, St. Francis College, Loretto; Adjunct Associate Professor, Physical Therapist Assistant Program, Community College of Allegheny County, Boyce Campus, Monroeville, Pennsylvania

Robert H. Whipple, M.A., P.T.

Assistant Professor, Department of Neurology, University of Connecticut Health Center, Farmington, Connecticut

Susan L. Whitney, Ph.D., P.T., A.T.C.

Departments of Physical Therapy and Otolaryngology, University of Pittsburgh; Director of the Balance and Vestibular Physical Therapy Service, CORE Network, LLC, Pittsburgh, Pennsylvania

Ann K. Williams, Ph.D., P.T.

Professor and Chair, Physical Therapy Department, The University of Montana, Missoula, Montana

Deborah C. Wojcik, M.Ed., M.P.T.

Assistant Professor, Programs in Physical Therapy, Hahnemann University, Philadelphia, Pennsylvania

FOREWORD

Functional capacity is the primary determinant of the day-to-day needs of older people. A question of major interest is, "What are the factors that deprive older people from achieving functional independence?" Clinicians of all kinds make effective judgments about treatment strategies based on anecdotal information. But it is clear that to understand thoroughly how to help older persons achieve functional independence requires understanding of the physiology and pathophysiology of aging. Although our understanding is presently limited, research over the past 50 years or so has allowed us some insight into the biology of aging.

Most authors regard the period of modern gerontological research to have begun about 1950, when systematic studies that described aging (senescence) changes in the structure and function of organs and tissues were carried out. The optimism that these studies engendered—that in a relatively short time science would sort out the underlying mechanisms by which aging changes occur—has not yet been realized fully.

In spite of the slow progress in understanding, the average life span of humans has increased more since 1900 than in the 5,000 years before 1900. In 1900 the average life span in the United States was about 47 years, whereas in 1995 it was 76 years. Between 1960 and 1994 the elderly population (i.e., those over age 65) in the United States doubled in size, while the population over age 85 increased 274%. In that same period, the entire U.S. population increased by only 45%. Mortality data as a function of age imply that a fundamental vulnerability develops in people as they get older so that there is a dramatic increase in the probability of dying of virtually any cause. Unfortunately, at the time of this writing, the mechanisms responsible for the change in vulnerability are still not understood.

Historically, a major impediment to aging research has been the inabilty of investigators to identify a global, crosscutting theory (or theories) of aging that could be tested directly. Although various global theories have been proposed, validation of these theories has not been possible. Aging is far too complex, is not one thing, and probably does not have a single cause. What's more, aging changes may be interdependent, so that investigators must deal with distinguishing primary from secondary changes. Superimposed on all this com-

plexity is the fact that random environmental damage combines with intrinsic processes to further modify the trajectory and obscure the mechanisms of the process.

Understanding aging and formulating coherent, testable hypotheses require that the various aspects of aging be dissected from each other and examined critically. This has proven to be a complex and discouraging task. No matter how complex, however, we cannot realistically ignore a process that occurs with essentially the same scenario in the somatic cells of most eukaryotes. Nor can we avoid the challenge of exploring the differing trajectories of aging in different species.

For the biologist, the compelling attraction of aging research is in discovering how so fundamental and universal a biological property works. To the rehabilitation specialist, however, the outcome of a better understanding of the process of aging means an improved armamentarium of treatment strategies for improving the quality of life of elderly people.

To summarize briefly what we know about aging, it is clear that aging is characterized by an increasing vulnerability to environmental changes. A consequence of this is that increasing chronological age brings with it an increasing probability of dying. Some biologists argue that the survivorship kinetics of biological aging may be an artifact of civilization, domestication, and zoos. In nature, populations of animals (including humans) only recently began to live long enough to show the kinetics characteristic of biological aging. Most species in the wild are killed by predators or die as a result of accidents long before they have a chance to show the increasing vulnerability that characterizes biological aging. In fact, we may ask why the biological aging process, characteristic of protected populations, should occur at all in nature. If we think of aging as a genetically programmed, purposeful process in which vulnerabilty to the environment increases with time, then we must consider how evolution would have selected for such a process. Why should evolution select for a negative property? Perhaps the most attractive set of ideas has been proposed by Medawar (1952) and Williams (1957). Both argue that optimization of reproduction is what is selected for. Medawar pointed out that deleterious genes associated with senescence may be delayed until the postreproductive period. Williams (1957) introduced the idea of antagonistic pleiotropy, which states that genes expressed early in life and associated with optimization of fecundity have deleterious effects later in life. Thus, aging may be the price we pay for mechanisms that ensure successful reproduction.

Perhaps the important biological question is not really about aging but rather about longevity. What are the mechanisms that provide the "assurance" that successful species live long enough to reproduce and to protect their offspring so that they in turn are able to reproduce? Once reproduction is ensured, the aging process has little or no evolutionary significance. Can longevity assurance mechanisms be tampered with?

In any case, maximum life span potential appears to be a species characteristic that implies there is a considerable genetic component to the mechanism controlling the rate of aging. For example, the mouse is a frequently used model for human physiology. Humans and mice have the same amount of DNA per cell, implying the same information potential. Yet mice age at 30 times the rate of humans, get cancer 30 times faster than humans, and presently no one knows why.

There are various classes of theories of the mechanisms of aging. Note that these theories, however classified, are not mutually exclusive and are global in nature.

One prominent theory is the somatic mutation theory of aging. This theory states that mutations in somatic cells (genetic damage), presumably resulting from background radiation and perhaps radiomimetic agents, will accumulate and eventually produce functional failure and ultimately death. The major experimental support for this theory was derived from the well-documented observation that exposure to ionizing radiation shortens life span. On logical grounds, however, life span shortening by radiation does not define whether the mechanism for this life span shortening bears any relationship to the normal mechanism of aging. There is not good evidence that it does.

Another theory, or group of theories, can be collected under the general heading of neuroendocrine theories of aging. This group of theories regards functional decrements in neurons and their associated hormones as central to the aging process. Given the major integrative role of the neuroendocrine system in physiology, this is an attractive approach. An important version of this theory proposes that the hypothalamic–pituitary–adrenal axis is the master timekeeper for the organism and the primary regulator of the aging process. Functional changes in this system are accompanied by or regulate functional decrements throughout the organism.

In the hypothalamus, for example, the cascade effect of functional decrements and their potential sequelae are evident. The neuroendocrine system regulates early development, growth, puberty, and control of the reproductive system, metabolism, and, in part, the activities of all the major organ systems in the body. Several lines of evidence have accumulated that support the neuroendocrine theory as a major participant in the aging process.

A third theory is the immunological theory of aging. This theory, as proposed by Walford (1981), is based on two observations: (1) that the functional capacity of the immune system declines with age, as seen in reduced T-cell function (Walford, 1969) and in reduced resistance to infectious disease; and (2) that the fidelity of the immune system declines with age as evidenced by the striking age-associated increase in autoimmune disease. Walford (1979) has related these immune system changes to the genes of the major histocompatibility complex in rats and mice. Decrements in the immune system clearly play an important role.

A fourth group of theories has to do with the role of free radicals in aging. These propose that most aging changes are due to damage caused by oxygen radicals. For example, auto-oxidation of lipids by free-radical pathways may lead to the formation of hydroperoxides, which then decompose to products such as ethane and pentane. Of course, other molecules may be damaged by free radicals, and reactive oxygen species may also operate to regulate gene expression directly. This is an attractive theory because it provides a mechanism for aging that does not depend on tissue-specific action but is fundamental to all aerobic tissues.

Modern gerontologists emphasize that the failures of aging tissues probably result from both genetic changes and environmental insults. A view that I find appealing is that the genetic component of aging is really the component that maintains the regulatory fidelity of the organism's physiology for a period consistent with reproductive success. These putative *fidelity assurance mechanisms* have a limited life span, after which they deteriorate, leaving the organism vulnerable to the random insults that result in dysregulation and ultimately death. Thus, as mentioned earlier, the important issue may be why we live as long as we do and what mechanisms exist to ensure that we do.

The concept of rehabilitation for older persons has a relatively short history. Addressing the problems of functional independence in the elderly developed in the wake of rehabilitation strategies for those with childhood diseases, those who had suffered trauma, and those who were to be returned to the workforce after injury. Antibiotics, vaccines, cardiac surgery, and antihypertensive drugs have now allowed new populations to emerge: those who have had functional impairments all their lives and have become elderly and those who have lost independence as a result of becoming elderly. These elderly challenge us to provide innovative, caring strategies to maintain their independence.

I have no doubt that, in the long term, the emerging understanding of the pathophysiology of aging will aid in the efforts of clinicians to maintain the independence of older people. In the short term, however, it will do little to provide interventions that delay the deteriorative cascades we recognize as aging. Nonetheless, the elderly are with us now and many need help.

The contributors to this volume are dedicated to caring for those with chronic problems, especially older individuals. They have presented state-of-the-art strategies for maintaining independence. Now it

is for the reader to implement these strategies to improve the quality of life of older persons.

VINCENT J. CRISTOFALO, PH.D.

REFERENCES

Medawar PB (1952). *An Unsolved Problem of Biology.* London: H. K. Lewis.

Walford RL (1969). *The Immunologic Theory of Aging.* Copenhagen: Munksgaard.

Walford RL, Bergmann K (1979). Influence of genes associated with the main histocompatibility complex on deoxyribonucleic acid excision repair and bleomycin sensitivity in mouse lymphocytes. *Tissue Antigens 14,* 336–342.

Walford RL, Jawaid S, Nalim F (1981). In vitro senescence of T-lymphocytes cultured from normal human peripheral blood. *AGE 4,* 67–70.

Williams GC (1957). Pleiotropy, natural selection and the evolution of senescence. *Evolution, 11,* 398–411.

PREFACE

The passage of time . . . aging . . . brings a plethora of experiences that constitute the psychosocial, economic, and medical milieu that our patients and we as health-care practitioners face every day. To provide quality health care for the older person in this robust arena, given the constraints of time and health-care payment systems, one must have easily accessible, comprehensive, and concise information. This text is written to enable the health-care provider to review or to learn quickly the pathology of a diagnosis or condition and to present treatment ideas, especially for rehabilitation, prevention (maintenance) care, and prognosis.

No two individuals experience life in identical fashion; thus, one hallmark of aging is the "uniqueness" of each person. Because aging may be viewed as an accumulation of microinsults that present as a collection of chronic diseases and one or more acute problems, the interactive relationships must be considered. This perspective is different from the isolated computerized model of labeling geriatric patients with the clean number listed in the *International Classification of Diseases,* 9th edition, *Clinical Modifications.* We as health-care providers must remain constantly vigilant to avoid this lure of simplification.

One of the issues encountered in geriatric patient care is that the symptoms and signs or responses to treatment may not be as clear as might be expected. The reward is recognizing this and determining an appropriate course of patient care in order to support each aging patient so that he or she has a sense of worth and control even in the presence of physical losses and illnesses. This textbook and, we hope, its readers will acknowledge the challenge and reward.

This book is for clinicians. Although not specifically designed to be a textbook for classroom instruction, students become practitioners; thus, it is also appropriate for the entry-level practitioner in the geriatric rehabilitation setting, including physicians, nurses, physical therapists, occupational therapists, speech pathologists, respiratory therapists, and social workers.

The text is written with a dual purpose for the seasoned practitioner who will benefit from reviewing the information and recognizing that he or she is giving proper care according to today's standards. Furthermore, the seasoned practitioner will also learn because of the breadth of information presented in this text.

For the health-care provider who is newly entering the field of geriatric care, this text will prove to be invaluable. It is clearly acknowledged that not every suggestion offered within the chapters has been put to the rigors of clinical research in order to validate efficacy; however, the suggestions are offered nonetheless because they represent potential treatment ideas, and they are the standard wisdom of the rehabilitation field at this time. Although some of the ideas have not been proven, they have not been refuted. If they had been refuted, they would no longer represent the standard wisdom that defines the ambits of care. These treatment ideas should be employed by thinking practitioners for individual patients.

Throughout the text, the reader should recognize different writing styles that also reflect different treatment approaches. The authors were encouraged to discuss the science of geriatric rehabilitation and to infuse the art of patient care, the soft underbelly of humane medical care for persons who are undergoing involution and are closing out a life. Some of the chapters in this text have references within the material presented. Other chapters have only selected readings at the end of the chapter. The editorial board encouraged each of the writers to minimize the references so that more treatment ideas, graphs, and clinical forms could be included. Readers are strongly encouraged to seek out further information from the lists of suggested readings.

The text is organized into seven separate areas. The first unit deals with some overview of geriatric care and the review of systems as they relate to aging. This should be helpful for classroom instruction and review of age-related changes. Chapter 1 specifically deals with the complexity of aging, pathology, and health care.

The second unit deals with aging pathokinesiology and is clearly directed at specific clinical conditions. It also parallels a rudimentary systems review, since the unit is subdivided into topics pertaining to musculoskeletal involvement, neuromuscular and neurologic involvement, neoplasms, cardiopulmonary diseases, and finally blood vessel, circulatory, and skin disorders.

The third unit deals with the aging and pathological sensorium, especially as it relates to vision, hearing, and communication. The following unit (Unit IV) presents a potpourri of common specific conditions, complaints, and problems and is followed by special considerations or physical therapeutic intervention techniques (Unit V). The sociopolitical, legal, and ethical considerations are addressed in Unit VI because they also impact on geriatric rehabilitation. It is important to recognize that the paradigm shifts at the end of life from the medical model to the dying model, which is more culture based. There is less concern about traditional rehabilitation constructs and greater emphasis on value of life and palliation to minimize suffering and to maintain quality for the dying patient and the family.

Unit VII, the final unit, elucidates the prominent members of the geriatric rehabilitation health-care team. I hope that health-care providers and others who use this manual will understand that:

1. Aging is not stagnant, dull, and/or unattractive.
2. Aging is very dynamic, perhaps too fluctuating, with a wide range of responses.
3. Aging is very diverse—a hallmark is the variability of individuals.
4. Aging is very challenging.
5. Aging is very complex.
6. The study of aging is the study of life—it starts in the uterus and our intervention must be life long.
7. Aging and living are synonymous.
8. ABOVE ALL ELSE, AGING IS VENERABLE AND VALUED.

Respectfully,
TIMOTHY L. KAUFFMAN, PH.D., P.T.

ACKNOWLEDGMENTS

A book of this breadth cannot be conceived, nurtured, and published without a host of persons making significant contributions. First of all, my associate editors have given freely of their time, talents, and energies, as have all of the contributing authors. Second, the Churchill Livingstone editors, especially Carol Bader; her associates Beth Zarret and Duy Linh Tu; and Leslie Burgess, who initiated this project, must be thanked for all of their prodding, patience, and assistance. Following the purchase of Churchill Livingstone by Harcourt Brace, a new team from the W. B. Saunders Company took over the reins, and their support has been incalculable, especially the guidance from Andrew Allen and the considerable editorial and publishing assistance from Christa Fratantoro, Suzanne Hontscharik, Denise LeMelledo, Tina Rebane, Selma Kaszczuk, Linn Jefferies, Karen O'Keefe, and Lynne Mahan. Larry Ward and Bernard Stolz are to be thanked for their excellent graphic art. Third, I must express immeasurable gratitude to my colleagues and staff who have supported me in this gargantuan endeavor. They include Wade Gamber, Wayne McKinley, Brian Hartz, Tony Dague, Ginny Weaver, Carolyn Gestewitz, John Oliveros, Heather Finkbiner, Ben Kauffman, Emily Kauffman, Dawn Simpson, Amy Sutton, Karen Ober, Dennis MacAdam, Mike Beiler, Susan Bedford, Mary Kuhn, Violet Sollenberger, Jessica Hess, and Mike Majsak.

Because of my concern for the environment, trees will be planted to replace those used to make paper for this book.

CONTENTS

Unit III

AGING AND THE PATHOLOGICAL SENSORIUM

Unit IV

SPECIFIC PROBLEMS

Unit V

SPECIAL PHYSICAL THERAPEUTIC
INTERVENTION TECHNIQUES

UNIT I

PHYSIOLOGICAL CONSIDERATIONS

Chapter 1

Wholeness of the Individual

Timothy L. Kauffman, Ph.D., P.T.
Osa Jackson, Ph.D., P.T.

INTRODUCTION

Aging is a wonderful and unique experience. That it includes only good things should not be inferred from the word "wonderful" but, instead, extraordinary and remarkable are implied. Aging starts in the uterus at the time of conception. It represents the passage of time, not pathology. By the age of 1, each individual's uniqueness is evident, and by the age of 5, the personality is well formed. Multiply the first 5 years of life 15 times and expand the environmental and life experiences, and one of the hallmarks of aging becomes clear—that is, individual uniqueness. No two persons age identically. Idiosyncracy is the norm, and it teaches the health-care provider to look at the wholeness of the individual geriatric patient as well as at the presenting chief complaint or primary diagnosis.

In today's health-care arena, the wholeness of the patient gets compressed into a computer number taken from the requisite International Classification of Diseases 9th Revision Clinical Modification (ICD-9-CM). Unfortunately, the number does not necessarily reflect the magnitude of the patient's condition but, instead, may reflect what pays the most or what allows the most hospital or rehabilitation days. In the United States, Medicare regulations establish these parameters.

The diagnosis of cerebral vascular accident (CVA) with the ICD-9-CM code of 436, with modifiers, may yield a variety of outcomes ranging from good to fatal, as follows: full recovery within 1 week; full recovery within 3 to 6 months; partial recovery; severe limitation in physical, cognitive, or communicative abilities; confined to chair, bed, or institution; or death. It is not just antecedent diagnoses such as chronic obstructive pulmonary disease, diabetes mellitus, or degenerative joint disease that are likely to affect the results of rehabilitation for the CVA; psychosocial factors must also be considered. For example, the grandmother of recent Russian immigrants may be labeled confused or poorly motivated when, in actuality, the language barrier is the major stumbling block in rehabilitation efforts.

Age alone is a factor to consider; however, chronological age based on date of birth is not always similar to physiological age, which is based on cross-sectional measurements and comparisons to age-estimated or established norms. For example, a specific 70-year-old male may have an aerobic capacity that is similar to that of the average 60-year-old; the older man is said to have a 10-year physiological age advantage. In Chapter 14 there is a photograph of three individuals ranging in age from 60 to 93; it clearly shows differences among the three, although generalizations can be cautiously extrapolated. But far too often that age span of 33 years is clumped together as if aging changes were monolithic. They are not. It is not common to compare a 10-year-old with a 43-year-old—which also presents an age span of 33 years. When dealing with a patient who has lived 7 decades or more, the person's individuality must be acknowledged by providers and administrators if optimal care is to be rendered.

VARIOUS MEDICAL MODELS OR PERSPECTIVES

The standard medical model of signs and symptoms equaling a diagnosis of a disease does not fit well with a geriatric population (Fig. 1–1). Fried et al. found this medical model to fit the actual cases in fewer than half of the geriatric patients that they studied. They developed several other models: the synergistic morbidity model, the attribution model, the causal-chain model, and the unmasking event model.

The synergistic morbidity model uses a scenario in which the patient presents with a history of multiple, generally chronic diseases (represented by A, B, C in Fig. 1–2) that result in cumulative morbidity. When this hypothetical patient loses functional capacity, medical attention is sought. This may also be viewed as a cascading effect.

The attribution model employs a scenario in which a patient attributes declining capacity to the worsening of a previously diagnosed chronic health

1

Medical

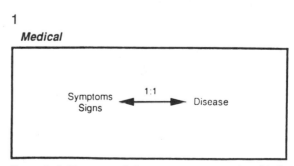

Figure 1–1 Diagnosis of illness presentation in the elderly: diagrammatic representation of the medical model. (From Fried LP, et al. Diagnosis of illness presentation in the elderly. *J Am Geriatr Soc* 1991; 39:117–123.)

2

Synergistic Morbidity

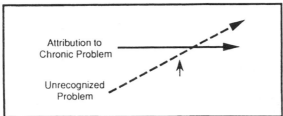

3

Attribution

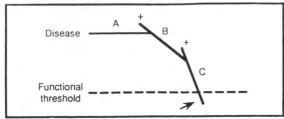

Figure 1–2 Diagrammatic representations of the synergistic morbidity model (2) and the attribution model (3) for diagnosis of illness presentation in a geriatric population. The description of each model is provided in the text. The arrow indicates the usual time of presentation for medical evaluation. (From Fried LP, et al. Diagnosis of illness presentation in the elderly. *J Am Geriatr Soc* 1991; 39:117–123.)

systems compensate for the deficient vestibular system. However, when walking on soft carpet or in a darkened room, this individual may have marked balance dysfunction which may lead to a fracture resulting from a fall.

Coming from a similar perspective, Besdine presented, in his introduction to *The Merck Manual of Geriatrics,* several important concepts that relate to the complexity of geriatric care. First he states that "the restriction of independent functional ability is the final common outcome for many disorders in the elderly." Like Fried et al. in their attribution and unmasking-event models, Besdine warns that "deterioration of functional independence in active, previously unimpaired elders is an early subtle sign of untreated illness characterized by the absence of typical symptoms and signs of disease." Additionally, he suggests that in geriatric medicine there is a "poor correlation between type and severity of problem (functional disability) and the disease problem list." Besdine warns further that finding a diseased organ or diseased tissue does not necessarily determine the degree of functional impairment that will be found. Another lesson he points out is that "the severity of illness as measured by objective data does not necessarily determine the presence or severity of functional dependency."

condition (see Fig. 1–2). But physical examination and workup reveal a new, previously unrecognized condition that is causing the declining health status. This possibility is especially important to consider when evaluating or caring for a patient labeled with a chronic disease such as multiple sclerosis, arthritis, or postpolio syndrome. Not all new complaints are attributable to the chronic condition.

The causal-chain model (Fig. 1–3) employs a scenario in which one illness causes another illness and functional declines. In this case, disease A causes disease B, which precipitates a chain of additional conditions that may worsen the other conditions. For example, a patient who has severe arthritis (disease A, as shown in Fig. 1–3) is unable to maintain good cardiovascular health, which leads to heart disease (disease B). The cardiac condition leads to peripheral vascular disease (disease C) which may lead to amputation (disease D).

The final model proposed by Fried et al. is the unmasking event model (Fig. 1–3). In this situation, a patient has an unrecognized and subclinical or compensated condition. When the compensating factor is lost, the condition becomes apparent and is often viewed as an acute problem. For example, a patient who suffers from vertigo may have functional balance because the visual and proprioceptive

4

Causal Chain

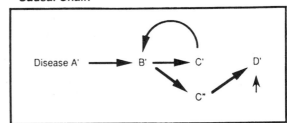

5

Unmasking Event

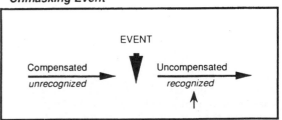

Figure 1–3 Diagrammatic representations of the causal chain model (4) and the unmasking event model (5) for diagnosis of illness presentation in a geriatric population. The description of each model is provided in the text. The arrow indicates the usual time of presentation for medical evaluation. (From Fried LP, et al. Diagnosis of illness presentation in the elderly. *J Am Geriatr Soc* 1991; 39:117–123.)

AGING CONSIDERATIONS AND REHABILITATION

Physical Exercise

Exercise, Fitness, and Aging

From a philosophical point of view, one might consider movement to be the most fundamental feature of the animal kingdom in the biological world. Thus, life is movement. Movement is crucial for securing not only basic needs such as food, clothing, and shelter, but also for obtaining fulfillment of higher psychosocial needs that involve quality of life. Maintaining independence in thought and mobility is a universal desire that is, unfortunately, not achieved by all individuals.

The value of exercise and fitness is that they help people to maintain the fullest vigor possible as time ages everyone. By exercising, one may, it is hoped, enhance the quality of life, decrease the risk of falls, and maintain or improve function in various activities. Fitness, however, is more than aerobic capacity. It is a state of mind, and it involves endurance (physical work capacity determined by oxygen consumption, $\dot{V}o_2$), strength, flexibility, balance, and coordination and agility.

The benefits of exercise are systemic and may be viewed as being favorable for all body systems and functions, provided the phenomena of overuse are abated before causing irreparable damage to the organism. The opposite is also true; the deleterious effects of immobility are profound, as Chapter 60 makes clear. Box 1–1 presents a number of the beneficial effects of exercise on the action of various cells, tissues, and systems and on the organism as a whole as judged by comparing the findings with those of sedentary people.

The beneficial effects of the systemic response to aerobic exercise by the cardiopulmonary and cardiovascular systems as well as by the musculoskeletal system are fairly well recognized. These are graphically presented in Figure 1–4, which compares typical linear senescence, disease, and levels of physical activity. Less well recognized is the association between fitness and mortality. A higher level of fitness is associated with a lower mortality rate. However, many exercise enthusiasts do not extol the benefits of exercise in order to lengthen lives. Rather, the emphasis is placed on experiencing a better quality of life by maintaining robust health and physical competence.

Exercise and Cancer

Over the past several decades the death rate from heart disease has been decreasing and the incidence of cancer deaths has been increasing. A favorable relationship is now being shown between exercise and lower cancer risk. The exact mechanism is not clear; however, it is possible that aerobic fitness exercise enhances the immune function, which reduces cancer risk. It appears that the favorable effect of exercise on cancer risk is found particularly in breast, prostate, and testicular cancers. Conversely, the risk of skin cancer increases for those who work and play in the sun without proper protection.

The benefits of exercise for cancer rehabilitation are not to be overlooked. Exercise may control or reduce nausea during chemotherapy. It reduces muscle loss and fatigue. It enhances satisfaction with life and improves psychosocial adjustment. The immune function may also be maintained or enhanced. The full relationship between exercise and cancer remains to be defined.

Exercise is extremely diverse, ranging from passive range-of-motion to strength training to enhance muscle hypertrophy and including balance and gait mobility and cardiovascular fitness. The multiple interactive physiological effects of exercise require recognition. However, the importance of looking at the whole individual goes beyond physical activity alone.

Confusion

Only several decades ago, the simple symptom of confusion was synonymous with aging and senility. Now it is well recognized that acute confusion may be caused by drugs (diuretics, tricyclic antidepressants, antihistamines, barbiturates, sleep-inducing hypnotic drugs); sleep deprivation; infection (typically, respiratory or urinary tract infections that are not always febrile); diet; dehydration; sunset syndrome; cardiac arrhythmia; environmental influ-

---

Box 1–1

Aging Declines Modified by Exercise

Blood lipid profile	Muscle strength
Blood pressure (systolic)	Osteoporosis
Cardiac capacity	Physical endurance
Glucose tolerance	Pulmonary reserve
Immune natural killer cells	Reaction time
Intelligence scores	Serum cholesterol
Memory	Social interaction
Muscle capillary density	Walking speed

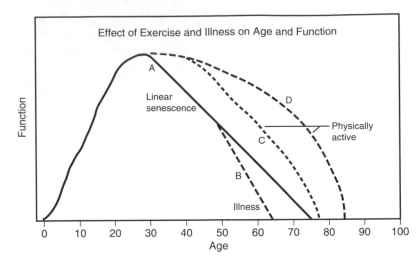

Effect of Exercise and Illness on Age and Function

Figure 1–4 The age-related declines have been described as linear senescence, shown in curve A. Illness such as heart disease or cancer may accentuate the decline, as shown in curve B. Physically active persons benefit by delaying the declines in function, as shown in curve C. Curve D represents a higher level of fitness and the absence of misfortune.

ences (heat, cold); and stress (psychosocial factors, depression, anxiety). Thus, to work with an acutely confused patient, one must look at a variety of potential, interactive causes.

Additional Considerations

In addition to a lifetime of experience yielding individual variations, other gerontological considerations influence rehabilitation care. For example, integrative functions decline to a greater degree than can be communicated by simple measurements. Nerve conduction velocity may show an insignificant decline in a 65-year-old when compared to that of a 25-year-old, but integrative activities such as responding to postural perturbation are likely to show a greater decline.

Within the aging individual, the physiological range of homeostasis is sometimes greater. As shown in Figure 1–5 the mean skin temperature is shown to be similar for various body parts when young and old are compared. However, note that the physiological range of measurements is greater in the aging individuals.

When rehabilitating the geriatric patient, it is vital to remember that multiple chronic diseases are common and many systems may be involved. Because of the greater physiological range of homeostasis and the multiple systems and diseases, the aging individual is more vulnerable to the stresses of rehabilitation.

A comprehensive functional assessment is crucial if treatment is to be effective. Because of the many concomitant conditions and diseases, improvement may manifest more slowly and with a greater variety of responses during the rehabilitation process. This uniqueness is not always acceptable

within the ambits of the present health-care delivery system and the classical medical model, as shown by Fried in Figure 1–1.

A NEW PARADIGM

Throughout this chapter the concepts of wholeness and uniqueness have been emphasized vis-à-vis the medical model of health-care and several alternative models. One additional paradigm requires discussion. This paradigm is best viewed as personal empowerment as described by the Feldenkrais Method and Landmark Education.

Many regions of the world contain small pockets of clinical practices that differ from the mainstream medical model of how a patient is described and related to. These innovative practices have some threads in common. Principally, they adhere to the concept that each individual is 100% responsible for his or her reactions in any particular situation or event. This individual responsibility allows for the enormous variety of functional changes or disturbances as a result of very similar pathological or psychosocial crises. The reality to be examined is the presence of a unique life experience that each individual patient brings to the health-care arena. The health-care provider, too, brings his or her own stories to that arena.

Self-awareness and the taking of personal responsibility make it possible for patients to explore ways of releasing the past and supporting themselves by using the traumatic event (illness, loss, or injury) as an opportunity to reinvent themselves and their personal visions of the future. The idea invites examination of the possible strategies of using the basic skills of communication not only to support the person in claiming a vision of hope and possibil-

Young Dermatomes			Old Dermatomes	
RANGE	MEAN		RANGE	MEAN
33.4 – 35.3	34.3		21.0 – 34.8	28.5
31.9 – 33.5	32.4		34.0 – 37.4	
32.4 – 33.9	33.2			
			32.4 – 37.0	
32.4 – 34.8	33.4			
			31.1 – 36.1 back	33.7
31.0 – 33.7	31.6			
			26.0 – 37.2 popliteal	32.1
30.0 – 31.9	31.0		21.2 – 36.4	30.4
29.6 – 31.9	31.0		20.0 – 37.2	26.8

Figure 1–5 A sample of skin temperatures of young and old adults. Measurements of skin temperature were made by various investigators with different instruments under resting conditions without extreme ambient temperatures or humidity. When possible, range and mean centigrade temperatures are reported. (From Kauffman T. Thermoregulation and the use of heat and cold. In: Jackson O, ed. *Therapeutic Considerations for the Elderly.* New York: Churchill Livingstone; 1987:72.)

ity but also to release the sense of tragedy and the perceptions of victimization and helplessness they might be feeling. All of these factors can minimize the depression that is a major clinical finding among older persons.

A model for recovery and rehabilitation must be developed. It should take the best components of all ideas presented to date and create a paradigm that ultimately supports the patient to choose and to make a commitment to self. The commitment will have to use all the advances and distinctions in psychoneuroimmunology. The patient will have to explore the possibility of being satisfied with life in whatever expression it may take for each individual. A key component of this paradigm is the exploration of how to participate in satisfying relationships with other people. A rehabilitation paradigm that takes this into account can support the inner sense of belonging and the core motivation to the commitment to live. In this model, age becomes functionally irrelevant for the average individual. The idea that each day presents a solid and isolated experience was suggested by William Osler early in this century. The technologies of the mind and the emotions are greatly altered when this idea is applied in the health-care arena. When put into clinical practice, the concept represents another possibility for rehabilitation.

A spinoff of the idea of present-tense living is the examination of the automatic reactions that each patient develops in order to make life work efficiently. The wholeness of the individual is represented by the myriad of habits that are developed over a lifetime. Every person has deeply ingrained habits of thinking, emotional response, sensation, breathing, and movement. When meeting the aging patient, the health-care worker must operate from an awareness of the patient's own habits. A primary and important distinction is that even though a patient has a habit of action he or she may not be aware of that habit. When the rehabilitation process begins, it is necessary—if the patient's reality is to be honored and respected—that all communication build from an awareness of the patient in terms of all relevant aspects of his or her life's history. In this paradigm, rehabilitation becomes a series of questions that help the health-care provider to identify the current preferred strategies of the patient in approaching a situation. It is important to learn what the patient is willing to examine and to explore new ways of being effective in particular situations. Examples of educational approaches that take these ideas and apply them to enhancing the quality of everyday living include the Feldenkrais Method and the Landmark Education. The entire world is searching for new ways of providing effective rehabilitative care for the aging patient. The master clinician will have to take into account the whole patient, including his or her unique life's experiences whenever rendering effective empathetic care.

SUGGESTED READINGS

Besdine R. Introduction. *The Merck Manual of Geriatrics.* Rahway, N.J.: Merck Sharp & Dohme Research Laboratories; 1990: 2–4.

Feldenkrais M. *Awareness Through Movement.* New York: Harper & Row; 1977.

Fried LP et al. Diagnosis of illness presentation in the elderly. *J Am Geriatr Soc* 1991; 39:117–123.

Fries J, Crapo L. *Vitality and Aging: Implications of the Rectangular Curve.* San Francisco: W.H. Freeman; 1981.

Iverson D. *Exercise in cancer prevention and cancer rehabilitation.* Presented at 4th International Congress on Physical Activity Aging and Sports. Heidelberg, Germany, 1996. Can Am Concepts, 360 Monroe St., Denver, CO 80209.

Kiningham RB. Physical activity and the primary prevention of cancer. *Prim Care* 1998; 25:515–536.

The Merck Manual of Geriatrics, 2nd ed. Whitehouse Station, N.J.: Merck; 1995.

Paffenbarger S Jr et al. Physical activity, all-cause mortality, and longevity of college alumni. *N Engl J Med* 1986; 314:605–613.

Sandvik M et al. Physical fitness as a predictor of mortality among healthy, middle-aged Norwegian men. *N Engl J Med* 1993; 328:533–537.

Thomas S. Exercise and activity programmes. In: Pickles B, Compton A, Cott C, Simpson J, Vandervoort A, eds. *Physiotherapy with Older People.* London: W.B. Saunders; 1995: 148–170.

Chapter **2**

Skeletal Muscle Function in Older People

Walter R. Frontera, M.D., Ph.D.
Lars Larsson, M.D., Ph.D.

INTRODUCTION

Impairment of neuromuscular performance evidenced by muscle weakness, slowing of movement, loss of muscle power, and early muscle fatigue is a prominent feature of old age in humans. As a result, many elderly men and women have functional limitations on walking, lifting, maintaining postural balance, and recovering from impending falls. These limitations lead to difficulties in performing activities of daily living, to functional dependence, and to disability. The mechanisms underlying these impairments, limitations, and disabilities are complex, but alterations in the components of the motor units play an important role (Table 2–1). By 80 years of age, 40% to 50% of muscle strength, muscle mass, alpha motoneurons, and muscle cells are lost. In many respects the motor unit is the final common pathway to both movement and disability, so it is of significant clinical importance to have detailed knowledge about the muscle-tissue–specific effects of aging. The independence associated with mobility is critical in achieving a high quality of life. Demographic information from around the world indicates an increasing number and percentage of elderly persons, and the social and economic consequences of this growth underscore the importance of understanding geriatric neuromotor performance.

This section reviews the aging of the motor unit and places specific emphasis on skeletal muscle structure and function. It should be remembered that many factors associated with aging, such as inactivity, undernutrition, and chronic disease, are also playing an important role in the age-related functional decline. However, the extent to which an active lifestyle and exercise training can alter the aging process is unknown. Discussions of the central and peripheral nervous systems, of obvious relevance to muscle cell adaptations, are included elsewhere in the text.

NEUROMUSCULAR PERFORMANCE

Muscle Strength

From a functional perspective, the most important age-related change in the neuromuscular system is the decline in static, dynamic, and electrically evoked muscle strength. This phenomenon has been reported to occur in both the upper and lower extremities of men and women. It must be noted, however, that the decline in eccentric strength seems to be less than that in the other types of muscle actions (i.e., static and concentric). In general, the decline in strength starts during the third decade of life and accelerates during the sixth and seventh decades. The overall rate of progression is approximately 8% per decade. Thus, in older persons, the level of force required to perform the activities of daily living may be relatively closer to their maximal capacity than it is in younger individuals. Therefore, additional impairments in muscle function associated with acute or chronic diseases, hospitalizations due to trauma or surgery, and inactivity may accelerate the decline in strength. The end result may be the early development of symptoms and signs of neuromuscular impairment, dysfunction, and disability. It must be noted that aging progresses at different rates in different individuals and that there is wide interindi-

Table 2–1 The Effects of Aging at Different Levels of the Human Motor Unit

Motor unit	↓ Number and ↑ size
Contractile properties	↑ Contraction and ½ relaxation times
Anterior horn	↓ Number of cells
Peripheral nerves	↓ Motor nerve conduction velocity
Neuromuscular junction	↓ More complex and irregular
Muscle	
Strength	↓ Upper and lower extremities
Contractility	slow contraction
Mass	↓ Segmental and whole body
Fiber number	↓ Types I and II
Fiber area	↓ Type II fiber area
Fiber type	no change; increased coexpression of myosin isoforms
Local muscular endurance	↓ Endurance; earlier onset of fatigue

vidual variability in the degree of functional loss with age.

Physiologically, muscle weakness may be due to a decline in the ability to activate the existing muscle mass, a reduction in the quantity of muscle tissue and therefore in the number of force-generating crossbridges interacting between thin and thick filaments, a decrease in the force developed by each crossbridge, or all three factors. It seems that the ability to activate maximally the remaining motor unit pool is well preserved in the aged. Muscle atrophy and loss of myofibrillar protein, on the other hand, are caused by a reduction in the number of motor neurons in the spinal cord and an incomplete reinnervation of denervated muscle cells that result in a decline in the number and size of muscle fibers. Substantial evidence supports the occurrence of quantitative changes in skeletal muscle during aging. In addition, there is some evidence that intrinsic qualitative properties of the contractile material, such as maximum force per cross-sectional area (specific force), are negatively affected by aging.

Speed of Contraction

Another important characteristic of neuromuscular performance is the time course of muscle actions. This characteristic can be studied by in vivo measurements of the speed of contraction of individual muscles or muscle groups and by in vitro studies in single muscle fibers of the maximal shortening velocity. This property is important because the velocity of movement and the power (force × velocity) generated by muscle can have greater relevance than absolute muscle strength to ability to perform a number of activities of daily living, to independence, and to functional capacity.

In the elderly, the in vivo muscle twitch (evoked by electrical stimulation) is characterized by prolonged contraction and one-half relaxation times. Thus, fused tetanic forces occur at lower stimulation frequencies, an adaptation that increases muscle efficiency. However, this adaptation also lengthens the time for muscle relaxation, thus impairing the ability to perform rapid and powerful alternating movements. Human studies have shown that the time to produce the same absolute and relative forces during voluntary contractions is lengthened, and therefore the ability to generate explosive force (power) and to accelerate a limb is reduced. These alterations have a negative effect on the protective reactions used before or during a fall.

Possible neural mechanisms underlying the effects mentioned above include undefined changes in the central nervous system, a delay in the conduction velocity of motor nerve fibers, a delayed transmission in the neuromuscular junction or all three. Also, changes in the proportions of motor units and myofibers of different types, particularly a decrease in the number or the relative cross-sectional area of type 2 fast fibers (see below), alterations in the sarcoplasmic reticulum and in calcium handling within the fibers, changes in the myosin isoform composition of different fibers, altered functional and enzymatic properties of myosin, an increased passive resistance of the connective tissue structures, or a combination of factors may contribute to altered contractile behavior.

In terms of the temporal relationship among these changes, it is relevant to point out that the prolongation of twitch contraction and relaxation times is already present in the third decade of life and that it precedes the loss of muscle strength.

Muscle Endurance

The effect of age on local muscular endurance is controversial and probably reflects different experimental approaches. According to some authors, but not all, a decline in muscular endurance is a feature of old age that contributes to functional loss and disability. Exercise performed at a given absolute intensity requires a higher percentage of the maximal capacity in older persons. Also, compared with younger adults, older individuals must activate a larger percentage of the reduced muscle mass to generate the same power. This may result in a greater metabolic stress and an earlier onset of fatigue.

Alterations in muscle with advanced adult age that may contribute to the decrease in muscle endurance include reduced blood supply and capillary density, impairment of glucose transport and therefore of substrate availability, lower mitochondrial density, decreased activity of oxidative enzymes, and decreased rate of phosphocreatine repletion.

Muscle Mass

A reduction with age in muscle cross-sectional area and volume that ranges from 10% to 40% has been demonstrated in studies using various techniques at the segmental, or limb, level (ultrasound, computerized tomography (CT), magnetic resonance imaging (MRI), morphometry of whole human muscles) and in studies using whole-body estimates (urinary creatinine excretion, whole-body potassium). In general, although there may be differences among individuals and muscles, the decline starts as early as the third decade of life and seems to accelerate after the age of 50. The loss of muscle tissue is accompanied by a significant increase in non-muscle tissue (fat and connective tissue) that ranges between 27% and 127%. These findings underline the limitations of limb-circumference measurement as a clinical index of muscle size. Finally, the relevance of loss of muscle tissue to weakness in older persons is demonstrated by the fact that when strength values are expressed per unit of muscle mass, the age- and gender-related differences tend to decrease or, in some cases, disappear.

The factors contributing to the loss of muscle mass with age seem to be (1) reduction in the number of both general types (I, slow, and II, fast) of muscle fibers and (2) decline in cross-sectional area predominantly of the type II fibers; the cross-sectional area of type I fibers seems to be well maintained. The combination of effects on type II fibers indicates that the relative area (percentage of type II fibers × mean fiber area of type II fibers) occupied by fast-contracting fibers is significantly reduced with age. This may contribute to the changes in contractile behavior mentioned above.

Motor Unit

The basic functional component of the human neuromuscular system is the motor unit. Each unit consists of an alpha motoneuron soma in the anterior horn of the spinal cord, its motor axon, and the muscle fibers innervated by the axon. The decline in motor performance with age is associated with profound alterations in the motor unit characterized by degeneration of the neural elements, reorganization of the remaining components, variations in the proportion of the different types of motor units, and changes in the properties of the individual motor units.

Histological studies in humans have shown that aging is associated with a reduced number of motor neurons in the anterior horn, a decline in the number of nerve fibers in ventral and dorsal roots at different levels of the spinal cord, accumulation of lipofuscin in the cell body of neurons (a sign of neuronal aging), and axonal degeneration in the peripheral nerves. The latter, together with segmental demyelination, may contribute to the reduction in motor nerve conduction velocity seen with advanced adult age.

Electrophysiological studies using different techniques—quantitative needle electromyography (EMG) of the motor unit action potential, single-fiber EMG, and methods based on the surface-detected motor unit action potential size—have consistently shown that the number of motor units decreases with age in the proximal and distal muscles of both upper and lower extremities. Some studies suggest that this process may accelerate after the seventh decade of life. Simultaneously, the size of the remaining motor units increases, probably as a result of reinnervation by the surviving axons of the fibers that had lost their nerve supply. On the other hand, age-related changes in contractile parameters of single motor units have been measured in muscles of the human hand and foot. The units in older subjects are characterized by prolonged contraction time, prolonged half-relaxation time, larger surface-detected action potentials, and a larger mean twitch tension, which is consistent with their larger size. These alterations in contractile behavior of single motor units correlate well with studies of whole-muscle contractile behavior in the elderly.

Finally, changes in the neuromuscular junction have not been extensively studied, but the existing evidence suggests that the end-plate in older human muscle is more complex and irregular, so synaptic transmission may be delayed.

Fiber Type Distribution

Many morphological, biochemical, and physiological properties of skeletal muscle are determined, or at least strongly influenced, by the proportion and distribution of the different fiber types. Thus, a loss or a transformation of fibers may have a significant effect on muscle function. Based on the studies with the available techniques, there is no definitive answer to the question of changes in the relative proportion of fiber types I and II during aging. It has already been mentioned that the relative area occupied by type I fibers increases in proportion to the relative area occupied by type II fibers.

LIMITATIONS OF THE SCIENTIFIC EVIDENCE IN HUMANS

Finally, it is important to recognize that there are limitations on the collection of data when studying human aging. Therefore, the evidence presented here should be interpreted judiciously and in the context of the following limitations. First, not all skeletal muscles are affected equally by the aging process. Thus, our conclusions are limited in application to those muscles that are accessible to study in humans such as some of the limb muscles, rather than, for example, the chronically active diaphragm.

Second, many human studies depend on the accumulation of indirect evidence and the use of whole-body (urinary creatinine excretion) or noninvasive techniques (computerized tomography). Contrary to animal studies, whole human muscles can be studied only postmortem, and the muscle biopsy can sample only a relatively small number of muscle cells.

Third, because of a longer life span as compared to some animals like rats and mice, human studies are usually cross-sectional in nature, and longitudinal studies are difficult to conduct. By definition, cross-sectional studies compare subjects of different genotypes, ages, habits, and causes of death. Also, older subjects represent the fittest, the group that survived to later years, and may not be representative of the entire aging population.

Finally, extrapolation from animal studies to the human condition should be done with caution. Species differences may explain some of the conflicting results in the literature such as those related to the change or lack thereof in number of muscle fibers with advancing age.

CONCLUSION

It has been proposed that the loss of muscle strength, muscle mass, and muscle fiber number is the result of a neurodegenerative process that involves denervation of motor units and subsequent reinnervation. If reinnervation fails to keep up, denervated myofibers may be lost and replaced by nonmuscle tissue. It should be noted, however, that the decline in muscle strength, muscle cross-sectional area, and muscle fiber number starts before a loss of motor neurons can be detected. On the other hand, the acceleration of muscle weakness and atrophy seems to coincide with the start of neuronal and motor unit loss during the sixth decade of life. It is possible that methodological problems and the inherent ethical limitations of human studies complicate the integration of the results of the different published reports. More studies are needed to define the temporal relationship between the various age-related adaptations in the components and characteristics of the motor unit. This may prove to be essential before proper preventive and rehabilitation programs can be implemented.

SUGGESTED READINGS

Booth FW, Weeden SH, Tseng BS. Effect of aging on human skeletal muscle and motor function. *Med Sci Sports Exerc* 1993; 26:556–560.

Chamari K, Ahmaidi S, Fabre C, Massé-Biron J, Préfaut Ch. Anaerobic and aerobic peak power output and the force-velocity relationship in endurance-trained athletes: effects of aging. *Eur J Appl Physiol* 1995; 71:230.

Doherty TJ, Brown WF. Age-related changes in the twitch contractile properties of human thenar motor units. *J Appl Physiol* 1997; 82:93.

Frontera WR, Meredith CN. Exercise in the rehabilitation of the elderly. In: Felsenthal G, Garrison SJ, Steinberg FU, eds. *Rehabilitation of the Aging and Elderly Patient*. Baltimore: Williams & Wilkins; 1993:35.

Hakkinen K, Pastinen U-M, Karsikas R, Linnamo V. Neuromuscular performance in voluntary bilateral and unilateral contraction and during electrical stimulation in men at different ages. *Eur J Appl Physiol* 1995; 70:518.

Jubrias SA, Odderson IR, Esselman PC, Conley KE. Decline in isokinetic force with age: muscle cross-sectional area and specific force. *Eur J Physiol* 1997; 434:246.

Lindle RS, Metter EJ, Lynch NA, et al. Age and gender comparisons of muscle strength in 654 women and men aged 20–93 yr. *J Appl Physiol* 1997; 83:1581.

Phillips WT, Haskell WL. "Muscular fitness"—easing the burden of disability for elderly adults. *J Aging Phys Act* 1995; 3:261.

Porter MM, Vandervoort AA, Lexell J. Aging of human muscle: structure, function and adaptability. *Scand J Med Sci Sports* 1995; 5:129.

Rogers MA, Evans WJ. Changes in skeletal muscle with aging: effects of exercise training. In: Holloszy JO, ed. *Exercise and Sport Science Reviews, XXI*. Baltimore: Williams & Wilkins; 1993:34.

Sonn U, Frandin K, Grimby G. Instrumental activities of daily living related to impairments and functional limitations in 70-year-olds and changes between 70 and 76 years of age. *Scand J Rehab Med* 1995; 27:119.

White TP. Skeletal muscle structure and function in older mammals. In: Lamb DR, Gisolfi CV, Nadel E, eds. *Perspectives in Exercise Sciences and Sports Medicine: Exercise in Older Adults VIII*. Carmel, Ind.: Cooper; 1995:115.

Chapter **3**

Effects of Aging on Bone

Mary M. Checovich, M.S.
Everett L. Smith, Ph.D.

INTRODUCTION

Bone is a tissue that gives form to the body, supporting its weight, protecting organs, and facilitating movement by providing attachments for muscles so they can act as levers. Although the general anatomy of the skeleton is genetically determined, skeletal strength and shape can be influenced by a variety of factors, including mechanical loading, pharmacological agents, and nutritional intake. The skeleton consists of specialized connective tissue made up of cells that produce, maintain, and organize the cellular matrix.

BONE STRUCTURE

Macroscopic Anatomy

Bones vary in their shape but can be broadly divided into two general categories: flat bones (skull bones, scapula, mandible, etc.) and long bones (tibia, femur, humerus, etc.).

Long bones are designed for bearing weight and consist of a thick and dense outer layer (cortex) of compact bone of which 90% by volume is calcified. The long bone is composed of the central diaphysis, or midshaft, the metaphysis, and the epiphysis, which is capped with articular cartilage.

Although there is only one mechanism of bone formation, it may occur within cartilage (endochondral), within an organic matrix membrane (intramembranous), or by means of deposition of new bone onto existing bone (appositional). The bones of the vertebral column, the base of the skull, and the appendicular skeleton (other than the clavicle) are formed by endochondral ossification. Most of the bones of the face, the vault of the skull, and the pelvis are formed by intramembranous ossification. The formation of periosteal bone and bone modeling and remodeling depend on the process of appositional bone formation. All three types of bone formation occur throughout life and can contribute to the repair of the skeleton after injury or disease or to the treatment of skeletal deformity.

The degree of bone mass attained is governed by hormonal, nutritional, and mechanical factors. At all ages, women have lower bone mass than men. With increasing age, this gap widens. For cortical bone, a slow loss of bone mass begins near age 40 in both sexes (~0.3% to 0.5% per year) and gradually decreases with age. Additionally, women generally experience an accelerated period of bone loss around menopause. Bone loss rates of 5% to 6% per year for up to 10 years are not unusual. This accelerated loss is associated with the withdrawal of estrogen.

Microscopic Anatomy

Gross inspection shows that there are two forms of bone tissue: cortical (compact) bone and trabecular (cancellous) bone. Cortical and trabecular bone have the same matrix composition and structure, but the mass of the cortical bone matrix per unit of volume is much greater.

Cortical bone constitutes about 80% of the mature skeleton. Dense cortical tissue forms the diaphysis (midshaft) of long bones and there is little or no trabecular bone in this region. The thick cortical walls of the diaphysis become thinner and increase in diameter as they form the metaphysis, where plates of trabecular bone orient themselves to provide support for a thin shell of subchondral bone that underlies the articular cartilage.

Trabecular bone is a network of mineralized bone that forms the greater part of each vertebral body and the epiphyses of long bones and is present at other sites such as the iliac crest. It constitutes 20% of the total skeletal mass. Trabecular bone provides a large surface area and is the most metabolically active part of the skeleton, with a high rate of turnover and a blood supply that is much greater than that of cortical bone. It acts as a reservoir for calcium; it is negatively affected by immobility and some pharmaceutical agents (e.g., glucocorticoids, corticosteroids, anticonvulsant therapy) and positively affected by other pharmaceutical agents (e.g., estrogen replacement therapy (ERT), calcitonin, bisphosphonates, alendronate).

Cortical bone fulfills mainly the mechanical and protective function and trabecular bone fulfills the metabolic function of the skeleton. In long bones, the thick, dense cortical bone of the diaphysis provides maximum resistance to torsion and bending. In the metaphyses and epiphyses, the thinner cortices allow greater deformation to occur under the same load.

Cortical or trabecular bone may consist of woven (primary) or lamellar (secondary) bone. Woven bone forms the embryonic skeleton and is replaced by mature bone. Fracture callus formation follows the same sequence. Woven bone is rarely present after the age of 4 years in humans. However, it can appear at any age in response to an osseous or soft-tissue injury. Woven bone is more flexible and more easily deformed than lamellar bone. For this reason, replacement of woven bone with mature lamellar bone is essential to restore the normal mechanical properties of bone tissue. Lamellar bone consists of highly oriented, densely packed collagen fibrils. These fibrils lend strength to bone.

To carry out the diverse functions of bone formation, bone resorption, mineral homeostasis, and bone repair, bone cells assume specialized forms characterized by morphology, function, and characteristic location. They originate from two cell lines: a mesenchymal stem cell line and a hematopoietic stem cell line. The mesenchymal stem cell line consists of undifferentiated cells, or preosteoblasts, osteoblasts, bone lining cells, and osteocytes. The hematopoietic stem cell line consists of circulating, or marrow, monocytes, preosteoclasts, and osteoclasts.

Undifferentiated mesenchymal cells that have the potential to become osteoblasts reside in bone canals, endosteum, periosteum, and marrow. These cells, under the right conditions, will undergo proliferation and differentiate into preosteoblasts and then mature osteoblasts. Osteoblasts never appear or function individually, but are always found in clusters along the bone surface. Active osteoblasts may follow one of three courses. They may remain on the surface of the bone, decrease their synthetic activity, and assume the flatter form of bone lining cells; they may surround themselves with matrix and become osteocytes; or they may disappear from the site of bone formation.

Osteoclasts are large multinucleated cells found on the surface of bone. They are the cells responsible for bone resorption. Specific hormones and growth factors influence their development. Osteoclasts are very efficient in destroying bone matrix. They begin by binding themselves to the surface of the bone, creating a sealed space between the cell and the bone matrix. Endosomes containing membrane-bound proton pumps transport protons into the sealed space, decreasing the pH from about 7.0 to about 4.0. The acidic environment solubilizes the bone mineral. Excess organic matrix is degraded by acid proteases secreted by the cells.

BONE REMODELING

Throughout life, physiological remodeling (removal and replacement) of bone occurs without affecting the shape or density of the bone. Remodeling occurs on the surface of the bone as well as within the bone. Remodeling includes osteoclast activation, resorption of bone, osteoblast activation, and formation of new bone at the site of resorption. Internal,

or osteonal, remodeling begins when osteoclasts create a tunnel through bone. These cutting cones create large resorption cavities. Within the cutting cones, groups of osteoblasts follow the advancing osteoclasts. Layers of osteoblasts arrange themselves along the surface of the resorption cavity behind the osteoclast and deposit successive lamellae of new bone matrix. These layers mineralize and fill in the canal. It appears that physiological remodeling serves to replace bone matrix in which defects may have developed because of normal use. It may also have a role in mineral homeostasis.

In normal adult bone, remodeling is usually a tightly controlled physiological process in which bone resorption equals bone formation. This may change under pathological conditions in which bone resorption and formation are stimulated. Primary osteoporosis is an uncoupling of the balance between resorption and formation. Imbalances of bone remodeling lead to persistent deficits of bone mass, which translate into fracture susceptibility.

CALCIUM AND MECHANICAL HOMEOSTASIS

Bone cells respond to changes in hormonal levels to maintain calcium homeostasis and to change in mechanical loading to maintain mechanical competence. Serum calcium is maintained through regulation of calcium absorption from the gastrointestinal tract, reabsorption by the kidney, and resorption from bone. Lowered calcium blood levels increase parathyroid levels, which draws calcium from the skeletal reservoir. Increased mechanical loading stimulates greater bone mass. Osteocytes appear to detect strain and transmit messages to the preosteoblasts and preosteoclasts to increase the bone-forming activities relative to the bone-resorbing activities. The response of the cells integrates these signals with messages generated by hormones and growth factors for the overall maintenance of skeletal integrity and calcium homeostasis.

CONCLUSION

The rapid increase in the understanding of the mechanisms that seem to control bone cell function has led to many advances in musculoskeletal research. The ability to manipulate formation and resorption of bone as needed will substantially improve the treatment of musculoskeletal disorders. Interventions that apply the knowledge of bone cell function offer the potential to treat numerous diseases.

SUGGESTED READINGS

Avioli LV, Krane SM, eds. *Metabolic Bone Disease and Clinically Related Disorders.* Philadelphia: WB Saunders; 1990.

Mazess RB. On ageing bone loss. *Clin Orthop* 1982; 165:239–252.

Mundy GR, Martin TJ, eds. *Physiology and Pharmacology of Bone.* New York: Springer Verlag; 1993.

Smith EL, Gilligan C. Dose-response relationship between physical loading and mechanical competence of bone. *Bone* 1996; 18:455–508.

Urist MR, ed. *Fundamental and Clinical Bone Physiology.* Philadelphia: JB Lippincott; 1980.

Chapter **4**

Effects of Age on Joints and Ligaments

Louis R. Amundsen, Ph.D., P.T.

INTRODUCTION

With the passage of time, many micro and macro changes take place in the axial and appendicular skeletal joint structures and periarticular connective tissue. The changes may be due to aging, trauma, pathological processes or, most likely, a combination of factors. These common and individually unique events may alter joint movement, posture, and function. It is important for the clinician to be cognizant of the typical changes in joints and ligaments and to modify treatment procedures accordingly.

JOINTS AND LIGAMENTS

Joints, or articulations, are the connections between bones of the skeleton. Some joints are designed to hold bones together without allowing movement, and others are designed for efficient movement. Joints (articulations or arthroses) are classified as synovial (diarthroses) or nonsynovial (synarthroses). The synovial joints allow maximal movement and minimal stability. Nonsynovial joints, classified as fibrous or cartilaginous, allow limited or no movement and a maximum of stability. Fibrous suture joints, which join the bones of the skull, generally become more stable with age and are often classified as truly immovable joints. As a person ages these fibrous joints become calcified, or coated with bone matrix. Fibrous joints (gomphosis joints), which hold the teeth in their sockets in the mandible or maxilla often become less stable with age because of changes in the bony sockets or in

the fibrous connective tissue. Fibrous syndesmosis joints, which hold the radius and ulna or the tibia and fibula together with interosseous ligaments, allow considerable movement. Stiffening of the ligaments limits the extent and speed of movement of these joints in the elderly. Cartilaginous joints include the synchondrosis joints (hyaline cartilage growth centers of adolescents) and the symphysis joints of the pubic symphysis, the manubriosternal joint, and the intervertebral joints between bodies of vertebrae. Changes in the cartilaginous intervertebral disks, such as loss of hydration, increased rigidity, and degeneration of collagen, contribute significantly to the loss of range of motion or mobility of the spine with age.

Synovial Joints

Diarthroses, or synovial joints, are designed to allow smooth, efficient movement by means of the hyaline cartilage at the ends of the articulating bones, the lubrication by synovial fluid, and the

Table 4–1 Changes in Normally Aging Articular Cartilage

Measurement	Aging
Tissue water content	Decreased
Glycosaminoglycans	
Chondroitin sulphate content	Normal or slightly decreased
Chondroitin sulphate chain length	Decreased
Ratio of chondroitin 4-sulphate:chondroitin 6-sulphate	Decreased
Keratan sulphate content	Increased
Hyaluronic acid content	Increased
Proteoglycans	
Extractability	Decreased
Aggregation	Normal
Size of monomers	Decreased
Rate of maturation of hyaluronate-binding region	Decreased
Tissue content of free hyaluronate-binding region	Increased
Link protein	Fragmented
Degradative enzyme activity	
Neutral proteoglycanase	Normal
Acid protease	Normal
Collagenase	Normal

Adapted from Brandt KD, Fife RS. Ageing in relation to the pathogenesis of osteoarthritis. *Clin Rheum Dis* 1986; 12:117–130.

flexible articular capsule enclosure. The inner linings, or synovial membranes, of the capsule are the source of synovial fluid. The outer layer of the capsule is a fibrous membrane that is attached to the articulating bones and that encloses the joint and offers limitation to the separation of the articulating bones. Fibrous thickenings of the capsule form ligaments, which are pliable but are designed to limit movement of the joint by preventing excessive separation of the articulating bones. Most joints of the upper and lower extremities are synovial joints, as are those between the ribs and vertebrae, between the ribs and costal cartilages and the sternum, and between the articular processes of adjacent vertebrae as well as the atlantooccipital joint, the medial and lateral atlantoaxial joints, and the temporomandibular joint. In general, the movement of synovial joints is limited by the tension of ligaments that do not stretch, by muscle tension, and by body structures, such as the thorax, the limbs, the pelvis, and so forth.[1-3]

Cartilage

In synovial joints, articular cartilage or hyaline cartilage covers the ends of articulating bones. The outer surface consists of collagen fibers arranged parallel to the surface; it looks like a moist, polished pearl. This smooth surface minimizes resistance to sliding and gliding. The outer surface is attached to a transitional layer of collagen fibers and eventually to the bone by calcified cartilage. The middle layer is relatively thick and will absorb shock. The cartilage itself has no nerve or blood supply. Pain and position, or proprioception, receptors are located in the capsule and in the ligaments of the joint. When compressed, the articular cartilage exudes fluid through pores in the outer layer, and when the compression ceases, synovial fluid is drawn back into the cartilage. This intermittent pressure is essential for nourishing the articular cartilage. Prolonged periods of compression or lack of compression cause deterioration of the articular cartilage. Social expectations of less physical activity, diminished sensation of pressure and pain, illness, hospitalization, decreased muscle strength and coordination, falls, and hip fractures, for example, cause elderly individuals to be less likely to move at optimal intervals and to be more likely to have deteriorated articular cartilage. Articular cartilage has a limited ability to repair damage to itself, and this capacity is further diminished in the elderly.

Table 4–2 Range of Motion for Selected Joints

Motion	Age	
	<40	75+
Shoulder abduction	184 ± 7[a]	118 ± 20[b]
Hip flexion	122 ± 12[c]	105 ± 10[d]
Hip extension	22 ± 8[c]	17 ± 8[e]
Knee flexion	134 ± 9[c]	100 ± 20[d]
Ankle dorsiflexion	25 ± 6[f]	8 ± 8[d]
Ankle plantar flexion	56 ± 6[a]	35 ± 15[d]
Cervical flexion	50 ± 9[g]	38 ± 9[g]
Cervical extension	82 ± 15[g]	50 ± 15[g]
Lumbar flexion	47 ± 7[h]	25 ± 10[h]
Lumbar extension	18 ± 10[h]	10 ± 6[h]

Created using data from the following sources:

[a]Boone DC, Azen SP: Normal range of motion of joints in male subjects. *J Bone Joint Surg* 61:756, 1979.

[b]Bassey EJ, Morgan K, Dallosso HM, Ebrahim SBJ: Flexibility of the shoulder joint measured as range of abduction in a large representative sample of men and women over 65 years of age. *Eur J Appl Physiol* 58:353, 1989.

[c]Roach KE, Miles TP: Normal hip and knee active range of motion: The relationship to age. *Phys Ther* 71:656, 1991.

[d]James B, Parker AW: Active and passive mobility of lower limb joints in elderly men and women. *Am J Phys Med* 68:162, 1989.

[e]Same as reference c, but the age range is 60 to 74 years.

[f]Greene WB, Heckman JD: *The Clinical Measurement of Joint Motion.* American Academy of Orthopedic Surgeons, Rosemont, IL, 1994.

[g]Youdas JW, Garrett TR, Suman VJ, et al: Normal range of motion of the cervical spine: An initial goniometric study. *Phys Ther* 72:770, 1992.

[h]Amundsen LR: The effect of aging and exercise on joint mobility. *Orthopaedic Physical Therapy Clinics of North America* 2:241, 1993.

Normal aging also causes a reduction in the amount and quality of synovial fluid, which contributes to the deterioration of articular cartilage (Table 4–1).

Joint Capsules and Ligaments

The joint capsules and ligaments become stiffer with age because of the increase in the formation of crosslinks in collagen fibers and the loss of elastic fibers. The stiffening of the capsules and ligaments has direct and indirect effects on the extent and quality of movement. This stiffening directly hampers joint motion which in turn causes a deterioration in the quality of afferent information from the joint receptors. The end result is slower and more uncertain or uncoordinated movements. This combination makes the elderly less likely to move spontaneously through complete range of motion.

CONCLUSION

With aging, the loss of range of motion is likely to result in diminished ability to perform basic activities of daily living and higher-level occupational and recreational activities. Loss of range of motion is likely to occur in the following joint movements: cervical flexion, extension, and lateral bending; thoracic and lumbar flexion, extension, and lateral bending; shoulder flexion, abduction, and rotation; elbow flexion and extension; forearm pronation and supination; all movements of the hand and wrist; hip flexion, extension, abduction, adduction, and rotation; knee flexion and extension; ankle dorsiflexion, plantar flexion; and all movements of the foot. Table 4–2 includes examples of range of motion to be expected from elderly subjects. Although adult women usually have greater range of motion than men, it is not consistent for all joints or within all age groups. For this reason no attempt was made to separate values by gender.

REFERENCES

1. Carola R, Harley JP, Noback CR. *Human Anatomy and Physiology*, 2nd ed. New York: McGraw-Hill; 1992.
2. Norkin CC, Levangie PK. *Joint Structure and Function*, 2nd ed. Philadelphia: FA Davis; 1992.
3. Digionvanna AG. *Human Aging: Biological Perspectives*. New York: McGraw-Hill; 1994.

Chapter 5

Aging and the Central Nervous System

Darcy Umphred, Ph.D., P.T.
Rosanne W. Lewis, M.S., P.T., G.C.S.

INTRODUCTION

Changes that occur in the nervous system with age can be discussed at a cellular level and at a subsystem level. Identification of specific changes can be found throughout the research literature and there exist differences that attain levels of statistical significance when older persons are compared to young adults. At the same time, these differences do not always reflect functionally significant differences when the activities of daily living of healthy older adults are analyzed. Thus, discussing the changes that occur with increasing age is difficult, and it is a controversial task. As humans age, their activity levels change, and their choices of activities vary tremendously, as do their nutritional intake and generalized health. All these factors relate directly to the function of the nervous system and to its ultimate control over the entire body. Genetic predisposition as well as environmental factors play roles in how the nervous system acts and reacts in an aging individual. As humans age they become more diverse rather than more homogeneous so it becomes difficult to compare one adult to another. There has been time in each life for many experiences—the accumulation of minor and major traumas, exposure to toxins, overuse and disuse of major body systems—all of which affect the functioning of the central nervous system (CNS). So difficulties arise when asking, What is expected with normal aging? Yet when one looks specifically at the nervous system, certain changes are observed with aging. These changes in and of themselves do not create disabilities, but their cumulative effect may dramatically influence an aging adult's ability to compensate and relearn once a specific pathology or disease has created functional loss.

NERVOUS SYSTEM CHANGES WITH AGING

In the brain there is an age-related decrease in weight and gyral thickness and an increase in ventricular size. But there is no research showing decline in function related to these changes in the healthy aging human.[1] Evidence exists that changes occur in neurotransmitters with aging but again, such changes are not related to dysfunction in the healthy aging human.[1] Loss of conduction velocity in sensory and motor neurons in the central and peripheral nervous systems and loss of myelin sheaths and large myelinated fibers occur with advancing age.[2] Although these losses might appear to explain a propensity for falling as a result of the slower entry of sensory information into the system, or a delayed motor response time, a connection between a deficiency in one part of the system and the overall function of an individual has not been proven. Further, it is not understood why some individuals can function well into very old age without falling.

Sensory Changes

Documented changes also occur in both the visual and auditory systems with age. Visual acuity declines with age gradually until the sixth decade, then decreases rapidly in many individuals between the ages of 60 and 80. Traditional testing of acuity is valid for reading but not for functional tasks such as observing a step in a darkened room.[1] For an individual to respond appropriately requires receiving the input, processing that input either perceptually and cognitively at an intellectual level or automatically at a motor level and, finally, selecting the motor response that best matches the environmental requirements. Thus, the client whose visual acuity is corrected with glasses for reading may be impaired when evaluated for motor function. An individual who wears bi- or trifocals and glances down for visually augmented feedback may see a distorted image, so inaccurate information is sent to the nervous system. Thus, the motor response may be appropriate for the input being received but inappropriate for the actual environment. The nervous system functions on consensus and thus will always use, if available, other sensory systems and prior learning to determine whether to respond to visual information. Similarly, an individual with visual impairment may respond adequately to environment demands and show no signs of motor limitations.

Hearing loss is also common among the elderly; the causes of such dysfunction are either peripheral or central deficits generally associated with disease. It is important for the therapist working with the geriatric patient to be aware of the client's hearing abilities before giving auditory cues. Whether the individual's auditory difficulty is caused by a peripheral conduction problem or an auditory processing problem plays a critical role in the selection of treatments and the methods of patient-clinician interaction. Although hearing loss itself does not lead to motor impairment, often when the auditory portion of the eighth cranial nerve is involved, the vestibular portion is also affected. This results in potential vertigo and balance impairment and increases an individual's risk of falling.

The processing of information in the cognitive and emotional areas of the CNS cannot be ignored when considering CNS changes with age, with or without pathology. Health-care providers must remember that when the processing or the learning of cognitive materials becomes a problem, that avenue for assistance in motor learning may be lost. Without cognitive assistance, procedural learning of motor programs will become the only avenue to regaining functional control over movement. The principles of motor learning then become paramount in optimizing the therapeutic environment for patient improvement.

Changes in the Limbic System

The health-care provider must also consider the emotional system in all patients, especially when looking at CNS function. Emotions are controlled and modified by the limbic system. This system has extensive connections to the hypothalamus, so emotion is often expressed through regulation of the autonomic nervous system as well as in the tone of the striated muscle system.

Many behavioral syndromes have been attributed to this area of the brain. The most pertinent to the elderly was described by Hans Selye in 1956 as the general adaptive syndrome (GAS).[3] Today it is considered a response to stress and it can be observed in any frail individual, such as a premature infant, an individual with severe CNS damage, or an elderly individual with fragile bodily systems. The GAS response is paradoxical to the anticipated response. Under stress, an individual generally becomes sympathetic, with an increase in heart rate and blood pressure and a fight-flight reaction. In the GAS, the same environmental conditions initially cause a sympathetic response but in time, and sometimes quickly, the individual switches to a parasympathetic reaction. The blood pressure drops, the heart rate decreases, the blood pools in the periphery, and the level of consciousness can drop.[3]

Research since 1956 has shown that concentrations of hormones occur with stress and that the amount of hormones elicited by stress increase with the age of the animal.[4] By virtue of advanced age, a patient may be very close to multiple-system failure. Such an individual would be considered frail. The hypothalamus regulates the areas of the brain stem that control the heart, the lungs, the internal organs, and the immune system.

A client may have recently developed a disease that adds stress to the already frail system. If treatment is interpreted by the individual as creating even more stress, the individual's system may flip into a GAS, which has the potential of evolving into a life-threatening situation. The patient's response may be to withdraw, and the health-care provider's reaction generally would be to increase the level of input in order to motivate or wake up the patient. In the GAS, the patient withdraws further and could potentially arrest. For this reason the health-care provider should evaluate the patient's emotional response to the environment and try to keep a homeostatic autonomic balance. This requires sensitivity to all systems of the body—respiration, blood pressure, and level of alertness as well as specific motor responses to treatment. All of these systems are ultimately under the control of the limbic system.

Changes in the Motor System

The motor system, with the guidance of prior learning and experience as well as the CNS's analysis of current needs, modulates the state of the motor pools in the brain stem and spinal cord in order to drive peripheral nerves and orchestrate synergistic interactions of muscle groups to create functional behavior and mastery of the environment. Ultimate control of that end product called functional behavior is the result of the consensus of a variety of areas within the motor system. Understanding how this motor system regulates and controls movement is the key to identifying motor impairments and understanding why an individual exhibits functional disabilities.

The areas typically considered to be part of the motor system are the frontal lobe, the basal ganglia (BG), the cerebellum (CB), the brain stem, and the spinal cord. The thalamus plays a key role as a relay and modulator, whereas the limbic, or emotional system has the ability, directly and indirectly, to alter the state of motor responses. Obviously, the sensory areas also guide and alter existing motor programs. Where the motor system begins and ends is not clear because there are so many interdependent systems that loop between one area and another; therefore, a linear analysis is not appropriate. There is no one area that controls motor output, yet certain areas, or nuclear masses, are responsible for specific aspects of motor function. When any one of these areas is diseased or injured, specific clinical symptoms manifest. Similarly, some motor components such as base tone in striated muscles are regulated by more than one area, so a deficit does not automatically reflect the involvement of a spe-

cific area. The CNS is made up of many connected neuronal loops, so a deficit in a neuronal loop might present a clinical problem that would make it appear as if a nuclear mass or system were damaged. Advanced age is not a reason for CNS problems; disease and injury are. Thus, CNS motor changes that occur with aging do not necessarily indicate functional motor deficits.

Research does show that the motor system changes with age.[1] For example, the influence of head-turning plays a greater role in electromyographic activity in synergistic upper- and lower-extremity muscle groups in an aging brain than in a young brain. This suggests that the CNS no longer has the refined regulating ability over preprogrammed synergistic patterning that might be called an asymmetrical tonic neck pattern. A child gains control over all preprogrammed movement patterns and refines that regulation; possibly an older adult begins to lose some of that refinement. Whether this is because of disuse or aging is not clear. Again, it must be emphasized that these changes, although statistically significant, do not represent measurable functional changes. The significance of these changes may be more meaningful following injury or disease. If the aging CNS loses some of its plasticity or ability to adapt, then it may take more time to learn new programs or alter existing ones. This might explain why aging adults seem to exhibit synergistic patterns very quickly following injury, whereas a younger adult may take more time. If new learning is impossible, then the need to create an environment that optimizes old learning should be clearly identified and used in the therapeutic environment to achieve optimal functioning.

A complete explanation of the specifics of the motor control system[5, 6] is not within the scope of this chapter, but a brief overview of the system might help the reader to understand and appreciate the complexity of the system. The frontal lobe of the brain not only helps process the motivation to move, it also modulates or regulates information that travels between primary motor centers such as the BG and CB. In addition, it plays a primary role in regulating fine motor function through the corticospinal and corticobulbar systems. Normal movement results from the coordinated work of multiple areas that influence the final common pathways of motor neurons.

The frontal lobe plays a primary but not a dictatorial role in the modulation of fine motor behavior. After summating and modulating messages from other areas of the CNS, the frontal lobe sends messages concurrently to the BG and the CB. In turn, these centers formulate new motor plans or draw upon existing plans to correctly modulate the motor system. If either center or the loops connecting them is damaged or diseased, then motor function may not be smooth, coordinated, effortless, or able to match the environmental context of the activity. The CB, unlike the BG, is simultaneously aware of the peripheral kinesthetic environment through the proprioceptors in the limbs and trunk and based on the position of the head in space as judged by the vestibular system. Similarly, it is aware of existing states of the motor pool via a variety of afferent tracts that send that information directly to the anterior lobes of the CB. For this reason, the CB is considered a synergistic programmer. Not only is it responsible for helping to write new programs, it also makes sure that the program being played matches the environmental context. The CB will run the desired program until it is told to do something else. If there is a mismatch between the desired movement sequence and the environment, it will try to readjust the synergistic patterns and run the program that matches the environment. For example, if an individual is walking on a level cement surface and suddenly the surface changes because of a crack or a hole, the CB will pull in appropriate synergistic muscle groups to allow the person to keep walking.

The basal ganglia are responsible for changing the plan of movement and initiating new programs, whereas the cerebellum, in preparation for the changes to take place, regulates the state of the motor generators (base tone) and controls the force, speed, and direction of movement. For example, if an individual is rising to a standing position and when vertical goes beyond his or her limits of stability and starts falling, the BG change the motor set from rising to falling. Both the BG and the CB play roles in modulating posture but the specific roles are different. The BG and aspects of the CB play key roles in the development of new motor programs and the refinement of existing ones. They relay specific motor programming to the frontal lobe by way of the thalamus, and they relay programming down through the brain stem to the motor generators of the cranial and spinal neurons. Therefore, changes in any of these structures or in the pathways between them that occur with aging could have critical effects on normal movement. The changes do not necessarily create identifiable alterations in motor performance although, along with other pathology, they could become cumulative, with the end result being loss of function. For example, a reported loss, with age, of Purkinje cells in the CB has not been related to loss of function.[1] Yet this change along with cerebellar degeneration or a cerebellar stroke would be cumulative and the result might be a greater deficit than would occur in a younger individual with only the diagnosed medical pathology.

In summary, the research shows changes in the anatomy and chemistry of the brain with aging, but they have not been shown to affect function directly in the healthy elderly human. Pathology and disease are the causes of functional limitations. Thus, structural or anatomical changes due to aging do not necessarily correlate with functional loss. Similarly, lack of structural or anatomical change does not necessarily reflect normal functional ability. The aging process may affect the potential of the nervous system to adapt with extreme plasticity but age is only one factor that influences potential, and it should never be considered the primary cause of functional disability.

MODELS OF DISABILITIES

A medical diagnosis of a disease is an important element in understanding a patient's health, but the medical diagnosis may or may not be a critical factor in understanding why that individual has functional limitations. For this reason, various impairment/disability/handicapped models have been developed to differentiate the reasons for functional limitations.

Impairment/Disability/Handicapped Model

Therapists are expected to identify the specific components that have led to functional problems, predict how long it will take to correct or compensate for the problem, and establish a treatment protocol that will get that patient functional in the shortest time. This responsibility of differential diagnosis closely interrelates with the concept of impairment/disability/handicapped or independence models (IDHIMs) (Fig. 5–1). Therapists evaluate functional skill as activities of daily living that directly correlate with the disability component of any IDHIMs. What allows an individual to demonstrate normal functional skills are the interactions of many body systems and their abilities to function adequately so as to allow for normal motor output. A breakdown in any portion of one of these systems can lead to an impairment that can be identified, evaluated, and treated, although all impairments do not automatically lead to disabilities. In the elderly, there exists the potential for problems in many systems and subsystems, such as joint changes, resulting in a smaller range of motion, muscular weakness or lack of endurance due to disease or disuse, cardiac insufficiency, pulmonary dysfunction, and central and peripheral nervous system impairments. It is the interaction of all these systems and impairment within them that ultimately lead to functional limi-

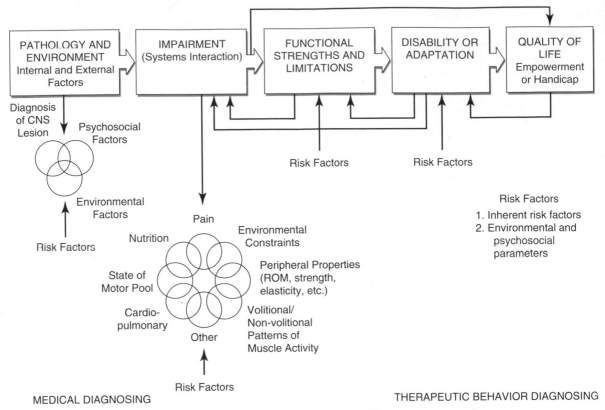

Figure 5–1 Behavioral model for evaluation and treatment of human movement performance.

tation. Many impairments that occur in aging adults originate in the nervous system.

THEORIES OF MOTOR CONTROL AND MOTOR LEARNING

Motor control as a system includes components that are differentiated into biomechanical, muscular/skeletal (power, strength, and muscle elasticity), and central (state of the motor pool, available synergistic programming, postural integrity, balance, force, speed, trajectory, and automatic versus anticipatory programming). All these components interact and must be evaluated within the context of the environment in which the activity is occurring, for that will determine whether the CNS can adapt or if the environment must be changed. Movement should not be analyzed on only a biomechanical, or muscular/skeletal or central basis. That would result in the exclusion of a large portion of the whole and would not lead to the most accurate prognosis and treatment. It is always the interaction of all the variables that determines the motor patterns observed and establishes whether they are caused by degeneration due to age, disuse over time, or dis-

ease. Table 5–1 illustrates the variables in motor control that are considered to originate in the nervous system and those that are not.

To understand the distinction between an impairment and a disability, it is necessary to understand how the various systems function together in the healthy individual. For the most part, the human body has been provided with large physiological reserves in all systems. Thus, a deficit in a portion of one system may have little or no effect on the whole organism because the reserves in other areas can substitute for small deficiencies. It has been postulated that with aging, many areas of physiological reserve may be close to a critical level of dysfunction. In this scenario the whole organism functions normally, using up its reserves over time, until the occurrence of an acute problem in one area. Then the other parts of the system do not have the ability to compensate for the lack, and function is lost. In some instances there can be improvement in impairments through therapeutic intervention, especially if some reserve is still available. If the therapist correctly relates that impairment to a certain function and creates an optimal environment for relearning, then even with depleted reserves, function often can be improved. In other instances

Table 5–1 Motor Control Components and System Interactions: Classification of System and Subsystem Impairments

Systems Traditionally Considered Central	Systems Traditionally Considered Peripheral or Environmental
1. *State of the motor pool* Hypotonicity Hypertonicity Rigidity Tremor 2. *Synergies (volitional or reflexive)* Pattern of motor program Flexibility over programming 3. *Postural integration* Agonist/antagonist coactivation Automatic prolonged holding against gravity in all spatial positions 4. *Balance* Limits of stability Sensory integration of somatosensory, visual, vestibular Interaction of ankle, hip, stepping synergies Interaction with postural function Interaction with task/environmental context 5. *Speed of movement* Ability to alter rate of movement throughout entire task Movement responses to speed demands 6. *Timing* Ability to start, stop, and change a motor plan Interaction with environmental context Timing of muscle sequencing relationship to task 7. *Reciprocal movements* Ability to change direction Rotary components present/absent Turnaround time/delay Smoothness of agonist/antagonist 8. *Trajectory or pattern of movement* Trajectory, velocity, acceleration curve Smoothness throughout range 9. *Accuracy* Placement of entire body or a component part at a specific point in space Changes with demand for speed, difficulty of task, direction, distance 10. *Task content* New versus old learning 11. *Emotional influences* Value placed on activity Differentiation of procedural and declarative learning Fear factor Motivation 12. *Sensory organization* Intact, deficient, compensation, conflict 13. *Perception/cognition* Interaction of sensory organization with perceptual processing Ability to use cognition to assist in motor learning Short, intermediate, long-term cognitive abilities 14. *Hormonal, nutritional, levels of consciousness* Daily biorhythms and levels of alertness throughout day Drug and nutritional interactions on central and peripheral function	1. *Range of motion* Specific joint limitation Causation within joint structure 2. *Muscle strength or power* Muscle endurance Muscle power 3. *Cardiac function* Output Pacing Endurance Interaction with respiratory system 4. *Respiratory function* Input/output Exchange Interaction with cardiac system 5. *Circulatory function* Ability to supply muscles with foodstuffs, oxygen, minerals, etc. Ability to eliminate waste 6. *Other organ and system interactions* Skin integrity and pliability Kidney, liver, intestinal function 7. *Environmental context* The specific task or functional activity Familiarity with existing task or environment (hospital versus home) 8. *Endurance* Differentiation of disuse from system failure or inefficiency 9. *Psychosocial factors* Family demands Ethnic, culture beliefs and stressors Past experiences and role identification Religious beliefs and their interaction with health-care delivery Individual's belief in and acceptance of a health-care system and its expectations

the therapist cannot change the impairment but can find an alternative way for the patient to use intact systems to perform the desired function. For example, an aging individual who chooses to become more sedentary over time may no longer need to keep his or her vestibular system at a high level of sensitivity. The lack of movement may lead to some joint limitation in the ankle and hip, which may decrease the limits of stability of balance. As the individual ages, his or her visual system may become compromised. None of these minor impairments necessarily leads to balance dysfunction or to falls. If an individual then suffers a vascular insult with acute residual motor impairments, the additional preexisting impairments become compounded and interact with the new problem.

SYSTEMS INTERACTIONS AND REHABILITATION

It is the total interaction of all systems that the therapist must consider. Some systems have changed over a long period of time and will probably not readapt quickly, such as the vestibular system. If range is regained, but power is not available, then a new impairment exists.

Some systems that have changed no longer have the ability to adapt—vision, for example. Still others, such as central motor control, may have undergone acute injury, and the therapist will have to determine through assessment which systems within the CNS are intact, which are trying to compensate for systems with deficits, thus showing dysfunction themselves, and which systems are permanently damaged and no longer have the ability to compensate and learn. The end result of this scenario is problems with balance and the potential for future falls. The disability leads to potential dysfunction in all activities that require standing balance and to the end result of high risk for falls and future impairment from a fall. The impairment category would be balance; the specific impairments would fall under muscle power and central. Central impairment may include state of the motor pool, synergistic patterning, or postural control. Each impairment can be evaluated as it is identified and quantitatively measured. The number and magnitude of impairments will determine prognosis and clearly direct the therapist toward intervention.

Motor learning,[7, 8] as differentiated from motor control,[9] is the way the motor system learns new programs and refines existing ones. When therapists are creating environments to help a patient regain motor function, a variety of motor learning principles must be considered. First, determination of the specific stage of motor learning will direct both the type of practice used and the reinforcement programs initiated.

There are three stages of motor learning: acquisition, refinement, and retention. Stage one, acquisition, requires extra reinforcement, which can be internally driven, through normal, inherent sensory feedback systems, or can be externally driven, through augmented feedback from someone else. As the individual increases skill in the activity, less feedback is necessary. Similarly, the type of practice schedule selected by the therapist can range from mass practice (daily and structured), to distributed (scheduled by the therapist or patient), to random (part of daily living). Acquisition of a skill requires mass practice, whereas retention depends more on random practice.

When the therapist introduces the activity, another concept must be considered. The task itself will determine whether it will be practiced as a cohesive activity, taught in separate parts and then put together as a whole, or taught as a progressive sequence of parts. This is the practice context. Simple and discrete tasks are more easily taught as whole activities, whereas a complex skill is generally learned best as an activity that is broken into parts and then reassembled as a whole. Intermediate skills and serial tasks are often best learned progressively.

Much of the research into motor learning has been done on normal people; it has not been determined how practice schedules, practice context, and reinforcement correlate with aging, let alone with the aging individual who has central processing problems. The interaction among all these conceptual areas along with the specific impairments of a particular elderly individual will create a map for the therapist to determine the specific pathway that will lead to motor learning by the patient in the shortest time with the most successful outcome.

CLINICAL EXAMPLES

In many instances, improvement of an impairment can be achieved through therapeutic intervention. If the therapist correctly relates the impairment to a certain functional ability, then corrects the impairment problem during the functional activity, the level of disability can be reduced. In other instances, the therapist cannot change the impairment but can find an alternative that allows the patient to use intact systems to perform the desired function, thus altering the level of disability. In the first scenario, the patient's ability to go beyond skill acquisition to skill retention and to carry over into other functional activities is high, whereas in the second scenario, the skill is activity-specific and has little carryover to other functional behaviors.

An example of the first instance is a patient who has recently had a cerebrovascular accident (CVA). The therapist works with that individual, putting him or her into postures and situations or activities that demand that the CNS respond. This response will activate the brain's plasticity and adaptability. Regaining strength in the hemiparetic side, modulating synergistic patterns, improving balance and postural control (all acute impairment) will lead to a return to normal functional activities such as sitting, transferring, and gait (potential disabilities). In this example, it is important for the therapist to conclude from initial testing that previously learned motor programs are intact but because of the CVA, certain impairments exist within the loop systems. If alternative loops or synaptic sensitivities exist, then recovery potential is high and the prognosis is good as long as the treatments are consistent with appropriate environmental contexts, practice scheduling, practice context, and the goals and expectations of the patient.

An example of the second scenario is an elderly client who has recently had an amputation following prolonged diabetic instability and eventual gangrene. The therapist is never going to change the general impairment of limb loss or the medical condition of diabetes. That impairment has in and of itself altered the state of the nervous system. The sensory system has changed, as has the posture, balance, and motor programming needed to ambulate with a prosthetic device. The inherent sensory feedback necessary to create new programs will have to be evaluated. There may be progressive impairment due to the diabetes. But if new learning can occur and new programs can be written, then this elderly individual may be able to run the programs, even with progressive sensory deterioration. Thus, the therapist will have to work with the patient in using a prosthesis to regain normal gait programming. Strengthening the residual limb muscles will not necessarily lead to functional strength when using the prosthesis. To match the context of the environment with the task, the programming necessary, and the patient-specific impairment, the therapist would want to work on standing and walking. Additional considerations such as skin integrity, pain, and range of motion should be interfaced with the practice environment. The therapist would potentially be optimizing the environment for early and maximal function. That is, the therapist must realize that this gait training is a new learning situation. The old programs for walking that the client learned as a small child and practiced for decades will no longer work as total programs. In this situation the therapist may have to allow the patient to concentrate on the task at first, but for the client to be truly successful in this new variation of ambulation he or she must practice it as an automatic task. That practice would first have to be performed at a mass practice level and finally as an activity of daily living and thus on a random schedule. The therapist will have to introduce variety into the gait training gradually, by varying the lighting or the surface and by distracting the client with conversation. Gait is a preprogrammed pattern that develops variability in relationship to different contexts, so practicing the pattern as a whole would be the context of choice. The therapist has created an environment that has changed the CNS, even though the original impairment was not centrally induced.

CONCLUSION

The nervous system is a complex conglomerate of nuclear masses that communicates with all bodily systems and expresses its thoughts, feelings, and desires to the world through motor behavior. Its goal does not change with advancing age, nor does a number imply that the nervous system is no longer functioning adequately or normally or that it has diminished ability to adapt and learn. Yet through life's experiences, age itself does potentially affect all bodily functions, including that of the nervous system. Whether those changes become functional impairments and disabilities is client-specific and is often directly correlated with disease, not with specific age. Therapists should evaluate the interactions of the various impairments and correlate them with functional behavior in order to identify the best treatment protocols, those that will lead to optimal performance in the shortest time. Application and synthesis of knowledge regarding motor control and learning play key roles in the effectiveness of a clinician.

REFERENCES

1. Craik RL. Sensorimotor changes and adaptation in the older adult. In: Guccione AA, ed. *Geriatric Physical Therapy*. St. Louis: Mosby; 1993:72.
2. Lewis CB, Bottomley JM. *Geriatric Physical Therapy: A Clinical Approach*. Norwalk, Conn.: Appleton & Lange; 1994.
3. Umphred, DA. Limbic complex. In: Umphred DA, ed. *Neurological Rehabilitation*, 3rd ed. St. Louis: Mosby-Yearbook; 1995.
4. Frolkis VV. Stress-age syndrome. *Mech Ageing Dev* 1993;69:92.
5. Kandel ER, Schwartz JH, Jessell TM. *Principles of Neural Science*, 3rd ed. New York: Elsevier; 1991.
6. Schmidt RA. *Learning and Performance from Principles to Practice*. Champaign, Ill.: Human Kinetics Books; 1991.

7. Shumway-Cook A, Woollacott M. *Motor Control: Theory and Practical Application*. Philadelphia: Williams & Wilkins; 1995.
8. Umphred DA. Introduction and overview, multiple conceptual models: frameworks for clinical problem solving. In: Umphred DA, ed. *Neurological Rehabilitation*, 3rd ed. St. Louis: Mosby-Yearbook; 1995:3.
9. Newton RA. Contemporary tissues and theories of motor control: assessment of movement and balance. In: Umphred DA, ed. *Neurological Rehabilitation*, 3rd ed. St. Louis: Mosby-Yearbook; 1995:81.

Chapter 6

Cardiac Considerations in the Older Patient

Meryl Cohen, M.S., P.T.

INTRODUCTION

Determination of health and wellness among young individuals is relative, varying from person to person. Similarly, the effects of an aging cardiovascular system vary among the elderly. Controversies exist in the literature regarding the application of a single model to the influence of aging on heart function. Structural changes that occur with aging are more consistent and more easily identifiable than are physiological changes. The latter findings are difficult to distinguish for several reasons, including the interrelatedness of dynamic variables contributing to myocardial performance, the pathophysiology and symptomatology of heart disease, and the concept of hypokinesis in American society, part of which the older person is considered to be entitled. In addition, comparison of studies is limited because of measurement inconsistencies and varying definitions of "elderly" and "heart disease." Many of the pioneering studies of the 1950s and 1960s should be reproduced using new definitions of "old" and paying more deliberate attention to the presence of heart disease in study populations.

Nevertheless, there is general consensus regarding the effects of aging on several factors that influence cardiac performance. These factors have been studied in older individuals who are healthy and in those with heart diseases, both at rest and during various levels of exertion. This chapter presents these findings as a model of declining cardiac performance with increasing age. Comparison is made to the baseline "young" model in an attempt at defining a "healthy older" model. The unique influences of exercise and disease on this model are then discussed, with an emphasis on the clinical implications of these physiological changes.

CARDIOVASCULAR STRUCTURE

Age-related changes in cardiovascular tissue can be found in cardiac contractile fibers, conducting tissue, and valvular structures. Although the actual number of myocytes decreases, the myocyte volume per nucleus increases in both ventricles. Commonly, the coronary microvasculature is unable to accommodate this increase in tissue volume, which raises the likelihood of myocardial ischemia. In addition, there is an increase in nondistensible fibrous tissue and an accumulation of senile amyloid deposits (see Box 6–1). The loss of pacemaker cells (sinoatrial node tissue) and the increase in fibrous tissue in conducting pathways combine to increase the risk of cardiac arrhythmias in the elderly.

Simultaneous age-related changes occur in coronary arteries and systemic vasculature. These

---

Box 6–1

Age-Related Changes in Cardiovascular Tissue*

Cardiac	↓	Number of myocytes (myofibrils and pacemaker cells)
	↑	Size of myocytes (myocellular hypertrophy)
	↑	Lipid deposition in myocytes
	↑	Lipofuscin deposition in myocytes
	↓	Mitochondrial oxidative phosphorylation
	↑	Amyloid deposition in the heart
	↓	Rate of protein synthesis in internodal tracts
	↑	Fibrosis and calcification of valves (especially the mitral annulus and aortic valve)
Vascular	↑	Endothelial cell heterogeneity (size, shape, axial orientation)
	↑	Nondistensible collagen, fibrous tissue, and calcium in media
	↑	Thickness of smooth-muscle cells in media

* ↑ = increase; ↓ = decrease

changes tend to increase the stiffness of the vessel walls (see Table 6–1; Fig. 6–1). Typically, proximal portions of the arteries change first, and the left coronary artery changes before the right. Together, the locations of the changes and the increased vessel rigidity cause an increase in peripheral vascular resistance. The heart attempts to adapt to this increased afterload (see discussion below) with myocellular hypertrophy, which probably accounts for the increase in myocyte volume previously mentioned. In addition, the alterations found in endothelial cells lining the arterial lumen cause a decrease in laminar blood flow, possibly establishing sites for lipid deposition.

CARDIOVASCULAR PHYSIOLOGY

The job of the heart is to pump blood rich with oxygen to body tissues. The ability of the heart to do this work efficiently is closely affected by three other systems: the lungs, the vasculature, and the blood. Age or disease-related changes occurring in these systems will directly affect cardiac function (see related Chapters 7, 8, and 42 to 49).

Cardiac output (CO), or the volume of blood pumped to body tissues each minute, depends on the frequency of cardiac contractions (heart rate) and the volume of blood ejected with each contraction (stroke volume). Heart rate (HR) can be influenced by many external factors; however, intrinsically, the HR depends on pacemaker tissue function

and autonomic nervous system stimulation. In addition to the loss of pacemaker cells in older people, there is also a decreased sensitivity to beta-adrenergic stimulation (see Box 6–2). These two age-associated changes in heart rate control may or may not affect the resting heart rate, but they do typically decrease the maximal exercise heart rate.

Cardiac output is maintained in the older individual if the stroke volume (SV) is able to increase and compensate for any blunted heart rate response. This is the case if the individual remains physically fit, but usually the resting and submaximum CO tend to decrease with aging owing to a decrease in SV. This reduction in SV may be a result of alterations in a number of variables (see Box 6–2).

Stroke volume is influenced by ventricular filling (preload), ventricular contractility, and peripheral vascular resistance (afterload). Ventricular filling occurs early during diastole and is rapid and mostly passive, with the last portion of filling attributed to atrial contraction. However, with aging, a prolonged contraction relaxation time and decreased myocardial compliance (due to increased nondistensible fibrous tissue) cause a greater dependency on slower, active atrial contraction for the majority of diastolic filling (see Fig. 6–2).

Myocardial contractility is directly affected by sympathetic nervous system stimulation, specifically, beta-adrenergic receptors. Older individuals are less responsive to catecholamine stimulation, which results in a blunted inotropic response. In

Table 6–1 Age-Related Cardiovascular Responses to Exercise[a]

	Due to Aging	After Exercise Training
Resting		
Oxygen consumption	↔	↔
Heart rate	↔	↔
Stroke volume	↔	↔
Arteriovenous oxygen difference	↑	?
Submaximal exercise		
Oxygen consumption	↔	↔
Heart rate	↔	↓
Stroke volume	↔	?
Arteriovenous oxygen difference	↑	?
Maximal exercise		
Oxygen consumption	↓	↑
Heart rate	↓	↔
Stroke volume	↓ or ↑	↑
Arteriovenous oxygen difference	↓ or ↔	↑ or ↔
Cardiac output	↔ (?) or ↑	↔

[a] ↑ = increase; ↓ = decrease; ↔ = no change; ? = insufficient data on elderly subjects.
(From Protas E. Physiological change and adaptation to exercise in the older adult. In: Guccione A. ed. *Foundation of Geriatric Physical Therapy.* St. Louis, Mo.: Mosby–Year Book; 1993: 38.)

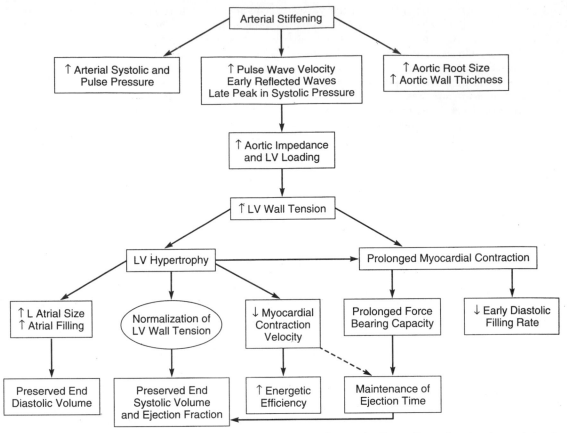

Figure 6–1 Cardiac consequences of age-associated increase in central arterial stiffness. (Reproduced with permission from Gerstenblith G, Lakatta EG. Aging and the cardiovascular system. In: Willerson JT, Cohn JN. *Cardiovascular Medicine*. New York: Churchill Livingstone; 1995.)

addition, if diastolic filling volumes are inadequate, contractile tension can be diminished due to the Frank Starling law of the heart, which states that the *energy of contraction is proportional to the initial length of the cardiac muscle fiber.*

The final component of stroke volume determination is cardiac afterload (opposition to left ventricular ejection). As discussed above, afterload increases with aging due to increased vascular rigidity. Vascular stiffness is a result not only of loss of elastic elements but also of decreased responsiveness to catecholamine stimulation, which enables prolonged vasoconstriction.

It is important to note that in the aging heart's attempt to maintain CO, the consequent left ventricular hypertrophy can account for the onset of myocardial ischemia independent of coronary atherosclerosis. On a purely physiological basis, several factors may contribute to the older heart's increased predisposition to developing ischemia:

• a disproportionate increase in myocyte size relative to the available circulation, resulting

in a demand by tissue for more oxygen than the blood can supply;

• an inability of aging coronary vessels to dilate due to increasing stiffness and prolonged sympathetic-mediated vasoconstriction, resulting in an inadequate blood supply for cardiac demand;

• the prolonged time for ventricular relaxation, which utilizes more energy and oxygen than does a rapid relaxation period, thus creating a supply-demand imbalance;

• myocardial ischemia caused by any of these physiological processes of aging, which further decreases myocardial compliance and worsens ischemia, ventricular filling, and, finally, systolic function.

AGE-RELATED CARDIOVASCULAR CHANGES AND EXERCISE

The decline in cardiac performance that occurs with aging reduces cardiac reserves. The healthy older

Box 6–2

Age-Related Changes in Cardiovascular Function*

- ↓ Beta-adrenergic responsiveness
- ↑ Afterload (vascular impedance)
- ↓ Early diastolic filling
- ↑ Dependency on atrial contraction
- ↑ Contraction-relaxation time (prolonged)
- ↑ Left ventricular end-diastolic pressure (rest and exercise)
- ↓ Ability to adjust to rapid volume shifts
- ↑ Vascular tone
- Left ventricular hypertrophy

* ↑ = increase; ↓ = decrease

individual is less able to accommodate to the added stress of exertion and fatigues more easily than does the healthy younger individual with comparable workloads. Maximal oxygen consumption ($\dot{V}O_2$ max), a measure of total body oxygen intake at exhaustion and an index of overall cardiovascular and pulmonary fitness, tends to decrease with aging. Oxygen consumption ($\dot{V}O_2$) can be expressed by the following formula (the Fick equation):

$$\dot{V}O_2 = CO \times A\text{-}\dot{V}O_2 \text{ difference}$$

oxygen consumption = cardiac output
× arteriovenous oxygen difference

The decline in $\dot{V}O_2$ max may be partially attributed to a decrease in cardiac output. The age-related decrease in skeletal muscle mass and consequent decrease in oxygen extraction may also contribute to the decrease in $\dot{V}O_2$ max (see Table 6–1).

Elderly individuals who exercise regularly show less of a decrease in $\dot{V}O_2$ max and may be able to reverse a number of age-associated changes in cardiovascular function (see Table 6–1). It is of interest to note that many of the benefits of exercise training enjoyed by older persons are similar to those found in the younger population. For example, compared to sedentary elderly individuals, older persons who are exercise-conditioned tend to have a lower resting HR and blood pressure, improved diastolic function, lower peripheral vascular resistance, and improved peripheral oxygen utilization. In addition, "trained" elderly demonstrate

lower rates of myocardial infarction, heart failure, and overall morbidity and mortality due to disease.

AGE-RELATED CARDIOVASCULAR CHANGES AND DISEASE

Increased morbidity is associated with advancing age. More than 50% of all individuals over 60 years of age have heart disease. The combination of age-related changes in the cardiovascular system and the impact heart disease has on cardiac performance make physiological responses during rest and exercise difficult to anticipate. Isolation of the effects of aging on the heart are inconclusive in the presence of heart disease. For example, myocardial scarring due to the chronic ischemia of coronary artery disease decreases ventricular compliance and

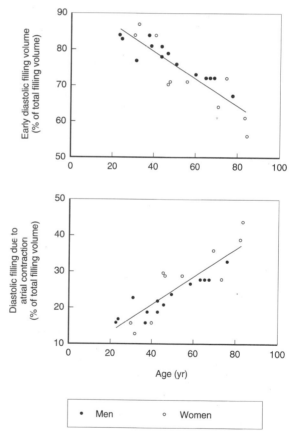

Figure 6–2 Age-associated decrease in early diastolic filling rate is compensated for by an increase in filling due to atrial contraction. (Based on data from Swinne CJ, Shapiro EP, Lima SD, Fleg JL. Age-associated changes in left ventricular diastolic performance during isometric exercise in normal subjects. *Am J Cardiol* 1992; 69:823–826. Reproduced with permission from *The Merck Manual of Geriatrics*, edited by William B. Abrams and Robert Berkow. Copyright 1990 by Merck & Co., Inc., Rahway, NJ.)

slows ventricular filling, eventually promoting diastolic dysfunction. As discussed previously, the senescent heart also exhibits increased myocardial wall stiffness, which slows ventricular filling and can similarly lead to diastolic dysfunction. Diastolic dysfunction is the primary cause of heart failure in elderly patients. More than 50% of patients older than 80 years who have heart failure have "normal" systolic function. Table 6–2 lists additional examples of the clinical consequences of age-related cardiovascular changes, some of which cannot be distinguished from preexisting disease. Clinical measures that may assist the practitioner in recognizing these changes are also listed in Table 6–2.

In addition, older individuals with comorbidities of the lung or circulation can show significantly reduced exercise capacities. Failure of the lungs to diffuse oxygen into the blood effectively or failure of the blood to transport oxygen and exchange it in the tissue creates a greater demand on cardiac efficiency. The older individual may not have the reserve capacity to increase either the heart rate or the stroke volume to meet this demand. This may stimulate compensatory mechanisms in cardiac performance such as ventricular hypertrophy or keep the individual from tolerating physical activity.

It is worth noting that the older individual typically takes medication for the management of heart disease or other illnesses. Many of these agents directly alter the physiological performance of the heart at rest or during exercise or both. Oftentimes, the prescribed dosage of a drug does not achieve the desired therapeutic outcome or the polypharmacy of the older person increases the risk of drug toxicity. For example, digoxin, a drug commonly prescribed for the management of congestive heart failure and atrial arrhythmias, can be toxic to an older individual. Digoxin tends to accumulate in the blood because of the reduced glomerular filtration rate through the kidneys, a common finding with aging. When quinidine, an antiarrhythmic drug, is taken in combination with digoxin, the serum digoxin level may double, further increasing the risk of digoxin toxicity, a potentially fatal condition. Hence, knowledge of the indications and pharmacokinetics of commonly prescribed drugs is essential for caregivers working with a geriatric population (see Chapter 13, "Pharmacology").

CONCLUSION

Cardiac performance is a dynamic interplay of compensatory mechanisms, some of which may not be available to the older individual. The senescent cardiovascular system, stressed by the presence of disease of the heart or other organs and commonly supported by pharmacological agents, appears vulnerable to decompensation. Although the aging process cannot be stopped, health-care providers are

Table 6–2 Clinical Consequences of Age-Related Cardiovascular Changes and Clinical Measurements

Age-Related Change[a]	Clinical Consequences	Clinical Measure/Symptom[b]
↓ β-adrenergic responsiveness	Blunted heart rate response to exercise	HR, BP, RR, RPE
	Orthostatic hypotension	HR, BP, lightheadedness, change in color
	Longer to reach steady state	HR, RR
	Longer to recover from exercise	HR, RR
↑ Vascular tone; ↑ vascular stiffness (↑ afterload)	Systolic hypertension	BP
	Signs of ventricular hypertrophy	Laterally placed PMI
	Symptoms of myocardial ischemia	RPP, ECG, chest pain, change in color
Pacemaker and conducting tissue cells	Arrhythmias (e.g., sss[c])	HR, BP, ECG, rhythm
	Conduction blocks	HR, BP, ECG, rhythm
↓ Ventricular compliance	Diastolic dysfunction, heart failure	S4, BP (may be normal)
↓ Early diastolic filling	Left atrial hypertrophy, atrial arrhythmias	HR, ECG, rhythm
Prolonged relaxation time	Symptoms of ischemia	RPP, ECG, chest pain, change in color

[a] ↑ = increase; ↓ = decrease
[b] HR = heart rate; BP = blood pressure; RR = respiratory rate; RPE = rating of perceived exertion; PMI = point of maximal impulse; RPP = rate-pressure product; S4 = fourth heart sound
[c] sss = sick sinus syndrome

challenged not only to help the healthy older individual to safely slow or reverse the progressive decline but also to consider these changes when implementing a demanding rehabilitation program. The value of an exercise program for older individuals should not be underestimated. Minimal improvements in cardiovascular and pulmonary fitness can enable an older person to continue to live independently.

SUGGESTED READINGS

Cohen M, Hoskins-Michel T. *Cardiopulmonary Symptoms in Physical Therapy Practice.* New York: Churchill Livingstone; 1988:15–41.

Forman DE, Wei JY. Age-related cardiovascular changes. In: Rich MW (ed). *Geriatric Cardiology.* Boston: Beth Israel Hospital, CVR&R 1994:47–51.

Kispert C. Measuring function in the elderly: cardipulmonary. In: Proceedings of the Eugene Michels Forum, Section on Research. American Physical Therapy Association. Washington, D.C. February 12, 1988:23.

Lakatta EG. Normal changes of aging. In: Abrams WB, Beer MH, Berkow R, eds. *The Merck Manual of Geriatrics,* 2nd ed. Rahway, N.J.: Merck, Sharp and Dohme Research Laboratories; 1995:429.

Protas E. Physiological change and adaptation to exercise in the older adult. In: Guccione A, ed. *Foundations of Geriatric Physical Therapy.* St. Louis, Mo.: Mosby–Year Book; 1993:33.

Shephard RJ, Sidney KH. Exercise and aging. *Exerc Sport Sci Rev* 1978; 6:1.

Wei JY. Cardiovascular anatomic and physiologic changes with age. 1986; 2(1):10–16.

Wei JY. Age and the cardiovascular system. *N Engl J Med* 1992; 327(24):1735.

Chapter **7**

Pulmonary Considerations in the Older Patient
Meryl Cohen, M.S., P.T.

INTRODUCTION

Age-related changes in the pulmonary system of a healthy individual are slow and progressive. Often, the decline in pulmonary function is not noticed until the person reaches 60, 70, or even 80 years of age. Unlike the cardiovascular system, the pulmonary system has large ventilatory reserves available to compensate for the structural and physiological consequences of aging. However, in the presence of pulmonary disease, these reserves are often inadequate and can impose severe limitations on the performance of physical activities (see Chapter 49

for a discussion of pathological lung conditions). In addition, exposure to environmental toxins over a lifetime can contribute to a more rapid decline in pulmonary function in the older person.

The age-related changes that occur in lung tissue and in the "musculoskeletal pump" are discussed in this chapter. A clear distinction among the effects of aging, subclinical disease, and prolonged exposure to air pollutants on the pulmonary system is difficult to establish, as all three cause similar structural and physiological abnormalities. General observations regarding the senescent lung and the effects of exercise and pulmonary disease on age-related changes in pulmonary function are also discussed. The clinical effects of aging on the pulmonary system and the implications for care-givers of older individuals are identified.

PULMONARY STRUCTURE

Age-associated changes can be found in the anatomical structures of the pulmonary system. Both the gas-exchanging organ—the lung tissue—and the musculoskeletal pump—the thoracic cage and its muscular attachments—show decline in the older individual when they are compared to the organs of a healthy younger person (see Box 7–1).

The Lung

Changes in the alveolar membrane, including loss of the alveolar-capillary interface, and increase in alveolar size due to the destruction of walls of individual alveoli, are the major forms of damage found in the aging lung. The general disintegration of the supporting fibrous network of the lung and of the septa of the alveoli is considered a consequence of aging, but these changes can also result from repeated inflammatory injuries caused by lifelong exposure to environmental oxidants and cigarette smoke.

The Musculoskeletal Pump

Many of the age-related changes in the thoracic cage result from the loss of mineral and bone matrix and the increased crosslinking of collagen fibers (see Chapter 25, "The Bony Thorax") which contribute to the characteristic thoracic kyphosis and barrel chest of the older individual. The decreased mobility of the bony thorax and the less efficient resting position of the muscles of respiration alter lung performance and further contribute to the decline in pulmonary function with age.

Box 7-1

Age-Related Changes in Pulmonary System Structure*

Airways
- ↑ Rigidity of trachea and bronchi
- ↓ Elasticity of bronchiolar walls
- ↓ Cilia

Replacement of smooth muscle fibers in bronchioles with noncontractile tissue

Lungs
- ↑ Mucus layer (thickening) and ↑ mucus glands
- ↑ Thinning of alveolar walls (↓ alveolar collagen)
- ↓ Functional respiratory surface resulting from destruction of alveolar septa (loss of fibrous supporting network)
- ↑ Alveolar diameter with a ↓ in alveolar surface area
- ↓ Alveolar-capillary interface (due to ↑ alveolar size and ↓ capillary bed)
- ↑ Lung compliance
- ↓ Lung parenchymal weight

Vascular walls stiffen as media and intima thicken
- Probable ↓ surfactant producing cells

Respiratory Muscles
- ↓ Contractile protein
- ↑ Noncontractile protein
- ↑ Connective tissue
- ↓ Capillary numbers relative to muscle fibers
- ↑ Contraction and relaxation times

Alteration in diaphragm position and efficiency

Skeleton
- ↓ Loss of bone mineralization
- ↓ Disc spaces
- ↓ Costal movements resulting from reduced sternal and costovertebral motion (↑ stiffness at joints)
- ↑ Anterior-posterior thorax diameter
- ↑ Kyphosis resulting from a decrease in thoracic length

* ↑ = increases; ↓ = decreases.

PULMONARY PHYSIOLOGY

The primary functions of the pulmonary system are to exchange gas between the blood and the atmospheric air and to protect the body from airborne invaders. Resting lung function results from a balance of elastic tissue forces pulling inward and musculoskeletal-pump forces pulling outward. This dynamic and mostly involuntary interplay between lung tissue and chest wall musculoskeletal components depends on the compliance of both. Age-related changes in lung tissue compliance result from structural changes in the alveoli. The decrease in efficiency of pulmonary function is not generally perceived in normal elderly people because compromise of other systems with less reserve usually accounts for the alterations in their activity patterns.

The decline in alveolar structure and the pulmonary capillary bed contributes to the changes seen in ventilation (movement of gas to and from the alveoli) and gas distribution. Effective diffusion of oxygen and carbon dioxide into and out of the blood stream depends on the integrity of the alveolar membrane and on adequate vascularity. Because alveolar membranes and capillary interfaces are compromised in the older individual, the ventilation-perfusion mismatching that is normally found in young individuals worsens with advancing age. As a result, there are larger ventilated areas relative to perfused portions of the lung (physiological dead space) which leads to a noticeable reduction in diffusing capacity (see Box 7–2).

The loss of elastic recoil in alveolar and conducting tissue and the disintegration of the fibrous supporting network also contribute to an increase in ventilation-perfusion imbalance. Smaller airways are unable to stay patent at low lung volumes (with expiration), leading to early airway closure. The resulting collapse of distal airways creates an imbalance in ventilation-perfusion. In addition, the excessive decrease in ventilation as compared to circulation causes a lowering of arterial oxygen pressure (Pao_2). See Box 7–3.

An increase in closing volume due to small airway collapse and poor lung emptying due to increased alveolar compliance and decreased elastic recoil help to account for the increase in functional residual capacity (FRC). This is the volume at which the lung comes to rest at the end of quiet expiration. Residual volume (RV), the volume that remains in the lung after maximal expiration, increases as well. The increases in lung volume tend to flatten the diaphragm, the major muscle responsible for inspiration, as it is unable to return to its original resting position. The altered diaphragm mechanics cause an increase in the anterior-posterior diameter of the rib cage. Changes in the position of

Box 7-2

Age-Related Changes in

Pulmonary Function[a]

- ↑ Ventilation-perfusion mismatch (less homogenous)
- ↓ Diffusing capacity
- ↑ Physiological dead space
- ↓ Lung emptying
- ↑ Respiratory muscle oxygen consumption (rest)
- ↑ Minute ventilation (rest)
- ↓ Inspiratory muscle strength

[a] ↑ = increases; ↓ = decreases.

the diaphragm and in the dimensions of the thorax increase the work of breathing, and the muscle primarily responsible for inspiration is at a mechanical disadvantage when it comes to performing the increased work (Fig. 7-1).

The progressive decrease in chest wall compliance and the consequent stiffness also increase the energy expended when breathing. More oxygen is consumed by the respiratory muscles, and the minute ventilation increases to meet this demand. In addition, there are age-related decreases in the strength and endurance of ventilatory muscles that are similar to those seen in skeletal muscle (see Chapter 3). Inspiratory and abdominal muscle weakness can also compromise cough efficacy. This becomes more significant with aging as the mucous layer of lung tissue thickens and a more forceful cough is required to mobilize secretions.

The decrease in thoracic mobility also results in decreased vital capacity (the maximum amount of air that can be exhaled following a maximum inhalation) and decreased maximal voluntary ventilation (the volume of air breathed when an individual breathes as fast and as deeply as possible for a given time). This decline in pulmonary function can negatively impact an older individual's ability to exercise.

AGE-RELATED PULMONARY CHANGES AND EXERCISE

In general, pulmonary responses to low and moderate exercise are the same in people of all ages. The pulmonary system can respond to the increased demands of exercise by increasing the minute ventilation (the amount of air moved into or out of the lungs per unit of time). Minute ventilation is dependent on the tidal volume (the volume of air normally inhaled and exhaled with each breath during quiet breathing) and the frequency of breathing (respiratory rate). In the older individual, initial increases in minute ventilation are achieved by increases in tidal volume. Dyspnea is perceived when the increase in tidal volume reaches 55% to 60% of vital capacity. As already discussed, vital capacity decreases with advancing age. Hence, the ability to increase minute ventilation may be reduced at higher intensities of exercise.

In addition, the older individual tends to perform work less efficiently, generating more blood lactate. The resultant acidosis is compensated for by an increased ventilatory effort to expire more carbon dioxide. Often, this results in early fatigue and a higher rating of perceived exertion (RPE) for a given workload by comparison to a younger or more fit older individual.

At low exercise workloads, an older individual continues to demonstrate ventilation-perfusion mismatching and decreased diffusing capacity. However, during vigorous exercise, pulmonary artery pressure increases. This tends to increase the alveo-

Box 7-3

Age-Related Changes in Pulmonary

Function Measures[a]

- ↑ Residual volume (RV)
- ↑ Functional residual capacity (FRC)
- ↓ or ↔ Total lung capacity (TLC)
- ↑ Closing volume
- ↓ Maximal voluntary ventilation (MVV); ↓ 30% between 30 and 70 years of age
- ↓ Vital capacity (VC); ↓ 25% between 30 and 70 years of age
- ↓ Forced expiratory volume (FEV_1)
- ↓ Arterial pressure of oxygen (PaO_2); 75 mmHg is normal for 70 years of age
- ↓ Oxygen saturation
- ↓ Diffusing capacity of carbon monoxide (DLCO)

[a] ↑ = increases; ↓ = decreases; ↔ = no change.

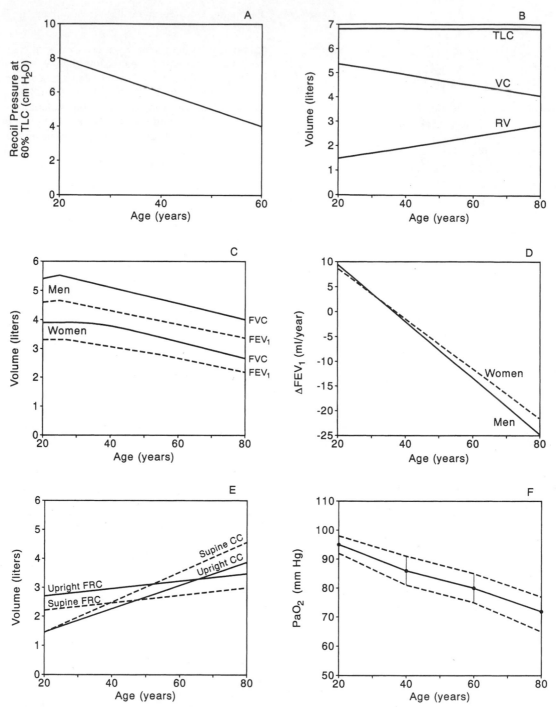

Figure 7–1 Representative changes in respiratory function with age. Curves show mean or generalized changes, and there may be considerable variation among individuals. Note the varying age scales on the horizontal axes. (A) Changes in lung elastic recoil with age. (Adapted from Murray JF, *The Normal Lung.* 2nd ed. Philadelphia: WB Saunders, 1986; 339–360.) (B) Changes in static lung volumes with age. TLC, total lung capacity; VC, vital capacity; RV, residual volume. (C) Changes in FVC (solid lines) and FEV₁ (dashed lines) with age in men and women. (Adapted from Burrows B, Cline MG, Knudson RJ et al, A descriptive analysis of the growth and decline of the FVC and FEV₁. *Chest* 1983; 83:717–724.) (D) Changes in the rate of loss of FEV₁ with age in men (solid line) and women (dashed line). (Adapted from Burrows B, Lebowitz MD, Camilli AE, Knudson RJ, Longitudinal changes in forced expiratory volume in one second in adults. *Am Rev Respir Dis* 1986; 133:974–980.) (E) Changes in CC (defined as RV plus CV) and in FRC with age. Solid lines, upright posture; dashed lines, supine posture. (F) Changes in PaO₂ (at sea level) with increasing age. Dashed lines represent ± 2 SD from the mean for the subjects studied. (Adapted from Sorbini CA, Grassi V, Solinas E, Muiesan G, Arterial oxygen tension in relation to age in healthy subjects. *Respiration* 1968; 25:3–13.) (Reproduced with permission from Pierson DJ. Effects of aging on the respiratory system. In: Pierson DJ, Kacmarek RM. *Foundations of Respiratory Care.* New York: Churchill Livingstone; 1992.)

lar capillary blood flow throughout the lungs. With improved perfusion, the ventilation-perfusion imbalance lessens and lung function and exercise tolerance improves.

With exercise training, an older individual is able to show some improvement in the pulmonary response to exercise (see Table 7–1). Most of the improved pulmonary function results from greater efficiency of ventilatory and skeletal muscle performance. This is evidenced by the decreased production of lactate and carbon dioxide when undertaking a given workload. The individual is able to work at a lower percentage of maximal voluntary ventilation and has an increased ventilatory response for a given oxygen uptake ($\dot{V}E/\dot{V}O_2$) and less perceived dyspnea. Improved pulmonary function may also be attributed to the increase in thoracic mobility typically seen after exercise training. Individuals who are initially sedentary show the greatest improvement in function. Measurements commonly used in the clinic to monitor pulmonary response to exercise are found in Box 7–4.

Exercise can also help to mobilize secretions because it increases minute ventilation. Secretion retention can predispose an older individual to disease, hence exercise may further prevent decline of pulmonary function.

AGE-RELATED PULMONARY CHANGES AND DISEASE

The weakening of pulmonary structure and the decline in performance that occur with advancing age tend to have minimal impact on the functional ability of the healthy older individual. In the presence of chronic lung disease, pulmonary performance may be the limitation to exercise. Although the physiological changes in chronic obstructive pulmonary disease (COPD) are similar to those observed with aging, any lung disease that alters alveolar cell function or thoracic cage mobility can negatively impact lung function.

The cumulative effects of COPD on the pulmonary changes normally seen with aging include a range of physiological outcomes. During rest, an individual may or may not show an increase in minute ventilation. At low workloads, an early increase in minute ventilation is observed as the lungs attempt to improve the ventilation-perfusion imbalance. Clinically, the older individual with COPD may be chronically short of breath but accepts it as a normal part of aging. As the intensity of work increases or as the disease progresses, the growing work of breathing causes an increase in the relative percentage of oxygen delivered to the respiratory muscles. Often, in the presence of thoracic cage

Table 7–1 Age-Related Pulmonary Changes with Exercise*

	Due to Aging	After Endurance Exercise Training
Submaximal exercise:		
Minute ventilation ($\dot{V}E$)	↑	↓
Carbon dioxide production	↑	↓
Blood lactate	↑	↓
Maximal exercise:		
Maximal exercise ventilation ($\dot{V}E_{max}$)	↓	↑
Maximal voluntary ventilation (MVV)	↓	↑
$\dot{V}E_{max}$/MVV	↓	↑

* ↑ = increase; ↓ = decrease
(Adapted from Protas E. Physiological change and adaptation to exercise in the older adult. In: Guccione A, ed. *Geriatric Physical Therapy*. St. Louis: Mosby–Year Book; 1993:42.)

rigidity and a significant loss of diffusing capacity, the extra energy required for pulmonary muscle function is obtained from inefficient anaerobic processes. This is seen clinically as a significant in-

Box 7–4

Clinical Monitors Used to Measure Pulmonary Responses to Exercise

Respiratory rate (RR)
Oxygen saturation (SaO_2)
Rating of perceived exertion (RPE)
Heart rate (HR)
Oxygen consumption ($\dot{V}O_2$)
Anaerobic threshold (AT)
Arterial blood gases (ABG)
　Oxygen tension (PaO_2)
　Carbon dioxide tension ($PaCO_2$)
　pH
Peak expiratory flow rate (PEFR)
Breath sounds
Cough
Color (lips, fingernails)

crease in dyspnea and heart rate and a decrease in arterial oxygen tension, which creates an even greater minute ventilation. In an attempt to meet this increased demand for oxygen, the heart tries to increase its performance. In some patients with compromised heart reserve, a decline in heart function can occur and, when combined with increased performance efforts, that can lead to heart failure and further compromise of the oxygen delivery system.

Age-related changes in the lungs may increase an older person's risk of developing pulmonary disease. The thickening of the mucous layer, the loss of cilia and ciliary function within airways, decreased cough effectiveness due to muscle weakness, and early airway closure combined with increased closing volume may contribute to the increased risk of pneumonia that is seen in the older population. In addition, the age-associated decline in the physiological performance of the immune system may further predispose senescent lungs to infection.

CONCLUSION

Age-related changes occur in lung tissue and in the musculoskeletal pump. Pathological conditions potentiate the effects of these changes.

Although the objective benefits of exercise training are difficult to measure, older individuals with pulmonary disease are able to recognize an improved physical work capacity and sense of well-being. Respiratory and peripheral muscle conditioning and increased thoracic cage mobility improve the mechanical efficiency of the musculoskeletal pump and of oxygen extraction by the tissues. This may interrupt the declining cycle of dyspnea, inactivity, and worsening dyspnea and enable an individual to remain independent and active. In addition, the improved strength and endurance of respiratory and abdominal muscles can facilitate cough effectiveness and assist in the management of retained secretions, thus decreasing the risk of pulmonary infection.

SUGGESTED READINGS

Brandstetter RD, Kazemi H. Aging and the respiratory system. *Med Clin North Am* 1983; 67(2):419–431.

Clough P. Restrictive lung dysfunction. In: Hillegass E, Sadowsky S, eds. *Essentials of Cardiopulmonary Physical Therapy.* Philadelphia: W.B. Saunders; 1994:189.

Cohen M, Hoskins-Michel T. *Cardiopulmonary Symptoms in Physical Therapy Practice.* New York: Churchill Livingstone; 1988:1–9.

Kispert C. Measuring function in the elderly: cardiopulmonary.

In: Proceedings of the Eugene Michels Forum, section on research. American Physical Therapy Association. Washington, D.C. February 12, 1988:23.

Patrick DF. Pulmonary rehabilitation of the geriatric patient. *Top Geriatr Rehabil* 1986; 2:55–69.

Protas E. Physiological change and adaptation to exercise in the older adult. In: Guccione A, ed. *Foundations of Geriatric Physical Therapy.* St. Louis: Mosby–Year Book; 1993:33–45.

Tockman MS. The effects of age on the lung. In: Abrams WB, Beer MH, Berkow RJ, eds. *The Merck Manual of Geriatrics*, 2nd ed. Whitehouse Station, N.J.: Merck Research Laboratories; 1995:423.

Zadai CC, ed. *Pulmonary Management in Physical Therapy.* New York: Churchill Livingstone; 1992.

Chapter **8**

Effects of Aging on Vascular Function

Deborah Wojcik, M.Ed., P.T.
Kristin von Nieda, M.Ed., P.T.

INTRODUCTION

The oxygen transport system is the biological system responsible for (1) bringing oxygen into the body from the ambient environment, (2) circulating the oxygen throughout the body, (3) supplying the tissue level with oxygen, and (4) ultimately removing the waste products created as a result of utilizing the oxygen. The vascular system is the part of the oxygen transport system that supplies the oxygen and nutrients to the working tissue and accepts the metabolic waste. By supplying a steady stream of oxygen-rich blood, the vasculature allows working tissue and muscle to function at optimal levels. In addition, the ability to shunt blood preferentially and to deliver oxygen to the areas of greatest metabolic demand makes the vascular system an important component of the oxygen transport system.

The vascular system is made up of three basic types of blood vessels: the arterial, the capillary, and the venous vessels. The normal structure of most blood vessels includes three layers. The outermost layer, the adventitia, consists of longitudinally oriented connective tissue. In the arterial vessels, the adventitia contains a significant number of elastic fibers. The middle layer, or the media, is a highly elastic, circumferentially oriented fibromuscular layer. The intima, the innermost layer, is composed of a single layer of longitudinally oriented endothelial cells. The thickness of each respective layer varies throughout the vascular system depending on the location and the function of the specific blood vessel. Figure 8–1 summarizes the relative differences among the arterial, capillary, and venous vessels.

The arterial aspect of the system contains a higher percentage of vessels whose walls are highly elastic and contain significant amounts of smooth muscle. Hence, the arterial system can accommodate the large volume of blood received as cardiac output and propel it forward using the property of elastic recoil. The presence of smooth muscle in the arterial system also allows it to control and direct the flow of blood throughout all parts of the vascular system via autonomic control and according to local metabolic demand.

The capillary beds are the sites of gas exchange between the arterial vasculature and the respective tissue. To accommodate such an important function, the capillaries consist of very thin walls that have little resistance to the diffusion of oxygen and other metabolic products. For this reason, the capillaries are single-cell layers of intima.

The capacitance vessels, or veins, serve as collecting tubules; they collect the blood as it exits the capillary beds. The veins have very little smooth muscle in the media but are the vessels responsible for propelling the blood from the periphery back to the central part of the circulatory system. This function is accomplished by a combination of venous smooth muscle contraction, external muscle compression, and a series of unidirectional internal venous valves. At any given time, the majority of the blood volume is located in the venous circulation. As venous return is the principal determinant of cardiac preload, adequate flow of blood from the venous circulation is necessary to ensure sufficient cardiac output. The large reservoir of blood maintained in the venous circulation also allows for an adequate reserve that can be readily tapped into during periods of increased oxygen demand. Therefore, the mechanisms responsible for propelling the venous circulation are essential.

STRUCTURAL CHANGES ASSOCIATED WITH AGING

Like all other parts of the oxygen transport mechanism, structural changes occur in the vasculature as an individual ages. Changes are noted in each of the three layers but are very different from layer to layer. Within the intima, the endothelial cells are no longer oriented in a uniform longitudinal fashion. The more irregular orientation of the intimal lining has a significant impact on the dynamics of and resistance to bloodflow. Generally, there is an increased thickness of the subendothelial layer of the intima as a result of the calcification of the vessels' structural components and the deposition of connective tissue and lipids in the vessel wall. This thickening of the innermost layer has a significant effect on the transport of oxygen and other nutrients. The ability of oxygen to diffuse readily from the vasculature to the working tissue may be impaired. Significant calcification also occurs in the media layer, thereby hindering the normal contraction capability of the vessels' smooth muscle. The adventitial layer is most affected by a decrease in the number of elastic fibers and an increase in collagen. This loss of elasticity prevents the vessel from readily accepting incoming bloodflow and, just as significantly, it does not allow for the occurrence of the elastic recoil which normally assists in propelling the blood forward into the vascular system.

PHYSIOLOGICAL CHANGES ASSOCIATED WITH AGING

The alterations in the structure of the blood vessels that result from aging have a physiologically sig-

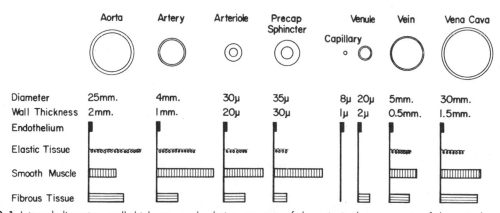

Figure 8–1 Internal diameter, wall thickness, and relative amounts of the principal components of the vessel walls of the various blood vessels that compose the circulatory system. Cross-sections of the vessels are not drawn to scale because of the huge range in size from aorta and vena cava to capillary. (Reproduced with permission from Berne RM, Levy MN. *Cardiovascular Physiology*, 4th ed. St. Louis: C.V. Mosby; 1981:2. Redrawn from Burton AC. *Physiol Rev* 1954; 34:619.)

nificant impact on the arterial system. Because of a significant loss in the elasticity of the large arteries and the aorta, the vessels become more rigid. This results in a decreased ability to accept the cardiac output as it is ejected from the heart. The vasculature attempts to compensate for this decrease in cardiac output into the vascular system by maintaining an increased state of resting vasodilation in the large proximal arteries. In addition, the higher collagen content in the vessels results in an increased hysteresis in the vessel walls, which causes further dilation. Hysteresis occurs as a result of the large proximal vessels stretching as much as possible to receive the cardiac output, but due to their loss of elastic recoil, the vessels are unable to return to their original size and shape. The net result is slightly increased resting dilation. This increased vasodilation is an attempt by the vascular system to restore the cardiac output lost as a result of the increased rigidity of the vessels. The loss of the elastic recoil, in turn, precipitates a decrease in the ability of the vessel to compress and propel the blood forward through the peripheral vascular system. An overall decrease in compliance as a result of the stiffening occurs throughout the vascular tree. Any decrease in arterial vessel compliance requires that an elevation in pressure be generated to move a given volume of blood through a vessel. Because the heart is the pump that generates the initial propelling force, a decrease in the compliance of the arterial system results in an increase in the workload being placed on the heart.

Venous changes also occur as a result of normal aging. These changes are similar to the arterial changes; they result in an overall stiffening of the venous system. In addition, the efficiency of the unidirectional venous valves lessens. The valves begin to lose their integrity, and that means the flow is no longer being propelled in one direction. It therefore becomes more difficult to maintain venous return, and there exists the potential for the occurrence of venous pooling and retrograde bloodflow. As the forward movement of blood from the venous circulation to the heart determines preload, any loss of forward flow may negatively impact cardiac output.

At the level of the arterioles and capillaries, alterations in structure (summarized in Box 8–1) result in alterations in function. There is a decrease in the overall responsiveness of the small arteries and capillaries. A variable pattern in the distribution of bloodflow at rest is noted. Much of this decrease in flow to muscle may be attributed to the diminished ability of the small arteries and arterioles to vasodilate. A net change toward vasoconstriction ensues in these vessels. The decrease in flow has significant impact on the diffusion capability of the

---

Box 8–1

Changes in the Vasculature
Associated with Aging

STRUCTURAL CHANGES:

Endothelial thickening
Smooth-muscle calcification
Decreased elastic fiber content
Increased collagen content
Loss of venous valve integrity

PHYSIOLOGICAL CHANGES:

Decreased elasticity
Decreased elastic recoil
Potential for impaired diffusion
Decreased compliance
Potential for venous pooling
Increased total peripheral resistance

---

vessel. This alteration in vascular diameter not only decreases flow to many areas of muscle but it also increases the turbulence of the flow that does exist. Turbulent bloodflow is nonuniform and highly random. Laminar flow, on the other hand, is streamlined and uniform. Because turbulent flow is significantly more resistive than laminar flow, the resistance to propelling the blood increases, and the workload required to overcome that increased resistance intensifies. The mere presence of a vasoconstricted, or narrowed, vessel diameter increases the resistance to bloodflow. Blood vessel diameter is well known to be the single greatest determinant of resistance to flow. It is not surprising to note that aging blood vessels demonstrate a decline in the ability to shunt blood preferentially from areas of lower metabolic activity to areas of greater metabolic demand. All of these peripheral changes combine to raise total peripheral resistance, as vasomotor tone is the factor that determines peripheral resistance. In addition, because diastolic blood pressure is a reflection of total peripheral resistance, the potential exists for elevation of diastolic blood pressure. A significant systemic result of a constant increase in total peripheral resistance and a constant decrease in arterial distensibility is increased afterload. This increased afterload is believed to be responsible for the higher resting systolic blood pressure associated with aging. In addition, the vascular changes noted with aging are postulated to precipitate the left ventricular hypertrophy seen with advancing age.

AUTONOMIC SYSTEM CHANGES WITH AGING

Cardiac and vascular activity is controlled by the autonomic nervous system as well as by a series of autonomically mediated cardiopulmonary reflexes. With aging, a decrease in β-adrenergic receptor sites is noted in the vasculature. The loss of β-receptor sites allows an α-adrenergic–mediated response to predominate. An α-mediated response, if unchecked, results in a state of greater resting vasoconstriction. This autonomically mediated vasoconstriction compounds the vasoconstriction resulting from the previously described mechanisms.

A significant decrease in the reactivity of cardiopulmonary reflexes, especially the reflex mediated by the baroreceptors, occurs with advancing age. Baroreceptor activity is directed by the stretch demanded of vascular walls in the aorta and the carotid arteries by the blood flowing through the vessels. A decrease in the stretch required and, thus, in baroreceptor activity normally results in messages ordering restoration of cardiac output to increase blood pressure. This reflex activity is essential to prevent the orthostatic hypotensive response (a drop ≥ 20 mmHg in systolic blood pressure) that could occur with movement from the reclining to the upright position. A decrease in overall baroreceptor activity coupled with a decrease stretch of the vessel wall as a result of rigidity hinders the short-term regulation that normally occurs in the cardiac and vascular systems as a result of body-position changes.

Failure of the baroreceptor to sense the venous pooling that occurs with the assumption of the upright position results in a significant and often symptomatic drop in systolic blood pressure. The symptoms associated with this orthostatic response are dizziness, syncope, and reflex tachycardia. Alterations in baroreceptor activity and declines in the responsiveness of the aged vascular system result in an exaggerated orthostatic response with advancing age. It is, therefore, very important that individuals of advanced age participate in dynamic standing exercises to limit the orthostatic response. Static exercises do not have the same ability to limit the orthostatic responses, as they do not provide as efficient an extravascular pumping mechanism as do dynamic activities. It is also important that health-care providers carefully monitor vital signs and symptoms of orthostatic hypotension when working with elderly patients.

Deconditioning is another physiological state that results in an exaggerated orthostatic response. It is created by a period of relative inactivity. Many elderly individuals are sedentary and therefore deconditioned. This state results in less efficient oxygen transport and poorly functioning skeletal muscle systems. A deconditioned person needs more energy to perform tasks and is less able to adapt quickly and efficiently to alterations in the body's homeostasis. Thus, the exaggeration of the orthostatic response during body position changes can be great. Any health professional working with an elderly patient must be aware of this potential for increased orthostatic response and know how to monitor and treat the response.

ALTERATIONS IN THE VASCULAR RESPONSE TO EXERCISE WITH AGING

The ability to adapt and respond to the changing needs of the body during exercise is an essential function of the vascular system. Box 8–2 summarizes the changes associated with the response to exercise in the elderly individual. It is the vasculature that transports oxygen from the central circulation to the metabolically active peripheral sites. Many of the changes previously discussed exhibit a significant effect on the ability of the vasculature to supply the tissues with the needed oxygen during exercise. This potential deficit often causes an older individual to reach fatigue quickly when exercising.

Under normal circumstances, exercise or any other period of increased activity is a sympathetically mediated state. Greater activity is associated with a rise in the release of the adrenergic mediators epinephrine and norepinephrine. Such a release raises the state of activity of most body systems, which allows cardiac output and oxygen transport to increase during exercise. However, because of having fewer and less sensitive adrenergic receptors, the aged vascular system is less responsive to this sympathetically mediated state and may be un-

Box 8–2

Alterations in the Response to Exercise

Decreased responsiveness to sympathetic outflow
Decreased oxygen delivery
Elevated systolic and diastolic blood pressure
Difficulty with thermoregulation
Inability to efficiently shunt bloodflow
Decreased A-VO$_2$ difference
Increased anaerobic metabolism during dynamic exercise
Earlier onset of fatigue

able to increase oxygen delivery in response to the demand being placed on the transport mechanism by autonomic mechanisms.

Alterations in the autonomic response to exercise can also result in higher-than-anticipated systolic and diastolic blood pressure responses with activity. With exercise, normal diastolic blood pressure shows no change or a slight decrease from resting levels. During exercise, slight elevations in diastolic blood pressure—no greater than 10 mmHg—although not technically normal responses are not considered clinically significant. An elevation of diastolic blood pressure of more than 10 mmHg, however, is considered abnormal. Systolic blood pressure should rise in proportion to the intensity of the activity being performed.

At a more local level, the peripheral vessels are less responsive to alterations in metabolic activity. Normally, increased metabolic activity in skeletal muscle results in vasodilation to meet the oxygen demand of the tissue. The stimulation of skeletal muscle vascular adrenergic receptors during exercise also results in vasodilation. Older individuals have less ability to vasodilate in response to greater metabolic activity. These same individuals also have decreased activity mediated through the adrenergic receptors, as mentioned previously. This inability to quickly increase blood supply with increased local metabolism coupled with a decreased ability to vasodilate, as a result of structural changes, prevents blood from being quickly shunted from areas of low metabolic activity to areas of more active muscle metabolism. Loss of this mechanism decreases an older individual's ability to do skeletal muscle work.

Older individuals, when exercising, have been shown to have a higher percentage of their cardiac output shunted to the skin and viscera and less directed toward working muscle. This is in part due to their decreased ability to thermoregulate. Normal thermoregulation relies on the processes of conduction, convection, and evaporation. Evaporation is the predominant mechanism for heat loss during exercise. As the process of evaporation is a sympathetically mediated function, older individuals have a decreased ability to utilize this mechanism for thermoregulation, which places them at higher risk for heat exhaustion. Older individuals attempt to compensate for this by shunting more cardiac output to the skin to improve heat loss via conduction and convection. Unfortunately, these two thermoregulatory mechanisms are not efficient mechanisms for adequate heat loss at rest or during exercise. This shunting also prevents the delivery of an adequate blood volume to skeletal muscle.

There also exists decreased muscle capillary density as one ages, further limiting the vascular supply. This decreased capillary to muscle-fiber ratio has a significant impact on an individual's ability to exercise, as less blood volume is delivered at any given time. Another important measure of the function of the oxygen transport system is the arteriovenous oxygen difference (A-Vo_2 diff) which is a measure of the utilization of oxygen by working muscle. Changes in skeletal muscle tissue structure, mitochondria, and metabolic enzymes result in a decreased A-Vo_2 diff. Therefore, less oxygen is being extracted from the capillary bed for use during exercise. Alterations in muscle fiber makeup in elderly muscles may also result in less efficient use of oxygen from the vasculature. Older individuals have a lower percentage of fast-twitch glycolytic fibers in skeletal muscles. Often, slow-twitch oxidative muscle fibers are preserved, as these are the muscles utilized daily for performing ADL activity. When a period of inactivity, a sedentary lifestyle, or an acute illness becomes superimposed upon aging, a decrease in slow-twitch oxidative fibers is also noted.

Biomechanical factors may also have an impact on vascular function during exercise. A loss of fast-twitch glycolytic muscle fibers with age results in a loss of the ability to generate high tension in a short time, as is often required during exercise. A resulting inefficiency in the performance of an activity requiring high force production is common. Often, an individual will attempt to perform or maintain an activity by performing a maximal contraction. Performance of a maximal contraction is known to result in external compression of the vasculature within the muscle, which causes ischemia. Ischemia in a working muscle results in an inability of the muscle to perform work. If the individual is also deconditioned, a loss of the more fatigue-resistant slow-twitch fibers results, further inhibiting the individual's ability to perform work. Poor biomechanical performance of an activity is also associated with an increased level of anaerobic metabolism and an earlier onset of fatigue. Skeletal muscles performing work in the elderly, therefore, are more susceptible to earlier fatigue and even, possibly, to ischemia.

CONCLUSION

Age-related changes occur in all of the various components of the oxygen transport mechanism, including the vasculature. In rehabilitation, it is important to note that strength and fitness training programs in the elderly have been shown to decrease the amount of decline in function of many bodily systems, including the vascular system. Although training will not entirely eliminate the inevitable decline that occurs with advancing age, the severity of the decline will be lessened.

SUGGESTED READINGS

Davies CTM. The oxygen-transporting system in relation to age. *Clin Sci* 1972; 42:1–13.

Lakatta E et al. Cardiovascular regulatory mechanisms in advanced age. *Physiol Rev* 1993; 86:2.

Martin A. Hypertension. In: Martin A et al. *Heart Disease in the Elderly*. New York: John Wiley & Sons; 1984:59.

Martin W et al. Effects of aging, gender, and physical training on peripheral vascular function. *Circulation* 1991; 84:654–664.

de Nicola P et al. Arterial hypertension. In *Cardiology and the Aged*. Stuttgart: Schattauer; 1985:184.

de Nicola P et al. Arterial hypotension. In *Cardiology and the Aged*. Stuttgart: Schattauer; 1985:200.

Zadai C et al. Cardiopulmonary rehabilitation of the geriatric patient. In: Lewis C, ed. *Aging and the Healthcare Challenge*, 3rd ed. Philadelphia: F.A. Davis; 1996:196.

Chapter 9

The Effects of Aging on the Digestive System

Ronni Chernoff, Ph.D., R.D., FADA

INTRODUCTION

Nutrient intake necessary to maintain health and prevent disease may be different from that required by the treatment of chronic medical conditions or for the recovery of health following an acute medical episode. The nutritional needs of an elderly individual who requires rehabilitation are unique and may change with alterations in physical condition over time. And, aside from the demands of disease or rehabilitation, older people have nutritional requirements that are affected by the normal aging process of the gastrointestinal tract.

The physiological changes associated with advancing age include loss of lean body mass and body protein compartments, decrease in total body water, reduction in bone density, and proportional gain in total body fat. These body composition alterations contribute to the functional changes that are noticeable in older adults. In the restoration or rehabilitation of function in elderly individuals, adequate nutrition is an important factor; therefore, an awareness of these physiological changes is key to nourishing and treating older patients adequately.

Some of the changes in the nutritional requirements of individuals can be accommodated if the clinician is alert to their presentations and causes. Distinguishing between age-induced changes and nutritional deficiencies may be difficult. Observing nutritional intake, physical strength, functional status, and physiological alterations that occur with time will yield important clues to potential nutritional problems in elderly people. The demands of chronic disease, the extraordinary needs of acute illness, and the basal requirements to maintain homeostasis make the provision of nutritional care to elderly, chronically ill patients a challenge for their caregivers.

NUTRITIONAL REQUIREMENTS OF THE AGING

Energy

The maintenance of health and the provision of adequate nutrition in elderly people requires an understanding of the impact of age on nutritional requirements. A well-documented change that occurs over time is the decrease in energy metabolism. The lessened energy requirement is related to a decrease in total protein mass rather than to a reduction in the metabolic activity of aging tissue.

Basal energy requirements reflect the energy needed for all the metabolic processes that are involved in maintaining cell function; the reduction of active protein (metabolic) mass results in lowered energy needs.

Protein

Protein requirements in elderly individuals might be expected to decrease to accommodate a lower total lean-body mass. However, studies appear to indicate that protein requirements may be slightly higher in older subjects. One explanation is that lower calorie intake contributes to reduced retention of dietary nitrogen; thus, the body requires more dietary protein to achieve nitrogen balance.

Protein needs are also affected by immobility, which contributes to negative nitrogen balance. Elderly people who are bedbound, wheelchairbound, or otherwise immobilized require higher levels of dietary protein to achieve nitrogen equilibrium. Surgery, sepsis, long-bone fractures, and unusual losses such as those that occur with burns or gastrointestinal disease increase the need for dietary protein.

Some clinicians have been wary of providing high levels of protein for fear of precipitating renal disease in elderly individuals. Research has produced no evidence that dietary protein induces deterioration of renal function in individuals who have no evidence of renal disease. For elderly patients who have a measurable decline in renal function, therapeutic regimens should be followed.

Fat

The major contribution of fat in the diet is energy, essential fatty acids, and fat-soluble vitamins. Because only small amounts of fat are needed to provide essential fatty acids, and fat-soluble vitamins are available from other dietary sources, the primary contribution of dietary fat is calories. For older people, restricting dietary fat and thereby reducing calorie intake is a reasonable strategy to maintain calorie balance without restricting intake of other nutrients. However, in some individuals overly rigid restrictions on dietary fat may contribute to energy deficits.

Recommendations to alter the type and amount of fat in the diet of older adults are somewhat controversial; major differences in opinion exist regarding the altering of dietary fat in adults over age 65 as a controllable variable in the reduction of risk for heart disease.

Carbohydrates

Carbohydrate intake in the diets of elderly people should be approximately 55% to 60% of the total caloric intake, with an emphasis on complex carbohydrates. The ability to metabolize carbohydrates appears to decline with advancing age. It is important to encourage complex carbohydrate intake in elderly people because it provides fiber, a constituent of the diet that enhances bowel motility, which tends to decrease over time. Fresh fruits and vegetables are difficult to chew if oral health is not optimal or dentures do not fit properly, and these foods are expensive when they are out of season. Cereal fibers should be encouraged as an alternative, but it is difficult to obtain adequate fiber from cereal foods alone.

Vitamins

Vitamin requirements for people over age 65 are mostly speculative at present, although there is much ongoing research. Vitamin deficiencies, particularly for some of the water-soluble vitamins, may exist subclinically in elderly persons. When the stress of an illness or an injury occurs, reserve capacity may not be able to compensate for rapid depletion of tissue stores and the individual may become overly deficient. Subclinical deficiencies may exist in people who have adequate but not excess dietary intake, because the absorption and utilization of these vitamins can be compromised by the use of multiple medications or single nutrient supplements or by the declining efficiency of the small bowel to absorb micronutrients.

The water-soluble vitamins that are often the focus of attention are vitamins C and B_{12}. Although there appears to be no age-related alteration in vitamin C (ascorbic acid) absorption, a deficiency of this vitamin is often linked with wound healing problems or easy bruisability. Vitamin C is an essential element in the manufacture of collagen, the protein matrix that holds cells together and is, therefore, necessary when new tissue is being made. The recommended daily allowance (RDA) of vitamin C is 60 mg, a level far exceeded in most American diets. With large doses of supplemental vitamin C, tissue saturation is reached rapidly and the excess vitamin is excreted in urine. Very large doses (greater than 1 g per day) may contribute to serious side effects in sensitive individuals, such as chronic diarrhea or the formation of kidney stones. There is little evidence that massive doses of vitamin C aid in wound-healing or ward off the common cold or cure cancer.

Many older adults may be at risk for a deficiency of vitamin B_{12}. The major dietary sources of vitamin B_{12} are red meat and organ meats, which many elderly people have chosen to forgo because of their fat and cholesterol content. In addition to dietary inadequacy, some older adults have a condition called atrophic gastritis in which the production of gastric acid lessens. Gastric acid is necessary for vitamin B_{12} to be released from a series of protein carriers and linked to an intrinsic factor that forms a complex with the vitamin and allows it to be absorbed. Production of the intrinsic factor also decreases with atrophic gastritis. Symptoms of vitamin B_{12} deficiency are generally nonspecific but include irritability, lethargy, and mild dementia.

It is not often that elderly people are found to be deficient in the fat-soluble vitamins A, D, E, and K because of the ability of the liver tissue to store fat-soluble vitamins. Vitamin D is at the greatest risk for deficiency, particularly in homebound or institutionalized people, as a result of limited exposure to sunlight, the use of sunscreens, and an inadequate intake of dairy products. It is also known that the amount of vitamin D precursor in skin, which is stimulated by sunlight, particularly ultraviolet rays, decreases with age. Dietary vitamin D goes through several conversions in the liver and kidney to become the active form of the vitamin; with advancing age, the kidney becomes less efficient in performing the final step of conversion. Vitamin D makes important contributions to bone mineralization and immune function, so it is wise to encourage the inclusion of foods rich in vitamin D in the diets of elderly individuals who may be at risk of deficiency.

The risk of vitamin A toxicity is greater than the risk of vitamin A deficiency. This is especially true of older people who are taking over-the-counter vitamin supplements, many of which have very high levels of vitamin A. Beta carotene, a vitamin A precursor, has received a great deal of attention in recent years because of its apparent protective effect against various types of neoplasms, but the long-term effects of high doses of beta carotene have not been adequately explored.

Minerals

Requirements for most minerals do not change with age, but iron is an exception. Need for iron decreases because of a tendency toward increased storage of iron in tissue and the cessation of menstrual blood loss in women. Calcium requirements have attracted much attention in recent years. Some investigators have suggested that dietary calcium intake recommendations be raised from 800 to 1200 or 1500 mg per day to reduce the risk of osteoporosis; however, many investigators do not think that requirements should be changed.

For most other major minerals, such as sodium and potassium, requirements are not changed by the aging process, although they are impacted by the presence of acute or chronic diseases and their treatments.

Water

Water is an important nutrient for older people. Inadequate fluid intake may lead to rapid dehydration and precipitate the associated problems of hypotension, elevated body temperature, constipation, nausea, vomiting, mucosal dryness, decreased urine output, and mental confusion. It is particularly noteworthy that these problems are rarely attributed to fluid imbalances, which are so easily corrected.

Fluid intake should be adequate to compensate for normal losses through kidneys, bowel, lungs, and skin and for unusual losses associated with increased body temperature, vomiting, diarrhea, or hemorrhage. A reasonable estimate of fluid needs is approximately 1 mL of fluid per kcal ingested, or 30 mL per kg of actual body weight. The minimum intake for all older adults regardless of their size or caloric intake should be approximately 1500 mL per day. Fluid needs can be met with water, juices, beverages such as tea or coffee, gelatin desserts, and other foods that would be liquid at room temperature. Tube feeding formulas contain approximately 750 mL of water to 1L of solution; it is wise to compensate for the solids displacement by adding 25% of the volume of the tube as additional free water. All health-care practitioners should be concerned about adequate hydration in their patients who live at home, especially if they exercise in hot, humid or cold, dry conditions and when patients are frail or live alone.

THE AGING GASTROINTESTINAL TRACT AND NUTRITION

The system most directly associated with adequate dietary intake is the gastrointestinal tract. The ingestion, digestion, and absorption of nutrients are essential processes that are part of the maintenance of nutritional status. The function of the gastrointestinal tract is, therefore, intricately involved in nutrition and a determinant of nutritional status.

The Oral Cavity

The changes associated with the aging process affect the structures of the mouth. Bone loss is a common problem, and in the oral cavity, where the alveolar bone is more prone to brittleness and fragility, there is an increased likelihood that tissue damage might occur due to oral trauma, periodontal disease, and loss of teeth. Nutritional deficiencies can manifest in periodontal and perioral tissue, causing impairment of chewing and of normal ingestion of food.

As lean body mass decreases, gum tissue may be lost due to disease and atrophy. This process, along with bone resorption, leads to an increased risk of root caries, periodontal disease, and loss of structure to support dentures. These changes, along with others in oral musculature and the mucous membranes, contribute to difficulty in chewing food adequately. Many individuals alter their dietary intake to compensate for their diminished efficiency in chewing, thereby putting themselves at risk for malnutrition. Malnutrition is associated with negative outcomes and adds an additional burden to the challenge of rehabilitation.

Other changes that can occur in the mouth and thus affect nutritional status include decreased taste and smell sensitivity, loss of the ability to taste and smell, and diminished salivary flow, which is associated with disease conditions and the effects of medications.

In chronically ill patients, changes in the oral cavity should be assessed so as to ensure that an individual is able to consume adequate nutrients to maintain or restore nutritional status through a period of rehabilitation.

The Esophagus

The esophagus is the conduit that transports food from the mouth to the stomach. While it may not seem to be a terribly important part of the gastrointestinal tract, esophageal dysfunction may have a profound impact on nutritional status and, therefore, on the recovery from an illness or other physiological problem.

The most common dysfunction is related to swallowing disorders. Problems in swallowing may be characterized by pain, choking, spitting, or vomiting. These symptoms are usually associated with an obstruction, a cerebrovascular accident, neurological disease, or degenerative muscular disease. Gastroesophageal reflux may be a secondary problem that results from weakness in the lower esophageal sphincter, failure of peristalsis, or an injury or illness in the stomach.

Diagnosis and correction of esophageal problems are key to safe ingestion of food and liquids. Depending on the cause and severity of the dysfunction, dietary modification may be the appropriate treatment. More severe problems require medical, pharmacological, or surgical interventions. In any case, consideration of nutrition status is important to ensure adequate nutrient intake.

The Stomach

The stomach serves several functions in the digestive process: it mechanically breaks up food; it digests food through chemical and enzymatic actions; and it serves as a reservoir to hold partially digested food until it can be released into the small intestine. There is no evidence that age has a significant effect on gastric function; however, age-related conditions and diseases may result in altered gastric function.

The gastric conditions most commonly seen in elderly individuals are atrophic gastritis, peptic ulcer disease, and gastroesophageal reflux disease. Atrophic gastritis may contribute to the perception of a food intolerance but, more importantly, it may also be a major factor in vitamin B_{12} deficiency, as gastric acid is required for the digestion process that allows this vitamin to be absorbed. Folic acid may also be malabsorbed in cases of atrophic gastritis.

Peptic ulcer disease is becoming more common among the elderly even though its incidence in the general population appears to be declining. Medications such as H_2-antagonists and antacids may have multiple side effects that can lead to other problems, including constipation, obstruction, osteomalacia, diarrhea, dehydration, and electrolyte disturbances.

Gastroesophageal reflux disease is usually associated with the incompetence of the lower esophageal sphincter. There is no evidence that this is an age-related condition but some older individuals do experience it.

The Pancreas

No strong evidence suggests that age affects the pancreas in any significant way, although the pancreas is smaller and lighter in individuals beyond the age of 70, and there appears to be a reduction in secretory output. This reduction is not considered clinically significant until pancreatic output is less than 10% of normal.

Diseases of the pancreas do occur in older people and are common among them. Acute pancreatitis occurs in older patients and it may have acute consequences that can result in sepsis and shock. An uncomplicated course may show a brief period of pain, nausea, and vomiting and tends to occur in individuals who have biliary tract disease. A more severe occurrence may show abscesses, other septic symptoms, or shock as its consequences and may require surgery and stress metabolism management.

Chronic primary inflammatory pancreatitis is a disease of older people. Symptoms include steatorrhea (passage of fat in feces), diabetes, pancreatic calcification, and weight loss. This is often a pain-free condition that is unpredictable in its response to therapy.

The Liver

The liver tends to get smaller in mass with advancing age, and that can lead to changes in its structure and functioning. These changes can have significant effects because many of the functions of the liver—synthesis, excretion, and metabolism—are crucial in the maintenance of health. Such functions are affected by systemic diseases and by liver diseases, both of which are common in elderly people.

Important changes that occur in the livers of elderly people include altered drug metabolism and a diminishing rate of protein synthesis. Both of these factors contribute to a weaker ability to respond appropriately to drug therapy or to the physiological insults associated with disease.

The Small Bowel

The gastrointestinal tract, beginning at the mouth and ending at the anus, is a large muscle that propels food and its digested products through the body. Food is ingested and almost immediately acted upon by digestive enzymes, chemicals, and mechanical actions. Many of the critical digestion and absorption functions occur in the small bowel, and age and disease can have an impact on the normal function of the small bowel. For example, one common disorder related to carbohydrate metabolism is disaccharidase intolerance, or deficiency of lactase. Lactase deficiency occurs with age and in common gastrointestinal diseases such as viral gastroenteritis, Crohn's disease, bacterial infections, and ulcerative colitis. Symptoms are associated with the ingestion of milk and milk products when such ingestion of lactose exceeds the production of lactase in the small bowel.

Celiac disease is a disorder with vague symptoms. It involves sensitivity to gluten, a protein often found in wheat products. The problem commonly results from an injury to the small bowel resulting from exposure to gluten, which contributes to malabsorption and steatorrhea. The treatment is to eliminate gluten from the diet. Replacement of malabsorbed nutrients (iron, folic acid, calcium, vitamin D) should be part of the therapy.

Another source of malabsorption in older individuals is bacterial overgrowth. This may be associated with the decrease in gastric acid production by the stomach and the age-related decrease in bowel motility. Generalized malabsorption may result from this condition; vitamin B_{12} is a nutrient that is at risk of being malabsorbed.

Other conditions that may damage the small bowel and impair its ability to digest and absorb essential nutrients include radiation enteritis and inflammatory bowel diseases. Radiation enteritis is often a consequence of treatment for cancer of the cervix, uterus, prostate, bladder, or colon. The cells in the small intestine, because of their rapidly dividing nature, are vulnerable to damage from radiation. Symptoms including diarrhea, nausea, cramping, and distention often occur years after the period of therapy and may go unreported. Malabsorption and dehydration are potential nutritional consequences.

Inflammatory bowel disease may occur but its symptoms may be attributed to other conditions, as it is more commonly seen in younger people. Careful diagnosis is important for early treatment and adequate nutritional intervention.

The Large Intestine

The primary function of the large intestine is the absorption of water, electrolytes, bile salts, and short-chain fatty acids. The major conditions of the large intestine that are commonly experienced by older people are colon cancer, diverticulosis, and constipation. If diagnosed early enough, colon cancer is treatable with surgery and radiation therapy. Diverticular disease may be asymptomatic in elderly patients until an infection occurs and the individual becomes symptomatic. Dietary treatment is the same for older and younger patients.

Constipation is a common complaint among older adults. It may occur as a result of a variety of conditions: neurological disease, drug effects, systemic disease, inadequate fluid intake, lack of dietary bulk, and physical inactivity. Treatment should be based on the cause of the condition and should be sure to include adequate hydration, dietary fiber, and physical activity.

CONCLUSION

The patient who is in rehabilitation should be encouraged to eat as much as possible. Underlying disease conditions should be treated first, of course, with nutritional adequacy encouraged as appropriate. Smaller, more frequent meals may be accepted more readily by elderly patients with smaller appetites and early satiety. The older patient with a moderate to severe kyphosis is likely to have a smaller abdominal cavity and thus would benefit from the same strategy. Oral liquid supplements can be added to solid food consumption if fluid overload is not a contraindication. The goal of refeeding should be to provide 35 kcal/kg of the patient's actual weight and at least 1 g of protein per kg. Our experience has demonstrated that only 10% of elderly people who have protein malnutrition can consume enough calories to correct their nutritional deficiencies; most subjects require more aggressive nutritional intervention. Aggressive nutritional interventions that should be considered if the malnourished patient cannot consume adequate calories orally are enteral or parenteral feeding.

SUGGESTED READINGS

Chernoff R, ed. *Geriatric Nutrition: The Health Professional's Handbook.* Gaithersburg, Md.: Aspen; 1991.
Holt PR, Russell RM, eds. *Chronic Gastritis and Hypochlorhydria in the Elderly.* Boca Raton, Fla.: CRC Press; 1993.
Lipschitz DA, ed. Nutrition, aging, and age-dependent diseases. *Clin Geriatr Med* 1995; 11:553–765.
Munro H, Schlierf G, eds. *Nutrition of the Elderly.* Nestlé Nutrition Workshop Series. New York: Raven Press; 1992.

Chapter **10**

Laboratory Assessment: Considerations for Aging Persons

Chris Stabler, M.D.

INTRODUCTION

Of all the people who have ever lived to age 65, more than half are alive today. This striking statement has implications for the ongoing care of the elderly.

The biology of aging is not completely understood. It is known that tissue cultures have a finite lifespan and that growth and replication slow with age. However, metabolic functions often remain constant after senescence occurs. Extrapolating this information from tissue culture to human beings is somewhat risky but is accurate in one aspect: aging is not marked by predictable biochemical changes. As people age they become more dissimilar, belying any stereotype of aging. Abrupt declines in any system or function must be attributed to disease and, therefore, not to normal aging. Finally, in the absence of disease or modifying risk factors, the concept of healthy old age is absolutely valid. This chapter on laboratory assessment will emphasize the fact that most healthy elderly people will maintain laboratory values considered normal for the rest of the adult population.

AGE-RELATED CONSIDERATIONS

Certain basic tenets apply when assessing the elderly patient. In the process of normal aging, there is a decline in the reserves of most organ systems, particularly the central nervous system, circulatory system, gastrointestinal system, and hemopoietic system. New disease in the elderly will generally affect these vulnerable systems more rapidly than it would in younger adults. Laboratory values may become abnormal more quickly in the early stages of disease in elderly patients. Likewise, the impaired physiological reserve of the hepatic and renal systems may make the elderly more susceptible to the side effects of commonly used pharmacological agents.

Although there are no syndromes of old age anemia, old age renal failure, or old age hepatic dysfunction as clinical entities in the absence of disease, there are a few laboratory findings that are common in the elderly and that would be considered

pathology in younger people. Impaired glucose tolerance, an elevation of blood sugar in response to the ingestion of a high simple carbohydrate load, can occur in the elderly. Likewise, bacteriuria in the absence of infection is also a commonly encountered laboratory finding in the elderly that would be considered pathological in younger adults.

In its scientific application, medicine has come to rely upon what is objective and measurable; Laboratory assessment of the elderly individual is a clear example. But interpretation of clinical tests still requires a physical assessment of the patient in order to fully understand the implications and diagnostic capabilities of laboratory testing.

Normal laboratory ranges are derived by studying what is considered to be a disease-free population. The distribution of laboratory values in what would be considered a normal group are identified. The mean value and standard deviations are calculated, and the mean value plus or minus two standard deviations yields the normal range for a specific laboratory test. The assumption that these populations are disease-free and representative of normal values for laboratory testing may be false, but established normals hold true.

Despite the drawbacks of available laboratory testing, it is an important adjunct to the assessment of the elderly patient. Numerous articles have been written in the recent past regarding the interpretation of abnormal laboratory values in the elderly. Chiari reported that acute inflammation had a significant impact on iron and nutritional status indices in older patients. Inflammation, measured by a high C-reactive protein (CRP) correlated inversely with albumin and prealbumin. Measures of nutritional status and elevated CRP also varied directly with serum ferritin, a measure of iron deficiency. Inflammatory processes such as rheumatological illness, infection, and nonhematological malignancies are common and accounted for 95% of diagnoses in patients with persistently elevated erythrocyte sedimentation rates (ESRs). The clinician evaluating a patient with an elevated ESR should look for a diagnosis, as standardized mortality ratios for patients with persistently elevated ESRs are strikingly high.

Elis found that idiopathic normocytic normochromic anemias did occur in a population of patients aged 80 and older. A small group of 31 patients with no identifiable explanation for their anemia were found to have normal bone marrow aspirates, and in follow-up tests they showed small but incremental increases in their hemoglobin, independent of treatment. In this small population in which iron deficiency or clinical illness was not found as a cause, idiopathic normocytic normochromic anemia was found to be an acceptable diagnosis in symptom-free patients. In rehabilitation, these patients may present clinically with fatigue, shortness of breath, confusion, agitation, and apathy. In cases of preexisting atherosclerotic heart disease, angina and peripheral edema may worsen. Miller et al. described apparent idiopathic hyponatremia in an ambulatory geriatric population. Their study demonstrated that a subset of healthy elderly with serum sodium less than 135 mEq/L had a syndrome of idiopathic antidiuretic hormone (SIADH). Their conclusions supported the hypothesis that aging is a risk factor for the development of SIADH-like hyponatremia in a subset of older patients who do not show an apparent underlying cause. They surmised that aging may be an independent cause of the development of hyponatremia in the old old. In rehabilitation, these patients may present clinically with lethargy, fatigue, and muscle cramps.

Assessment of nutritional status has been studied extensively. In normal, healthy, ambulatory adults, nutritional status assessed by anthropometric and biochemical methods shows that there is no significant difference in serum protein and amino acids between elderly subjects and young adults. The historic assumption that the elderly show declining serum protein and albumin levels seems inconsistent with these data. Decreases in serum proteins and albumin as well as prealbumin are directly related to states of nutritional deficiency or inflammatory conditions previously addressed.

INDICATIONS FOR LABORATORY ASSESSMENT

When is laboratory assessment necessary? Routine laboratory testing should be determined by a patient's presentation, history, and current medication use. For example, a patient who must use diuretics requires regular assessment of serum electrolytes, especially serum potassium. Simple alterations in diet such as the inclusion of increased sodium may cause potassium-wasting in the elderly kidney and precipitate hypokalemia, a cause of muscle weakness in the elderly. A patient on anticholesterol medication such as the HMGCoA reductase inhibitors requires regular assessment of liver functions. A patient receiving ticlopidine (Ticlid), a platelet inhibitor used in patients with transient ischemic attacks and stroke requires a regular blood count.

Laboratory assessment is especially important in the evaluation of a patient who presents with new physical findings. The workup for dementia and delirium is particularly vital. Neurosyphilis, vitamin B_{12} and folic acid deficiencies, and acute infection can be detected by means of laboratory assessment and are precipitants of acute delirium and dementia.

Radiological findings and other physical diagnostic tests such as a lumbar puncture can quickly identify reversible causes for a patient's neurological changes.

Lethargy and altered levels of consciousness may also be presenting symptoms in a patient with abnormal laboratory values. Hypoglycemia, hyponatremia, acidosis, hypoxia, and hypocalcemia are direct causes of central nervous system depression and can be identified through commonly used laboratory tests. Neuromuscular irritability, tetany, and muscle spasms may present in severe cases of hypocalcemia.

A patient who presents with peripheral, sensory, or motor deficits may be suffering from a disease identifiable by blood chemistries. Peripheral neuropathies are caused by diabetes mellitus (hyperglycemia), heavy metal ingestion, and medication toxicities. Biochemical assessment can identify these problems.

Deteriorating renal function as evidenced by elevations of serum creatinine and blood urea nitrogen may place the patient at greater risk for medication toxicity. Frequent assessment of medication serum levels and adjustment of doses is the hallmark of safe continued usage in the face of renal insufficiency. Abnormalities in thyroid hormone levels may present differently in the elderly than in younger adults. Cardiac arrhythmias and weight loss may be the presenting symptoms of hyperthyroidism in the elderly. Hypothyroidism may present more insidiously, with the typical symptoms of myxedema occurring less frequently. Alterations in

Table 10–1 Selected Normal Laboratory Values

Serum Electrolytes	Normal Values
Carbon dioxide	23–31 mEq/L
Chloride	98–107 mEq/L
Potassium	3.5–5.1 mEq/L
Sodium	136–145 mEq/L
Metabolic Indicators	*Normal Values*
Calcium	8.6–10.0 mg/dL
Cholesterol	158–276 mg/dL Recommended <200 mg/dL
Creatinine	0.8–1.5 mg/dL
Free thyroxine (FT_4)	0.8–2.3 mg/dL
Glucose fasting	82–115 mg/dL
Glucose, 2 h postprandial	<120 mg/dL
Protein Total	6.0–8.0 gm/dL
Albumin	3.5–5.5 gm/dL
Globulin	2.0–3.5 gm/dL

Table 10–2 Effect of Aging on Laboratory Values

Increased	Unchanged	Decreased
Serum copper	Hemoglobin	Creatinine clearance
Serum ferritin	RBC count	Serum calcium
Serum immunoreactive	WBC count	Serum iron
parathormone	Serum vitamin A	Serum phosphorus
Serum cholesterol	Leukocyte zinc	Serum thiamine
Serum uric acid	Serum pantothenate	Serum zinc
Serum fibrinogen	Serum riboflavin	Serum 1,25-dihydroxycholecalciferol
Serum norepinephrine	Serum carotene	Serum vitamin B_6
Serum triglycerides	Erythrocyte sedimentation rate	Serum vitamin B_{12}
Serum glucose	Serum IgM, IgG, IgA	Plasma vitamin C
Prostate-specific antigen (PSA)	Blood urea nitrogen	Serum selenium
	Serum creatinine[a]	Plasma gammatocopherol (vitamin E)
	Serum alkaline phosphatase	Triiodothyronine (T_3)
		Serum testosterone
		Dihydroepiandrosterone

[a]Serum creatinine may be normal, even though creatinine clearance is decreased with aging as a result of an age-related decrease in creatinine production. (Source: *The Merck Manual of Geriatrics,* edited by William B. Abrams, Mark H. Beers, and Robert Berkow. Copyright 1995 by Mercer & Co., Inc.; Whitehouse Station, NJ.)

---

mental status, lethargy, weight gain, and thought disorders may be caused by hypothyroidism in the elderly.

Tables 10–1 and 10–2 indicate normal values and possible age-related effects of routinely used laboratory assessments of the elderly. Significant deviations may indicate disease or deterioration of organ systems in these patients.

CONCLUSIONS

In summary, clinical use of laboratory testing for the assessment of geriatric patients is a useful tool when combined with physical assessment. Laboratory values, although traditionally derived from middle-aged populations, can be applied to elderly populations, with rare exceptions. Abnormal laboratory values should be investigated for the presence of disease states and not attributed to age alone. Reductions in physiological reserves account for the earlier presence of abnormal values in asymptomatic disease states in the elderly.

SUGGESTED READINGS

Chiari MM. Influence of acute inflammation on iron and nutritional status indexes in older patients. *J Am Geriatr Soc* 1995; 43:767–771.

Elis A. A clinical approach to idiopathic normocytic-normochromic anemia. *J Am Geriatr Soc* 1996; 44:832–834.

Fried LP, Williamson J, Bundeen-Roch K, et al. Functional decline in older adults: expanding methods of ascertainment. *J Gerontol* 1996; 51A:M206–M214.

Miller M, et al. Apparent idiopathic hyponatremia in an ambulatory geriatric population. *J Am Geriatr Soc* 1996; 44:404–408.

Robbins J, et al. Hematological and biochemical laboratory values in older cardiovascular health study participants. *J Am Geriatr Soc* 1995; 43:855–859.

Tietz NW, et al. *Clinical Guide to Laboratory Tests*, 3rd ed. Philadelphia: W.B. Saunders; 1995.

Verdery RB. Failure to thrive in older people. *Geriatric Med Clin* 1997; 13(4):613–794.

Chapter **11**

Thermoregulation: Considerations for Aging Persons

John Sanko, Ed.D., P.T.

INTRODUCTION

Internal body temperature is a relatively stable physiological function and one of the most frequently measured vital signs. Core temperature normally does not vary by more than $\pm 0.55°C$ ($\pm 1°F$) unless a febrile illness develops. Healthy, unclothed persons experimentally exposed to ambient temperatures as low as 12.6°C (55°F) and as high as 59.4°C (140°F) were able to maintain near constant core temperatures in spite of these extreme environmental conditions.[1-5]

Humans are classified as homeotherms, which means they must maintain their internal temperature within a very narrow range.[2] The critical temperature range, which hovers near 37°C (98.6°F), must be maintained for the life-sustaining biochemical processes and other bodily functions to proceed at the appropriate rate, frequency, and duration. Internal temperatures above 45°C to 50°C (113°F to 122°F) destroy the protein structure of various enzymes, which results in biochemical breakdown, tissue destruction, severe illness, and death (Fig. 11–1). Body temperatures below 33.9°C (93°F) slow metabolism to dangerously low levels and disrupt nerve conduction, which, in turn, results in decreased brain activity. Life-threatening cardiac arrhythmias begin to appear at temperatures near 30°C (86°F) (see Fig. 11–1).

In essence, all warm-blooded animals, including human beings, live out their entire lives within a few degrees of death.[3, 4] Core temperatures falling outside the normal range are indicative of some pathology or the failure of the thermoregulatory system to maintain thermal balance. The complexity of the physiological mechanisms involved in thermoregulation is shown in Figure 11–2.

HYPERTHERMIA

Hyperthermia is the condition in which internal core temperature exceeds the normal range. Hyperthermia can be caused by infections, brain lesions, environmental conditions, or heavy exercise. When caused by an infection, the responsible microorganisms release toxins called pyrogens into the bloodstream; they reach the temperature control centers of the brain and raise the thermal setpoint. This state, known as fever, is actually beneficial and is part of the immune system's response. Higher core temperatures adversely affect the invading microorganisms' ability to replicate. This generally limits the extent of the infection and leads to its suppression.

In the older adult, the fever response is often diminished or absent, which may explain the increased morbidity and mortality rates associated with infections in the elderly.[5]

When the ambient temperature rises above 30°C (86°F), progressive vasodilation of the cutaneous vasculature commences and is followed by sweating and evaporation.[2] Factors such as high humidity and physical activity magnify the effects of ambient temperature, taxing the thermoregulatory mecha-

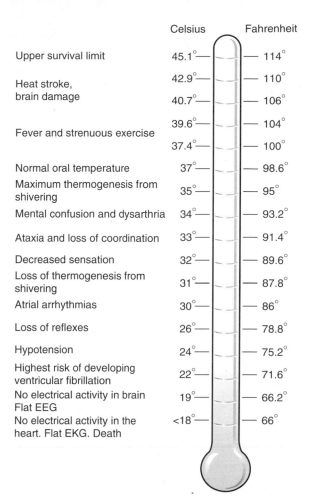

Figure 11–1 Physiological consequences of variations in core temperature. Core temperature has a direct effect on physiological function. Extreme core temperature will seriously challenge homeostasis, which can have fatal consequences. (Data from Guyton AC. *Textbook of Medical Physiology*, 7th ed. Philadelphia: W.B. Saunders, 1986:849; and Rhoades RA, Tanner GA. *Medical Physiology*. Dubuque, Iowa: Brown and Benchmark, 1994:245.)

nisms. This is an especially important factor in home health-care when treating debilitated patients. Unlike fever, nonfebrile rises in body temperature are not beneficial and threaten homeostasis. If normal thermal regulation is in any way impaired, these increases can reach dangerous levels. With core temperatures above 40.7°C (106°F), heat stroke and irreversible brain damage become imminent (see Fig. 11–1).

If the internal core temperature drops below 34.1°C (94°F), the ability of the hypothalamus to regulate body temperature is also severely impaired.[1-5] If the body temperature continues to fall unchecked, loss of motor control, sensation, and consciousness will be followed by ventricular fibrillation and death (see Fig. 11–1).

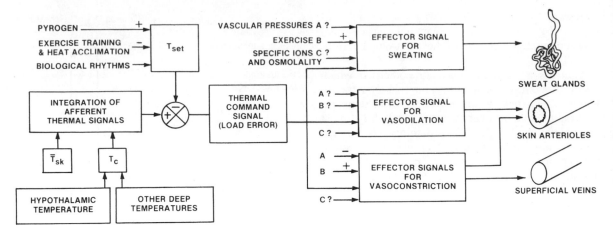

Figure 11–2 Physiological mechanisms for maintaining thermoregulatory homeostasis. Breakdown or impairment in any of the thermoregulatory mechanisms can lead to serious problems in maintaining homeostasis. (From Pandolf KB, Sawka MN, Gonzalez RR, eds. *Human Performance Physiology and Environmental Medicine at Terrestrial Extremes.* Indianapolis: Benchmark; 1988:106. With permission from the McGraw-Hill Companies.)

HYPOTHALAMUS AND THERMAL REGULATION

The hypothalamus normally acts as the body's thermostat, initiating heat-dissipating, heat-conserving, or heat-generating mechanisms in relation to internal core and body surface temperatures.[1-5] The temperature-reduction mechanisms include vasodilation, sweating, inhibition of shivering, and decreased chemical thermogenesis.[1-5] When body temperature begins to rise, sympathetic outflow from the hypothalamus to the cutaneous vasculature is inhibited, allowing for vasodilation and increased heat transfer from the skin to the external environment. This mechanism is capable of increasing heat dissipation through the skin by as much as 800%. Sweating and evaporative loss further enhance the skin's ability to dissipate heat. When the challenge of cold is presented to the body, the hypothalamus conserves or generates body heat by measuring sympathetic tone, which results in vasoconstriction of the cutaneous circulation, piloerection, shivering, and increased metabolism through the secretion of thyroxine.[1-5]

MOBILITY AND PSYCHOSOCIAL FACTORS

In spite of the exquisite physiological mechanisms for dealing with temperature change, behavioral modification may be human beings' greatest defense against environmental challenges to thermoregulatory homeostasis. When our surroundings become too warm or too cold, we try to avoid such conditions by moving to a more comfortable location. In addition, we may add or remove clothing as conditions warrant. Because 30% to 40% of the body's heat can be lost through the head, the simple act of wearing or not wearing a hat can have a profound influence on the thermoregulatory process.[6] The very young and the elderly are at the greatest risk when exposed to extremes of environmental conditions.[2] This may be due in part to their inability to recognize the magnitude of the situation and take appropriate action.

Older adults often find themselves dependent upon others for their well-being, commonly as a result of deficits in physical or cognitive function. The incidence of chronic disease increases dramatically with age. Over 50% of those beyond 65 years of age report some limitation in mobility due to arthritis, and another 16% have other orthopedic problems that limit their ability to carry out the normal activities of daily living (ADLs).[7] Musculoskeletal and neurological conditions often reduce the older adult's functional level to a point where he or she becomes partially, if not fully, dependent upon others to carry out the ADLs. Thermoregulatory stress may be one of many reasons why elders who are dependent on others for help with ADLs have a four times greater chance of dying within a 2-year period than those who are totally independent.[7] In addition, approximately 15% of the population over 65 years of age are in some way cognitively impaired.[7] The incidence of cognitive impairment rises rapidly with age. Some deterioration in mental function is seen in nearly 50% of those individuals 85 years of age and older.[7] These physical and mental impairments, as well as others, combined with a reduction in the functional capacity of various organ systems makes the older adult particularly vulnerable to thermoregulatory stress.

Thermal Injury

Heat stroke, heat exhaustion, and hypothermia are most prevalent among the elderly and are inversely related to socioeconomic status. When elderly individuals on fixed incomes turn the heat down in the winter because they can't pay high heating bills, they are certainly predisposing themselves to hypothermia. Conversely, elderly persons unable to afford air conditioning are 50 times more likely to die of heat stroke than those who have access to air conditioning.[8] Although it has been stated that numerous predisposing physiological factors share responsibility, many temperature-related threats to health could undoubtedly be prevented if elderly individuals just stayed indoors, turned the heat or air conditioning up or down, and dressed more appropriately.[2, 3] In cases in which economic status or physical or mental condition makes these actions impossible, those involved should be referred to the appropriate agencies for the protection of their welfare.

PHYSIOLOGICAL FACTORS

Skin Receptors and Circulatory Response

Even when healthy and mentally alert, the elderly are less able to sense changes in skin temperature, and this makes them more susceptible to thermoregulatory problems.[2, 9] Thermoreceptors for both hot and cold are found in the skin, the spinal cord, and hypothalamus itself.[3] Skin temperature, unlike core temperature, is extremely variable. Receptors in the skin provide the hypothalamus with important feedback regarding the need to dissipate, conserve, or generate heat.[4] Numerous bare nerve endings just below the skin are sensitive to heat and cold. They are classified as warm- or cold-receptors, depending on their rate of discharge when exposed to variations in temperature. Receptors responding to cold are about 10 times more numerous.[4] It is not known whether the effectiveness of these thermoreceptors declines with age. However, because their function depends on an adequate oxygen supply, it seems reasonable to assume that any age-associated impairments in cutaneous circulation would reduce the effectiveness of thermoreceptors.[10] It is known that the dermis becomes thinner and less vascularized with age.[11]

The changes in skin thickness and circulation along with reduced autonomic nervous system function alter the effectiveness of the vasomotor response. The vasomotor mechanism can alter cutaneous blood flow from near zero when exposed to extreme cold to increases of 500% to 1000% when exposed to vigorous warming. The evaporative loss of sweat from the skin surface helps to dissipate heat in the cutaneous circulation. A study that compared men 45 to 57 years old with men 18 to 23 years old indicated that the older men required twice as long before the onset of sweating during moderate intensity exercise. "Subsequent studies of older women showed even greater impairments in the sweating mechanism." The number of sweat glands does not appear to change significantly with aging.[11] Therefore, it is reasonable to assume that the decline in autonomic nervous system function reduces the performance of sweat glands and alters the body's ability to dissipate excess heat. In addition, the hypothalamus appears to become less sensitive to temperature variations, and there is evidence of age-correlated reductions in autonomic nervous system function.[1]

It is unclear how much of the thermoregulatory impairment seen in the elderly is age-related and how much is the result of chronic disease processes and a sedentary lifestyle. Several investigators have found little or no difference in thermoregulation during exercise in physically fit younger and older subjects.[3, 12] The efficiency of the cardiovascular system's ability to dissipate body heat is enhanced by aerobic fitness. Resistive exercise has been found to be particularly beneficial in maintaining or retarding muscle loss in the elderly and should be considered when not contraindicated. Muscle is a significant tissue not only for heat generation, but also for the mobility needed for thermoregulation.

Other Physiological Factors

The ingestion of food, alcohol, and medications to control blood pressure, cardiac function, depression, and pain all exert influence on thermal balance and regulation. A sufficient, well-balanced diet is essential to provide the calories needed to generate heat and maintain adequate levels of metabolically active muscle. Muscle, which is the major organ of metabolism and heat generation, can decrease by 10% to 12% in the older adult. One-third of the U.S. population over 65 has some form of nutritional deficit, often eating inappropriate quantities of foods low in nutritional values. Because 80% of the calories consumed go toward the maintenance of body temperature, this deficit can further contribute to the thermoregulatory inadequacies experienced by some older adults. The shivering mechanism, which can increase metabolism and heat generation by 300% to 500%, is also adversely affected by the loss of muscle tissue.[2–4]

POSSIBLE EFFECTS OF MEDICATION

Although there is still a great deal to be learned regarding the effects of aging on the thermoregulatory function, it appears that physical conditioning and adequate nutrition help to preserve this function in healthy older adults. All older individuals are, however, not healthy or physically fit. Many have chronic conditions that interfere with their abilities to deal with even mild variations in temperature. In addition, various medications can interfere with the normal physiological responses necessary to maintain thermal homeostasis. Dehydration may occur in individuals taking diuretics for the management of congestive heart failure or hypertension. A loss as small as 1% of an individual's total body fluid can lead to consequential increases in core temperature, decreased sweating, reduced cardiac output, and a diminution in skin blood flow. In one study, a diuretic-induced 3% loss of body fluid resulted in a significant reduction in plasma volume and a 15 to 20 beat per minute increase in heart rate.[13]

Beta-antagonists are another category of medication commonly prescribed for elderly individuals with heart disease and hypertension. In a Swedish study, 54% of patients taking beta-blockers complained of cold hands and feet, and 35% of patients on diuretics complained of this problem.[13] Additionally, individuals using beta-blockers were found to rate their perception of exertion for a given workload significantly higher then would be predicted for that workload.

Although the use of illicit drugs is lowest among the elderly, the misuse of prescription drugs is a major problem for this group. In one survey of elderly persons living independently in the community, 83% reported they were using two or more prescription drugs, with an average of 3.8 medications per person.[14] Many elderly have been found to misuse prescription and nonprescription over-the-counter drugs. Surveyed individuals reported taking two to three times the recommended dosages of aspirin, laxatives, and sleeping pills.[14] Misuse of laxatives could further increase the rate and severity of dehydration, and sedatives defeat the autonomic nervous system's ability to react to environmental conditions.

Alcohol also inhibits the body's ability to regulate temperature by interfering with the vasomotor system and altering cutaneous blood flow, which impairs the body's ability to dissipate or conserve heat. The dehydrating effects of alcohol can also contribute to an inadequate thermoregulatory response by reducing plasma volume and decreasing the sweat response. Combined with prescription and nonprescription medications, alcohol can create serious problems for any individual, particularly the elderly. It has been estimated from surveys and information gained during hospital admissions, that between 2% and 10% of all older persons living in the community misuse alcohol.[15]

POSTSURGICAL CONSIDERATIONS

A number of geriatric patients receiving physical therapy in acute- and extended-care facilities are postsurgical patients. The tremendous advancements and successes in joint replacement surgery have made these procedures relatively commonplace. Plasma lost during surgery may result in some degree of dehydration, but anesthetics present the greater challenge to thermoregulation for these patients. Most anesthetics and sedatives impair the body's ability to maintain core temperature by blocking the normal heat-generating activity. There are some benefits of mild hypothermia for the surgical patient, but there are also increased risks for the elderly. A 2°C (3.6°F) drop in core temperature has been shown to substantially increase blood loss during hip arthroplasty surgery. The incidence of ischemic myocardial events increases for a 24-hour period following intraoperative hypothermia. Higher rates of wound infections, delayed healing, and immunosuppression are also seen following anesthesia-induced hypothermia. The elderly appear to be at the greatest risk for developing one or more of these complications because of their predisposition to hypothermia, even when exposed to only moderately cold conditions.[16]

CLINICAL CONSIDERATIONS

In spite of the fact that numerous age-correlated alterations in thermoregulation have been identified, the ability to regulate internal core temperature appears to remain within acceptable limits in the healthy, fit older adult. Furthermore, few of the changes seen in autonomic, circulatory, and thermal function are solely the result of biological aging. Reduced physical work capacity, body composition changes, chronic illness, the use and misuse of various medications, and alterations in cognitive function become more prevalent with advancing age and influence the function of various body systems involved with thermoregulation.

Whenever treating any individual with exercise or thermal modalities, age should be a consideration. Ideally, the ambient temperature in exercise areas should be 19.8°C to 22°C (68°F to 72°F) with a relative humidity of 60% or less. When exercise is to be performed outdoors, appropriate clothing is a necessity. Planning outdoor activities during moderate weather is also important. It would not be prudent to exercise in midafternoon on a hot summer day or late in the evening on a cold winter day. Because older adults may build up heat more quickly and take longer to dissipate it than their younger counterparts, frequent rest periods in well-ventilated areas should be incorporated into any exercise regimen.

CONCLUSION

The safe and effective use of exercise, heat, cold, or hydrotherapy requires thorough assessment of

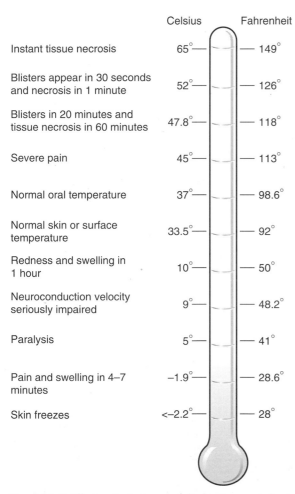

Figure 11-3 Effect on body tissues of direct exposure to heat and cold. Surface temperature may be very different from core temperature. Extremes in local tissue temperature will lead to cell death and tissue necrosis, regardless of core temperature. Local thermoregulatory impairments can lead to systemic consequences if not corrected. (Data from Guyton AC. *Textbook of Medical Physiology*, 7th ed. Philadelphia: W.B. Saunders, 1986:849; and Rhoades RA, Tanner GA. *Medical Physiology.* Dubuque, Iowa: Brown and Benchmark, 1994:245.)

Box 11-1
How to Avoid Hyperthermia

- Wear loose-fitting, light clothing during periods of high heat and humidity.
- Take cool baths or showers during periods of high heat and humidity.
- Drink adequate amounts of fluids, even when not thirsty.
- Use air conditioning or fans to cool and circulate the air.
- Avoid excessive exercise during peak temperatures of the day, especially when humidity is high and fans and air conditioning are not available. This is particularly important in the home health-care setting.
- When performing physical activity or exercise outdoors, use caution. Avoid working in direct sunlight on hot days. Take frequent breaks in cool or shady areas.

the individual's condition, medical history, and ability to withstand thermal or cryogenic stress. A past medical history of hypersensitivity to heat or cold, Raynaud's disease, urticaria, wheals, diabetes, or heart disease requires further consideration prior to treatment. Pain and temperature sensation should be assessed.

The normal effects of direct heating and cooling

Box 11-2
How to Avoid Hypothermia

- Wear several layers of loose-fitting clothing and a hat.
- Stay dry.
- Maintain an adequate, balanced diet.
- Drink adequate amounts of fluids, but limit alcohol consumption.
- Be sure to turn the heat up when the weather is cool.
- Frequently check on elderly individuals in the community who live alone.
- When performing physical activities or exercise outdoors, use caution. A great deal of heat loss can occur even when the temperatures are only moderately cool. Always consider windchill.

Table 11–1 Heat-Related Emergencies

Condition	Signs and Symptoms	Treatment
HEAT EDEMA	Swollen feet and ankles	Have the person elevate the lower extremities and wear support stockings. If symptoms are a consequence of a cardiovascular condition, drug therapy may be required.
HEAT CRAMPS	Severe muscle spasm, particularly in the lower extremities	Allow patient to rest in a cool place, cool down with moist towels, and drink electrolyte replacement fluids.
HEAT SYNCOPE	Pooling of blood in veins causing decreased cardiac output; symptoms ranging from lightheadedness to loss of consciousness; typically cool and wet skin	Have patient lie down, rest, and drink electrolyte fluids. This condition is caused by physical exertion in a warm environment by an individual not acclimatized to the environment.
HEAT EXHAUSTION	Loss of volume in the circulatory system caused by excessive sweating; cool and clammy skin; nausea, headache, confusion, weakness, and low blood pressure	Rest and fluid replacement are called for with this condition. Fluids with electrolytes may be necessary. Unconsciousness occurs rarely.
HEAT STROKE	High skin and core body temperature; loss of consciousness; possible convulsions; dry skin, indicating loss of the sweating mechanism for cooling	This is the most severe heat-related condition. Cool the body as rapidly as possible. Seek immediate medical care.

Data from Judd RL, Dinep MM. Environmental emergencies. In: Judd RL, Warner CG, Shaffer MA, eds. *Geriatric Emergencies.* Rockville, Md.: Aspen Publishers, 1986:255.

Table 11–2 Cold-Related Emergencies

Condition	Signs and Symptoms	Treatment
CHILBLAINS	Skin lesions that occur after prolonged exposure of the skin to temperatures below 15.4°C (60°F)	Protect the injured area and prevent reexposure.
TRENCH FOOT	Swollen body part (usually foot); waxy, mottled appearance of skin; complaints of numbness; caused by prolonged exposure to cool water	Remove wet shoes and socks. Gently rewarm. Cover any blisters with sterile dressings.
FROST NIP	Reddened skin that becomes blanched; numbness or tingling; ears, nose, lips, fingers, and toes most commonly affected	Gently warm the involved area. If the condition does not resolve itself, treat the individual for frostbite.
FROSTBITE	Waxy appearance or skin; may turn mottled	Gently warm but do not rub or squeeze the injured part. Transport patient immediately for advanced medical treatment.
HYPOTHERMIA	Shivering in early stages; drowsiness and lethargy; slow breathing and bradycardia; possible loss of consciousness	Gently rewarm the individual in mild cases. Immediately transport for advanced medical care in moderate to severe cases.
COLD ALLERGY	Urticaria, erythema, itching, and edema; systemic reactions, including hypotension, tachycardia, syncope, and gastrointestinal dysfunction	Gently warm and acclimatize the individual.

Data from Judd RL, Dinep MM. Environmental emergencies. In: Judd RL, Warner CH, Shaffer MA, eds. *Geriatric Emergencies.* Rockville, Md.: Aspen Publishers; 1986:255.

of the tissues may be altered in some elderly individuals (Fig. 11–3). Vital signs should be monitored along with skin temperature, sensation, color, sweat rate, and rate of perceived exertion (RPE). Additional care should be taken with individuals on medication and those who have impaired cognitive and mental function.

Should a thermoregulatory crisis occur, standard emergency and medical procedures should be followed (Tables 11–1 and 11–2). A few simple precautions can help to prevent many of these crises (Boxes 11–1 and 11–2). Additional research in the area of thermoregulation and aging is needed to resolve the many contradictory findings. Until these questions have been answered, the clinician must carefully consider the use of modalities and exercises with persons of various ages, based on the current body of knowledge, experience, and common sense.

REFERENCES

1. Guyton AC. *Textbook of Medical Physiology*, 7th ed. Philadelphia: W.B. Saunders; 1986:849.
2. Downey JA, Lemons DE. Human thermoregulation. In: Downey JA, Myers SJ, Gonzalez EG, Lieberman JS, eds. *The Physiological Basis of Rehabilitation Medicine*, 2nd ed. Boston: Butterworth-Heinemann; 1994:351.
3. Powers SK, Howley ET. *Exercise Physiology: Theory and Application to Fitness and Performance*, 2nd ed. Dubuque, Iowa: Brown and Benchmark; 1994:245.
4. Rhoades RA, Tanner GA. *Medical Physiology*. Boston: Little, Brown; 1995:588.
5. McCance, KL, Huether, SE. *Pathophysiology: The Biologic Basis for Disease in Adults and Children*, 2nd ed. St. Louis: Mosby; 1994.
6. McArdle WD, Katch FI, Katch VL. *Essentials of Exercise Physiology*. Malvern, Penn.: Lea & Febiger; 1994:423.
7. Guccione A. Implications of an aging population for rehabilitation: demography, mortality, and morbidity in the elderly. In: Guccione A, ed. *Geriatric Physical Therapy*. St. Louis: Mosby–Year Book; 1993:3.
8. Wongsurawat N. Temperature regulation in the aged, In: Felsenthal G, Garrison SJ, Steinberg FU, eds. *Rehabilitation of the Aging and Elderly Patient*. Baltimore: Williams & Wilkins; 1994:73.
9. Kauffman T. Thermoregulation and use of heat and cold. In: Jackson OL, ed. *Clinics in Physical Therapy* XIV. New York: Churchill Livingstone; 1987:69.
10. Collins K, Dore C, Exton-Smith A, et al. Accidental hypothermia and impaired temperature homeostasis in the elderly. *Br Med J* 1977; 1:353.
11. Finch CE, Schneider EL, eds. *Handbook of the Biology of Aging*, 2nd ed. New York: Van Nostrand Reinhold; 1985.
12. Drinkwater BL, Horvath SM. Heat tolerance and aging. *Med Sci Sports Exerc* 1979; 1:49.
13. Claremont AD, Costill DL, Fink W, et al. Heat tolerance following diuretic-induced dehydration. *Med Sci Sports Exerc* 1976; 8:239.
14. Hooyman NR, Kiyak HA. *Social Gerontology: A Multidisciplinary Perspective*, 3rd ed. Boston: Allyn and Bacon; 1993.
15. Sessler DI. *Perioperative Thermoregulation in the Elderly*. University of California, Unpublished manuscript.
16. Judd RL, Dinep MM. Environmental Emergencies. In: Judd RL, Warner CG, Shaffer MA, eds. *Geriatric Emergencies*. Rockville, Md.: Aspen Publishers; 1986:255.

Chapter **12**

The Aging Immune System
Gordon Dickinson, M.D.

INTRODUCTION

Humans possess an elaborate array of host defenses against the many potential pathogens in their environment. Among these protective mechanisms are important mechanical and physiological guards such as skin and mucosal barriers, valvular structures like the epiglottis and the urethral valves, cleansing fluids (tears and respiratory tract mucus), and activities such as coughing. These defenses are, however, frequently breached, and it is the immune response that forms the final and most potent protection. "Immune response" generally refers to internal cellular and humoral defense mechanisms, especially those that are acquired.

INNATE AND ACQUIRED IMMUNITY

Immunity can be categorized as innate or acquired. The components of innate immunity are generally present from birth and do not require exposure to a pathogen for their development. Innate immunity includes the macrophage-phagocyte cell lines, which act as nonspecific scavengers within the body, engulfing and killing invaders that have breeched the skin or mucosal barriers. To assist the macrophages, there are substances in the serum called complement and acute-phase reactants that facilitate the attachment and ingestion of pathogens. The macrophages, as well as the complement and acute-phase reactants are poised to function as an immediate response system against virtually all bacteria. Even in the presence of complement and acute-phase reactants, however, phagocytic cells often have difficulty promptly and efficiently ingesting pathogens. Some bacteria such as *Streptococcus pneumoniae* and *Haemophilia influenzae*, for example, form a polysaccharide capsule that shields them from these defenses. Moreover, many pathogens are either too large for ingestion by macrophages (e.g., parasites) or thrive in an intracellular location (e.g., viruses, mycobacteria, and an assortment of other pathogens). To bolster these defenses, an acquired immune system has evolved, which is extremely potent and pathogen-specific, but which must be primed by a first-time exposure to the pathogen. Once in place, acquired immunity is permanent. The term "immunity" generally refers to the activity of the acquired immune system.

T and B Lymphocytes

The principal components of the acquired immune system are the T and B lymphocytes. All lymphocytes originate from progenitors in the bone marrow. Some evolve into B lymphocytes, so called because in birds these cells originate in the bursa of Fabricius. The B lymphocytes become antibody factories when activated by helper-inducer T lymphocytes. T lymphocytes circulate through the thymus gland and develop special powers enabling them to recognize foreign matter (an antigen), retain memory of the antigen, and influence B lymphocytes to produce antibodies against this antigen. These highly specific antibodies attach to the invader, either killing it directly or facilitating the process of phagocytosis, and ultimately cause the destruction and clearance of the invader from the body. Because the lymphocytes retain memory of the invader, the next exposure to this invader prompts a specific, immediate response. This ability of the immune system to develop and maintain a highly effective, specific response is the basis of vaccination.

The T-lymphocyte family also includes natural killer cells, which, when activated, have the ability to select and destroy abnormal host cells (i.e., malignant cells) and to destroy intracellular pathogens such as viruses by destroying the cells harboring them. Other T lymphocytes, the T-suppressor lymphocytes, have the ability to down-regulate and turn off the immune response once an invader is repelled. The macrophages and lymphocytes interact with one another by secreting soluble products known as cytokines. There are more than a dozen unique cytokines, and presumably others will be discovered.

IMMUNE FUNCTION CHANGES AND RISK OF INFECTION

The aging process is associated with changes in immune function, particularly in those functions directed or carried out by the lymphocyte system. Although some research has suggested that the aging process itself may be the result of the immune system's turning against the body, at present such a theory remains speculation. Most observations of age-associated altered immune function concern

failure of or deficiency in function. The increased incidence of malignancies is due, in part, to a loss of the immune system's surveillance and eradication of abnormal cells as they arise. Aging also is associated with increased activity in or loss of control of some aspects of the immune system. For example, the incidence of monoclonal gammopathies (multiple myeloma) rises in the older population, and the frequency of both anti-idiotypic (antibodies directed against other antibodies) and autoimmune antibodies increases as a person ages. Long before our understanding of the intricacies of the cellular immune system and the specialized properties of its various components, it was known that the thymus gland progressively atrophies until it becomes virtually a vestigial organ in later life.

Investigation of immune function suggests that most dramatic changes occur within the cellular arm of the immune system and that those cells involved in production of antibodies ("humoral immunity"), the B lymphocytes, function relatively well even in the very old. Specific changes in immune function that have been described as being associated with aging are listed in Box 12–1.

Box 12–1

Changes in Immune Function Associated With Aging

- Atrophy of the thymus with decreased production of thymic hormones
- Decreased in vitro responsiveness to interleukin-2
- Decreased cell proliferation in response to mitogenic stimulation
- Decreased cell-mediated cytotoxicity
- Enhanced cellular sensitivity to prostaglandin E-2
- Increased synthesis of anti-idiotype antibodies
- Increase in autoimmune antibodies
- Increased incidence of serum monoclonal immunoproteins
- Decreased representation of peripheral blood B lymphocytes in men
- Diminished delayed hypersensitivity
- Enhanced ability to synthesize interferon-gamma, interleukin-6, tumor necrosis factor-alpha

Clinically, however, the aging person is at increased risk both for infection and for an untoward outcome of infection. Some of this risk suggests an origin in diminished immune function. For example, the incidence of pneumococcal pneumonia, low throughout adolescence and most of the adult years, rises dramatically in persons over the age of 65, as does the mortality rate for pneumococcal pneumonia. The severity of influenza is also enhanced in the elderly, and there is a strikingly increased risk for death. Primary varicella (chickenpox) is a dreaded infection in older persons because of the potential for severe pneumonitis and encephalitis, which often have fatal outcomes in this population. The elderly are also at risk for reactivation of latent infections. For example, varicella zoster and reactivation tuberculosis are seen with increased frequency in older persons.

Other Pathologies Increase Risk of Infection

Not all of the increased risks for infection are attributable to changes in immune function. Indeed, many diseases afflicting the elderly create increased vulnerability to infection unrelated to changes in the immune system. For example, the pulmonary edema of congestive heart failure is frequently a contributing factor to the development of pneumonia, presumably because the edema enhances bacterial growth and compromises clearance mechanisms. Peripheral vascular disease causes ischemic breakdown of skin and soft tissue, allowing direct invasion of microbes while impairing the blood flow necessary to carry host defenses to the site. Another example is a cerebral vascular accident that leaves the patient with an impaired cough mechanism and malfunctioning epiglottic closure, with an attendant risk for aspiration. What is usually transient colonization with aspirated oral bacterial flora is not cleared, but progresses to cause bronchitis or pneumonia. Malignancies, which occur more frequently in the elderly, increase the risk for infection by means of a number of mechanisms. They can interfere with the cleansing effects of body fluids by interrupting normal flow—as is seen with endobronchial carcinoma or laryngeal carcinoma, for example—thereby setting the stage for entrapment of bacteria normally swept away by mucus flow. Malignancies also frequently erode normal cutaneous or mucosal barriers, providing a direct invasion route into soft tissues and body cavities. The inanition that frequently accompanies metastatic malignancy is, moreover, associated with impaired cellular immunity.

All of these diseases may contribute to the risk for infection indirectly simply because the patient is hospitalized in a facility where the opportunity to acquire a virulent multidrug-resistant pathogen is much increased.

IMPLICATIONS OF IMMUNE DYSFUNCTION

As noted above, the major clinical significance of immune dysfunction in the elderly is an increased risk for infection and, all too frequently, severe morbidity when an infection occurs. A number of infections are recognized to occur more frequently in the elderly (Box 12–2). The implications for health professionals are obvious. Because infections may rapidly overwhelm the immune defenses and initiate an irrevocable course, clinicians must monitor patients closely. Early warning signals may be subtle: a sensation of being unwell, a change in mentation (lethargy, confusion), a decrease in appetite, or a diminution of physical activity. Such clinical signs and symptoms of infection may be muted in the older patient; crucial clues may be easily overlooked or attributed to other conditions. Fever, the hallmark of infection, may be subdued or even replaced by a drop in temperature in the older patient, and chills may be absent. Caregivers should pay attention to subtle clinical hints and investigate, first by questioning and examining the patient, then by following the bedside evaluation with laboratory and radiographic studies, as appropriate. Because the elderly patient frequently has other diseases that may cause these signs and symptoms, a timely, accurate diagnosis is often difficult to establish.

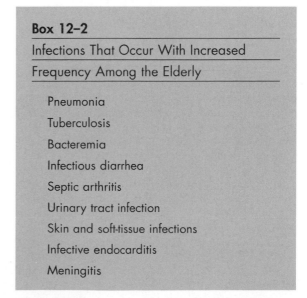

Box 12–2

Infections That Occur With Increased Frequency Among the Elderly

Pneumonia

Tuberculosis

Bacteremia

Infectious diarrhea

Septic arthritis

Urinary tract infection

Skin and soft-tissue infections

Infective endocarditis

Meningitis

Therapeutic Intervention

Because bacteriological studies to detect the causative pathogen take hours or days, empiric treatment is frequently necessary to avoid undue morbidity and mortality associated with serious infections. The decision to initiate empiric antimicrobial treatment is often problematic when the presence of an infection has not yet been proven and the causative organism is not known. To diagnose and choose treatment, the clinician must weigh all available evidence, searching carefully for clues at typical sites for infection: respiratory tract, urinary tract, pressure sores on the skin, catheter insertion sites, and the biliary and gastrointestinal tracts. If a decision is taken to initiate empiric treatment, knowledge of a patient's prior infections and recent experiences with nosocomial pathogens within the facility will help the physician choose appropriate antibiotics. This process of determining the probable causative organism and starting empiric treatment is particularly difficult in the extended-care facility and the home-care setting and when the patient is being transferred among various treatment facilities. Effective and timely communication among the health-care team members is a necessity if patients in such circumstances are to receive optimal care. As in all areas of health care, prevention is greatly preferred to treatment. Of primary importance is attention to the seemingly mundane details of daily care to avoid situations that are known to place a patient at risk for infection. Malnutrition exacerbates the frailty of the elderly, so monitoring the patient's nutritional needs and intervening to assure they are met are important. Such nutritional intervention may require no more than assistance with meals. Although nutritional supplements are commercially available, balanced meals prepared to accommodate the patient's taste and any impairment of mastication are usually sufficient. Measures to avoid skin breakdown also should be followed meticulously: frequent turning of the immobile patient, cleaning of skin soiled by incontinence, and attending to bowel and urinary habits to minimize incontinence. Discontinuation of unnecessary medical devices such as intravenous catheters and urinary catheters also eliminates two of the greatest iatrogenic sources of serious infection.

Basic to the prevention of nosocomial infections is strict attention to good infection control practices that are universally recommended but seldom scrupulously followed. In many centers, the problem of nosocomial spread of pathogens has been exacerbated by the emergence of multidrug-resistant pathogens, a phenomenon likely to continue in the future. Outbreaks of infection within hospitals and nursing homes caused by methicillin-resistant *Staphylococcus aureus*, multidrug-resistant *Enterobacteriaceae*, streptococci, and even *Mycobacterium tuberculosis* have been documented. However, most, if not all, outbreaks are avoidable.

Vaccines

No discussion of preventive medicine for the elderly is complete without mention of vaccination against two important pathogens: influenza and *S. pneumoniae*. Influenza vaccines are updated yearly to include antigens from the most recent endemic strains and are typically given in the autumn of the year to elicit antibodies in the recipient in time for the winter influenza epidemic. The pneumococcal vaccine, containing type-specific antigens from 23 of the most prevalent *S. pneumoniae* capsular types, is recommended for all persons over the age of 65.

The pneumococcal vaccine is not, however, without its critics. In elderly recipients, particularly among subgroups with liver, renal, and other chronic diseases, response is suboptimal. Moreover, the component antigens can vary considerably in their immunogenicity, with some eliciting very low antibody responses or none at all, and others producing predictably good antibody titers. The emergence of penicillin-resistant *S. pneumoniae* in the past decade has, however, enhanced the potential benefit of vaccination against this pathogen. Since antibody levels produced tend to wane with time, some authorities now recommend revaccination every 5 to 10 years.

CONCLUSION

Changes in the immune systems of aged persons add to the complexity and the challenge of providing good health care to the elderly. Comorbidities further complicate this problem. Because an elevation in body temperature is not always seen, clinicians and care providers must be aware of the subtle manifestations of infection such as a sense of being unwell, lethargy, confusion and diminished appetite or physical activity. The choice of medical intervention is not always clear-cut, but good nutrition and infection control are necessary. Vaccinations are helpful, although their use is not without controversy.

SUGGESTED READINGS

Adler WH, Nagel JE. Clinical immunology and aging. In: Hazzard WR, Bierman EL, Blass JP, Ettinger WH Jr., Halter JB, eds. *Principles of Geriatric Medicine and Gerontology*, 3rd ed. New York: McGraw-Hill; 1994.

Ben-Yehuda A, Weksler ME. Host resistance and the immune system. *Clin in Geriatr Med* 1992; 8:701–710.

Levin MJ, Murray M, Rotbart HA, Zerbe GO, White CJ, Hayward AR. Immune response of elderly individuals to a live attenuated varicella vaccine. *J Infect Dis* 1992; 166:253–259.

Paganelli R, Quinti I, Fagiolo U, et al. Changes in circulating B cells and immunoglobulin classes and subclasses in a healthy aged population. *Clin Exp Immunol* 1992; 90:351–354.

Schwab EP, Callegari PE, Johnson JJ, Williams WV, Schumacher HR Jr. How aging impacts the immune system. IM. 1992; 13:34–41.

Thoman ML, Weigle WO. The cellular and subcellular bases of immunosenescence. *Adv Immunol* 1989; 46:221–261.

Weigle WO. Effects of aging on the immune system. *Hosp Pract* 1989; 24:112–119.

Chapter **13**

Pharmacology Considerations for Aging Persons

Charles D. Ciccone, Ph.D., P.T.

INTRODUCTION

Elderly people receiving physical rehabilitation services are commonly taking medications to help resolve acute and chronic ailments. These medications are intended to improve the patient's health but they frequently cause side effects that can have a negative impact on the patient's response to physical rehabilitation. Likewise, older adults are more susceptible to adverse effects of drugs because of many factors, including excessive drug use, declining function in various physiological systems, and altered drug metabolism and excretion. It follows that therapists should be aware of the primary medications being taken by their elderly clients and how those medications can affect patients' participation in rehabilitation.

Some of the primary medications used to treat conditions commonly seen in older adults are addressed here. This discussion is not meant to be all-inclusive but should help clinicians to recognize and understand how medications taken by the elderly can affect their response to rehabilitation.

TREATMENT OF PAIN AND INFLAMMATION

Opioid Analgesics

Opioid (narcotic) medications such as morphine and codeine (Table 13–1) are powerful analgesics that bind to neuronal receptors in the spinal cord and brain. These medications reduce synaptic activity in pain-transmitting pathways, thereby decreasing pain perception. Common side effects of opioids include sedation, respiratory depression, constipation, and postural hypotension. Therapists should also be aware that older adults are more susceptible to opioid-induced psychotropic reactions such as confusion, anxiety, hallucinations, and euphoria/dysphoria. This reaction is especially common in elderly patients recovering from surgery.

Nonopioid Analgesics

Nonsteroidal anti-inflammatory drugs (NSAIDs) are the primary group of nonopioid analgesics. NSAIDs include aspirin, ibuprofen, and similar agents (see Table 13–1) and these drugs are often effective in treating mild to moderate pain. These medications actually produce four clinically important effects: decreased pain, decreased inflammation, decreased fever, and decreased blood coagulation. All of these effects are mediated through inhibition of the biosynthesis of lipid compounds called prostaglandins. Certain prostaglandins, for example, mediate painful sensations by increasing the nociceptive effects of bradykinin. NSAID-mediated inhibition of prostaglandin synthesis therefore helps reduce painful sensations in a variety of clinical conditions. The primary problem associated with NSAIDs is gastrointestinal distress, including gastric irritation and ulceration. These medications may also cause damage to the liver and kidneys, especially in older adults who have preexisting hepatic or renal dysfunction.

Acetaminophen, the active ingredient in Tylenol and other products, is another type of nonopioid analgesic. This agent is different from the NSAIDs in that it does not produce any appreciable anti-inflammatory or anticoagulant effects. Likewise, acetaminophen does not produce gastrointestinal irritation, but this medication can cause severe hepatotoxicity in people with liver disease or when patients overdose on this drug.

Anti-inflammatory Medications

Treatment of inflammation consists primarily of the NSAIDs and anti-inflammatory steroids. As indicated earlier, NSAIDs inhibit the synthesis of prostaglandins and this inhibition reduces the proinflammatory effects of certain prostaglandins. NSAIDs tend to be effective in treating a variety of conditions that exhibit mild to moderate inflammation. More severe inflammatory conditions often require the use of anti-inflammatory steroids known

Table 13–1 Analgesic and Anti-inflammatory Medications

Category	Common Examples	
	Generic Name	Trade Name
Opioid analgesics	Hydromorphone	Dilaudid
	Meperidine	Demerol
	Morphine	Many trade names
	Oxycodone	Roxicodone
	Propoxyphene	Darvon
Nonopioid analgesics		
NSAIDs[a]	Aspirin	Many trade names
	Ibuprofen	Advil, Motrin, others
	Ketoprofen	Orudis
	Ketorolac	Toradol
	Naproxen	Aleve, others
	Piroxicam	Feldene
Acetaminophen	—	Tylenol, others
Glucocorticoids	Cortisone	Cortone, others
	Dexamethasone	Decadron
	Hydrocortisone	Many trade names
	Methylprednisolone	Medrol
	Prednisone	Deltasone, others

[a]Nonsteroidal anti-inflammatory drugs.

as glucocorticoids. Medications such as prednisone, cortisone, and so on (see Table 13–1) inhibit a number of the cellular and chemical aspects of the inflammatory response, often producing a dramatic decrease in the symptoms of inflammation. Glucocorticoids, however, cause many severe side effects including breakdown of collagenous tissues, hypertension, glucose intolerance, gastric ulcer, glaucoma, and adrenocortical suppression. Tissue breakdown (catabolism) can cause severe muscle wasting and osteoporosis, especially in older people who may already be somewhat debilitated.

PSYCHOTROPIC MEDICATIONS

Antianxiety Drugs

Treatment of anxiety has traditionally consisted of benzodiazepines, including Valium and similar agents (Table 13–2). These drugs work by increasing the inhibitory effects of an endogenous neurotransmitter, γ-aminobutyric acid (GABA), in areas of the brain that control mood and behavior. The primary side effect of benzodiazepine antianxiety agents is sedation. These drugs may also cause tolerance and physical dependence when used continually for prolonged periods (more than 6 weeks). Benzodiazepines also have extremely long meta-

bolic half-lives in older adults, which means that it takes a very long time to metabolize and eliminate these drugs. As a result, benzodiazepines can accumulate in older patients and reach toxic levels evidenced by symptoms of confusion, slurred speech, dyspnea, incoordination, and pronounced weakness.

A newer type of nonbenzodiazepine antianxiety medication has been developed, and it is known as buspirone (BuSpar). This agent, chemically classified as an azapirone, increases serotonin activity in the brain, thus decreasing symptoms of anxiety. Buspirone has been used increasingly in older adults because this agent does not appear to produce sedation or cause tolerance and physical dependence.

Antidepressants

Several different types and categories of antidepressant medications exist (see Table 13–2). These drugs all share the common goal of trying to increase activity in the brain at synapses that use amine neurotransmitters including catecholamines (norepinephrine), 5-hydroxytryptamine (serotonin), and dopamine. Depression is supposedly caused by increased sensitivity of postsynaptic receptors at these synapses, and a drug-mediated increase in synaptic activity is intended to produce a compensa-

Table 13–2 Psychotropic Medications

Category	Common Examples	
	Generic Name	Trade Name
Antianxiety drugs		
Benzodiazepines	Alprazolam	Xanax
	Chlordiazepoxide	Librium, others
	Diazepam	Valium
	Lorazepam	Ativan
Azapirones	Buspirone	BuSpar
Antidepressants		
Tricyclics	Amitriptyline	Elavil, others
	Doxepin	Sinequan, others
	Imipramine	Tofranil, others
	Nortriptyline	Pamelor, others
MAO inhibitors	Isocarboxazid	Marplan
	Tranylcypromine	Parnate
Second-generation drugs	Amoxapine	Asendin
	Fluoxetine	Prozac
	Maprotiline	Ludiomil
	Paroxetine	Paxil
	Sertraline	Zoloft
Antipsychotics	Chlorpromazine	Thorazine
	Clozapine	Clozaril
	Haloperidol	Haldol
	Prochlorperazine	Compazine, others
	Promazine	Sparine, others
	Thioridazine	Mellaril

tory decrease (downregulation) in receptor sensitivity. Most antidepressants are nonselective and cause increased activity at synapses that use norepinephrine, serotonin, and dopamine. Certain antidepressants, however, have received considerable attention because these agents are more selective for serotonin pathways than other amine synapses. There is considerable controversy over whether serotonin-selective drugs such as Prozac, Zoloft, and Paxil are more effective than their nonselective counterparts. This debate remains unresolved at this time, with certain practitioners believing these selective drugs are more effective while critics question whether these drugs may actually produce more dangerous side effects in certain patients.

The primary side effects of antidepressants are sedation, postural hypotension, and the results of decreased acetylcholine function (anticholinergic effects) such as dry mouth, urinary retention, constipation, tachycardia, and confusion. These side effects are often much more pronounced in older people because of age-related declines in various physiological systems combined with the fact that these drugs have much longer metabolic half-lives

in older adults. Another primary concern about antidepressants is that there is typically a 4- to 6-week time lag between initiation of drug treatment and improvement of depression. Depression may actually worsen in some patients during this period, and therapists should be especially careful to note any increase in depressive symptoms while waiting for these drugs to take effect.

Antipsychotics

Psychosis seems to be caused by increased activity in certain brain dopamine pathways. As a result, antipsychotic medications block postsynaptic receptors in these pathways to help normalize dopaminergic influence. Common antipsychotics are listed in Table 13–2. These agents typically cause side effects such as sedation, postural hypotension, anticholinergic effects, and movement disorders including tardive dyskinesia, pseudoparkinsonism, severe restlessness (akathisia), and various other dystonias and dyskinesias. Tardive dyskinesia is characterized by oral-facial movements such as extending the tongue, grinding the jaw, puffing the cheeks, and various other fragmented movements of the neck, trunk, and extremities. This problem is often regarded as the most serious side effect of antipsychotic medications because symptoms of tardive dyskinesia may take several months to disappear or may remain indefinitely after the antipsychotic drug is discontinued. It follows that therapists should be especially cognizant of any aberrant movement patterns in patients taking antipsychotic medications, especially symptoms of tardive dyskinesia.

NEUROLOGICAL DISORDERS

Parkinson's Disease

The motor symptoms of Parkinson's disease (bradykinesia, rigidity, resting tremor) are related to the loss of dopaminergic neurons in the basal ganglia. The primary method of drug treatment is levodopa (L-dopa), which is the metabolic precursor to dopamine. Although dopamine will not cross the blood-brain barrier, levodopa will enter brain tissues where it is subsequently converted to dopamine, thus helping to restore the influence of dopamine in the basal ganglia. Levodopa is often administered with carbidopa, a drug that prevents premature conversion of levodopa to dopamine in the peripheral circulation. Combining levodopa with carbidopa in preparations such as Sinemet allows levodopa to reach the brain before undergoing conversion to dopamine.

Levodopa is associated with several side effects, including gastrointestinal irritation, hypotension, and psychotic-like symptoms. Other movement problems, including dyskinesias and dystonias, may also occur, especially at higher dosages. The most devastating problems, however, are typically related to a decrease in the long-term effectiveness of this medication. Patients who respond well to levodopa initially commonly experience progressively diminishing benefits from this medication after 4 or 5 years of continual use. This phenomenon is probably related to a progressive increase in the severity of Parkinson's disease; that is, drug therapy cannot adequately resolve the motor symptoms because of the advanced degeneration of dopaminergic neurons in the basal ganglia. Helping patients and their families to deal with the physical as well as psychological impact of decreased levodopa effectiveness is one of the more difficult tasks therapists face.

Several other types of medications are used to supplement drug therapy in Parkinson's disease (Table 13–3). These agents are typically used to supplement levodopa therapy, or they serve as the primary agent when levodopa is poorly tolerated or no longer effective. A common strategy is to combine several agents in low to moderate doses to obtain optimal benefits while avoiding the excessive side effects that would occur with large amounts of any single drug.

Antiseizure Medications

Some medications commonly used to control seizure activity are listed in Table 13–3. These agents act on the brain to selectively reduce excitability in neurons that initiate seizures. It is often difficult, however, to reduce excitation in these neurons without producing some degree of general inhibition throughout the brain. This is especially true in the older patient who has had a previous cerebral injury such as a cerebrovascular accident. As a result, older patients taking antiseizure medications are especially prone to side effects such as sedation, fatigue, weakness, incoordination, ataxia, and visual disturbances. Therapists should pay particular attention to patients taking antiseizure medications because they are in a position to help determine whether dosages of these medications are too high (as indicated by excessive side effects) or too low (as evidenced by an increase in seizure activity).

Treatment of Alzheimer's Disease

Tacrine (Cognex) and donepezil (Aricept) are two medications that were developed fairly recently to help improve cognition and intellectual function in patients with Alzheimer's disease. These drugs are cholinergic stimulants (see Table 13–3); they decrease acetylcholine breakdown at synapses in the brain, thereby helping to maintain acetylcholine influence in areas of the brain that are undergoing the neuronal degeneration associated with Alzheimer's disease. These drugs do not cure Alzheimer's disease, but preliminary evidence indicates that these medications may help patients retain more intellectual and functional ability during the early stages of this disease. The primary side effects associated with these drugs include loss of appetite and gastrointestinal distress (diarrhea, nausea, and vomiting).

CARDIOVASCULAR DRUGS

Antihypertensive Medications

Several drug categories (Table 13–4) are used to treat high blood pressure in older adults and reduce the chance of hypertensive-related incidents such as stroke, myocardial infarction, and kidney disease.

Table 13–3 Neurological Medications

Category	Examples	Rationale for Use
Treatment of Parkinson's disease		
Dopamine precursors	Levodopa (Sinemet)[a]	Are converted to dopamine in the brain; help resolve dopamine deficiency
Anticholinergic drugs	Benztropine (Cogentin) Biperiden (Akineton)	Normalize acetylcholine imbalance caused by dopamine loss
Dopamine agonists	Bromocriptine (Parlodel) Pergolide (Permax)	Directly stimulate dopamine receptors in brain
MAO_B[b] inhibitors	Selegiline (Eldepryl)	Decrease dopamine breakdown
Antiseizure medications		
Barbiturates	Phenobarbital (Solfoton) Mephobarbital (Mebaral)	Increase inhibitory effects of GABA[c] in brain
Benzodiazepines	Clonazepam (Klonopin) Clorazepate (Tranxene)	Increase inhibitory effects of GABA in brain
Carboxylic acids	Valproic acid (Depakene)	May increase GABA concentrations in brain
Hydantoins	Phenytoin (Dilantin) Ethotoin (Peganone)	Decrease sodium entry into hyperexcitable neurons
Iminostilbenes	Carbamazepine (Tegretol)	Similar to hydantoins
Succinimides	Ethosuximide (Zarontin) Phensuximide (Milontin)	May decrease calcium entry into hyperexcitable neurons
Treatment of Alzheimer's dementia		
Cholinergic stimulants	Donepezil (Aricept) Tacrine (Cognex)	Increase acetylcholine influence in the brain

[a]Sinemet is the trade name for levodopa combined with carbidopa.
[b]MAO_B, monoamine oxidase type B.
[c]GABA, gamma-aminobutyric acid.

Angiotensin-converting enzyme (ACE) inhibitors prevent the formation of angiotensin II, which is a powerful vasoconstrictor and stimulant of vascular smooth muscle growth. Agents such as alpha-blockers, beta-blockers, and other sympatholytic drugs decrease sympathetic nervous system stimulation of the heart and vasculature, thereby decreasing myocardial contraction force and peripheral vascular resistance. Calcium-channel-blockers reduce myocardial contractility and vascular smooth muscle contraction by limiting calcium entry into these tissues. Diuretics increase sodium and water excretion, thereby decreasing blood pressure by reducing fluid volume in the vascular system. Certain direct-acting vasodilators (see Table 13–4) reduce vascular resistance by inhibiting vascular smooth muscle contraction.

Elderly people with hypertension are treated routinely with diuretic agents because these drugs are fairly safe and well tolerated. ACE inhibitors have also been used increasingly in older patients because these agents reduce blood pressure and prevent adverse structural changes in the heart and

vasculature. In contrast, sympatholytics and vasodilators tend to produce a variety of unfavorable side effects in older patients so these drugs are typically used only in severe cases. Calcium-channel-blockers were gaining acceptance for use in older adults but recent studies have indicated that certain agents (such as the short-acting form of nifedipine) may actually increase the risk of myocardial infarction in certain patients. There is likewise some concern that calcium-channel-blockers may increase the risk of cancer. Hence, use of calcium-channel-blockers in older patients with hypertension requires further study.

Antihypertensive drugs produce various side effects, varying with the specific agent. Therapists must realize, however, that hypotension and postural hypotension are always possible whenever blood pressure is reduced pharmacologically. That is, blood pressure may fall more than 10 to 20 mmHg, especially when older patients sit up or stand up suddenly. Likewise, physical therapy interventions that cause extensive peripheral vasodilation (the Hubbard tank, the therapeutic pool) must

Table 13–4 Cardiovascular Medications

Category	Common Examples	Rationale for Use
Antihypertensive drugs		
ACE inhibitors	Captopril (Capoten) Enalapril (Vasotec)	Decrease angiotensin II synthesis; promote vasodilation and increased vascular compliance
Alpha-blockers	Doxazosin (Cardura) Prazosin (Minipress)	Promote vasodilation by decreasing sympathetic stimulation of vasculature
Beta-blockers	Metoprolol (Lopressor) Nadolol (Corgard) Propranolol (Inderal)	Decrease myocardial contractility by decreasing sympathetic stimulation of the heart
Calcium-channel-blockers	Diltiazem (Cardizem) Nifedipine (Procardia) Verapamil (Isoptin)	Promote vasodilation and decreased myocardial contractility by limiting calcium entry into vasculature and heart
Diuretics	Chlorothiazide (Diuril) Furosemide (Lasix) Spironolactone (Aldactone)	Decrease intravascular fluid volume; reduce workload on heart
Vasodilators	Hydralazine (Apresoline) Minoxidil (Loniten)	Promote vasodilation by inhibiting contraction of vascular smooth muscle
Treatment of congestive heart failure		
Digitalis glycosides	Digitoxin (Crystodigin) Digoxin (Lanoxin)	Increase myocardial contractility by increasing calcium entry into heart muscle
Others	Diuretics, ACE inhibitors Vasodilators	See above

be used very cautiously because these interventions add to the hypotensive drug effects and produce dangerously low blood pressure in older adults. Finally, certain antihypertensive agents such as the beta-blockers blunt the cardiac response to exercise and this effect may limit physical work capacity during activities that require high cardiac output, such as climbing stairs, exercise training, and so on.

Treatment of Congestive Heart Failure

Congestive heart failure (CHF) occurs commonly in older adults and is characterized by a progressive decline in myocardial pumping ability. The primary medications used to treat CHF are the digitalis glycosides such as digoxin (see Table 13–4). These agents increase calcium entry into myocardial tissues, thereby increasing contraction force. Digitalis drugs often produce temporary hemodynamic improvements that decrease the symptoms of CHF, but these agents do not alter the progression of this disease or decrease the rather high morbidity and mortality associated with heart failure. These agents, too, have a small safety margin and digitalis

drugs can accumulate rapidly in the bloodstream, causing toxicity in older patients. Digitalis toxicity is associated with symptoms such as gastrointestinal distress, confusion, blurred vision, and cardiac arrhythmias. Therapists should be alert for these symptoms because digitalis-induced arrhythmias can be quite severe or fatal.

Because of the problems related to digitalis, other medications have been used alone or with digitalis drugs to help treat patients with CHF. Diuretics and vasodilators have been used to decrease the workload on the failing heart by reducing fluid volume or decreasing vascular resistance, respectively. More recently, ACE inhibitors have been recognized as being very beneficial in patients with CHF. These agents decrease angiotensin II-mediated vasoconstriction and vascular hypertrophy so that cardiac workload is reduced. Unlike digitalis drugs, ACE inhibitors appear to improve the prognosis of patients with heart failure and decrease the morbidity and mortality associated with CHF. ACE inhibitors are also tolerated fairly well by older adults and have relatively minor side effects such as a mild allergic reaction (skin rash) or a dry persistent cough that occurs in some patients. As a result, ACE inhibitors continue to gain acceptance as a primary treatment of CHF in the elderly.

CONCLUSION

Medications often produce favorable as well as adverse responses in elderly patients receiving rehabilitation. Therapists must be aware of the types of medications commonly taken by older adults and of the possible side effects and adverse effects associated with these medications. Geriatric patients are more susceptible to adverse drug effects, and clinicians often play an important role in helping to identify untoward drug responses in the elderly. Likewise, therapists must be able to plan and modify rehabilitation strategies to capitalize on beneficial drug effects while minimizing or avoiding adverse drug effects.

SUGGESTED READINGS

Atkin PA, Shenfield GM. Medication-related adverse reactions in the elderly: a literature review. *Adverse Drug React Toxicol Rev* 1995; 14:175.

Ciccone CD. Current trends in cardiovascular pharmacology. *Phys Ther* 1996; 76:481.

Ciccone CD. *Pharmacology in Rehabilitation,* 2nd ed. Philadelphia: F. A. Davis; 1996.

Ciccone CD. Geriatric pharmacology. In: Guccione AA, ed. *Geriatric Physical Therapy.* St. Louis: Mosby; 1993:171.

Cutson TM, Laub KC, Schenkman M. Pharmacological and nonpharmacological interventions in the treatment of Parkinson's disease. *Phys Ther* 1995; 75:363.

Forman WB. Opioid analgesic drugs in the elderly. *Clin Geriatr Med* 1996; 12:489.

Jenike MA. Psychiatric illnesses in the elderly: a review. *J Geriatr Psychiatry Neurol* 1996; 9:57.

Moncur C, Williams HJ. Rheumatoid arthritis: status of drug therapies. *Phys Ther* 1995; 75:511.

Scheuer ML, Cohen J. Seizures and epilepsy in the elderly. *Neurol Clin* 1993; 11:787.

Shammas E, Dickstein K. Drug selection for optimal treatment of hypertension in the elderly. *Drugs Aging* 1996; 11:19.

II

PATHOKINESIOLOGICAL MANIFESTATIONS AND THERAPEUTIC INTERVENTION

MUSCULOSKELETAL INVOLVEMENT

Chapter **14**

Posture

Timothy L. Kauffman, Ph.D., P.T.

INTRODUCTION

Posture is the alignment of body parts in relationship to one another at any given moment. Posture involves complex interactions among bones, joints, connective tissue, skeletal muscles, and the nervous system, both central and peripheral. The complexity of these interactions is compounded when one considers the near infinitesimal variety of human balance, motor control, and movement in relation to gravity. Furthermore, with the passage of time, each organism undergoes change from microtrauma, frank injuries, and pathology to the connective tissues, muscles, and neural control mechanisms, which result in the unique variations of aging posture.

Posture is commonly assessed using a grid or a plumb line, with the patient in a static standing position; however, within the aging population this becomes more difficult because of the age-associated increase in postural sway. The postural control mechanisms affect minor shifts in weight in order to avoid fatigue, excessive tissue compression, and venostasis. Thus, posture is truly a relative condition requiring full body integration and both static and dynamic balance control, as shown in Figure 14–1.

Multiple factors are involved in common age-related postural changes. These factors may be pathological, degenerative, or traumatic, or may be due to primary musculoskeletal changes, primary neurological changes, or a combination of diminutions in the neuromusculoskeletal system.

Degenerative joint disease is a common age-related pathology involving bony and joint surface changes. (See Chapters 20, 26, and 27.) The osteophytes that result from arthritis may prevent normal joint motion, cause pain, and possibly encroach on nerves with a subsequent radiculopathy that includes muscle weakness and imbalance. Postural adjustments may be the result of attempts to unload weight from an osteophyte in order to reduce pain or to accommodate a radiculopathy.

AXIAL AND APPENDICULAR SKELETAL CHANGES

The common postural changes in the axial skeleton and the clinical implications associated with aging are enumerated in Table 14–1 and may be seen in Figures 14–2 and 14–3. It should be noted, however, that not all these changes should be classified as faulty or abnormal. Some of the changes may be normal compensatory changes resulting from other neuromusculoskeletal alterations in the spine, extremities, or central control mechanisms. For example, the head-forward position, especially when there is an increased extension of the upper cervical spine, may result as the body attempts to counter a dorsal kyphosis caused by wedged thoracic vertebrae.

Spinal spondylosis is found in the vast majority of persons by the age of 55. These changes may include deterioration of the spinal facet joints, loss of vertebral height, narrowing of the spinal canal or neural foramina, loss of intervertebral disc space, anterior lipping, bony bridges, and calcification of the periarticular connective tissue. Clinically, these changes may cause pain and reduction in spinal motions, especially the subtle rotation motions involved in segmental rolling and the normal reciprocal pattern of the extremities in normal gait. The sit-to-stand motion may be more difficult because of the loss of coordinated spine flexion and extension.

In the appendicular skeleton, numerous combinations of changes occur as a result of a lifetime of wear and tear, habit, trauma, and pathology in the neuromusculoskeletal system. These changes result in the unique postural features of aging individuals. The common age-associated extremity changes and clinical implications are enumerated in Table 14–2 and may be seen in Figures 14–2 and 14–3.

SOFT TISSUE

Postural changes caused by soft-tissue alterations may be a result of previous injuries that have lengthened or tightened tendons, ligaments, and joint capsules. Collagen is a major component of skin, tendon, cartilage, and connective tissue and it may become increasingly stiff due to crosslinkage

Table 14–1 Age-Associated Postural Axial Skeletal Changes and Their Clinical Implications

Axial Skeletal Changes	Clinical Implications
Head forward	Shifts center of mass forward; may increase dizziness due to compromising the basilar artery
Dorsal kyphosis	Reduces trunk motions for breathing and motor responses; encourages scapular protraction; may provoke shoulder pathologies
Flat lumbar spine	Reduces trunk/hip extension for gait strides
Occasional kyphosis of lumbar spine	Results from compression of vertebral bodies; not reversible
Least common increased lordosis	Tightness of trunk/hip extensors; weakened abdominals
Posterior pelvic tilt	Results from prolonged sitting; reduces trunk/hip extension for gait strides
Scoliosis	May alter balance, breathing, and extremity motions

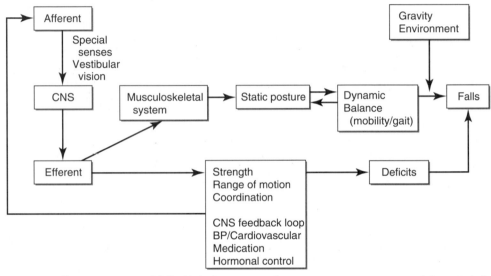

Figure 14–1 Factors affecting posture and falls. Multiple interactive forces govern static posture and dynamic balance. (From Kauffman T. Impact of aging-related musculoskeletal and postural changes on falls. *Top Geriatr Rehabil* 1990;5:34–43.)

Table 14–2 Age-Associated Postural Extremity Changes and Their Clinical Implications

Extremity Skeletal Changes	Clinical Implications
Scapular protraction or abduction	Alters normal scapulohumeral rhythm, leading to painful shoulder conditions
Tightness/contractures in elbow flexion, wrist ulnar deviation, finger flexion	Reduces reach and hand function
Hip flexion contractures (loss of hip extension to neutral or 0°)	Reduces stride length; may increase energy cost of mobility and may increase postural control requirements, especially if change is unilateral
Knee flexion contractures (loss of knee extension to neutral or 0°)	Reduces stride length and gait push-off; may increase energy cost of mobility and may increase postural control requirements, especially if change is unilateral
Varus/valgus changes at hip, knee, ankle	Reduces stride length and gait push-off; may increase energy cost of mobility; and may increase postural control requirements especially if change is unilateral. Usually is a cause of pain due to mechanical deformation and strain on musculoskeletal tissues.

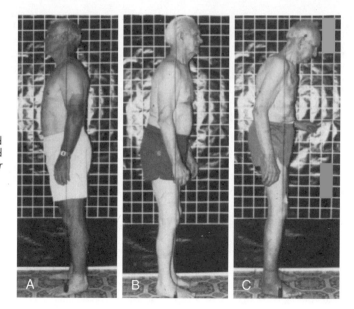

Figure 14–2 Lateral posture of (a) a 60-year-old man, (b) a 78-year-old man, and (c) a 93-year-old man. (From Kauffman T. Posture and age. *Top Geriatr Rehabil* 1987;2:13–28.)

between collagen fibers. Elastin is another major fibrous component of connective tissue that is found in the skin, ligaments, blood vessels, and lungs. With increasing age, elastin is supplanted by pseudoelastin, which is a partially degraded collagen or faulty elastin protein.

Additional soft-tissue changes that may affect postural alterations may be found in the muscle. The muscle length may be increased or shortened. There is a loss of muscle fibers, which is likely to result in reduced strength. The type I and type II muscle fiber relationship may be altered, which may influence postural control responses and mecha-

nisms. Also there is an increase in noncontractile tissue due to deposition of fat and collagen, which causes the muscle to be increasingly stiff. Muscle tone may increase, decrease, or vary because of changes in nervous system control. A more extensive discussion of these nervous system changes may be found in Chapter 5.

CLINICAL CONSIDERATIONS

In the geriatric population, posture should be assessed not only in the standing and sitting positions

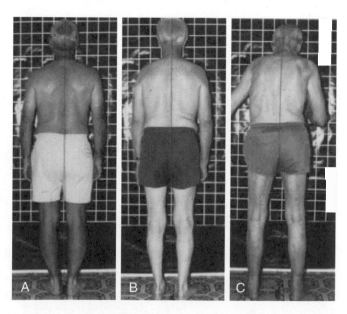

Figure 14–3 Posterior posture of (a) a 60-year-old man, (b) a 78-year-old man, and (c) a 93-year-old man. (From Kauffman T. Posture and age. *Top Geriatr Rehabil* 1987;2:13–28.)

Box 14–1

Clinical Intervention for Postural Changes
Causing Pain or Dysfunction

1. Brace, support, immobilize, protect

2. Heat, cold, electrical stimulation

3. Therapeutic exercise to enhance functional muscle strength, tone, length, coordination, and balance between agonist and antagonist

4. Medications

5. Surgery

but also in bed, especially in a patient who is confined to bed because of an injury or illness. It is especially important to prevent pressure areas, and special care should be taken to avoid muscle imbalances resulting from prolonged positioning. Areas of particular importance are the triceps surae, hip and knee flexors, and hip abductors and adductors, especially after hip surgery. It is common for the patient to assume a supine but side-bent posture that may lead to muscle imbalance. The patient who side-bends toward the operative side will suffer a contralateral hip abductor lengthening and an ipsilateral hip abductor shortening. The converse is true for the patient who side-bends away from the operative side. These muscle imbalances will become significant during rehabilitation when the patient attempts to regain independent ambulation and they may contribute to a Trendelenburg gait. See Chapter 16, "Stretch Weakness," for further discussion of muscle lengthening and stretch-weakness changes.

Clinical intervention should be undertaken in the case of such postural changes if the changes cause pain, impair function, or are likely to lead to future impairment. Typical interventions are listed in Box 14–1. These clinical interventions are not listed in order of importance. One or all of the interventions may be appropriate, depending upon the clinical assessment and the individual patient's condition and prognosis.

CONCLUSION

It is crucial to note that postural changes occur with increasing age and their characteristics are unique to each individual. Although not present in a young healthy adult, the new traits are not necessarily

faulty. As noted above, they may indicate normal compensation for a degradation in the neuromusculoskeletal alignment or control in any of its component parts. Many of these changes have taken place slowly over decades and may not be ameliorated easily, if at all.

SUGGESTED READINGS

Kauffman T. Posture and age. *Top Geriatr Rehabil* 1987; 2:13–28.

Kauffman T. Impact of aging-related musculoskeletal and postural changes on falls. *Top Geriatr Rehabil* 1990; 5:34–43.

Kendall FT, McCreary EK. *Muscles: Testing and Function*. Baltimore: Williams & Wilkins; 1983.

Moncur C. Posture in the older adult. In: Guccione A, ed. *Geriatric Physical Therapy*. St. Louis: Mosby; 1993:219–236.

Neuman DA. Arthrokinesiologic considerations in the aged. In: Guccione A, ed. *Geriatric Physical Therapy*. St. Louis: Mosby; 1993:219–231.

O'Brien K, Culham E, Pickles B. Balance and skeletal alignment in a group of elderly female fallers and nonfallers. *J Gerontol A Biol Sci Med Sci* 1997; 52A:B221–B226.

Chapter 15

Muscle Weakness and Therapeutic Exercise

Timothy L. Kauffman, Ph.D., P.T.

INTRODUCTION

The term "sarcopenia" has been coined to describe the less than normal strength of muscle that is associated with aging. Weakness has long been connected with aging; however, the role of muscle involves more than just providing strength. Obviously, muscle is involved with movement, which is crucial for joint nutrition as well as for cardiopulmonary health. Also, muscle is related to the circulatory system, as smooth muscle supports the walls of arteries and skeletal muscle is involved in the return of venous blood. Muscle is also involved in bone health and density. It is an impetus, as well, to the nervous system as it also has an afferent response with the muscle spindle. A principal source of body heat comes from muscle. Additionally, it provides a cushion of compressible tissue that helps to absorb impact in the event of trauma.

DEFINITIONS

Principally, however, muscle is noted for its roles in strength and movement. Strength may be defined as the tension that is generated by contracting muscle. It is best expressed as a force. Torque, a result of angular displacement, is the product of force and perpendicular distance from the line of force's action to the axis of rotation. Time is also a consideration for the tension that is generated and thus should be considered power.

The generation of muscle tension is determined largely by the cross-sectional area of the muscle and the recruitment of motor units. Other biomechanical factors such as muscle length and angle of displacement and physiological factors such as metabolism and muscle fiber type also influence strength. Insufficient strength to perform a functional motor task should be considered weakness.

There are various types of muscle contractions. When there is no change in muscle length, a static contraction occurs, which is also referred to as isometric (same length). Dynamic contractions are a lengthening or shortening of a muscle, also called, respectively, eccentric and concentric contractions. Isotonic (same tone) contractions involve movement of a constant weight through a motion. Normally, raising a weight is a concentric contraction and lowering it is an eccentric contraction. When a mechanical device resists the tension generated by the contracting muscle, thereby controlling the speed of the limb's movement, an isokinetic (same speed) contraction occurs. Isokinetic devices are essential for assessing torque at various speeds, which is clinically important because of the age-related loss of fast-twitch type II muscle fibers. This loss is one of several factors that probably contribute to the increasing inability to recover from a stumble which results in greater risk for injury.

ASSESSMENT

Assessment of muscle strength can be performed using a manual muscle test (MMT). Although the MMT is an ordinal scale measurement, it is invaluable because it can be performed in nearly every treatment setting. When using the manual muscle test, it is crucial to specify the type of contraction being performed. The original MMT was designed as an assessment of strength throughout the available range of motion, but it has been modified in many circumstances to a "make" test, in which the patient performs an isometric contraction at a specific joint position. This is a requisite modification of the MMT, especially for patients who have painful arcs or restrictions in motion. Clarity in documentation is enhanced when these specifics (type of test and position) are recorded.

In contrast, a "break" test is used when the patient is asked to hold the joint in a specific posi-

tion and the evaluator attempts to break the tension that is generated. This changes it from an isometric to an eccentric contraction. It should be noted that in healthy muscle, the highest tension is generated with an eccentric contraction followed by an isometric contraction, and the least tension is generated with the isotonic type of contraction. As noted above, lowering a weight is an isotonic eccentric contraction and may be a helpful technique for strength-training patients. For example, lowering a flexed upper extremity that is weight-loaded may be effective for increasing the strength of the lower trapezius, rhomboids, and deltoids.

Caution should be used when attempting to measure strength with the manual muscle test in aging people because of the frequent necessity of modifying the test positions. The test positions as enumerated in the standard manuals may have to be modified because of injury or disease in the aging patient. Also, a more functional position may be necessary because areas of weakness may be found only in certain positions of the joint's range of motion. These areas of weakness may be due to joint surface irregularities or changes in periarticular connective tissue and muscle length.

Hand-held and isokinetic dynamometers are very useful for assessing strength. Caution must be used to avoid pain in and injury to swollen areas and ulcerated or atrophied skin; the verbal extolling that frequently accompanies this testing may have to be restrained. Also, greater risk of joint injury due to age-related changes in periarticular connective tissue (see Chapters 4 and 65) should be considered when dynamometers are being used.

Another strength-assessment technique that is gaining popularity is the 1 RM or 10 RM technique. The "RM" stands for repetition maximum: a 1 RM test measures the maximal weight (dynamic and isotonic) that can be moved through the range of motion (ROM) one time, and 10 RM is the maximal weight moved 10 times. Some guessing must be involved in determining the starting test weight, which may be too heavy or too light, and weight adjustments must be made accordingly.

Perhaps more important than a frank measurement of the force of a muscle contraction is a functional assessment of motor performance, such as the ability to ascend and descend a flight of steps or to raise a 2-pound can of food onto the second shelf of a cupboard. Noting that the patient was able to ascend 6 steps before catching a toe or failing to elevate the lower extremity would be a functional parameter of muscle performance. Endurance is an important consideration, too, especially as it relates to functional outcomes. It is one factor in the 10 RM test and is frequently measured with isokinetic devices. In activities of daily living, endurance is always a consideration; for example, carrying a full 1-gallon jug (8 pounds) of water from the refrigerator to the kitchen table requires muscular strength and endurance.

STRENGTH TRAINING

Strength-training research has shown that the potential to increase strength is maintained in older persons. The benefits of strength training with isometric, isotonic, and isokinetic routines have been shown. Simple calisthenics without the use of machines are efficacious. Also, hypertrophy occurs even in persons up to the age of 90 years and above, although hypertrophy in and of itself is not necessarily a primary objective of care. Functional outcomes are related to strength and motor performance and should be the objective of rehabilitation.

Modifying Strength Training

When planning a strength-training routine for geriatric patients, it is crucial to consider the need to modify the training regimen in order to accommodate pathology in the cardiopulmonary and cardiovascular systems as well as in the neuromusculoskeletal system. Guidelines for exercise by patients with heart disease are presented in Chapter 42. The aging person is more susceptible to skin tears as well as injuries to muscles, joints, and ligaments. Fatigue, poor physical work capacity, and deconditioning are important considerations, especially in the frail elderly who have multiple diagnoses. The Valsalva maneuver must be avoided. Isometric exercises are safe provided that the hold time is no more than 5 to 10 seconds, the standard isometric contraction. Blood pressure has been shown to be adversely affected by isometric contractions longer than 30 seconds in duration.

Aging patients who need an exercise program benefit from individualized instruction that is tailored to meet functional goals. Some individuals are fully cognitive and capable of engaging in standard strengthening and fitness exercises. Others do not have the same physical, cognitive, or communicative abilities, so to be effective, the exercise program must be modified.

Monitoring response to exercise is requisite. This is achieved by observing and recording pulse rate, respiratory rate, perceived exertion, and quality of movement. For example, asynchronous muscle contractions or obtaining full range of motion for only the first 6 repetitions and not all 10 would be indicative of low quality of movement.

Blood pressure should be taken before, during, and after exercise, especially for patients with known or suspected cardiovascular, cardiopulmonary, or cerebrovascular disease. However, this is cumbersome in most outpatient clinics and in home health care with the use of a sphygmomanometer. An oxygen pulsimeter is used to measure oxygen levels and may be helpful for establishing safe exercise parameters. Clinically, the talk test is beneficial. This is a simple safeguard that avoids overloading the patient beyond capability by talking with him or her during the exercise routine. When overexercised, the patient will become dyspneic and be unable to talk in 2 to 3 word sentences.

Training Considerations

The overload principle is necessary but care must be taken to avoid excessive overload. Some patients with cognitive or communicative difficulties may benefit from gestures or range-of-motion exercises, including passive, active assistive, active, and resistive exercises, as well as proprioceptive neuromuscular facilitation. Physical contact may assist not only in attaining a desired movement but may also establish a trusting rapport between patient and care provider. Also, the benefit of sensory stimulation to muscle activation has been recognized, especially in work with children and individuals with neurological conditions.

With a weight training technique it is common to start the therapeutic exercise routine with 5 to 6 contractions, using only 50% of the maximal voluntary contraction (MVC). Successive sets of 5 to 6 repetitions are performed using 60%, 70%, and 80% of the MVC. The same technique of progressive resistive exercise may be done after a strength assessment with a hand-held dynamometer.

Functional activities done repeatedly, such as a sit-to-stand 10 times, not only will strengthen muscles, but also will enhance coordination, endurance, and motor learning. Practice is important for skill acquisition (see Chapter 5, "Aging and the Central Nervous System").

Some patients are too deconditioned to effectively undergo typical exercise routines such as progressive resistive exercise and standard weight-loading programs but they may benefit from a graded circuit routine using a combination of chair exercises and, if possible, ambulatory activities. For example, with supervision, a patient may perform bilateral shoulder flexion 10 times, followed by 10 repetitions of long-arc quads, followed by 2 repetitions of sit-to-stand, followed by 10 repetitions of hip flexion. Pulse rate should be monitored before and after exercise. The talk test may be employed as well. The speed and number of repeti-

Box 15–1

Sample Circuit Exercises for the Severely Deconditioned or Chairbound Patient

1. Check pre-exercise pulse and respiratory rate.

2. Raise both arms over head 10 times.

3. Straighten each knee 10 times (alternate sides).

4. Abduct both arms 10 times.

5. Flex each hip 10 times.

6. Repeat above routine or expand to additional exercises such as wheelchair push-ups, elbow flexion/extension, sit-to-stand; shoulder shrugs, gluteal squeezes; deep inspiration and forced exhalation; resistive exercise with or without elastic tubing; and walking, if possible. Length of exercise should vary based on the patient's ability and limitations. These more exertional exercises are best performed after the easier warm-up exercises in 2 through 5.

7. Check post-exercise pulse.

8. Rest until heart rate returns to approximately pre-exercise rate, after which repeat the routine, if appropriate.

tions of these simple exercises can be increased or decreased according to the patient's response to exercise. Also, walking exercises can be added. Some individuals may be able to exercise for only 1 minute with this circuit type of routine and others may be able to advance to 3 or 4 minutes. A rest of 1 to 5 minutes should occur before repeating the routine. It is safe to start the routine again when the pulse rate has returned to the pre-exercise level. A sample is provided in Box 15–1.

Exercise machines clearly have their benefit for some patients. Weight-training units, bicycles, stair-steppers, and rowing machines are all beneficial. As mentioned above, simple calisthenics and walking are mainstays in the exercise armamentarium for aging patients. Use of low weights at the ankles and wrists can increase the physical work during simple walking exercises.

WHEN STRENGTH TRAINING IS NOT EFFECTIVE

When an aging patient is undergoing a strength-training routine and there is no marked improve-

ment in strength despite the attempts to improve it, a number of factors may reduce the patient's potential to improve muscular performance. First of all, adequate nutrition is critical. Sufficient calorie and protein intake is necessary if any exercise routine is to be performed. However, malnutrition is common among the elderly; frequently, ill health precedes it. Decreased physical activity may also contribute to malnutrition. Bereavement, depression, dementia, and living alone are factors in decreased appetite. Changes in the gastrointestinal tract (see Chapter 9, "The Effects of Aging on the Digestive System") and medications may all diminish food and fluid intake. Vitamin D deficiency is a factor in osteoporosis that can contribute to back pain and subsequent weakness.

Dehydration is an important consideration when conducting exercises with patients, especially in the home-health setting. Adequate hydration is a concern not only during hot humid months but also during cold dry periods. Dehydration can alter mental status and thus decrease receptiveness to exercise. Lightheadedness, syncope, and orthostatic hypotension may also present as findings in the dehydrated elderly patient.

Blood Chemistry Imbalances

Iron deficiency anemia is not likely to occur in aging individuals with a sensible, balanced diet; however, it may be found in persons with neoplasm and gastrointestinal bleeding. This may manifest as decreased hemoglobin or hematocrit levels in the blood chemistry. The patient may present with fatigue and weakness.

Magnesium is a mineral important to normal muscle contraction, and a deficiency is commonly found with low serum levels of calcium, potassium, and phosphate. Hypomagnesemia is associated with muscle excitability, hyperreflexia, tetany, seizures, ataxia, tremors, and weakness.

Faulty calcium regulation may also contribute to changes in muscle performance. Hypercalcemia is often associated with primary hyperparathyroidism but may also be found after immobilization in patients with Paget's disease or with malignancies with bone metastases. The elevated calcium levels depress nervous system responses and muscle actions become sluggish and weak.

Hypocalcemia is a low serum calcium or low extracellular fluid concentration of calcium ions. It is associated with hypoparathyroidism, renal disease, and vitamin D deficiency. This may increase the excitability of the neuronal membrane, leading to spontaneous discharging and tetany contractions, possibly manifesting as carpopedal spasm. Trous-

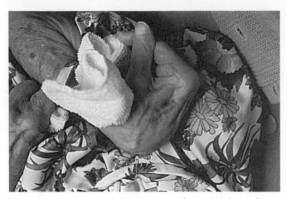

Figure 15–1 Carpopedal spasm manifests with hyperflexion at the wrist and at the metacarpal phalangeal and proximal joints of the third through fifth fingers.

seau's sign is an evaluative procedure to determine the presence of tetany from hypocalcemia by inducing carpopedal spasm 3 to 4 minutes after reducing blood flow to the hand with the use of a tourniquet on the arm. Carpopedal spasm is a condition usually found in confused, aging individuals. It manifests as hyperflexion at the wrist and the metacarpal phalangeal and proximal interphalangeal joints on the third through the fifth fingers (Fig. 15–1). The distal interphalangeal joints of these three fingers are commonly hyperextended as they come in contact with the palm. The thumb and the index finger are usually in opposition and pointing. This condition can lead to tissue maceration and ulceration of the palm and the hands.

Reversal of Trousseau's sign is simple, but treatment of longstanding carpopedal spasm is frustrating and often not effective. The goal is to prevent further injury. Range-of-motion exercises in or out of water may be helpful. Use of padding, washcloths, or finger spreaders may be tried. Electrical stimulation to the wrist and finger extensors and splinting may be considered.

Hypokalemic myopathy results from decreased serum potassium which is often secondary to the chronic use of diuretics. Muscle weakness develops slowly over days to weeks. It may be the result of hyperpolarization of nerves and muscles, or tetany.

Hypophosphatemia is a low-serum phosphate. Phosphate is normally stored in bone as hydroxyapatite and contributes to energy metabolism and cell membrane function and regulation. Phosphate loss may lead to muscle weakness.

Hyponatremia is decreased serum sodium and excess water relative to the sodium. It is common to patients suffering from diarrhea, vomiting, or suctioning. Use of diuretics may also contribute to this condition. Hyponatremia may present with fatigue, muscle cramps, and depressed deep tendon reflexes. Hypernatremia is an increased serum sodium and it may present with symptoms of weakness, lethargy, and orthostatic hypotension.

Hormonal Imbalances

Hyperthyroidism can cause acute myopathy in elderly patients. It may also cause myokymia, which is a continuous quivering or undulating muscle movement. Proximal limb muscle weakness and muscle fatigue may be present.

Hypothyroidism may present with impaired energy metabolism within muscles and decreased contractile force. Fatigue, muscle weakness, and muscle cramps may be seen, resulting from impaired calcium uptake by the sacroplasmic reticulum.

Prolonged use of corticosteroids for chemotherapy or for conditions such as myasthenia gravis or Cushing's disease may cause a corticosteroid myopathy. Muscle atrophy may be present and may involve most skeletal muscles, but weakness usually occurs first in the hip and quadriceps muscles. Mild aching in the muscles is not uncommon.

Asthenia

Asthenia is an ill-defined condition characterized by generalized weakness and usually involving mental and physical fatigue. The patient undergoing radiation or chemotherapy may suffer from asthenia and thus may not tolerate the rigors of rehabilitation as defined by the Medicare system (twice-a-day treatments as inpatients in rehabilitation units or a minimum of three times weekly in the home or outpatient setting). Other factors that may contribute to asthenia include anemia, malnutrition, infection, metabolic disorders, and medications such as Aldomet, Bactrim, Cardizem, Decadron, Donnatal, Elavil, Inderal, Lanoxin, Lopressor, Novahistine, Phenergan, Relafen, Sinemet, and Xanax. The International Classification of Diseases 9th Revision of Clinical Modifications breaks down asthenia into several different categories, including cardiovascular, psychogenic, hysterical, psychoneurotic, senile, tropical, and anhidrotic. The code for asthenia, 780.7, described it as malaise and fatigue. This does exclude unspecified debility. It is included in the section "Symptoms, Signs and Other Ill-Defined Conditions." Generalized weakness is given the same ICD-CM Code of 780.7. Asthenia is a factor in rehabilitation for many frail patients.

Other factors that may limit muscle responses to exercise include poorly oxygenated blood due to chronic lung disease and faulty or reduced cardiac responses. Beta-blockers and pacemakers often reduce the ability of the heart to respond to the increased demands from exercise, thereby circumscribing the effects of exercise. See Chapters 6, 7, 8, and 42 for more complete details.

CONCLUSION

The loss of muscle strength and muscle tissue in aging persons is an important, yet reversible, condition that influences health, function, and quality of life.

Humane rehabilitative care requires paying attention to medical diagnoses, nutrition, and blood chemistry as well as to the typical muscular evaluation. Recognizing the potential limitations of the muscular system when exercising allows realistic treatment goals and outcomes to be established.

SUGGESTED READINGS

Bassey E et al. Leg extensor power and functional performance in very old men and women. *Clin Sci* 1992; 82:321–327.

Frontera W et al. A cross-sectional study of muscle strength and mass in 45- to 78-yr-old men and women. *J Appl Physiol* 1991; 71:644–650.

Holloszy J. Workshop on sarcopenia: muscle atrophy in old age. *J Gerontol A Biol Sci Med Sci* 1995; 50A.

Kiel D. Laboratory evaluation of the geriatric patient in the planning of a rehabilitation program. In: Guccione A, ed. *Geriatric Physical Therapy.* St. Louis: Mosby; 1993.

Lexell J et al. Heavy-resistance training in older Scandinavian men and women: short- and long-term effects on arm and leg muscles. *Scand J Med Sci Sports* 1995; 5:329–341.

Merck Manual of Geriatrics, 2nd ed. Abrams W, Beers M, Berkow R, Fletcher A, eds. Whitehouse Station, N.J.: Merck Research Laboratories; 1995.

PDR Guide to Drug Interactions, Side Effects, Indications, 50th ed. Mehta M, ed. Montvale, N.J.: Medical Economics Company; 1996.

Porter M, Vandervoort A, Lexell J. Aging of human muscle: structure, function and adaptability. *Scand J Med Sci Sports* 1995; 5:129–142.

Skelton D et al. Strength, power and related functional ability of healthy people aged 65–89 years. *Age Ageing* 1994; 23:371–377.

Chapter **16**

Stretch Weakness
Timothy L. Kauffman, Ph.D., P.T.

INTRODUCTION

Stretch weakness is a clinical problem that results when a muscle remains in one position for too long a time. It is thought that weakness manifests as the muscle remains stretched beyond its normal physiological resting length. However, the exact physiology and morphology are not clearly known, and the concept is not universally accepted. Nevertheless, it remains a tenable theory.

The cause of stretch weakness is a combination of factors, including change in sarcomere length and sarcomere number, length of noncontractile musculotendinous structures, muscle spindle bias, joint structure and range of motion (ROM), motor control, habitual postures, gravity, and pain. Often a muscle imbalance between agonist and antagonist results. It is unclear how long it takes for these changes to occur, but most likely it is gradual over months and years unless paralysis or surgery is involved.

THE RISK IN PROLONGED SITTING

An example is a patient who spends an excessive amount of time sitting in a chair, possibly even sleeping in the chair at night. This posture involving hip and trunk flexion is likely to lead to increased resting-muscle length of the knee vastus muscles and the hip extensors. Additionally, periarticular connective tissue may shorten anteriorly at the hip and posteriorly at the knee. Bony and cartilaginous changes may also occur at these joints and in the connective tissue.

Typically, a patient in this circumstance stands with hips and knees flexed, a position that has a higher energy cost when compared to normal erect posture with 0-degree extension at the hips and knees. When tested in the seated position for hip extension, strength on the manual muscle test is likely to register in the good (4 out of 5) range. However, if the patient is placed prone, the standard test position, the stretch-weakened hip extensors are in a shortened position and are likely to grade in the fair (3 out of 5) range. The same may be found in knee extension; that is, good strength in the midrange and fair strength at terminal extension. An extensor lag may or may not be present. Some patients are capable of performing a locking isometric muscle contraction, which grades as good (4 out of 5) or even normal (5 out of 5), but a dynamic contraction in the terminal range may reveal less than good strength.

Stretch weakness is commonly seen in postural malalignment and is often associated with arthritic and osteoporotic changes, as can be seen in Table 16–1.

TREATMENT CONSIDERATIONS FOR STRETCH WEAKNESS

Treatment should be directed toward (1) improving muscle strength throughout the joint's range of motion, especially working the stretch-weakened mus-

Table 16–1 Common Areas of Stretch Weakness

Muscles Involved	Contributing Factors or Manifestations	Related Conditions
Scapular retractors or adductors	Dorsal kyphosis and head forward, prolonged sitting	Shoulder dysfunction, DJD,[a] vertebral collapse, rib fracture
Gluteus maximus	Prolonged sitting, flat or kyphotic lumbar spine, loss of erect bipedal posture	Spinal DJD, vertebral collapse, hip DJD
Trunk extensors	Prolonged sitting, loss of erect posture, dorsal kyphosis	Faulty postural control, vertebral collapse
Knee extensors	Prolonged sitting, loss of erect posture, extensor lag at full knee extension	DJD
Gluteus medius	Hip fracture, trunk side-bent in bed, compensated or uncompensated gluteus medius limp	Scoliosis, leg-length shortening, hip DJD
Ankle dorsiflexors	Prolonged sitting or bedrest with feet resting in plantar flexion position; no heel strike or poor clearance of toes during swing phase of gait	Heel cord shortening, gait/balance disturbance

[a]DJD, degenerative joint disease

cles in the functionally appropriate physiological range; (2) creating greater physiological balance between agonists and antagonists; (3) achieving closer to normal postural alignment, both resting and active; and (4) preventing further losses in strength and function.

Use of modalities such as moist heat, deep heat, and electrical stimulation may be helpful in relieving pain and facilitating the stretching of shortened musculoskeletal structures. Positioning and use of splints and braces should be considered to encourage normal resting length of the muscles and to prevent further stretching, or lengthening, of muscles and connective tissues. Emphasis should be placed on motor and postural control and active muscle actions of the agonist as well as on the stretching of tightened antagonists and soft tissue. Care-givers and families must be taught about the dangers of prolonged sitting and immobility. Simple sit-to-stand and range-of-motion exercises, especially in the antigravity muscles, are valuable.

In the above case of the prolonged sitting posture, terminal knee extension and the fully erect posture may be gained by working on static quad sets, static weight-loading with weights at 0 degrees of knee extension, extensor thrust exercises, bilateral and unilateral toe raises (plantar flexion), and gentle knee bends emphasizing return to full knee extension. Passive range of motion may be needed to attain full extension; trunk extension strengthen-ing exercises are also likely to be beneficial. These exercises should be considered not only for the additional ROM and strengthening they produce but also for their proprioceptive and kinesthetic input into the postural control mechanism and their ability to teach the patient the necessary motion. By gaining good to normal (4 or 5 out of 5) strength in terminal hip and knee extension, fully erect, energy-efficient posture may be attained—but not always. The automatic postural control mechanism of this postural set may not be reprogrammable.

CONCLUSION

Stretch weakness is a clinical condition that has yet to be fully investigated and defined. It clearly involves more than the length of the muscle and thus should be considered a neuromusculoskeletal problem. These neuromusculoskeletal changes may negatively impact posture, mobility, and quality of life and should be considered when evaluating the aging patient. Amelioration is possible in some, albeit not all, cases.

SUGGESTED READINGS

Connelly DM, Vandervoort AA. Improvement in knee extensor strength of institutionalized elderly women after exercise with ankle weights. *Physiother Canada* 1995; 47:15–23.

Grossman M, Sahrmann SA, Rose SJ. Review of length-associated changes in muscle. *Phys Ther* 1982; 62:1799–1807.

Kendall FP, McCreary EK, Provance PG. *Muscle Testing and Function*, 4th ed. Baltimore: Williams & Wilkins; 1993.

Chapter **17**

Contractures

Reenie Euhardy, M.S., P.T., G.C.S.

INTRODUCTION

Contracture is defined as the lack of full passive range of motion (ROM) resulting from joint, muscle, or soft-tissue limitations. Joint flexibility is inversely related to age. Generally, there is a systemic decrease in active and passive motion of all joints with age, with the decline becoming more pronounced during the ninth decade. However, not all elderly individuals experience a decline in joint flexibility as they age, and significant increases in joint ROM can be achieved through regular exercise and stretching programs.

MECHANISMS OF CONTRACTURE

Usually several factors combine to play a role in limiting full passive range of motion in the elderly. The normal effects of aging, a decline in physical activity, and, often, disease and pathology all occur simultaneously to contribute to joint contracture. Contractures can be divided into three categories according to the anatomical location of the pathological changes: (1) arthrogenic, including intra-articular adhesions; (2) periarticular, including connective tissue and joint capsule stiffness; and (3) myogenic, including shortened skeletal muscles of which there are two types, myostatic and pseudomyostatic. Other classification systems for identifying restricted joint motion involve intra-articular, periarticular, and extra-articular structures.

Myostatic contracture represents structural adaptation of muscle in response to changes in position of the corresponding joint. Muscles with myostatic contracture are shorter than their normal physiological length and show a reduction in the number of sarcomere units but no decrease in individual sarcomere length, as is found with pseudomyostatic contracture (Fig. 17–1). Myostatic contracture can be the result of bracing or casting or any restriction of joint movement, such as limited activity or bedrest.

Pseudomyostatic contracture is the loss of myofibril extensibility secondary to a decrease in individual sarcomere length; it is not accompanied by structural changes in the sarcomeres. Pseudomyostatic shortening may follow a tetanic muscle contraction such as a muscle spasm. Myofascial trigger points may be local areas in muscle where actin and myosin filaments remain chemically locked.

NORMAL EFFECTS OF AGING

Normal age-related changes that affect joint flexibility include increases in the viscosity of the synovium, calcification of articular cartilages, and stiffness of capsular and ligamentous tissues. Stiffness is measured by the stress-strain relationship of fibers. As the force (stress) on tissue is increased, the length (strain) of the tissue increases in a linear relationship, once the slack is taken out, until the length at which the tissue ruptures is reached.

Other factors associated with contracture formation that may be age-related include previous injury and abnormal postural patterns (see Chapters 14, "Posture," and 65, "Stiffness"). Repetitive-motion stresses resulting from occupational or leisure activities may predispose to osteophyte formation and the remodeling of the joint surfaces, which limits joint flexibility related to contractures.

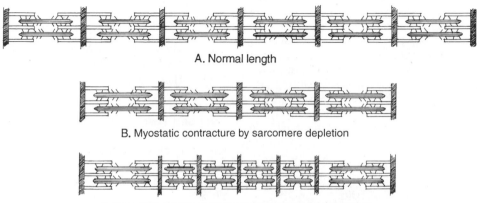

A. Normal length

B. Myostatic contracture by sarcomere depletion

C. Pseudomyostatic contracture by sarcomere shortening

Figure 17–1 Subclassifications of contractures. (Modified from Henry JA: Manual therapy of the shoulder. In: Kelley MJ, Clark WA, eds. *Orthopedic Therapy of the Shoulder.* Philadelphia: JB Lippincott, 1995.)

Activity Level

The interaction between aging and activity level and joint contracture is not well understood. Why some individuals do not experience even slight reductions in joint range of motion as they age is an important question that has not been answered; however, a decline in physical activity is typically related to joint contracture. Three components related to physical activity that play a role in the development of contracture are limb position, duration of immobilization, and habitual movement patterns. The type and amount of physical activity people engage in changes with age. Older adults often do not move their joints to the same extent and with the same frequency as younger persons do. Bedridden and extremely inactive or frail elderly persons are particularly prone to the development of contracture. Some degree of muscular shortening is present in sedentary persons even if they are healthy, especially in muscles that cross multiple joints.

PATHOLOGY

Arthrogenic contractures are usually the result of inflammation, infection, degenerative joint disease, or repeated trauma. Pain due to synovial effusion, which is associated with inflammation or arthritis, often culminates in voluntary and involuntary joint splinting and immobility. As joint movement is curtailed, contractures may develop. Osteoarthritic disease resulting in the deformity and remodeling of joint surfaces and rheumatic processes resulting in the scarring of the synovium contribute not only to intra-articular but also to periarticular joint contracture.

Neuromuscular dysfunction appears to be the most common cause of extra-articular physiological joint restriction, probably the consequence of spinal segment and supraspinal inputs that result in a shortening of the muscle fibers' resting length. Muscle spindle bias may be a factor. Pathology such as stroke, multi-infarct dementia, and diseases causing changes in neurotransmission such as Parkinson's may cause spastic posturing. Spastic posturing presents with a dynamic imbalance of muscle control in the involved extremities and results in myogenic contracture. Medications with extrapyramidal side effects such as antipsychotics may also contribute to contractures.

FUNCTION WITH CONTRACTURE

The functional significance of reduced joint ROM is determined by the amount of limitation, the overall physical condition and activity level of the individual, and the location of the involved joint. It has been suggested that a 30-degree knee flexion contracture is associated with a loss of ambulation ability. Contracture of hip flexion impacts on gait by reducing pelvic rotation, shortening stride, and increasing the energy cost of mobility. The ability to negotiate curbs and steps may be impaired. No guidelines have been established to determine what degree of shoulder contracture has a significant impact on function.

INCIDENCE

With aging, the upper extremity joints remain more flexible than the lower extremity joints. Men tend to lose range of motion more rapidly than women. Hip abduction is the lower extremity motion most commonly limited with age. Limited full hip extension (10 degrees hyperextension beyond 0 degrees, or neutral) is also common in the elderly. It is postulated that prolonged sitting is related to hip and knee flexion contracture. Hip flexion declines the least, with a significant reduction becoming apparent only after the age of 85.

TREATMENT

Prevention

Maintaining an active lifestyle and following a stretching exercise routine are the keys to preventing joint contractures in the elderly. Position is critical in the prevention of contracture in patients who have limited mobility. In the supine position the feet may have to be positioned in neutral dorsiflexion. The lower extremities should rest in neutral rotation, with the hips and knees extended. Shoulders should be in neutral protraction-retraction. Considerations relating to joint position and tissue length are crucial when placing patients in seated and sidelong positions. Muscles and joints should be stretched to their optimal range, ideally on a daily basis.

Heat and Passive Stretching

Contractures can often be reduced by selectively heating the fibrous tissues that limit motion. Stretching should be performed immediately after, or, if possible during, heat application, with temperatures brought to tolerance levels. Ultrasound may be the modality of choice for selectively heating contracted tissues because ultrasound allows deep penetration to between 3 and 5 cm. Diathermy may also be beneficial in heating deep tissues. Muscle temperature can be raised to 104° to 109°F, which influences the viscous properties of connective tissue and maximizes the effects of stretching. Small joints can be heated by immersion in paraffin wax. Moist heat is often used for generalized superficial heating; it assists with muscle relaxation but does not penetrate deeper than several millimeters.

Prior to applying heat, a careful clinical evaluation of the patient is necessary in order to rule out any persisting acute or subacute process or degenerative joint disease, and to determine whether range limitation results from bone spurs. The use of selective heating in conjunction with stretching, range-of-motion exercises, or other joint mobilization techniques may aggravate persistent inflammatory reactions and would be ineffective in the presence of bone spurs.

Massage and Stretching

Soft-tissue procedures that can reduce connective tissue and myogenic contractures include massage and stretching. Massage can produce gains in length when pseudomyostatic shortening of a muscle has occurred. When contracture develops following prolonged immobilization, muscle and connective tissues lose up to 80% of their tensile strength. Care must be taken not to use abrupt or vigorous stretching forces; prolonged, low-load stretching is needed. Guidelines for prolonged, low-load stretching include positioning the joint in its most extended position while applying superficial heat and a light static weight to cause tension on the distal part of the joint lever arm for 5 minutes. Active exercise of the antagonist muscles should be encouraged, especially in the terminal range.

Soft-tissue mobilization, a type of massage, employs forceful passive movement of the musculofascial elements, beginning with superficial layers and progressing to deeper tissues. Massage can restore independent mobility of muscle, fascia, and skin in the areas of fascial thickening and binding that occur in response to chronic postural deformity. Individual subjective response can serve as an indicator to gauge the appropriate amount of pressure to be applied. The technique is described as a "good hurt" when applied correctly. The use of too much force is revealed by involuntary muscle contraction, voluntary withdrawal, or reports of pain.

Deep Friction Massage

Deep friction massage is the application of concentrated, repetitive stroking that is directed perpendicular to the fiber orientation in a localized area of tendon, muscle, fascia, or ligament at the site of contracture. Clinically, it is used to restore mobility between otherwise freely moving structures; however, research substantiating the effectiveness of friction massage is limited. Deep friction massage can be a potentially harmful treatment for acute and chronic stages of rheumatoid arthritis or for joints with active or acute inflammation.

Myofascial Release

Myofascial manipulation applies firm mechanical forces in the direction of restricted motion to break up abnormal crosslinkages and restore independent mobility to fascial compartments. Myofascial release techniques involve the application of traction or elongation combined with some degree of simultaneous shearing, twisting, and, often, compression. All soft-tissue techniques must be applied judiciously because of skin and circulatory changes commonly present in older persons that increase the risk of injury.

Neuromuscular Techniques

Neuromuscular techniques promote muscle relaxation preceding passive stretching, which facilitates effective reduction of myostatic contractures. Therapeutic approaches include muscle energy, hold-relax, and contract-relax proprioceptive neuromuscular facilitation and post-isometric relaxation. Muscle relaxation and passive stretching are components of many of these techniques. Passive stretching is distinct from passive range of motion in that the latter stops at the first feel of a barrier to further movement, whereas passive stretching, or overstretching, is a process in which additional load is applied in order to elongate the tissues.

Manually resisted exercise in the available range preceding stretching or joint mobilization can enhance the effectiveness of treatment. When it is possible to use them, submaximal contractions against resistance that are performed through the available range are effective through several mechanisms: (1) they warm the tissues, (2) they increase afferent stimuli and thus reduce guarding, and (3) they fatigue the muscle, which limits resistance to passive stretching. Active contraction and passive stretching performed in tandem are thought to enhance muscle lengthening. A strong voluntary contraction is immediately followed by a brief refractory period when the muscle cannot contract, providing a moment when the muscle can be elongated.

Optimal passive stretching (overstretching) can occur only with muscle relaxation, so the participation of the patient is necessary to enhance treatment effectiveness. With cognitively impaired patients, relaxation as well as voluntary muscle contractions are often difficult to achieve; therefore, neuromuscular stretching techniques may not be useful.

Joint Mobilization

A loss of accessory, or joint-play movement, the movement normally present in the joint but not under voluntary muscle control, is often found with arthrogenic contractures. Particular techniques of joint mobilization that will impact joint dysfunction vary from one school of practice to another. Regardless of the particular technique used, the end result is to aid in restoring joint mobility by normalizing accessory movements. Oscillations, traction, and distractions with glide may all be used. Care must be taken when applying these techniques in the elderly because of the osseous and soft-tissue changes that have occurred in addition to any underlying pathology a patient may have.

Splinting and Casting

Several studies have demonstrated improvement in contractures with the use of splinting or casting. Serial casting is especially helpful for stretching plantar flexors, biceps, wrist flexors, and hamstrings, muscle groups that commonly contract in older persons with neurological pathology. However, neither splinting nor casting has been shown to be helpful in permanently reducing spasticity or posturing. Customized, adjustable orthoses molded to the individual limb can be changed at intervals to promote slow stretching. The devices may be removed for skin monitoring. Use of commercially available splints or braces has been reported to successfully reduce knee, ankle, and elbow contractures in some cases.

CONCLUSION

Determination of the underlying cause and of the structures implicated in a contracture guides the type of treatment approach employed. Because several factors typically contribute to contracture formation, a variety of approaches to treatment may have to be used either individually or simultaneously to improve range of motion. Caution must always be exercised when using these techniques with elderly individuals. Therapists must be sensitive to the frailty of aged tissues and should be cognizant of the coexisting pathologies elderly patients so commonly exhibit, for they can affect outcomes.

SUGGESTED READINGS

Currier DP, Nelson RM. *Dynamics of Human Biologic Tissues.* Philadelphia: F. A. Davis; 1992.
Henry JA. Manual therapy of the shoulder. In: Kelley MJ, Clark WA, eds. *Orthopedic Therapy of the Shoulder.* Philadelphia: JB Lippincott; 1995:285.
Jansen CM, Windau JE, Boutti PM, Brillhart MV. Treatment of a knee contracture using a knee orthosis incorporating stress-relaxation techniques. *Phys Ther* 1996; 76:182–186.
Kottke FJ, Lehmann JF. *Krusen's Handbook of Physical Medicine and Rehabilitation*, 4th ed. Philadelphia: W. B. Saunders; 1990.
Moseley AM. The effect of casting combined with stretching on passive ankle dorsiflexion in adults with traumatic head injuries. *Phys Ther* 1997; 77:240–247, discussion 248–259.
Neumann DA. Arthrokinesiologic considerations in the aged adult. In: Guccione AA, ed. *Geriatric Physical Therapy.* St. Louis: Mosby; 1993:47.

Chapter 18

Postpolio Syndrome
Susan Rush, M.H.E., P.T., G.C.S.

INTRODUCTION

Thirty years after an acute episode of poliomyelitis, approximately half of the 1.6 million survivors have presented to health-care professionals with a list of complaints that is led by overwhelming fatigue and weakness (Box 18–1). Various combinations of neuromusculoskeletal, cardiorespiratory, psychosocial, and general medical problems reported by polio survivors have been labeled as postpolio syndrome (PPS). Initially, it was postulated that the polio virus may have been reactivated in the body or that a form of amyotrophic lateral sclerosis (ALS) was affecting the polio survivors. Time and research determined that the symptoms constituted an entity unique to those who had had a documented case of acute poliomyelitis, had achieved and maintained a relatively high level of function for at least 30 years, and had subsequently found themselves plagued with new weakness and loss of function. Overworked muscles, terminal axonal degeneration, impaired neuronal transmission, premature aging of polio-damaged cells, increased vulnerability of polio-affected motor neurons, reduced size of the anterior horn-cell pool resulting from the original

Box 18–1

Common Complaints of People with Postpolio Sequelae

- Fatigue
- Weakness
- Muscle pain
- Joint pain
- Increased falling
- General instability
- Feeling "brain dead"
- Muscle cramps
- Muscle fasciculations
- Sleep disorders
- Respiratory distress
- Dysphagia/choking
- Diminished endurance
- Hypersensitivity to cold
- Delayed strength recovery after exhaustion
- Psychosocial problems
- General medical problems

respiratory difficulty, swallowing problems or choking, or orthopedic-type problems may warrant referral to the respective specialist for evaluation and testing. Individuals using crutches, canes, or manual wheelchairs are predisposed to maladies such as carpal tunnel syndrome, tendinitis, impingement syndromes, or other repetitive-motion injuries. Increasing changes in the spine due to osteoporosis may predispose to severe respiratory distress. Lower extremity weakness, pelvic asymmetry, muscle imbalance, or leg-length discrepancy may precipitate back or lower extremity pain. Radiculopathies and spondylolisthesis should not be overlooked in the PPS individual. Careful musculoskeletal and nervous system evaluation by the therapist can be crucial in identifying any of these problems. The geriatric-trained therapist will note similarities between normal age-related changes in older patients and complaints registered by PPS patients. In the past, PPS was considered to be premature aging.

THERAPEUTIC INTERVENTION

Therapeutic intervention is a tremendous challenge for all health-care professionals who deal with PPS clients. Ideally, all members of the health-care team would have a basic understanding of PPS when working with the postpolio survivor. It is essential to remember that these individuals have lived with disability for many years and are intimately acquainted with their bodies and how they function. They know what is happening to them and their ability to function, and they remember all too well the years of struggle with rehabilitation they endured to achieve a remarkable level of independence in spite of tremendous losses. These survivors are typically very strong-willed, type A individuals who have lived through abusive, painful, and often humiliating circumstances following the acute illness to achieve "normalcy" and escape the stigma of being "crippled." The PPS client may not be particularly responsive to many proposed therapeutic interventions that are reminiscent of past treatment or devices that were forced upon him or her. It is crucial that the PPS client be an active participant in setting goals in order to retain functional independence for as long as possible and to have more energy to enjoy the fun, happier times of life. The polio survivor also needs to participate in adopting proposed treatment; otherwise compliance will be negligible. The health-care worker should allow long periods of time (in some cases, over a year) for the PPS individual to accept and incorporate suggestions that are reminiscent of a painful past. The provider should remember that undoing 30-plus years of conditioning cannot occur quickly.

polio, and general systemic deconditioning caused by other symptoms were possible reasons for the functional losses. These factors may make the elderly patient who has a history of polio particularly likely to be experiencing PPS when a functional loss cannot be attributed to other causes.

SIGNS AND SYMPTOMS OF PPS

There are no definitive tests for diagnosing PPS. Electromyography (EMG) and muscle biopsy can indicate chronic and ongoing denervation, but the diagnosis of PPS is made chiefly on the above subjective clinical findings (see Box 18–1). Postpolio syndrome is defined as two or more of these signs and symptoms, especially new muscle weakness in previously involved or previously noninvolved areas and diminished endurance.

It is important to listen carefully as the PPS individual relates current problems to ensure that no comorbidities are being overlooked. Reports of

It may be helpful to explain that acceptance of interventions now will preserve function and independence for the future.

Therapeutic interventions include implementing techniques of energy conservation and work simplification, assessing for or modifying existing adaptive equipment and orthotics, weight loss, assistive breathing, counseling, behavior modification, food or swallowing modifications, and a carefully monitored, highly structured exercise routine. Exercise should be designed to maintain strength, prevent muscle tightness and joint contractures, and improve endurance to enable the performance of the activities of daily living. Any exercise program must not cause pain or initiate or increase fatigue. It must be low-intensity training utilizing isotonic, isokinetic, concentric, eccentric posture; dynamic and static bipedal balancing; coordination; and stretching exercises interspersed with mandatory, frequent (every 2 to 5 minutes) rest periods. It is recommended that PPS subjects work at submaximal work rates in 15 to 30 minute sessions three to five times a week. Exercycling and swimming are recommended types of exercise that promote general cardiovascular conditioning without putting undue stress on already overworked muscle groups. No matter what form of exercise is prescribed, frequent monitoring is required to ascertain specific adherence to the designated, carefully designed protocol. Without close monitoring, the PPS patient is likely to overwork and cause overwhelming exhaustion from which it is difficult to recover.

CONCLUSION

Following these general guidelines will prove rewarding for therapist and patient alike in that strength, endurance, and flexibility may be improved. Heavy resistive exercise for body-building or strengthening may yield desired results over the short run but may be contraindicated or at least should be done with precaution because of the possibly deleterious long-term effects of systemic loss of strength and function.

PPS clients are now appearing in clinics with many symptoms compatible with overuse injuries. Treatment for these individuals would be the same as for the non-PPS individual—that is, heat, cold, modalities (i.e., ultrasound, electrotherapies, contophoresis, phonophoresis, whirlpool, massage, and trigger point therapy; see Chapters 68 and 69 for further discussion of these treatments), exercise, and aquatics, with caution about avoiding exhaustion or overwork.

SUGGESTED READINGS

Agre JC, Rodriquez AA, Tafel JA. Late effects of polio: critical review of the literature on neuromuscular function. *Arch Phys Med Rehabil* 1991; 72:923–931.

Aston JW. Post-polio syndrome. *Postgrad Med* 1992; 92:249–260.

Ciocon JO, Potter JF. Post-poliomyelitis sequelae in the elderly. *J Am Geriatr Soc* 1989; 37:256–258.

Dean E, Ross J, MacIntyre D. A rejoinder to "Exercise Programs for Patients with Post-Polio Syndrome: A case report." *Phys Ther* 1989; 69:695–698.

Twist DJ, Ma DM. Physical therapy management of the patient with post-polio syndrome: a case report. *Phys Ther* 1986; 66:1403–1406.

Orthopedics 1985; 8: entire issue.

Orthopedics 1991; 14: entire issue.

Chapter 19

Osteoporosis

Diane Krueger, B.S.
Mary M. Checovich, M.S.
Neil Binkley, M.D.

INTRODUCTION

Osteoporosis, which literally means "porous bone," is one of the most common diseases to occur with advancing age. This bone-weakening disease leads to fractures, which are increasing in incidence as our population is aging. Fractures of the proximal femur (hip) are associated with more functional impairment and higher mortality rates than all other osteoporotic complications combined.

DEFINING OSTEOPOROSIS

A recent National Institutes of Health (NIH) consensus-development conference defined osteoporosis as "a systemic skeletal disease characterized by low bone mass and microarchitectural deterioration of bone tissue, with a consequent increase in bone fragility and susceptibility to fracture."[1]

Several aspects of this definition are worthy of emphasis. First, osteoporosis is a *disease*. Osteoporotic fractures are too often incorrectly viewed simply as part of the normal aging process rather than as a preventable and treatable disease. Second, this definition requires only the *susceptibility* to fracture rather than the occurrence of a fracture, as was required by prior definitions. This allows diagnosis and treatment of osteoporosis to occur in an asymptomatic state—before it presents with fracture.

Chapter 19 • Osteoporosis **83**

Box 19-1

World Health Organization Classification of Skeletal Status

- Normal: bone mineral density that is not more than one standard deviation below the young adult mean value

- Low bone mass, or osteopenia: bone mineral density that lies between 1 and 2.5 standard deviations below the young adult mean value

- Osteoporosis: a value of bone mineral density that is more than 2.5 standard deviations below the young adult mean value

- Severe osteoporosis: a value of bone mineral density more than 2.5 standard deviations below the young adult mean value and the presence of one or more fragility fractures

---

Thus, the approach to the treatment of osteoporosis is analogous to hypertension in that both are asymptomatic diseases in which the likelihood of catastrophic presentation (fracture and stroke, respectively) can be reduced by early diagnosis and treatment.

The World Health Organization (WHO) has recommended the utilization of bone mass measurement (Box 19-1).[2] Categories are defined by comparing an individual's bone mass to that of the average young adult. These guidelines define "osteopenia" as a state of low bone mass. Individuals with this condition are at somewhat increased risk for fracture, so it is ideal that steps toward dietary and behavioral modification be taken to prevent future bone loss. People with more pronounced reduction in bone mass but no history of fracture are said to have osteoporosis. These individuals are at increased risk for fracture with minimal or no trauma. The most severe category, those people with both markedly low bone mass and a history of fracture, are described as having severe osteoporosis. These guidelines help to identify individuals at different stages of the disease process, thus directing the aggressiveness of therapy.

EPIDEMIOLOGY AND ECONOMIC AND FUNCTIONAL IMPACT

It is estimated that osteoporosis affects about 25 million U.S. citizens and causes approximately 1.5 million fractures annually, usually of a vertebra, hip, or wrist.[3] Based on these numbers, it is expected that nearly two in every five females and one in eight males will sustain an osteoporotic fracture in their lifetimes. Furthermore, a typical 50-year-old woman has a 50% chance of sustaining an osteoporotic fracture in her remaining lifetime.[4] Not surprisingly, the medical care costs of osteoporotic fractures are significant; they are estimated to be about $13.8 billion annually.[5] Given demographic trends, it is projected that by the year 2020, the treatment of osteoporosis sequelae will cost $30 to 60 billion per year.[6] These numbers highlight the need for effective prevention and treatment strategies.

The economic costs are extreme, and the personal and functional costs are likewise significant. Specifically, of those who sustain a hip fracture—about 250,000 people annually in the United States—the 1-year mortality rate is from 12% to 20%.[6] Furthermore, the functional morbidity is substantial, as nearly half of the persons able to walk prior to hip fracture subsequently do not regain functional ambulation.

CLINICAL EVALUATION

The clinical approach to an individual with suspected osteoporosis begins with the history and physical examination. Important historical information includes family history of osteoporosis, calcium and vitamin D intake, and the presence or history of diseases, medications, and behavioral factors (alcohol, caffeine, tobacco, physical inactivity) associated with bone loss. In addition, it is necessary to consider the occurrence and circumstances of falls as well as the overall past medical history.

The physical examination should focus upon exclusion of recognized causes of bone loss such as malignancy and other systemic illnesses, including hyperthyroidism and Cushing's syndrome. It is also important to assess risk of falling by utilizing orthostatic pulse and blood pressure, visual acuity testing, and identification of diseases associated with balance impediment, such as Parkinson's disease, prior stroke, peripheral neuropathy, and postural/musculoskeletal impairments.

Subsequent laboratory evaluation should include serum chemistries (to evaluate hepatic and renal function and exclude secondary hyperparathyroidism), a complete blood count and sedimentation rate (to assess for multiple myeloma), and assessment of thyroid function. A multitude of other laboratory tests such as markers of skeletal turnover are available but not recommended for routine clinical use at this time.

A spine x-ray is indicated when a patient presents with back pain, posture change (kyphosis), or asymptomatic height loss. Since not all back pain is the result of osteoporotic fracture, it is important to establish the presence or absence of vertebral compression fractures to rule out other causes of pain. Although standard x-rays are indicated in this setting, they are not sensitive measures of the amount of bone present, as significant bone loss can occur without being detectable by the eye.

Measurement of bone mass is required to detect small changes in bone. It is well established that low bone mass, as measured by a variety of techniques, is predictive of future fracture risk; however, when the measurement should be made remains a point of controversy. Reasonable indications for bone mass measurement are listed in Box 19–2. A number of methods exist for the measurement of bone mass, including radiogrammetric absorptiometry, dual-energy x-ray absorptiometry (DXA), quantitative CT scanning, and ultrasound. Currently, DXA is the most widely used technology because it is very precise, capable of measuring a number of skeletal sites, and reasonably inexpensive, and it produces very low radiation. These instruments measure bone mineral density and report these values in g/cm^2 as well as in the form of a T score. The T score can be thought of as the number of standard deviations below the young/normal mean and can be directly applied to the WHO recommendations (see Box 19–1). For instance, an individual with a reported T score of -2 is two standard deviations below young/normal and would be classified as osteopenic. It is probable that both DXA and ultrasound will be used widely for such measurements in the immediate future.

Box 19–2

Clinical Indications for Bone Mass Measurement

- Perimenopausal women: as baseline to discuss initiation of ERT therapy
- Radiography suggesting osteopenia: as confirmation of diagnosis
- Corticosteroid therapy: as documentation of baseline and subsequent bone loss
- Implementation of osteoporosis therapy: to determine effectiveness of therapy
- Diagnosis of osteoporosis: as a tool to assess disease severity

PREVENTIVE STRATEGIES

At this time, it is impossible to restore osteoporotic bone to normal. This means that prevention is of the utmost importance. Approaches to prevention include maximizing peak bone mass and reducing subsequent postmenopausal and age-related bone loss.

To maximize peak skeletal mass, adequate calcium and vitamin D intake, as well as exercise, are important during the adolescent years when the greatest skeletal growth occurs. Subsequently, a small amount of additional bone mass is accrued until approximately age 30, when peak bone mass is attained.

Skeletal mass then remains relatively stable until the time of menopause. However, during this time, skeletal insults such as amenorrhea and prolonged immobilization may lead to irreversible bone loss. Following estrogen deprivation at menopause, approximately 10 to 15% of the average woman's skeletal mass is lost during the ensuing 5 to 7 years. This loss can be prevented by the use of estrogen replacement therapy at the time of menopause. Estrogen replacement leads to preservation of bone mass and reduction of fracture incidence. The use of this treatment requires detailed consideration of the potential risks versus the potential benefits and must be decided on an individual basis (see Chapter 61, "Estrogen Replacement Therapy"). Other pharmaceutical agents such as alendronate[7] (see following Treatment section) and raloxifene[8] are effective in the prevention of bone loss at the time of menopause. Raloxifene is the first of a new class of medications designed to mimic the effect of estrogen on the skeleton without the estrogen-like side effects.

Following the phase of bone loss caused by estrogen deprivation, age-related bone loss of about 1% per year usually occurs. This loss can be combated by optimizing calcium and vitamin D intake. In essence, if the calcium intake or its absorption from the intestine (which is facilitated by vitamin D) is inadequate, the body uses the skeleton as a calcium reservoir so it can maintain the blood's calcium level. Over the course of years, ongoing withdrawals from the "skeleton bank" result in bone loss and, potentially, in osteoporosis.

A recent NIH consensus conference and the National Osteoporosis Foundation recommend that the optimal calcium intake for postmenopausal women is 1500 mg/day, a 500-mg increase over premenopausal women. The same calcium intake amounts are recommended for males—1000 mg when between the ages of 25 and 65 and 1500 mg after the age of 65 (Box 19–3).

It is ideal to obtain the full amount of calcium

Box 19–3

Optimal Calcium Requirements

Group	Optimal Daily Intake (in mg of calcium)
Infants	
Birth–6 months	400
6 months–1 year	600
Children	
1–5 years	800
6–10 years	800–1200
Adolescents/Young Adults	
11–24 years	1200–1500
Men	
25–65 years	1000
Over 65 years	1500
Women	
25–50 years	1000
Over 50 years (postmeno- pausal)	
On estrogens	1000
Not on estrogens	1500
Over 65 years	1500
Pregnant and nursing	1200–1500

From NIH Consensus Statement: Bethesda, MD, National Institutes of Health, Office of the Director; 1994:12(4).

from the diet, but it is common for postmenopausal women to consume less than half of the recommended amount. For the average woman ingesting 600–700 mg of calcium, the addition of 600 to 800 mg of calcium in supplement form is often recommended. However, it is important to realize that the recommendations noted above are *elemental* calcium and that all calcium supplements contain only a percentage of the elemental form. For instance, the common calcium supplements, calcium carbonate and calcium lactate, contain 40% and 22% elemental calcium, respectively.

Vitamin D facilitates calcium absorption in the intestine, so optimal intake of it is important in osteoporosis prevention. As vitamin D intake in the diet is typically inadequate, daily supplementation with a multiple vitamin containing 400 IUs of vitamin D is usually recommended as a part of osteoporosis treatment and prevention programs.

The effect of ingesting optimal amounts of calcium and vitamin D, although a seemingly simple intervention, should not be underestimated. The provision of adequate calcium and vitamin D is the foundation of osteoporosis treatment and has been demonstrated to reduce hip fractures in elderly women by about 30%.[9]

Finally, a program of weight-bearing exercise is important in the prevention of osteoporotic fractures. "Heel strike," that is, weight-bearing exercise, is an important factor in bone maintenance. An optimal exercise regimen has not been established, but a walking program of 2 to 3 miles three days per week is recommended. Exercise may also reduce the risk for falls and result in a reduction of fractures.

TREATMENT OF OSTEOPOROSIS

Treatment of osteoporosis can range from simple behavior modification to extensive drug therapy; ideally, a multidisciplinary approach should be used. Patient education may be performed by members of a multidisciplinary team or by the individual clinician. Its purpose is to facilitate an informed therapeutic decision, so such education must provide an improved understanding of the disease process and its prognosis, information about behavior modification (in terms of alcohol and tobacco consumption and the risk of falls), nutritional instruction, and information regarding available treatment options. A standard treatment regimen should include calcium and vitamin D optimization, an exercise program, and the avoidance of excessive tobacco and alcohol use. Depending on the individual, additional treatment may include prevention strategies, physical therapy interventions, and medications.

None of the currently approved medications for the treatment of osteoporosis can return bone mass to normal. However, they do increase or stabilize bone mass and reduce the risk for future fracture by approximately 50%.

Estrogen replacement therapy (ERT) remains the standard for both the prevention and the treatment of osteoporosis. When ERT is started at the time of menopause, it reduces the occurrence of osteoporotic fracture by up to 50%. Treatment with ERT prevents further bone loss, so it can still be beneficial even after significant bone loss has occurred. However, ERT therapy may not be well accepted, as some women are unwilling to use it because of unwanted side effects, such as vaginal bleeding and the potential of increased risk for breast cancer. It is currently estimated that up to 25% of prescriptions for ERT go unfilled.

Calcitonin was the first FDA-approved alternative to ERT therapy in the treatment of osteoporosis. It is a naturally secreted hormone that decreases bone resorption, thereby decreasing bone loss. Calcitonin is available as a subcutaneous injection and a nasal spray. It maintains bone mass, reduces fracture risk and, in some people, has an analgesic effect on the pain of osteoporotic fracture. Side effects, including nausea and flushing, are quite common with injectable calcitonin but rare with the nasal formulation.

Alendronate is the most recent drug to receive approval for osteoporosis treatment. It too increases bone mass by decreasing bone resorption, which leads to approximately a 50% reduction in the occurrence of new fractures.[10, 11] This treatment is available in oral form and has fewer side effects than ERT for many women. However, there is a strict regimen to follow for ingestion: consumption on an empty stomach one half hour prior to eating and remaining upright during that period. There have been reports of esophageal irritation and abdominal pain associated with alendronate.

THE ROLE OF PHYSICAL THERAPY IN OSTEOPOROSIS TREATMENT

As the major morbidities following osteoporotic fractures are pain and functional impairment, it is to be anticipated that the role of physical therapy in the treatment of patients with osteoporosis is extensive.

The implementation of an exercise and conditioning program to increase muscle strength, endurance, and balance offers benefits at most stages of the disease by reducing the risk of falls and helping to maintain mobility and function. Treatment of individuals who have sustained vertebral fractures may include strict bedrest lasting approximately 1 week. This is generally a powerful intervention that can relieve severe, acute, and subacute back pain associated with vertebral compression fractures. As pain recedes, patients can be introduced to exercise specifically tailored for them individually. The exercise program should include stretching and back extensor strengthening exercises. Generalized strengthening programs will aid in coordination and should help in the prevention of falls. A long-term program of physical activity should also include weight-bearing and aerobic exercises.

In addition, protecting the skeleton while maintaining and increasing physical activity is very important. Guidelines for safe movement such as good body mechanics may reduce pain following osteoporotic fracture. In some cases, the implementation of an assistive device may be indicated to maintain mobility and decrease risk of falls. Balance assessment and specific balance-retraining exercises are important, especially for the patient who has fallen.

In addition to exercise and general behavior modification, physical measures may also be used to decrease the amount of pain medication required by patients. Alternatives to narcotics may include heat and cold therapy, TENS, and orthoses. They not only decrease dependency on pain medication but may reduce the risk of falling by eliminating the side effects that pain medication has on the central nervous system.

CONCLUSION

The optimal approach to prevention and treatment includes evaluation of diet, with the optimization of calcium and vitamin D intake, lifestyle modifications, if indicated, use of pharmaceutical therapies, and a physical therapy program designed for the individual. This approach can prevent many osteoporotic fractures and allow patients to maintain active and independent lives.

REFERENCES

1. Consensus Development Conference on Diagnosis, Prophylaxis, and Treatment of Osteoporosis. Report of the Hong Kong Conference. *Am J Med* 1993; 94:646–650.
2. Kanis JA, Melton LJ III, Christiansen C, Johnston CC, Khaltev N. The diagnosis of osteoporosis. *J Bone Miner Res* 1994; 9:1137–1141.
3. Cummings SR, Kelsey JL, Nevitt MC, O'Dowd KJ. Epidemiology of osteoporosis and osteoporotic fractures. *Epidemiol Rev* 1985; 7:178–208.
4. Melton LJ III, Chrischilles EA, Cooper C, Lane AW, Riggs BL. Perspective: how many women have osteoporosis? *J Bone Miner Res* 1992; 7:1005–1010.
5. Ray NF, Chan JK, Thamer M, Melton LJ III. Medical expenditures for the treatment of osteoporotic fractures in the United States in 1995: report from the National Osteoporosis Foundation. *J Bone Miner Res* 1997; 12:24–35.
6. Cummings SR, Rubin SM, Black D. The future of hip fractures in the United States: numbers, costs, and potential effects of postmenopausal estrogen. *Clin Orthop* 1990; 52:163–166.
7. Hosking D et al. Prevention of bone loss with alendronate in postmenopausal women under 60 years of age. *N Engl J Med* 1998; 338:485–492.
8. Delmas P, et al. Effects of raloxifene on bone mineral density, serum cholesterol concentrations, and uterine endometrium in postmenopausal women. *N Engl J Med* 1997; 337:1641–1647.
9. Chapuy MC, Arlot ME, Duboeuf F, et al. Vitamin D_3 and calcium to prevent hip fractures in elderly women. *N Engl J Med* 1992; 327:1637–1642.
10. Black DM et al. Randomized trial of effect of alendronate on risk of fracture in women with existing vertebral fractures. *Lancet* 1996; 348:1535–1541.
11. Libermen UA et al. Effect of oral alendronate on bone mineral density and the incidence of fractures in postmenopausal osteoporosis. *N Engl J Med* 1995; 22:1437–1443.

Chapter **20**

Rheumatic Conditions

June Hanks, M.S., P.T.
David Levine, Ph.D., P.T.

INTRODUCTION

Joint pain may be caused by many articular and nonarticular diseases. A diagnosis of arthritis may be established following careful attention to clinical manifestations, laboratory tests, radiographic and imaging studies, and responses to drug therapy. Although arthritis can affect anyone, certain types of arthritis are commonly associated with aging. Discussed are the pathophysiology, medical management, and recommended therapy for the following rheumatic conditions: osteoarthritis, rheumatoid arthritis, systemic lupus erythematosus, gout, pseudogout, polymyalgia rheumatica, bursitis, and tendinitis.

OSTEOARTHRITIS

Osteoarthritis (OA), also called osteoarthrosis or degenerative joint disease, is a common condition involving cartilage degeneration, the remodeling of subchondral bone, and overgrowth of bone at joint margins. Joint effusion and thickening of the synovium and capsule also may occur. OA affects both males and females, becomes more prevalent with increasing age, and accounts for much of the lower extremity disability present in the elderly. OA may affect any synovial joint, but typically, it affects the knee, hip, spine, carpometacarpal joints, and distal interphalangeal joints of the hand (Table 20–1). See Table 4–1 for normal aging changes in articular cartilage.

The term "primary OA" is given to OA that develops without a predisposing condition. When OA results from some other local or systemic factor such as trauma, developmental deformity, or infection, it is termed secondary OA.

The disease process of OA affects the entire joint, including the articular cartilage, synovium, subchondral bone, and surrounding supportive connective tissues. However, the most marked changes in OA involve the articular cartilage. In an unaffected joint, the articular cartilage provides a smooth, almost frictionless weight-bearing joint surface that spreads and minimizes local loads. Repeated excessive loading of normal cartilage and subchondral bone or normal loading of biologically deficient cartilage and subchondral bone may lead to the development of OA. As the cartilage degenerates and thins, it is less able to redistribute forces, resulting in a greater force transference to the subchondral bone, which causes reactive hardening. Osteophyte formation (bone spurs) may develop at joint margins. As the joint surface deteriorates, capsular laxity may occur, leading to joint instability.

On radiographs, OA is evidenced by decreased joint space, osteophyte formation, subchondral sclerosis, and subchondral trabecular fractures. Radiographic evidence of OA is present in most individuals over 65 years of age, although not all individuals are symptomatic. Generally, however, a positive correlation exists between clinical and radiographic findings.

Clinical Findings

Clinical characteristics include joint pain, stiffness, tenderness, instability, and enlargement. Periarticular muscle atrophy and weakness occur, contributing to disability. Early in the disease course, pain is worsened by activity and relieved by rest. As the disease progresses, pain is often present even at rest. Articular cartilage is devoid of nerve endings, so the pain associated with OA arises from innervated intrarticular and periarticular structures. In the spine, bony overgrowth may encroach on emerging nerve roots, causing pain. Stiffness, usually oc-

Table 20–1 Commonly Involved Joints

Joints	RA	SLE	OA	GOUT
Temporomandibular	X			
Spine	C[a]		CL[a]	
Sacroiliac				
Shoulder	X	X		
Elbow	X	X		X
Wrist	X	X		X
MCP		X	X[b]	
PIP	X	X	X	
DIP			X	
Hip	X		X	
Knee	X	X	X	X
Ankle	X			X
Subtalar/midtarsal	X			X
MTP/IP	X			X

Modified from Banwell BF, Gall V, eds. *Physical Therapy Management of Arthritis.* New York: Churchill Livingstone, 1988; 45.

RA, rheumatoid arthritis; SLE, systemic lupus erythematosus; OA, osteoarthritis, Gout (acute); MCP, metacarpophalangeal; PIP, proximal interphalangeal; DIP, distal interphalangeal; MTP/IP, metatarsalphalangeal/interphalangeal

[a]C, cervical; L, lumbar
[b]First metacarpal

curring in the mornings and following periods of rest, is relieved by movement. Motion limitation may be caused by irregular joint surface movement due to cartilage degeneration, muscle spasms due to pain, muscle weakness due to disuse, and osteophyte formation. Crepitus, a clicking or crackling sound, may occur as the joint is moved. Joints may enlarge due to synovitis, joint effusion, connective tissue overgrowth, or osteophyte formation. Joint deformity may occur, as forces are inappropriately distributed among joint structures.

Inflammation is not a typical characteristic of OA but may occur as a result of trauma or irritation to the synovium. In erosive inflammatory OA, a variant form of OA, episodic inflammation occurs and affects primarily the proximal and distal interphalangeal joints of the hand.[1]

Treatment Considerations

Typical therapeutic interventions for OA include education, rest, pharmacological agents, exercise, and possibly surgery. Patients should be instructed in joint protection and energy-conservation techniques to help prevent acute flare-ups and to help minimize joint stress and pain. Regularly administered pharmacological agents include analgesics and nonsteroidal anti-inflammatory drugs (NSAIDs). Intra-articular corticosteroid injections may benefit acute joint inflammation.

Rehabilitation should include appropriate weight-bearing and nonweight-bearing exercises. An individually designed program of strengthening, range-of-motion, and cardiovascular fitness exercises should be implemented. The design of the strengthening program should include low weight and much repetition so as to minimize stress on the joints. Resistive exercise that produces increased joint pain during or after exercise probably indicates that too much resistance is being used, stress is being placed at an inappropriate part of the range of motion, or the exercise is being performed incorrectly. Stretching exercises incorporating a low load, prolonged stretching performed three or more times a day will lead to a more appropriate length-tension relationship for the muscles surrounding the affected joints and may lead to decreased stress in the intra-articular and periarticular joint structures. Home exercise programs must be carefully planned and monitored. The physical modality of heat may decrease pain and stiffness, and cold may decrease pain and inflammation. Splints, braces, and gait devices, such as crutches, walkers, or rolling walkers, may be helpful in decreasing joint stress. Weight loss may prevent the onset of symptoms and may alleviate symptoms.

Surgical interventions such as arthroscopy, arthroplasty, and angulation osteotomy may provide symptomatic relief, improved motion, and improved joint biomechanics. The most common major orthopedic procedure performed in the elderly is hip surgery, the indications being fracture or pain due to OA. More than 70% of hip and knee joint replacements are performed because of OA.[2] Elderly patients are at higher risk for complications than younger patients, but most have a satisfactory outcome and significant relief of pain.

RHEUMATOID ARTHRITIS

Rheumatoid arthritis (RA), one of the most common of the rheumatic diseases, is a chronic, systemic, inflammatory autoimmune disorder. The hallmark feature of RA is chronic inflammation of the synovium, peripheral articular cartilage, and subchondral marrow spaces. In response to the inflammation, granulation tissue (pannus) forms and results in the erosion of articular cartilage. Inflammation in tendon sheaths may lead to tendon fray or rupture. RA is a systemic connective tissue disease, and although systemic and extra-articular pathological changes can occur, such changes are less frequent and less severe than joint changes. Systemic and extra-articular manifestations include muscle fibrosis and atrophy, vasculitis, pericarditis, fatigue, weight loss, generalized stiffness, fever, anemia, pleural effusion, increased susceptibility to infection, and neurological compromise leading to sensory or motor loss or both. Subcutaneous, nontender nodules may occur on the extensor surface of the forearm or other pressure areas. RA may be mild, resulting in only occasional pain and discomfort and slightly decreased function. Severe RA leads to significant pain, decreased function, and joint deformity.

The prevalence of RA increases with age, with a prevalence of greater than 10% in persons over age 65. The overall female-to-male ratio is 3:1, but female predominance is less marked when onset occurs beyond age 60.[1] The onset of RA may be acute but is usually insidious. The clinical course of RA is variable and unpredictable. In the initial stages, joint pain and stiffness are prevalent, especially in the mornings. As the disease progresses, motion becomes more limited and ankylosis may develop. Treatment effectiveness may be difficult to determine because of spontaneous exacerbations and remissions. Testimonials of "cures" with unproven remedies are common, as certain treatment approaches may have been initiated during the initial stages of a spontaneous remission.

The cause of RA is unknown. There is evidence of a genetic predisposition for the disease that can be triggered by bacteria or viruses. The pathogenesis of RA is better understood than the cause. The characteristic chronic inflammatory process begins

Table 20–2 Common Peripheral Joint Deformities in Rheumatoid Arthritis

Joint	Position of Contracture or Deformity
Shoulder	Adduction, internal rotation contracture
Elbow	Flexion pronation contracture → deformity
Wrist/Carpal	Radial deviation, volar subluxation
MCP/PIP/DIP	MCP ulnar drift, swan-neck deformity, boutonnière deformity, mallet deformity, rheumatoid thumb deformity[a]
Hip	Flexion contracture → deformity, adduction contracture, leg-length discrepancy— soft tissue or bony
Knee	Flexion contracture → deformity, patella subluxation, genu varus/ genu valgus
Ankle	Plantar flexion contracture
Subtalar/Midtarsal	Pronation
MTP/IP	Lateral subluxation, hallux valgus → rigidus, hammer toes/cock-up toes

From Banwell BF, Gall V, eds. *Physical Therapy Management of Arthritis.* New York: Churchill Livingstone, 1988; 53.
[a] Nalebuff classification according to joint of initial involvement

with synovitis and develops as microvascular endothelial cells become swollen and congested. As the disease advances, the synovium becomes progressively thickened and edematous, with projections of synovial tissue invading the joint cavity. Pannus, a tumor-like thickened layer of granulation tissue, infiltrates the joint, destroying periarticular bone and cartilage. Fibrotic ankylosis may eventually occur, with bony malalignment, visible deformities, muscle atrophy, and subluxation of joints. In advanced RA, bony ankylosis and significant disability may occur.

A definitive diagnosis is based on a combination of clinical manifestations and laboratory findings, as there is no laboratory test that is specific for RA. Common laboratory findings in persons with RA include decreased red blood cell count, increased erythrocyte sedimentation rates, and positive rheumatoid factor (RF). A positive test of RF is not diagnostic, as RF is found in a small percentage of normal individuals. However, RF is found in the serum of 85% of adults with RA, and the concentration of RF in persons with RA is higher than in normal individuals with RF.[1]

Clinical Findings

Joint manifestations occur bilaterally, affecting principally the small joints of the hands and feet, ankles, knees, wrists, elbows, and shoulders (see Table 20–1). Typically, the metacarpophalangeal and proximal interphalangeal joints of the hand are affected, but the distal interphalangeal joints are spared. RA can affect the hip, knee, ankle, and small joints of the foot. In axial involvement, the upper cervical spine is most commonly affected. Tenosynovitis of the transverse ligament of the first cervical vertebra and disease of the facet joints may lead to instability and cord compression.

Joint deformities result from synovitis, pannus formation, cartilage destruction, and voluntary joint immobilization due to pain (Table 20–2). The change in joint mechanics that results from cartilage degeneration and the erosive effect of chronic synovitis may lead to ligament laxity. The changed mechanics result in abnormal lines of pull from tendons, leading to joint deformity. Additionally, tenosynovitis may occur, causing an obstruction of tendon movement within the tendon sheath or causing tendon rupture. Synovitis can lead to compression of nerves, particularly in the carpal tunnel and, less commonly in the tarsal tunnel. The ulnar nerve may be compressed at the elbow or in the hand. (See Chapter 36, "Localized Peripheral Neuropathies.")

Common deformities of the hand include radial deviation of the wrist, ulnar deviation at the metacarpophalangeal joints, and deformities in the fingers. Flexion deformity of the elbow and loss of shoulder motion is common. Because of the weight-bearing nature of the lower extremities, major disability can result, particularly in the toes and ankles.

Treatment Considerations

Effective treatment of RA attempts to reduce the inflammation, provide pain relief, maintain and restore joint function, and decrease the development of joint deformity. Medications include NSAIDs, corticosteroids, slow-acting antirheumatic drugs, and disease-modifying antirheumatic drugs, such as antimalarials (e.g., chloroquine), gold, penicillamine and methotrexate.[1] Patients must balance activity and rest. Fatigue may be decreased with appropriate rest, which may include 8 to 10 hours of sleep at night and an afternoon nap. Energy should be conserved for daily activities. Prolonged bedrest has not proven to be beneficial. Therapeutic exercise cannot alter the course of the disease but can help to prevent deformity and loss of motion and muscle strength. Active and passive range-of-motion exercises, pain-free isometrics, and proper positioning and posture should be performed regularly to achieve these goals. Joint-stressing activities should be avoided. Splints and assistive devices should be used as needed to protect the joints. During active inflammatory periods, exercise should be performed carefully, taking special care to protect the joints. Heavy resistive exercise should be avoided, as the joint compression that occurs with this kind of exercise could increase pain and contribute to joint damage. Because the limitation of motion is caused by distended joint capsules and not to adhesions, forceful stretching should be avoided. During times of remission, non-impact or low-impact aerobic conditioning such as swimming or stationary bicycling can be performed within the patient's tolerance. Gentle stretching can be performed. Relaxation exercises often help to decrease muscle tension and stress. Surgical procedures may be performed with the goal of reducing pain, improving function, and correcting instability or deformity. Common surgical procedures include tenosynovectomy, tendon repair, synovectomy, arthrodesis, and arthroplasty.

SYSTEMIC LUPUS ERYTHEMATOSUS

Systemic lupus erythematosus (SLE) is an autoimmune disease that affects primarily young women. The peak incidence of SLE occurs between the ages of 15 and 40, but it may affect both younger and older persons, with a female-to-male ratio of approximately 5:1. In older persons, the female-to-male ratio is approximately 2:1. SLE is more prevalent in blacks and Hispanics than in Caucasians.

The cause of SLE is unknown, but it may involve immunological, environmental, hormonal, and genetic factors. The prime causative mechanism is thought to be autoimmunity. Immunity is suppressed and tissues are damaged as antibodies are produced against many body tissues and tissue components such as blood vessels, red blood cells, lymphocytes, and various organs. Antibodies directed against components of the cell nucleus, the antinuclear antibodies (ANA), are found in most SLE patients. Two ANA molecules, ANA-DNA and ANA-Sm, are unique to SLE and are used as diagnostic criteria. The kidneys and skin are commonly affected, and biopsies are used to assess the disease course and to confirm diagnosis. These organs demonstrate inflammation and degeneration. The central nervous system and heart are commonly affected. Venous and arterial thrombosis occurs commonly. Persons with longstanding SLE may develop atherosclerosis, osteonecrosis, and neurodegeneration. Studies indicate that immune-system abnormalities in SLE are genetically determined. Disease-triggering events include infectious agents, stress, hormonal changes, diet, toxins, and sunlight.

As with most rheumatic diseases, the diagnosis of SLE is made after laboratory testing and careful examination of clinical manifestations. The most common clinical manifestations include malaise, fever, weight loss, arthritis, arthralgia, pericarditis, pleurisy, Raynaud's phenomenon, vasculitis, lymphadenopathy, lesions of the skin, and involvement of the central nervous system, kidney, and gastrointestinal systems.

The "butterfly rash" is the most typical skin manifestation, occurring as a red, raised lesion in a malar distribution. The rash is usually precipitated by exposure to the sun. The arthritis associated with SLE may be symmetrical or nonsymmetrical and typically affects the knees and the small joints of the hands and wrists (see Table 20–1). Typically, the arthritis is nonerosive, but it can lead to deformities. Common neurological and psychiatric manifestations include intractable headache, seizures, motor and sensory peripheral neuropathy, psychoneurosis, organic brain syndrome, and psychosis. Gastrointestinal manifestations include diffuse abdominal pain, nausea and vomiting, and anorexia. While the short-term prognosis has improved in recent years, the long-term outlook for patients with SLE is generally poor, with complications that result from the disease itself or as a consequence of treatment. Late complications of SLE include end-stage renal disease, atherosclerosis, pulmonary emboli, venous syndromes, avascular necrosis, neuropsychological dysfunction, and shrinking lung syndrome.[1]

Treatment Considerations

Treatment of SLE is determined by disease activity and severity. Drugs that reduce inflammation and interfere with immune function are commonly prescribed. Nonsteroidal anti-inflammatory drugs may be used to treat musculoskeletal complications. Skin lesions may be treated with corticosteriods and anti-malarial agents. Corticosteriods are used in the treatment of systemic symptoms of SLE such as pericarditis, nephritis, vasculitis, and CNS involvement. In some patients, cytotoxic drugs such as methotrexate, azathioprine, and cyclophosphamide are prescribed. Patients must be monitored closely for side effects.[1]

Patient education is paramount in the treatment of SLE. The patient must understand that periods of remission and exacerbation are typical. Many SLE patients are photosensitive and must be reminded to avoid or reduce sun exposure whenever possible. SLE patients are at increased risk of infection and should be informed of the importance of prompt evaluation of unexplained fever. The patient should be urged to get adequate rest.

Physical therapy and occupational therapy can be helpful in increasing strength and motion and to provide splinting of affected joints. Heat may be used to relieve joint pain and stiffness. Regular active exercise may prevent contractures.

GOUT

Gout is a metabolic disease characterized by the deposition of monosodium urate crystals in connective tissues, which results in painful arthritis. The hyperuricemia associated with gout may be caused by a variety of factors, including a genetic defect in purine metabolism that results in an overproduction or undersecretion (or both) of uric acid. Other associated factors include obesity, diet, lifestyle, and hemoglobin levels.[1] Diurctics lead to an under-excretion of uric acid and may play a role in the pathogenesis of gout, particularly in the elderly.[3] Primary gout typically occurs in men older than age 30 and in postmenopausal women. Secondary gout occurs primarily in the elderly and results from the hyperuricemia associated with diseases such as diabetes mellitus and hypertension. The mechanisms are not fully defined but are probably related to diminished renal function, dehydration, decreased tissue perfusion, and the use of certain drugs that cause uric acid overproduction or underexcretion. Gout is relatively common in organ transplant recipients because of the use of cyclosporine and reduced renal function, regardless of the organ transplanted.[1]

The clinical course of gout typically follows four stages: asymptomatic, acute, intercritical, and chronic. An asymptomatic period of urate crystal deposition in connective tissue often appears prior to the first episode of gouty arthritis. The initial episode of gout is usually sudden, occurring during the night. The patient awakes with severe unexplained joint pain and swelling. The first metatarso-phalangeal joint is often affected (see Table 20-1). The ankle, tarsal joints, and knee are also commonly involved. Acute attacks may be precipitated by trauma, alcohol, drugs, or acute medical illness. The intercritical stage is characterized by symptom-free periods that may last for months or years. Crystal deposition persists during these asymptomatic periods. Gout's chronic stage is characterized by tophi, large masses of urates within the subarticular bone or surrounding soft tissues. Less commonly, tophi form in the internal organs. Tophi deposits precipitate joint erosion and tendon rupture.

The kidney is the organ most commonly involved in gout. The deposition of urate crystals in the kidney and its associated structures may lead to urate nephropathy, acute obstructive renal failure, or uric acid stones. Approximately 20% of persons with chronic gout die of renal failure.[4]

Not all persons with hyperuricemia develop gout. The presence of monosodium urate crystals in synovial fluid is generally considered necessary to establish a definitive diagnosis. Even during asymptomatic periods, monosodium urate crystals may be demonstrated in synovial fluid aspirated from previously involved joints as well as from joints that have never been involved.

Treatment Considerations

Treatment of gout is aimed at terminating acute attacks, reducing hyperuricemia, preventing recurrence, and preventing erosive joint damage and kidney complications. During acute attacks, oral or intravenous colchicine, NSAIDs, corticosteroids, or adrenocorticotrophic hormone may be used.[1] Included in the treatment regime are bedrest, joint immobilization, and local cold application to inflamed joints. Attack frequency may be decreased by certain dietary and lifestyle changes. Recommended dietary modifications include the avoidance of alcohol and a restriction of purine-rich foods, such as liver, kidneys, shellfish, salmon, peas, beans, and spinach. Weight loss and the avoidance of repetitive trauma are helpful prophylactic measures that can enable the avoidance of drug therapy during intercritical periods. Drug therapy for hyperuricemia may be necessary. Infected or ulcerated tophi may require excision.

Practical considerations include the use a bed cradle to keep bed covers off inflamed joints, the intake of plenty of fluids to prevent the formation of kidney stones, prompt treatment of acute attacks, and rapid attention to the side effects of drug therapies. Assistive devices may also be used to decrease stress on inflamed joints.

PSEUDOGOUT

Pseudogout (PG), a chronic recurrent arthritis similar to gout, results from calcium pyrophosphate dihydrate (CPPD) crystal deposition in articular and periarticular structures. The presence of CPPD crystals in joint tissue is common in the elderly, and there is only a weak correlation with joint pain. In contrast, with early onset CPPD, the disease often progresses to severe degenerative OA.[5] The pattern of joint involvement is symmetrical, though possibly more advanced on one side. Acute PG is characterized by self-limited attacks of acute joint pain and swelling. Any synovial joint may be affected, but the knee is the most common. Calcification from CPPD crystal deposits is characteristically demonstrated on well-exposed radiographs of the knees, pelvis, and hands. Acute attacks may be provoked by surgery, trauma, or severe illness. Joint inflammation and destruction may occur simultaneously or independently, thus resembling other rheumatic diseases. Diagnosis is made through the demonstration of CPPD crystals, radiographic manifestations of typical calcifications, acute arthritis, and chronic arthritis in the knees, hips, wrists, carpal joints, elbows, shoulders, and mctacarpophalangeal joints. Acute attacks are managed through joint aspiration to relieve pressure, injection of steroids, administration of analgesics and NSAIDs, the use of oral or intravenous colchicine, and treatment of any underlying metabolic or endocrine disorder.[1]

Persons with PG may experience multiple joint involvement, with low-grade inflammation lasting for weeks or months. The morning stiffness, fatigue, synovial thickening, and flexion contractures associated with PG may lead to a misdiagnosis of RA. The pattern of joint degeneration in PG is distinct from that of OA in that symmetrical involvement is the rule. Rehabilitation of persons with pseudogout should focus on joint protection during acute attacks, maintenance of range of motion and energy conservation practices.

POLYMYALGIA RHEUMATICA

Polymyalgia rheumatica (PMR) is, second to RA, the most common inflammatory rheumatological disorder in the elderly.[6] PMR is characterized by the gradual development of persistent pain, weakness, and stiffness in proximal muscles, in combination with systemic signs and symptoms of fever, weight loss, and high erythrocyte sedimentation rates. More common in women than men, PMR occurs mostly in those over 60 years of age. Symptoms are usually symmetrical, and onset may be abrupt. Stiffness is typically worse in the morning.

Tenderness and limited shoulder motion are the primary physical findings. Radiographs and muscle biopsies are normal, but shoulder synovitis is commonly present. Differentiating PMR from OA, RA, influenzal syndromes, inflammatory myopathies, malignancies, infections, and fibromyalgia may be difficult.

Polymyalgia rheumatica responds dramatically to prednisone therapy; thus, the response is used in diagnosis as well as treatment. The syndrome may be self-limited but more typically requires long-term treatment. Polymyalgia rheumatica is related to giant-cell arteritis, with both conditions frequently occurring in the same patient, though not necessarily simultaneously.[2] In the acute phase of PMR, prednisone is the most effective treatment. Later in the course of the disease, stretching and strengthening exercises may be helpful. Modalities such as ice and electrical stimulation may be used to decrease pain. The use of assistive devices may decrease the risk of falls.

BURSITIS

Bursae are small sacs, synovial-like membranes that contain a fluid that is indistinguishable from synovial fluid. They lie in areas of potential friction and commonly are located between bones and ligaments, skin, or muscles, an example being the ischial bursa, which lies between the ischial tuberosity and the gluteus maximus. Bursitis is defined as an inflammation of a bursa, with the most commonly affected bursae being the subdeltoid (subacromial), olecranon, ischial, greater trochanteric, and prepatellar. As a response to the stimulus of inflammation, the lining membrane may produce excess fluid, causing distension of the bursa.

Bursitis may be caused by an acute trauma such as a direct blow to the area, for example, trochanteric bursitis developing as a result of a fall onto the greater trochanter. Chronic trauma may be a cause, as is seen with overuse syndromes such as olecranon bursitis resulting from leaning on the elbow for extended periods. Infection secondary to a puncture wound, as well as other miscellaneous disease processes such as rheumatoid arthritis, gout, tuberculosis, and syphilis also may cause bursitis.[7] Septic bursitis should be considered a possibility when the cardinal signs of inflammation are present and the patient has a history of trauma to the area with puncture or abrasion of the skin. The bursal fluid may be aspirated and cultured to determine whether infection is present.

Clinical characteristics may include joint distension (effusion), pain, redness, increased temperature, and loss of function at the involved joint. Pain is usually worsened by activity at the involved joint and relieved by rest; however, pain may continue to be present at rest, but with less severity. Both active range of motion (AROM) and passive range of motion (PROM) are usually normal, with increased pain at the end of the range in the direction of stress to the bursa (e.g., elbow flexion with olecranon bursitis). Range of motion may be limited due to pain if the condition is very acute or the bursa becomes pinched during the movement, as with shoulder flexion or abduction that causes the subacromial bursa to be pinched under the acromion process. Resistive testing is usually negative, as the bursa is a noncontractile tissue, but discomfort may be caused by the contraction of neighboring muscles encroaching on the swollen bursa. Palpation directly over the area is typically painful.

Treatment Considerations

Therapeutic interventions for acute bursitis include protecting and resting the area, ice, anti-inflammatory medications, iontophoresis, and phonophoresis. Relieving the cause of the bursitis by altering postures or modifying environmental factors is helpful. For example, wheelchair armrests can be padded or protective elbow pads can be worn to reduce trauma to the olecranon bursa. Overhead work can be discontinued, as that position may further aggravate an inflamed subdeltoid bursa. Oral NSAIDs and local corticosteroid injections may be beneficial in reducing the inflammation and pain. As the acute inflammation subsides, pain-free AROM is encouraged to help to increase metabolism in the area and decrease swelling. In cases of chronic bursitis, determining the cause of the problem becomes the most important factor in successful treatment. A patient with chronic trochanteric bursitis may benefit from stretching a tight iliotibial band. Surgical intervention is uncommon and depends on the extent of the disease process. Surgery usually has the goal of creating more area for structures to move, such as an acromioplasty or removal of osteophytes from the undersurface of the acromion process and acromioclavicular joint.

TENDINITIS

Tendinitis is defined as the inflammation of a tendon; tenosynovitis is defined as inflammation of a tendon and tendon sheath. A tendon may become inflamed in many areas and as a result of several mechanisms. Inflammation may occur within the tendon itself, at the place where the tendon fuses with the muscle (the musculotendinous junction),

or where the tendon attaches to bone (the tenoperiosteal junction). Determining the exact location of the lesion is extremely important, as successful treatment must be directed to the exact lesion site. A common cause of tendinitis is anatomical or biomechanical constraint to the tendon, such as supraspinatus tendon impingement by the coracoacromial arch. Other common mechanisms include microtrauma due to repeated overload, such as the flexor tendons of the hand undergoing repeated contractions in a keyboard operator, and macrotrauma to a tendon. Calcific tendinitis occurs when calcium deposits form in the tendon, resulting in decreased blood supply to the tendon. Commonly affected tendons are the Achilles, rotator cuff, bicipital, patellar, common extensor group of the wrist, and posterior tibial. In the geriatric population, pain from Achilles or posterior tibial tendinitis must be differentiated from pain of vascular origin, such as thrombosis or thrombophlebitis. A common test is the Homan's sign in which the examiner squeezes the patient's gastrocnemius while forcefully dorsiflexing the ankle. Tenderness associated with increased firmness in the gastrocnemius suggests the presence of deep-vein thrombophlebitis. This test can be objectified by inflating a blood pressure cuff around the calf. In the absence of pathology, high pressures can be tolerated, whereas persons with deep-vein thrombophlebitis usually cannot tolerate pressures greater than 40 mmHg.[8]

Clinical characteristics may include pain, edema, redness, increased temperature, and loss of function at the involved joint. Symptoms are typically worsened by use of the involved tendon, especially with eccentric loading of the tendon as when going down stairs with patellar tendinitis. Use of the tendon in a range of motion in which it is likely to be impinged (painful arc) also will reproduce the patient's pain. An example is the painful arc produced by overhead abduction with supraspinatus tendinitis. Although commonly relieved by rest, pain may be present even at rest, if it is acute. AROM may be painful with muscle contraction of associated tendons. Passive motions may be painful, especially those resulting in full elongation of the tendon, such as full shoulder extension, elbow extension, and pronation in the case of bicipital tendinitis. Resistive testing is the key clinical diagnostic test; the tendon is strong and painful upon resistance. Palpation directly over the tendon is typically painful. In the case of a partial tear of the tendon, the resisted motion will characteristically present as weak and painful.

Treatment Considerations

Typical therapeutic interventions for acute tendinitis include protection and rest of the area, ice, and anti-inflammatory medications. Also essential is relieving any possible causes of the tendinitis by altering or modifying work or environmental factors that may be contributing to the problem, such as an office worker with extensor carpi ulnaris tendinitis who may further aggravate the condition by continuing to type or the patient using an assistive device for mobility who may need a modification of grip or a change in a platform device. Corticosteroid injections into the tendon or tendon sheath may be beneficial. However, it is important to remember that injection of steroids near the tendon may weaken it for 2 to 6 weeks.[9]

As the acute inflammation subsides, pain-free AROM is encouraged to help provide nutrition to the area and decrease swelling. In cases of chronic tendinitis, determining the cause of the problem becomes the most important factor in successful treatment. If a patient has a chronic supraspinatus tendinitis, the cause—such as weak shoulder external rotators or a bone spur on the inferior side of the acromion—should be identified. Chronic tendinitis is usually the result of poor blood flow to the injured area combined with continued stress on the area that does not allow for adequate maturation of the healing tissues. Transverse friction massage may be used in chronic tendinitis to increase the mobility of the scar and to stimulate the healing of the scar tissue with normal fiber alignment. Surgical intervention is performed only when conservative measures have not improved the condition. These procedures usually have the goal of creating more area for structures to move, such as an acromioplasty or removal of osteophytes from the undersurface of the acromion process and acromioclavicular joint in chronic subdeltoid bursitis.

CONCLUSION

Aging and arthritis are closely associated, and the resultant pain and deformity often impact negatively on the mobility and quality of life of elderly persons. In conjunction with medical and surgical interventions, successful management of the common arthritic diagnoses includes rehabilitative services such a proper therapeutic exercises, joint protection, use of assistive devices, and physical modalities for pain and swelling.

REFERENCES

1. Schumacher RH, ed. Primer on the Rheumatic Diseases, 10th ed. Atlanta, Ga.: Arthritis Foundation; 1993.
2. Felson DT. Weight and osteoarthritis. Am J Clin Nutr 1996; 63:430–432.
3. Wordsworth BP, Mowat AG. Rapid development of gouty tophi after diuretic therapy. J Rheumatol (Canada) 1985; 12:376–377.
4. Kumar V, Cotran R, Robbins SL. Basic Pathology, 5th ed. Philadelphia: W.B. Saunders, 1992; 103.
5. Baldwin CT, Farrer LA, Adair R, Dharmavaram R, Jimenez S, Anderson L. Linage of early-onset osteoarthritis and chondrocalcinosis to human chromosome 8q. Am J Hum Genet 1995; 56:692–697.
6. Wilske KR, Healey LA. Polymyalgia rheumatica and giant-cell arteritis: the dilemma of therapy. Postgrad Med 1985; 77:243–248.
7. Schoroeder E. Current Medical Diagnosis and Treatment. Stamford, CT: Appleton & Lange; 1992.
8. McCulloch JM. Evaluation of patients with open wounds. In: McCulloch JM, Kloth LC, Feedor JA, eds. *Wound Healing: Alternatives in Management.* Philadelphia: FA Davis, 1995; 126.
9. Zachazewski JE, Magee DJ, Quillen WS. Athletic Injuries and Rehabilitation. Philadelphia: W.B. Saunders; 1996.

Chapter 21

Dense Mineralized Connective Tissue: Osteomalacia and Paget's Disease of Bone

Katie Lundon, Ph.D., P.T.

INTRODUCTION

Osteomalacia and Paget's disease are two major bone-deforming diseases that can manifest in elderly people. Osteomalacia is a metabolic bone disorder with varied causes that affects the adult skeleton by means of abnormal mineralization and results in skeletal deformity. Paget's disease is a bone-remodeling disorder of unknown cause that affects primarily the elderly.

OSTEOMALACIA

Osteomalacia is a bone disease that involves the failure of newly formed or remodeling bone to mineralize, which results in an excess of unmineralized bone matrix (osteoid). Osteomalacia refers to the adult form of this condition, whereas rickets is the same disease process but it specifically targets the epiphysis in the growing skeleton. Osteomalacia is a consequence of inadequate or delayed mineralization of mature cortical and spongy bone because of loss, altered intake, or altered metabolism of 1,25 dihydroxyvitamin D_3 (vitamin D_3) and phosphate.

Causes

The gross histopathological and radiological abnormalities of osteomalacia are the common result of a number of different diseases. In general, osteomalacia is considered to be most commonly caused by altered metabolism of vitamin D_3 or phosphate or both, a condition for which the elderly population is at particular risk. Recent advances in understanding the biochemistry of vitamin D_3 metabolism have provided new insight into this condition. In developed countries, older people, particularly the housebound or institutionalized, are vulnerable to osteomalacia.

In general, vitamin D_3 deficiency occurs in those whose vitamin D_3 intake is close to zero and who, in addition, have minimal or no exposure to ultraviolet radiation. Vitamin D_3 deficiency may be caused by an inadequate intake of vitamin D_3 or there may be defective intestinal absorption of vitamin D_3, as is observed in malabsorption syndromes such as jejunoileal bypass. In addition, there may be an age-related diminished response by the intestine to vitamin D_3. In normal individuals, the main source of vitamin D_3 is dermal synthesis. There is an age-related decline in the dermal synthesis of 7-dehydrocholesterol, the precursor of vitamin D_3. A deficiency can also occur if there is a defect in vitamin D_3 metabolism. Most diseases are not caused by simple vitamin D_3 deficiency but involve abnormal production or regulation of its synthesis in the liver or kidneys. The ultimate consequence is the inability to produce sufficient quantities of this vitamin.

Renal disorders are the main cause of difficulty in metabolizing phosphate. When phosphate depletion is a causative factor, the serum phosphorus is markedly depressed. In osteomalacic patients it is common to find very low plasma phosphate levels. Alimentary phosphate deficiency is additionally aggravated by vitamin D_3 deficiency. Vitamin D_3 promotes jejunal phosphate absorption and renal phosphate reabsorption. Disorders that affect phosphate absorption in the intestines or reabsorption in the kidneys include certain conditions for which large amounts of phosphate-binding antacids have been administered. Such circumstances are of particular importance considering that these agents may be employed to manage other age-related disorders such as osteoporosis.

Pathogenesis

Osteomalacia is associated with many clinical, radiographic, and biochemical abnormalities, none of which is entirely pathognomonic of the disorder. Histological examination of a bone biopsy is often essential to establish a definitive diagnosis.

Histological Features

Osteomalacia is a state of high bone turnover and is characterized primarily by excessive amounts of inadequately mineralized osteoid (unmineralized bone tissue). Specifically, this increase in osteoid is associated with prolonged mineralization time. In cancellous bone, this osteoid presents in the form of large seams that coat the trabeculae and contribute to overall preserved bone volume. In cortical bone, intracortical bone resorption, or tunneling, as well as increased amounts of osteoid lining the haversian canals may be observed.

Biochemical Features

Mineralization of newly formed bone requires the deposition of adequate concentrations of calcium and phosphate. In general, the combination of moderate hypocalcemia and clear hypophosphatemia are hallmarks of adult osteomalacia.[1] Where there is vitamin D_3 deficiency because of dietary considerations or malabsorption, the serum calcium is low, the serum phosphorus is very low (due to decreased intestinal phosphate absorption and increased renal phosphate clearance caused by secondary hyperparathyroidism induced by the low serum calcium levels), and urine calcium excretion is also very low. There may also be elevated alkaline phosphatase and osteocalcin (also known as bone-Gla protein or BGP) levels.

Radiographic Signs

Confirmation of osteomalacia by roentgenographs can be difficult because of the many nonspecific changes such as osteopenia that are common to other diseases. These disease states include senile or postmenopausal osteoporosis, hyperparathyroidism, hyperthyroidism, and multiple myeloma.[2] Looser-Milkman pseudofractures (Looser's zones) are characteristic of osteomalacia (although they may also be seen in Paget's disease) and are a type of insufficiency fracture. Pseudofractures may be present where arteries cross bone surfaces at sites such as the pubic rami and femoral necks, the ribs, the metatarsals, the border of the scapula, the pelvic brim, or the medial aspect of the humeral head. Looser's zones are focal accumulations of osteoid that occur at right angles to the long axis in compact bone and that are often symmetrical in distribution. While Looser's zones may indicate partial insufficiency fractures, they can proceed to full lateral fractures with time because of the weakened underlying structure.

Osteomalacia is a major bone disease that may present with the x-ray appearance of osteopenia because of the thinning and apparent loss of mineralized secondary trabeculae. As osteopenia occurs in both osteomalacia and osteoporosis, sometimes a differential diagnosis can be made only by examining the histological features and pathogenesis characteristic of each underlying condition.

Clinical Presentation

Patients may have vague, generalized bone pain, multiple fractures, thoracic kyphosis and loss of height due to multiple vertebral compression fractures, and deformity of the lower limbs due to the malunion or bowing associated with pseudofractures. This condition can affect bone turnover to the extent that fractures occur in situations that otherwise might constitute only minimal to moderate impact stress. Lumbar scoliosis may develop because of the altered biconcave shape of affected vertebral bodies. The patient may complain of generalized bone pain of a dull, aching nature and muscle weakness, particularly in the proximal muscle groups in the lower extremities (also referred to as pelvic girdle myopathy) and back. This diffuse skeletal pain is typically exacerbated by physical activity, and tenderness may be elicited by palpation. Muscle weakness is a common accompaniment to prolonged vitamin D_3 deficiency, although the mechanism is unknown. A characteristic waddling gait manifests with this condition, and generalized muscle atrophy may be evident. Functional activities such as climbing stairs and ambulation may become difficult, making requisite the use of gait aids for support. In the extreme case, the composite presentation of weakness and muscle atrophy, skeletal deformities, and fracture incidence may even lead the affected individual to become wheelchair-bound or bedridden.

Management

In most cases, the stereotypical presentation of osteomalacia can be cured or at least improved with appropriate therapy for the specific underlying abnormality. Although there may be different underlying causes of this skeletal disorder, most signs and symptoms resolve with supplementation of vitamin D_3, which aims to restore plasma calcium and phosphate levels to normal. Bone pain should disappear promptly. Concurrent with appropriate pharmacological therapy, physical management strategies should include postural and peripheral muscle-strengthening exercises and gait retraining in order to attain maximal functional status. There are no apparent contraindications, but sound judgment should be used and proper precautions taken when treating a patient who has osteomalacia with ultrasound, electrical stimulation, heat, or cold or when loading the bone with weight-bearing and resistive exercises.

PAGET'S DISEASE OF THE BONE

Paget's disease, also known as *osteitis deformans,* is a common bone disorder among the elderly; it rarely affects people below the age of 40. Approximately 60% of those affected with this condition are male. Paget's disease is a chronic, asymmetrical, focal bone disease that features increased osteoclastic bone resorption and aberrant secondary osteoblastic bone formation.

Paget's disease is most prevalent in people with northern European ancestry and is common in the United Kingdom as well as in western Europe, Australia, and New Zealand. It is rare in Scandinavia, Asia, and Africa. The incidence of Paget's disease in North America appears to be comparable to that of Europe, with its prevalence ranging between 1 to 3% of adults over 40 years of age.

Etiology

There is no conclusive evidence to support the idea that Paget's disease is a disorder related to hormonal regulation of bone metabolism, a benign neoplasm, or a chronic inflammatory condition affecting bone. Osteoclasts in patients with Paget's disease contain characteristic intranuclear inclusion bodies, strongly suggesting infection with members of the paramyxovirus family. There is extensive evidence linking paramyxoviruses, notably measles and respiratory syncytial virus, with Paget's disease of the bone. Another paramyxovirus that has been inconclusively implicated in the development of Paget's disease is the canine distemper virus, a paramyxovirus of the morbillivirus family. Despite this association, any efforts to link Paget's disease with previous dog ownership have remained inconclusive. Despite the morphological findings suggestive of viral infection as a cause of Paget's disease, no virus has yet been definitively identified.

Pathophysiology

The pathophysiology of Paget's disease will remain speculative until a specific causative agent has been found. Paget's disease is a localized condition of excessive but disordered bone remodeling. The primary event of the disease is increased resorption followed by subsequent bone formation, with skeletal remodeling reaching 20 times the normal rate. Bone formation processes are typically excessive, irregular, and incomplete, creating a mixture of immature woven collagen matrix and lamellar bone. Although bone formation processes appear to be altered, the osteoblasts and fibroblasts look morphologically normal; this response is considered a consequence of prior increases in bone resorption. The disease front may proceed through bone, particularly the long bones and the skull, at a steady rate of about 1 cm per year. There is also an increase in vascular fibrous tissue in the marrow cavity.

The greater vascularity of pagetic bone is associated with increased arteriovenous shunting and increased local blood flow through the bone, which causes the typical increase in local warmth over affected bones. Because of arteriovenous shunting through bone, a high cardiac output state may be induced which, in some patients with underlying cardiac disease, may precipitate cardiac failure.

Biochemistry

Measurements of urinary hydroxyproline and serum alkaline phosphatase remain the most useful markers of disease activity. There is a rise in markers of bone resorption such as urine hydroxyproline as well as deoxypyridinoline crosslinks. An increase in the levels of serum alkaline phosphatase may be noted as it is a reflection of new bone formation. In patients with Paget's disease, serum calcium and phosphate levels are typically normal.

Histological Features

The overall structure of the bone demonstrates a mosaic pattern in which packets of bone are laid down subsequent to a phase of osteoclastic bone resorption. The bone that becomes enclosed in individual packets consists of true woven bone as well as lamellar bone. There is marked net bone formation that is essentially normal. Bone biopsy remains important for the differentiation between malignancy and the pagetic bone.

The Cells

The primary abnormality in Paget's disease is the osteoclast. Bone resorption is performed by the osteoclast, a multinucleated cell of hematopoietic origin. The pagetic osteoclast has a characteristic phenotype. The osteoclasts are very large and contain greater numbers of nuclei. The pagetic osteo-

clast presents in increased numbers, size, and activity, contains viral nuclear inclusions, expresses viral antigens, and is known to contain viral transcripts. It demonstrates increased tartrate-resistant acid phosphatase activity compared to normal osteoclasts. In addition, the pagetic osteoclast is hypersensitive to certain hormones such as calcitonin and vitamin D_3.

There is a secondary marked increase in osteoblastic activity, with deposition of increased amounts of matrix. As there is no mineralization defect, mineralization proceeds as normal.

Radiographic Signs

Unlike osteomalacia, Paget's disease offers x-rays and bone scans that are definitive in revealing an active disease process, so these methods are useful in the diagnosis of the disease. The typically focal nature of Paget's disease and the extent of spread in individual bones makes the bone scan useful in differentiating Paget's disease from other bone diseases, including metastatic carcinoma. A bone scan demonstrates an increased uptake of isotopes at diseased sites, reflecting the activity of bone formation.

Specific patterns of radiographic changes are featured in Paget's disease. A typical presentation includes radiolucent areas of patchy arrangement that indicate increased bone resorption, as well as evidence of regional bone formation processes represented by cortical and cancellous thickening and sclerosis and uneven widths of affected bones. Patchy areas of resorption typical of Paget's disease are referred to as *osteoporosis circumscripta*. In the pelvis, there may be evidence of sclerosis along the iliopectineal line. In the vertebrae, cortical thickening and expansion are characteristic, but this appearance may be difficult to distinguish from osteoblastic metastasis, which occurs without cortical thickening.

Clinical Presentation

Approximately 90% of individuals affected by Paget's disease are asymptomatic. Diagnosis is usually made by reports of bone pain or deformity, by x-ray, or by inadvertent detection of elevated serum alkaline phosphatase levels that are found upon routine biochemical testing. The most common complaints reported are pain, skeletal deformity, and change in skin temperature. Other clinical manifestations include diminished mobility and unsteady gait. In more severe cases of Paget's disease, pathological fractures may manifest. The major clinical features are outlined in Table 21–1.

Table 21-1 Major Clinical Features of Advanced Paget's Disease

Specific Bones	Clinical Features
Skull	Headaches, deafness, expanded skull size, cranial palsies
Facial bones	Deformity, dental problems
Vertebrae	Root compression, cord compression
Long bones	Deformity determined by stresses to bone, e.g., bowing of tibia (anterior) or femur (lateral)
	Secondary osteoarthritis
	Incremental fissure fractures
	Excessive operative bleeding
General	Bone pain
	Malaise
	Immobility
	Deformity
	Bone sarcoma
	Heat over affected bones
	High-output cardiac failure

Reproduced from Anderson DC, Richardson PC. Paget's disease of bone. In: *Textbook of Geriatrics and Gerontology.* New York: Churchill Livingstone; 1992:783–791.

The most common complaint in symptomatic patients is pain. Some pagetic lesions are not painful, but pain of varying degrees of severity can occur and is most commonly experienced at the site of the lesion, as supported by bone scan or x-ray findings.[4] Bone pain is often nocturnal and is thought to be the result of increased pressure on the periosteum or associated hyperemia. Other causes of pain may be nerve root compression or nerve entrapment if the diseased bone involves a nerve foramen or canal. The deep-rooted pain of Paget's disease is often unresponsive to simple analgesics, and is more likely to be experienced when at rest than during movement. The efficacy of physical modalities in treating pagetic pain in unclear and is best applied on an individual basis. Mixed sensorineural and conductive hearing loss is a common clinical manifestation of Paget's disease. Auditory nerve compression occurs when Paget's disease involves the petrous temporal bone and encroachment on the internal auditory meatus may cause compression of cranial nerve VIII, leading to hearing loss. Conduction deafness may be due to otosclerosis or indirect involvement of the cochlea or ossicles and is also a common finding in patients with Paget's

disease. Other cranial nerves may be affected as well. It is rare to find an extensive enough narrowing of the spinal canal to compromise the spinal cord.

Affected Sites

The bones most commonly involved in Paget's disease include the vertebrae, cranium, pelvis, sternum, and proximal ends of the long bones (e.g., the tibia), although any bone may be affected. The lumbar and sacral regions are commonly affected but are often asymptomatic. In some cases, as many as 20 or 30 bones may be simultaneously targeted by Paget's disease; however, the number of bones involved does not reflect the severity with which an individual bone may be affected. After initial diagnosis, the occurrence of lesions at new sites is unusual.

Skeletal Deformity

Because of abnormal bone remodeling processes inherent in the Paget's disease process, bone architecture becomes distorted in patients in advanced stages of the disease. Deformity develops in a slow and progressive manner, depending on the bone site affected. It appears that weight-bearing exacerbates the development of deformity, and pathological fractures occur most commonly in the long weight-bearing bones of the lower extremities—in the femoral neck and the subtrochanteric and tibial regions. An increase in skull size, lateral bowing of the long bones (especially the tibia, femur and humerus), and dorsal kyphosis are typical deformities in the Paget's patient. When compared with age- and gender-matched controls, patients who had Paget's disease of the bone involving the tibia, femur, or acetabular portion of the ilium demonstrated clinically and statistically significant functional and mobility impairments (measured using a mobility skills protocol of a 10-foot walk time, number of steps to complete a 360-degree turn, and a 6-minute walk distance).[5]

Fracture

A fracture is the most common complication of Paget's disease. It is likely to occur in weight-bearing bones such as the femora and tibiae under minimal to moderate conditions of stress. Malunion and nonunion are not uncommon tendencies in spite of the extensive blood supply to the bone in patients with Paget's disease.

Joint Arthroplasty

The metabolic activity of Paget's disease subsequent to total hip arthroplasty surgery was observed to have no effect on the clinical outcome, regardless of the location of the disease, in a 7.8-year follow-up study. For the femur, failure rates were similar for prostheses implanted in pagetic or non-pagetic bone, with cemented total hip arthroplasty (THA) being the most viable option for these patients.[6]

Management

Pharmacological interventions with any proven efficacy are those that act to inhibit bone resorption by the osteoclast. The strongest focus is on calcitonin and the bisphosphonates. The goal of these pharmacological therapies is to control the disease activity, to normalize biochemical parameters, and to ameliorate the symptoms. Given that the relief of bone pain, immobilization, hypercalcemia, and high-output cardiac failure associated with Paget's disease are related to the extent to which biochemical control is regained, pharmacological efforts are critical.

Subcutaneous, intramuscular, or intranasal administration of salmon or human calcitonin can be efficacious in its palliative effects. Calcitonin, in the short term at least, exerts its biological effects by inhibiting osteoclastic bone resorption by causing the osteoclast to shrink in size and decrease its bone-resorbing activity. Response to this therapy is monitored by evaluation of serum alkaline phosphatase, urinary hydroxyproline, or urinary deoxypyridinoline crosslinks. Calcitonin is associated with side effects that include headaches and flushing and, although it is still used in the treatment of this disease, it has largely been replaced by the more efficacious bisphosphonates.

The advent of potent new bisphosphonates (diphosphonates) enables the restoration and maintenance of normal bone turnover in the majority of patients with Paget's disease. Disodium etidronate is a first-generation bisphosphonate that is a potent inhibitor of osteoclastic bone resorption, but its effectiveness is known to be limited because of evidence of defective mineralization or development of osteomalacia and increased susceptibility to fracture with high dosages (10 to 20 mg/kg/day). Newer diphosphonates, such as clodronate and pamidronate (APD), unlike etidronate, do not impair mineralization and are promising agents in the control of this disease.

CONCLUSION

Goals of treatment in Paget's disease are to reduce pain and encourage the maintenance of or appropriate increases in mobility. The use of assistive devices for ambulation must be prescribed on an individual basis and must take into consideration issues such as degree of pain, deformity, leg-length discrepancies, and secondary arthritis in joints near active disease sites. Many of the problems such as the development of bony deformities are difficult to treat once established, but with early diagnosis and attention to prophylactic (pharmacological and physical) therapies, the progression of deformity may be delayed if not entirely prevented. This attention will ensure optimal prevention of disability and dependency.

REFERENCES

1. Hutchison RN, Bell NH. Osteomalacia in rickets. *Semin Nephrol* 1992; 12:127–145.
2. Pitt M. Rickets and osteomalacia are still around. *Radiol Clin North Am* 1991; 29:97–118.
3. Anderson DC, Richardson PC. Paget's disease of bone. In: Brocklehurst JC, Tallis RC, Fillit HM, eds. *Textbook of Geriatrics and Gerontology*. New York: Churchill Livingstone; 1992:783–791.
4. Hamdy R, Moore S, LeRoy J. Clinical presentation of Paget's disease of the bone in older patients. *South Med J* 1993; 86:1097–1100.
5. Lyles K, Lammers J, Shipp K, et al. Functional and mobility impairments associated with Paget's disease of bone. *J Am Geriatr Soc* 1995; 43:502–506.
6. Ludkowski P, Wilson-MacDonald J. Total arthroplasty in Paget's disease of the hip. *Clin Orthop* 1990; 255:160–167.
7. Delmas PD, Meunier PJ. Drug therapy: the management of Paget's disease of bone. *N Engl J Med* 1997; 336:558–566.
8. Papapoulos WE. Paget's disease of bone: clinical, phatgentic and therapeutic aspects. *Clin Endocrinol Metab* 1997; 11:117–139.

Chapter **22**

The Shoulder
Edmund M. Kosmahl, P.T., Ed.D.

INTRODUCTION

Elderly people are commonly affected by shoulder pain and dysfunction. Authorities suggest that from 20 to 34% of the geriatric population suffers from shoulder disorders.[1] Shoulder disorders in the elderly can lead to significant disability, and functional disability is correlated with shoulder dysfunction, especially loss of range of motion (ROM).[2] Important activities such as feeding, dressing, and taking care of personal hygiene can be compromised. Physical dysfunction can combine with intermittent or constant pain to diminish the quality of life. The purpose of this chapter is to review rehabilitation concepts for the following four geriatric shoulder problems: (1) degenerative rotator cuff, (2) fracture of the proximal humerus, (3) total shoulder arthroplasty, and (4) shoulder pain in hemiplegia.

DEGENERATIVE ROTATOR CUFF

Rotator cuff pathology is the most common affliction of the shoulder.[3] The rotator cuff comprises the musculotendinous insertions of the supraspinatus, infraspinatus, teres minor, and subscapularis muscles. These structures are important for nearly all shoulder functions, but they are most important for the activities that require overhead arm function.

Advancing age is correlated with pathology of the rotator cuff. A lifetime of activity can lead to degeneration of the rotator cuff in association with osteoarthritis of the glenohumeral and acromioclavicular joints. Degeneration frequently causes partial- or full-thickness tears in the cuff.

Degeneration of the rotator cuff is often associated with subacromial impingement syndrome. It is important to evaluate thoracic spinal and scapular posture when assessing the geriatric patient with degenerative rotator cuff. Subacromial impingement can be induced by excessive thoracic kyphosis and protracted scapulae. These postural malalignments place the glenoid and acromion in a downward and forward position. This position encourages subacromial impingement when the arm is elevated. When these postural malalignments are present, the treatment program should include exercises aimed at establishing a more normal postural alignment. Exercises for degenerative rotator cuff should be designed to avoid making a subacute inflammatory process worse. This involves designing exercises that avoid pain associated with positions that cause subacromial impingement. Table 22–1 summarizes rehabilitation treatment for degenerative rotator cuff without tear.

The history and presentation of the geriatric degenerative rotator cuff tear are typical. The patient usually does not report trauma. A typical scenario involves the sudden inability to raise the arm overhead during some functional activity. Pain may or may not be reported. Examination shows that the patient cannot hold the arm in the 90-degree abducted position (failure of the drop-arm test). Because of the poor condition of the degenerated tissues, operative repair of tears of the geriatric rotator cuff is not often considered. The metaphor of "trying to anastomose cooked spaghetti" is sometimes helpful in conceptualizing the rationale for nonoperative management of the geriatric rotator cuff tear.

The success of nonoperative management of rotator cuff tear is associated with the initial amount of ROM and strength.[4] For this reason, it is unreasonable to expect full functional return for the geriatric patient with rotator cuff tear who cannot actively raise the arm above the head at initial evaluation. Treatment should be aimed at decreasing inflammation and pain (when present), maintaining full passive ROM, and maximizing strength and functional ability. The treatments for degenerative rotator cuff summarized in Table 22–1 are also appropriate for the geriatric rotator cuff tear patient. Because the restoration of full and active overhead mobility is unlikely, assisted ROM exercises must be continued indefinitely in most cases. They are important to prevent additional dysfunction such as adhesive capsulitis.

FRACTURE OF THE PROXIMAL HUMERUS

Nondisplaced fracture of the proximal humerus is a common injury among geriatric patients. A fall on

---

Table 22–1 Treatments for Degenerative Rotator Cuff

Problem or Purpose	Treatment
Pain and inflammation	Rest, modalities (ice, heat, ultrasound, electrical stimulation)
Excessive thoracic kyphosis	Thoracic spinal extension exercises
Protracted scapulae	Scapular retraction exercises
Maintain or improve ROM	Passive and assisted ROM exercises (assistance from noninvolved upper extremity, overhead pulley, wand)
Maintain or improve strength	Isometrics, side-lying isotonics for internal and external rotators, assisted eccentric lowering of arm from overhead
Maximize function	Gradual introduction: touch top of head, back of neck, low back; adapt activities of daily living to functional capabilities

the outstretched arm is the usual mechanism of injury. These fractures are sometimes labeled pathological because generalized osteoporosis has weakened the bone enough that relatively minor trauma is sufficient to cause a fracture.[5] Metastatic bone disease can also lead to pathological fracture.

Nondisplaced or minimally displaced fractures account for approximately 85% of fractures at the proximal humerus.[6] There is generally no need for operative fixation of these fractures. Management usually involves sling or hanging cast immobilization. Movement of the shoulder should be avoided until there is initial formation of bone callus, which usually takes about 3 weeks. This period of immobilization is necessary to stabilize the fracture fragments.[7] One can expect loss of function of the joint capsule and muscles around the shoulder during this period of immobilization. This is primarily a function of the development of fibrous adhesions in response to bleeding in the capsule.

When callus formation allows it, active motion exercise should begin. It is unwise to apply passive motion exercises until there is x-ray evidence of fracture union (usually about 6 weeks). External resistance exercises should also be avoided during this period. Isometric exercises may be considered from the time of injury, provided there is no risk of displacing the fracture fragments by muscle contraction. This is a concern whenever the fracture involves the greater or lesser tuberosities. Submaximal isometric exercise may be appropriate to encourage muscle contractility without risking displacement of fracture fragments. An outline of general exercise procedures for nonoperative proximal humeral fracture appears in Table 22–2.

About 15% of fractures of the proximal humerus involve displacement that is greater than 1 cm or angulation that is more than 45 degrees. The four important fracture fragments are (1) the humeral head, (2) the greater tuberosity, (3) the lesser tuberosity, and (4) the humeral shaft. These fractures usually require operative reduction and internal fixation (ORIF) to allow fracture healing and return of function. More serious fractures can interrupt the blood supply to the humeral head. This interruption can lead to necrosis.

Rehabilitation following ORIF varies depending on the classification of the injury (Table 22–3) and the stability of fixation. Close communication with the surgeon can facilitate proper progression of the rehabilitation program without risking a delay in healing or reinjury. Some geriatric patients may not be candidates for ORIF. Certain patients cannot reasonably expect to tolerate (or survive) anesthesia. In other cases, osteoporosis may reduce bone stock to the point at which hardware fixation cannot be achieved. Complete restoration of function is an unrealistic goal for these patients. Still, every attempt should be made to maximize functional outcomes so dressing and grooming are possible.

TOTAL SHOULDER ARTHROPLASTY

Realizing a successful functional outcome following total shoulder arthroplasty requires a well-coordinated and consistent effort by patient, surgeon, and therapist. Significant functional loss preoperatively, especially as related to coexisting degenerative rotator cuff disease, may necessarily limit ex-

Table 22–2 Exercises for Proximal Humeral Fracture (Nonoperative)

Purpose	Exercise	Timeline
Maintain or improve ROM	Assisted ROM (wand, wall climbing, pendulum)	X-ray evidence of callus, usually 3 weeks
	Passive ROM, stretching (overhead pulley)	X-ray evidence of union, usually 6 weeks
Maintain or improve strength	Submaximal isometrics	No risk of fragment displacement, usually immediately
	Full active ROM against gravity	X-ray evidence of union, usually 6 weeks
	External resistance isotonics	Ability to perform full active ROM against gravity, x-ray evidence of union, usually 6 weeks
Maximize function	Touch top of head, back of neck, low back	Assisted: x-ray evidence of callus, usually 3 weeks
		Unassisted: x-ray evidence of union, usually 6 weeks

Table 22–3 Neer Classification of Proximal Humeral Fractures

Category	Description
One-part	Nondisplaced or minimally displaced
Two-part	One part displaced > 1 cm or angulated > 45°
Three-part	Two parts displaced and/or angulated from each other and from remaining part
Four-part	Four parts displaced and/or angulated from each other
Fracture-dislocation	Displacement of humeral head from joint space with fracture

Adapted from Neer CS II. Displaced proximal humeral fractures: I. Classification and evaluation. *J Bone Joint Surg* 1970; 52A:1077.

pectations of functional outcomes.[8] At a minimum, pain-free performance of eating, dressing, and personal hygiene activities should result. Failure rates for this procedure range from 9.6 to 25%.[9] Because of the relatively high potential for complications, the rehabilitation program should be carefully designed to advance the patient through progressive stages of tissue healing, joint mobilization, and muscle strengthening.[10] The focus of the rehabilitation program should be on ROM and strengthening exercises and the restoration of functional capabilities. Thermal, electrical, and acoustical modalities should play an adjunctive role only.

Ideally, the therapist should meet with the patient and the primary care-givers in the home preoperatively. ROM, strength, and functional abilities should be measured and documented. These findings, along with postoperative exercises, precautions, and activities should be demonstrated and discussed. The patient should understand that pain and stiffness are to be expected, but that they will resolve with diligent performance of the postoperative program. The patient should begin practicing the exercise program immediately to promote ease of performance postoperatively. The therapist should discuss preoperative findings with the surgeon. This preoperative consultation provides the opportunity to establish specific modifications that may be required on a case-by-case basis.

Postural Concerns

Geriatric patients often exhibit excessive thoracic kyphosis and protracted scapulae. These postural malalignments put the glenoid fossa in a downward and forward position, and this position can complicate the postoperative restoration of shoulder elevation ROM. For these patients, the exercise program should include spinal extension and scapular retraction exercises. Normally, these exercises are accomplished most easily in the sitting position. The exercise program should also include exercises to maintain or improve elbow, wrist, and hand ROM and strength. Submaximal isometric exercises may play an important part in the early postoperative strengthening program. Still, care must be taken to avoid overstressing the healing musculotendinous structures. Communication with the surgeon can clarify whether isometric tension can be applied safely.

Postoperative Rehabilitation

Early Stages

The postoperative program can begin as early as the day of surgery. Because contemporary shoulder arthroplasty systems do not rely on soft tissues for joint stability, early motion can be allowed. It is unwise to delay initiation of the program longer than 48 hours. Initial treatment begins with three or four assisted ROM exercise sessions per day. These sessions should be short (about 5 minutes) and can be preceded by the application of modalities or analgesics. Assisted ROM exercise should include pendulum, supine elevation, supine external rotation, overhead pulley elevation, and supine abduction with external rotation (hands clasped behind neck). Exercises should be designed so the patient can assist with the unaffected arm. Each exercise should be held in the position of maximum available ROM for 15 seconds and should be repeated three or four times. The use of slings and immobilization devices should be minimized or eliminated.

If all has gone well, ROM should improve to about 140 degrees of elevation and 40 degrees of external rotation by the time sutures are removed (10 to 14 days postoperatively). Exercise frequency can be decreased to twice daily, and duration of exercise can be increased to 10 minutes. Each exercise should be held in the position of maximum available ROM for 30 seconds and should be repeated three or four times. Add assisted internal rotation ROM exercise to the program (hands behind back, uninvolved hand pulls involved hand up the back). Progress the assisted external rotation exercise so the patient stands and uses a doorway for assistance. Advance the assisted elevation exercise to the standing position using a wand or the doorway for assistance.

Once elevation range reaches 160 degrees and

external rotation reaches 60 degrees (usually within 3 to 6 weeks postoperatively), elevation, external rotation, and internal rotation stretching exercises should increase in vigor. Stretching into the direction of horizontal adduction should be added. All exercises should be held in the position of maximal available stretch for 60 seconds and repeated two or three times. Elevation, external and internal rotation, and horizontal adduction stretching exercises should be continued indefinitely.

Stages of Strengthening

Active strengthening exercises normally should be initiated 10 to 14 days after surgery. The exercise program should consist of 10 repetitions of each exercise performed twice daily. Depending on the initial level of strength, easier exercises may be unnecessary. In the case of associated rotator cuff repair, the surgeon should be consulted before beginning gravity-resisted exercises.

Supine elevation is initiated as follows: have the patient lie supine with the arm at the side and the elbow flexed to 90 degrees. Have the patient reach for the ceiling by flexing the shoulder and simultaneously extending the elbow. If this cannot be accomplished actively, have the patient assist with the uninvolved arm. Then the patient should lower the elbow toward the supporting surface, causing an eccentric contraction of the shoulder flexors (the elbow should simultaneously flex). There should be no assistance for this eccentric exercise. Once the patient can do 10 unassisted repetitions both concentrically and eccentrically, a ½-lb weight should be added to the wrist or hand. When the patient can do 10 repetitions, the weight should be increased in ½-lb increments until 5 lbs can be lifted.

When supine elevation can be completed for 10 repetitions with 5 lbs, upright eccentric elevation is begun. Have the patient sit in a sturdy chair. The patient should use the uninvolved arm to elevate the operative arm as far above the head as possible. The patient should balance the arm above the head without assistance, then *slowly* lower the arm while simultaneously flexing the elbow. When this can be completed 10 times, a ½-lb weight should be added to the hand or wrist. The weight should be increased in ½-lb increments each time 10 repetitions can be completed. Weight should be increased until the patient can do 10 repetitions with 5 lbs. This type of submaximal eccentric exercise may stress the healing tissues less than maximal concentric exercise.

When the patient can complete 10 repetitions of the upright eccentric elevation exercise using 5 lbs of resistance, exercises using elastic tubing should be instituted. The elastic band or tubing exercises are not started initially because they introduce a chance of suddenly snapping back and causing injury. Exercises for shoulder flexion, extension, abduction, and internal and external rotation should be used. These are best done with the patient sitting in a sturdy chair. Flexion, extension, and rotation exercises are accomplished by looping the tubing around a nearby doorknob and positioning the patient appropriately. The abduction exercise is done by holding the tubing in both hands and stretching the operative arm away from the uninvolved arm. Have the patient pull the tubing as far as possible, hold for 5 seconds, then slowly return to the starting position. The patient should do 10 repetitions twice daily. These exercises should be continued indefinitely. Some patients may also require strengthening exercises aimed specifically at improving function of the scapulothoracic musculature.

SHOULDER PAIN IN HEMIPLEGIA

In the preface to his 1980 book, Cailliet stated, "The hemiplegic patient can improve his ambulation, communication, balance, and self-care through treatment, but in the overall picture of functional return, the shoulder remains an enigma."[11] Unfortunately, the intervening years have added little in the way of an understanding about the causes of and effective treatments for the painful hemiplegic shoulder. The purpose of this section is to review the incidence and suspected causes of and reported treatments for hemiplegic shoulder pain.

"Shoulder pain is probably the most frequent complication of hemiplegia."[12] In spite of this statement, reports about the incidence of this problem vary from 5 to 84%.[13] Operational definitions used for patient selection may account for these differences. For example, "pain," "tenderness," "mild shoulder discomfort," and "adhesive capsulitis" are all terms that have been used to identify patients with hemiplegic shoulder pain. Perhaps the definitive frequency study was conducted by Van Ouwenaller and colleagues. They followed 219 patients with cerebrovascular accident (CVA) for 1 year. The group found that 72% of patients had at least one incidence of shoulder pain during the recovery period.[12] This figure agrees exactly with later reports by Roy and colleagues[14] and by Bohannon and colleagues.[15] Roy and colleagues followed 76 patients for a period of 12 weeks after the onset of CVA. They found the greatest incidence of shoulder pain (24% at rest and 58% with movement) at 10 weeks after onset. The smallest incidence (12% at rest and 35% with movement) occurred during the first week after onset.

Table 22–4 Factors Associated with Hemiplegic Shoulder Pain

Factor	Statistically Significant
Prolonged hospital stay	x
Poor return of function	x
Glenohumeral subluxation	x
Reflex sympathetic dystrophy	x
Capsulitis	
Rotator cuff degeneration and tears	
Tendinitis	
Bursitis	
Spasticity	
Flaccidity	
Loss of external rotation ROM	x
Severity of CVA	
Time since onset of hemiplegia	x

Possible Mechanisms of Pain

The causes of hemiplegic shoulder pain are poorly understood. Some associated factors are listed in Table 22–4. Unfortunately, there is little empirical evidence to support or refute any of these suggested causes. Still, it appears that there is a statistically significant relationship between hemiplegic shoulder pain and the following associated factors: loss of external rotation ROM,[14,15] time since onset of hemiplegia,[15] prolonged hospital stay,[14] poor return of function,[14] glenohumeral subluxation,[14] and reflex sympathetic dystrophy.[14] It is important to note that "a statistically significant relationship" does not imply causality. Whether therapeutic interventions aimed at decreasing these suggested causes will reduce the incidence of hemiplegic shoulder pain remains to be proven.

In the absence of a clear understanding about the causes of hemiplegic shoulder pain, treatment should be directed by clinical observations. Evaluation and reevaluation of signs, symptoms, and responses to treatment interventions must continually be used to reformulate the treatment plan. Patients should be evaluated for signs of musculoskeletal problems (capsulitis, rotator cuff degeneration and tears, tendinitis, bursitis, and so forth). Treatment for such problems should be similar to treatment regimens used for nonhemiplegic patients who exhibit musculoskeletal shoulder problems. Preventing the loss of external rotation ROM as a result of capsulitis appears to be a particularly important therapeutic goal. The intelligent use of exercise and modalities should have a beneficial effect on musculoskeletal causes of hemiplegic shoulder pain.

Glenohumeral Subluxation

Glenohumeral subluxation as a cause of hemiplegic shoulder pain is a multidimensional problem. Theoretically, inferior subluxation places abnormal stresses on periarticular structures and leads to pain. The tension created by inferior subluxation can lead to ischemia, and ischemia is thought to cause inflammation and pain. One treatment approach suggests the use of various types of slings to reduce the glenohumeral subluxation. Although a sling can accomplish reduction, it may also delay return of voluntary muscle control. Because flaccidity is also a suspected cause of hemiplegic shoulder pain, the anticipated gains afforded by reduction of the subluxation may be derailed by a delay in the return of voluntary muscle control. Some slings are designed to reduce the subluxation while simultaneously allowing functional use of the extremity. These are preferable to slings that prevent voluntary use.

Another approach to the glenohumeral subluxation problem focuses on return of voluntary muscle control. The muscles that upwardly rotate the scapula (the trapezius and serratus anterior) and elevate the humeral head (the supraspinatus and deltoid) are the targets of this approach. The scapular muscles are important for maintaining a vertical position of the glenoid fossa. The humeral elevators can maintain the humeral head in the glenoid fossa as long as the fossa is not rotated downward. The requisite synergy between these muscle groups dictates that if any of these muscles is dysfunctional (flaccid or spastic), subluxation is likely to occur. Therapeutic interventions for this problem include exercise, electromyographic biofeedback, and functional electric stimulation. Interventions should be designed to restore normal voluntary control of these muscles.

Another issue worth mentioning is that of poor positioning and handling of the affected upper extremity. Although not established empirically, many feel that poor handling produces trauma and causes pain. This is thought to be more of a problem for patients with flaccid paralysis. Until proven otherwise, prudence dictates that health-care workers use the utmost care when positioning and handling the affected upper extremity. Also, the rapid restoration of voluntary motor control should be high on the list of therapeutic goals.

Hemiplegic shoulder pain is poorly understood. Possible treatment interventions are variable because of the lack of understanding about causes. Patients with hemiplegic shoulder pain should be evaluated for the presence of all of the suspected possible causes. Treatment should be directed at reducing possible causes that can be identified on a case-by-case basis.

CONCLUSION

Shoulder pain in elderly persons is a common cause of dysfunction and it requires appropriate treatment intervention. The choice of physical modalities and graded therapeutic exercise is related to the signs, symptoms, and temporal sequence of healing and rehabilitation. Education of the patient and communication with the orthopedist are important, especially after fracture or surgery. When treating the geriatric patient with shoulder dysfunction, the alignment of the trunk and the scapulae must be considered. With meticulous evaluation and treatment, there is good prognosis for recovery.

REFERENCES

1. Black JS, Agarwal AK, Rice EM. Painful shoulder in the elderly: a diagnostic challenge. *Emerg Med* 1991; 23:33.
2. Chakravarty K, Webley M. Shoulder joint movement and its relationship to disability in the elderly. *J Rheumatol* 1993; 20:8.
3. Cofield R. Rotator cuff disease of the shoulder. *J Bone Joint Surg* 1985; 67A:974.
4. Itoi T, Tabata S. Conservative treatment of rotator cuff tears. *Clin Orthop* 1992; 165:275.
5. McKinnis L. The shoulder joint complex. In: McKinnis L, ed. *Fundamentals of Orthopedic Radiology.* Philadelphia: F.A. Davis; 1997:325.
6. Skinner HB, Diao E, Gosselin R, et al. Musculoskeletal trauma surgery. In: Skinner HB, ed. *Current Diagnosis and Treatment in Orthopedics.* East Norwalk, Conn.: Appleton & Lange: 1995:51.
7. Malone TR, Waser-Richmond G, Frick JL. Shoulder pathology. In: Kelley MJ, Clark WA, eds. *Orthopedic Therapy of the Shoulder.* Philadelphia: J.B. Lippincott; 1995:104.
8. Iannotti JP, Williams GR. Diagnostic tests and surgical techniques. In Kelley MJ, Clark WA, eds. *Orthopedic Therapy of the Shoulder.* Philadelphia: J.B. Lippincott; 1995:185.
9. Wirth MA, Rochwood CA. Complications of shoulder arthroplasty. *Clin Orthop* 1994; 307:47.
10. Brems JJ. Rehabilitation following total shoulder arthroplasty. *Clin Orthop* 1994; 307:70.
11. Cailliet R. *The Shoulder in Hemiplegia.* Philadelphia: F.A. Davis; 1980.
12. Van Ouwenaller C, Laplace PM, Chantraine A. Painful shoulder in hemiplegia. *Arch of Phys Med Rehabil* 1986; 67:23.
13. Roy CW. Shoulder pain in hemiplegia: a literature review. *Clin Rehabil* 1988; 2:35.
14. Roy CW, Sands MR, Hill LD. Shoulder pain in acutely admitted hemiplegics. *Clin Rehabil* 1994; 8:334.
15. Bohannon RW, Larkin PA, Smith MB, et al. Shoulder pain in hemiplegia: statistical relationship with five variables. *Arch Phys Med Rehabil* 1986; 76:514.

Chapter **23**

Total Hip Replacement
Mark Brimer, Ph.D., P.T.

INTRODUCTION

The total hip replacement (THR) is an orthopedic procedure performed more than 120,000 times annually in the United States. The presence of severe and continuing pain and disability and the inability to perform one's job or participate in social and leisure activities generally make the decision to undergo the surgery easier for the patient and surgeon.

INDICATIONS FOR THR

The primary indications for a total hip replacement are:

- severe osteoarthritis
- rheumatoid arthritis
- avascular necrosis
- traumatic arthritis
- certain hip fractures
- benign and malignant bone tumors
- arthritis associated with Paget's disease
- ankylosing spondylitis
- juvenile rheumatoid arthritis.

There are relatively few contraindications to the total hip replacement procedure other than active local or systemic infection and other medical conditions that increase the risk of perioperative complications or death. Hemiarthroplasty, or partial reconstruction of the hip, is performed when the acetabular cartilage is intact and joint pathology is limited to the femoral side of the joint.

Previously, obesity had been considered a contraindication to surgery because of a reported high mechanical failure rate in heavier patients. The prospect of long-term reduction in pain and disability for heavier patients may, however, offset the risk associated with potential mechanical failure.

Data indicate that 62% of all THR procedures performed in the United States are performed in women, with two-thirds of those procedures being performed in persons older than 65 years of age. The highest age-specific rate of THR in men is between the ages of 65 and 74 years. For women, the highest age-specific rate is between 75 and 84 years.

If the patient desires to undergo bilateral hip

replacement sequentially, it is recommended that he or she wait at least 6 weeks between operations to avoid increased risk of complications from the presence of an occult venous thrombus from the first procedure. Otherwise, the bilateral procedure poses no increase in frequency of postoperative complications.

Historically, aseptic loosening of implanted components was identified as a major problem with THR. This problem was especially prevalent in younger and more active patients and in those who had undergone revision surgery. In the past 2 decades, however, the number of complications involving mechanical loosening has declined significantly. The incidence of mechanical loosening has decreased, as a result of improved fixation techniques, to the point where more than 90% of all total joints are never revised.

THE SURGICAL APPROACH FOR THR

The primary surgical approaches used for THR are the anterolateral and the posterior approaches. The choice of surgical approach often depends upon the surgical training of the physician. Many of the difficulties associated with using the anterolateral approach are related to the anterior third of the gluteus medius muscle, which partially obstructs the insertion of the stem of the component into the femur. This has become a more critical element with the introduction of cementless technology. The anterolateral approach does, however, provide excellent exposure of the acetabulum, which is why some surgeons prefer that approach.

Regardless of the approach taken, difficulties are occasionally encountered. When using the posterior approach, there is a tendency to place the femoral component in less than normal anteversion, thereby leading to less postoperative external rotation because of the presence of an intact anterior capsule. A patient who undergoes the anterolateral approach commonly demonstrates less internal rotation postoperatively and a weaker hip abductor that is associated with surgical interference with the function of the abductor muscle.

The Cement and Noncement Techniques

There are two available surgical mechanisms that can be used to properly secure the acetabular and femoral stem components. The cement technique adheres one or both of the replacement components to the surface of the bone with the use of polymethylmethacrylate bone cement. The cementless technique relies upon bone growth into porous or onto roughened surfaces for fixation.

The choice of which component to use with a particular patient may be based upon the individual's level of strenuous physical activity, age, health and well-being, and bone density. Surgical revision of both component types, as evaluated by the use of modern techniques, has been reported to be less than 5% for the cemented femoral component over a 10-year period. The number of uncemented acetabular components requiring revision in a 7-year follow-up is approximately 2%.

Of primary concern in the cementless implants is the importance of the precise mechanism of load transfer to the bone. If the fit in the proximal femur is too loose and the distal end is too tight, then the proximal part of the component will be stress-shielded which could cause increased porosity or bone loss. If the proximal segment is well fitted but the distal end underfills the medullary cavity, then the patient may exhibit distal toggling while under load, which causes persistent thigh pain.

REHABILITATION

Inpatient Postoperative Rehabilitation Considerations

The primary concern following THR is to have the patient begin to walk. Patients with uncomplicated THRs are generally encouraged to ambulate beginning on postoperative day 1. Although ambulation may be brief in duration, the role of the therapist is to encourage mobility, self-care, and proper weight-bearing and gait and to teach the patient how to get into and out of bed in the proper manner. (See Table 23–1 for gait training and ROM guidelines.)

In the initial stages, most orthopedic surgeons recommend that the patient not exceed 90 degrees of hip flexion after surgery. Especially if the posterior approach has been used, it is important to instruct the patient to avoid internal rotation and adduction of the hip. Any of these motions, singularly or in combination, may produce a dislocation of the replacement. The complication of hip dislocation is more likely to occur in a patient who presents with a neurological disorder or is mentally confused. A common mechanism to prevent dislocation is the use of an abduction pillow. Abduction pillows are, as a general rule, used for a 1-month period or until sufficient scar tissue build-up can be seen on x-ray (Box 23–1).

The hospital rehabilitation department that is preparing the patient for home or skilled-nursing placement should address the environment in which the patient will be placed. For example, a patient

Table 23–1 THR Gait Training and ROM Guidelines

Arthroplasty	Conventional (Cemented THR)	Bipolar Osteonics Ingrowth	Porous Coated	Trochanteric Osteotomy[a]
Mobilize (out of bed)	Postoperative day (POD) 1–2	POD 2	POD 2	POD 2–5
Ambulation weight-bearing	Partial weight-bearing (PWB) to weight-bearing as tolerated at discharge	(Porous coated stem, bipolar head) PWB 40–50 lbs	PWB 40–50 lbs	PWB
Range of motion of hip flexion	Same criteria for all: POD 2 up to 30 degrees, POD 4–6 up to 60 degrees, POD 6–10 up to 90 degrees			
Precautions	Applies to all: Avoid dislocation forces at hip, which are a combination of hip flexion, adduction, and internal rotation; no hip flexion greater than 90 degrees No resisted abduction of hip Initially walk with a slightly abducted gait			

[a]No active abduction.

From K. Lawrence, orthopedic team supervisor of Physical Therapy Department, Medical College of Virginia, Richmond, Va., with permission.

Box 23–1

THR Postoperative Concerns

Therapists are advised to individualize these programs by adding or subtracting exercises depending on the patient's postoperative condition. Additional preoperative instructions to the patient may address the following immediate postoperative concerns:

1. Most THR procedures require the presence of an abduction pillow or wedge placed between the legs when the patient is in bed or in a wheelchair.

2. Patients are cautioned not to exceed 90 degrees of flexion of the operative hip.

3. Passive or forcible movement of the hip that causes pain is contraindicated.

4. Internal rotation and adduction are contraindicated.

5. The patient is encouraged to perform active ankle exercises (rhythmic active dorsal and plantar flexion) frequently during the first few days postoperatively to prevent thrombophlebitis.

6. No weight-bearing or standing should take place unless under the direct supervision of the physical therapist.

7. Transfers and log-rolling should be performed away from the operative side, with the leg supported by a staff member.

From Echternach J. *Physical Therapy of the Hip.* New York: Churchill Livingstone; 1990.

Box 23–2

Home Care Instructions for THR Patients

FIRST 6 WEEKS POSTOPERATIVELY

DO NOT	DO
DO NOT sit in low chairs or sofas.	DO use help for putting on shoes and stockings.
DO NOT cross your legs.	DO use your compression stockings.
DO NOT force your operated leg to flex (bend) or rotate at the hip.	DO exercise as instructed.
DO NOT sit down on the floor of a bath tub.	DO sleep on your back.
DO NOT lean forward or raise your knee higher than your hip.	DO place a pillow between your knees when sitting or sleeping.
DO NOT discard the walking assistive device until instructed to do so.	DO use caution when sitting and reaching toward floor or toward phone/table on operative side. These motions encourage hip flexion and adduction, which are motions to be protected on the operative side.
DO NOT drive until permitted.	
DO NOT force hip abduction, external rotation, or extension if your doctor has performed an anterolateral surgical approach.	DO use caution getting into and out of bed and on and off of toilet seat. Avoid hip adduction, internal rotation, and flexion beyond 90° if your doctor has performed a posterolateral approach.

Box 23–3

Self-Administered Hip-Rating Questionnaire

Which hip is affected by arthritis? (Circle one)
    Left   Right   Both

Please answer the following questions about the hip(s) you have just indicated.

1. Considering all of the ways that your hip arthritis affects you, mark an X on the scale to indicate how well you are doing.

    0   25   50   75   100
    very well   well   fair   poor   very poor

    Circle one response for each question. (The score here is determined by subtracting the number marked from 100, with the number being interpolated if the mark is between printed numbers. The result is divided by 4, and the answer is rounded off to the nearest integer. The maximum is 25 points.)

2. During the post month, how would you describe the usual arthritis pain in your hip? (maximum, 10 points)
   A) Very severe (2 points)
   B) Severe (4 points)
   C) Moderate (6 points)
   D) Mild (8 points)
   E) Not present (10 points)

3. During the past month, how often have you had to take medication for your arthritis? (maximum, 5 points)
   A) Always (1 point)
   B) Very often (2 points)
   C) Fairly often (3 points)
   D) Sometimes (4 points)
   E) Never (5 points)

Box 23-3

Self-Administered Hip-Rating Questionnaire *Continued*

4. During the past month, how often have you had severe arthritis pain in your hip? (maximum, 5 points)
   A) Every day (1 point)
   B) Several days per week (2 points)
   C) One day per week (3 points)
   D) One day per month (4 points)
   E) Never (5 points)

5. How often have you had hip arthritis pain at rest, either sitting or lying down? (maximum, 5 points)
   A) Every day (1 point)
   B) Several days per week (2 points)
   C) One day per week (3 points)
   D) One day per month (4 points)
   E) Never (5 points)

6. How far can you walk without resting because of your hip arthritis pain? (maximum, 15 points)
   A) Unable to walk (3 points)
   B) Less than one city block (6 points)
   C) 1 to <10 city blocks (9 points)
   D) 10 to 20 city blocks (12 points)
   E) Unlimited (15 points)

7. How much assistance do you need for walking? (maximum, 10 points)
   A) Unable to walk (1 point)
   B) Walk only with someone's help (2 points)
   C) Two crutches or walker every day (3 points)
   D) Two crutches or walker several days per week (4 points)
   E) Two crutches or walker once per week or less (5 points)
   F) Cane or one crutch every day (6 points)
   G) Cane or one crutch several days per week (7 points)
   H) Cane or one crutch once per week (8 points)
   I) Cane or one crutch once per month (9 points)
   J) No assistance (10 points)

8. How much difficulty do you have going up or down one flight of stairs because of your hip's arthritis? (maximum 5 points)
   A) Unable (1 point)
   B) Require someone's assistance (2 points)
   C) Require crutch or cane (3 points)
   D) Require banister (4 points)
   E) No difficulty (5 points)

9. How much difficulty do you have putting on your shoes and socks because of your hip arthritis? (maximum, 5 points)

   A) Unable (1 point)
   B) Require someone's assistance (2 points)
   C) Require long shoehorn and reacher (3 points)
   D) Some difficulty but no devices required (4 points)
   E) No difficulty (5 points)

10. Are you able to use public transportation? (maximum 3 points)
    A) No, because of my hip arthritis (1 point)
    B) No, for some other reason (2 points)
    C) Yes, (3 points)

11. When you bathe—either a sponge bath or in a tub or shower—how much help do you need? (maximum, 3 points)
    A) No help at all (3 points)
    B) Help with bathing one part of your body, like back or leg (2 points)
    C) Help with bathing more than one part of your body (1 point)

12. If you had the necessary transportation, could you go shopping for groceries or clothes? (maximum, 3 points)
    A) Without help (taking care of all shopping needs yourself) (3 points)
    B) With some help (need someone to go with you to help on all shopping trips) (2 points)
    C) Completely unable to do any shopping (1 point)

13. If you had household tools and appliances (vacuum, mops, and so on), could you do your own housework? (maximum, 3 points)
    A) Without help (can clean floors, windows, refrigerators, and so on) (3 points)
    B) With some help (can do light housework, but need help with some heavy work) (2 points)
    C) Completely unable to do housework (1 point)

14. How well are you able to move around? (maximum 3 points)
    A) Able to get in and out of bed or chairs without the help of another person (3 points)
    B) Need the help of another person to get in and out of bed or chair (2 points)
    C) Not able to get out of bed (1 point)

This is the end of the Hip-rating Questionnaire. Thank you for your cooperation.

Johanson NA, Charlson ME, Szatrowski TP, et al. A self-administered hip-rating questionnaire for the assessment of outcome after total hip replacement. *J Bone Joint Surg* 1992; 74A: 587–597.

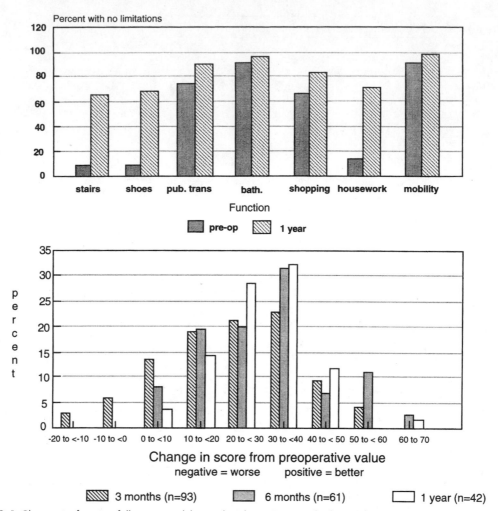

Figure 23-1 Change in function following total hip arthroplasty. Top graph shows changes in ADL. Bottom graph shows changes in functional scores at 3, 6, and 12 months postoperatively. (From Johanson NA, Charlson ME, Szatrowski TP, et al. A self-administered hip-rating questionnaire for the assessment of outcome after total hip replacement. *J Bone Joint Surg* 1992;74A: 587–597.)

returning home should be thoroughly informed about the proper use of an elevated toilet seat, the possibility of encountering steps or stairs, and how to deal with carpeted surfaces and the surfaces encountered outside the home. It is particularly important that a patient understand the proper positions for sleeping and what types of chairs are considered too low for comfortable and safe seating. A patient who plans return visits to the physician in the office must be instructed on how to properly enter, sit in, and exit from a car to avoid excessive hip flexion.

Activities of daily living should be discussed with the patient and immediate care-givers. Because a large majority of THR procedures are performed in the geriatric population, special consideration should be given to visual, balance, and endurance losses that may have occurred. A patient should be encouraged to use safe ambulation procedures until outpatient rehabilitation gait training needs can be addressed.

Outpatient and Home Health-Care Rehabilitation Considerations

In the outpatient, or home health-care, environment, the focus is on restoring normal activities of daily living and safe walking techniques (Box 23–2). In the initial stages (0–6 weeks), the patient should be advised to follow all dislocation precautions. These include the avoidance of excessive hip flexion and, in the case of the posterior approach, adduction and internal rotation. The patient should continue the use of elevated chairs and toilet seats until cleared by the surgeon to do otherwise.

In the 6 weeks following surgery, rehabilitation should focus on hip abduction and mild hip flexor and extensor strength. The patient may progress to walking with full weight-bearing, as ordered by the physician. A patient who has undergone the cementless technique may be required to maintain limited weight-bearing until sufficient new bone growth can be seen by the physician on x-ray.

Desired Rehabilitation Outcomes for the THR Patient

Most patients who undergo THR require limited outpatient physical therapy once a normal gait pattern can be resumed. The use of home programs as well as general conditioning exercises allow the patient to resume normal activities quickly. Gait may progress from using a walker to using a cane and then to using no assistive devices, as tolerated by the patient. Differences in leg length should be assessed and a shoe insert recommended if gait abnormalities persist. Once component stability has been obtained and dislocation potential has lessened, many surgeons encourage their patients to gain additional range of motion in the hip. Patients are generally encouraged to resume physical activities such as golf, tennis, bicycle riding, and walking in moderation.

The Self-Administered Hip-Rating Questionnaire shown in Box 23–3 has been used to assess patients' perspectives on outcomes after THR. As can be seen in Figure 23–1, most benefits were obtained in 6 months, and some favorable changes took place after 6 months. The greatest functional improvements occurred in stair climbing, wearing normal shoes, and performing housework well.

CONCLUSION

When rehabilitating a patient who has received a THR, it is important to understand the specific procedures and to implement properly the specific guidelines for mobility, weight-bearing, and range of motion. Normal recovery timelines and progressions must be followed, with special attention to physician recommendations. Favorable functional outcomes are expected in 6 to 12 months.

SUGGESTED READINGS

Garvin K, Hanssen A. Current concepts review: infection after total hip arthroplasty, past, present, future. *J Bone Joint Surg* 1995;77:1576–1588.

National Institutes of Health. Consensus Conference. Total hip replacement. *JAMA* 1995;273:1950–1956.

Neuman L, Freund K, Sorensen K. Total hip arthroplasty with the Charnley prosthesis in patients fifty-five years old or less. *J Bone Joint Surg* 1996;78:73–79.

Peters C, Rivero D, Kull L, Jacobs J, Rosenberg A, Galante J. Revision total hip arthroplasty without cement: subsidence of proximally porous-coated femoral components. *J Bone Joint Surg* 1995;77:1217–1226.

Chapter **24**

Total Knee Replacement
Mark Brimer, Ph.D., P.T.

INTRODUCTION

Total knee replacement (TKR), also referred to as total knee arthroplasty (TKA), is one of the most common surgical procedures performed for patients with advanced arthritis of the knee. Although there are well over 150 brand-name implants currently on the market and available for use, they may be divided into three categories: the linked prosthesis, the resurfacing implant, and the conforming implant.

THE THREE CATEGORIES OF IMPLANTS

In the linked prosthesis, the femoral and tibial components are physically fastened together at the time of manufacture or at some point during the surgical procedure. The linked prosthesis may be fully constrained, thereby permitting only flexion and extension, or it may permit flexion, extension, and limited axial rotation. Used primarily in the 1970s, the linked prosthesis is no longer commonly used because of the loosening of components that occurs when stresses are applied to the tibial side of the joint. They may, however, be appropriate for patients who have markedly unstable knees or after failure of one or more previous arthroplasties.

A resurfacing implant has a flat polyethylene tibial surface that articulates with the metallic femoral condylar component. A resurfacing implant requires proper balancing of the collateral and cruciate ligaments and, therefore, is not indicated in a case in which either the cruciate or the collateral ligament is absent or deficient. Because a large number of patients with advanced arthritis have a missing or attenuated cruciate ligament and compromised soft-tissue balancing, which is necessary for the procedure to succeed, resurfacing implants are not the primary choice of many physicians.

A conforming implant consists of a metallic femoral condylar component and a polyethylene tibial component. Designed to resist some of the translatory and shear stresses, they currently are used in 95% of all TKR procedures. The design of the conforming implant requires surgical sacrifice of the anterior cruciate ligament and, in some cases, depending upon the design of the particular implant, of the posterior cruciate ligament as well. The posterior cruciate is almost always removed in cases in which the patient presents a fixed varus or valgus contracture of 15 to 20 degrees and the associated fixed flexion deformity.

FIXATION OF THE IMPLANT

Surgical fixation of all of the knee components is accomplished through one of two methods. The first involves the use of polymethylmethacrylate bone cement; one or both of the components are cemented to the bony surfaces. In the second method, the implants are inserted and one or both of the components are attached in a cementless manner. Although cemented knee components are still utilized, the preferred mechanism for attachment is cementless. Some of the problems that have been identified with the use of cemented components include the following:

1. The polymethylmethacrylate bone cement is known to be brittle. If the cement fragments in the joint, it can become trapped between components, which results in excessive component wear.

2. As the polymethylmethacrylate hardens, it is known to become thermotoxic to adjacent bony cells. It has also been known to decrease leukotaxis and thereby increase the risk of infection at the implant site.

3. The use of bone cement is known to make surgical revision more difficult.

The cementless technique relies upon bone growth into porous or roughened surfaces for firm fixation. Proper and precise surgical placement of cementless components is essential if firm component attachment is to be obtained. Studies indicate that bone will not grow across gaps greater than 1 to 2 mm.

The choice of component may be based upon the patient's level of strenuous physical activity, age, health and well-being, and bone density. The primary contraindication to the use of cementless components is severe osteoporosis.

Monitoring for potential infection is particularly important in TKR because a large amount of foreign material has been implanted in a superficial joint. Although a TKR is a relatively safe orthopedic procedure, wound-healing difficulties can occasion-ally be seen, including problems such as marginal wound necrosis, skin sloughing, sinus tract formation, and hematoma formation. The presence of any of these complications may adversely affect the outcome. This is especially true with regard to range of motion in cases in which therapy must be stopped until the problem can be resolved.

REHABILITATION

Inpatient Postoperative Rehabilitation Considerations

The primary concern after a TKR is to see that the patient begins to walk. A patient with an uncomplicated TKR is generally encouraged to walk on postoperative day 1, even if ambulation time is brief. The role of the therapist is to encourage mobility, self-care, proper weight-bearing and gait, and getting into and out of bed in the proper manner.

During the first few days after surgery, many surgeons ask their patients to use a continuous passive motion device (CPM) to maximize range-of-motion results. These devices are used in conjunction with physical therapy exercises and range-of-motion and gait-training sessions two or three times a day. Patients are often encouraged to remain in the CPM device unless attending a physical therapy session or resting.

When a hospital rehabilitation department is preparing a patient to go home or to a skilled-nursing facility, staff members should consider the environment into which the patient is being discharged. For example, a patient returning home should be thoroughly trained in how to negotiate steps and flights of stairs, carpeted surfaces, and surfaces that might be encountered outside the home. It is particularly important that the patient understand the proper positioning of the knee during sleep in order to prevent unwanted contractures.

Performance of the activities of daily living should be discussed with the patient and the immediate care-givers. Because a large majority of TKR procedures are performed in members of the geriatric population, special attention should be paid to any impairments in vision, balance, or endurance that may have occurred. Patients should be encouraged to monitor the integrity of the wound site on a daily basis and to use safe ambulation procedures until outpatient gait-training needs can be addressed.

Outpatient and Home Health-Care Rehabilitation Considerations

In the outpatient or home health-care rehabilitation environment, the focus is on restoring the ability to

Box 24–1

Knee Society Clinical Rating System

Patient Category
  A. Unilateral or bilateral (opposite knee successfully replaced)
  B. Unilateral, other knee symptomatic
  C. Multiple arthritis or medical infirmity

PAIN	POINTS	FUNCTION	POINTS
None	50	Walking	
Mild or occasional	45	Unlimited	50
Stairs only	40	> 10 blocks	40
Walking and stairs	30	5–10 blocks	30
Moderate		< 5 blocks	20
Occasional	20	Housebound	10
Continual	10	Unable	0
Severe	0	Stairs	
Range of motion		Normal up and down	50
(5 degrees = 1 point)	25	Normal up; down with rail	40
Stability (maximum movement in any position)		Up and down with rail	30
Anteroposterior		Up with rail; unable down	15
< 5 mm	10	Unable	0
5–10 mm	5	Subtotal	____
10 mm	0	Deduction (minus)	
Mediolateral		Cane	5
< 5 degrees	15	Two canes	10
6–9 degrees	10	Crutches or walker	20
10–14 degrees	5	Total deductions	____
15 degrees	0	Function score	____
Subtotal	____		
Deductions (minus)			
Flexion contracture			
5–10 degrees	2		
10–15 degrees	5		
16–20 degrees	10		
> 20 degrees	15		
Extension lag			
< 10 degrees	5		
10–20 degrees	10		
> 20 degrees	15		
Alignment			
5–10 degrees	0		
0–4 degrees	3 points each degree		
11–15 degrees	3 points each degree		
Other	20		
Total deductions	____		
Knee score	____		
(If total is a minus number, score is 0.)			

Insall JN, Dorr LD, Scott RD, et al. Rationale of the knee society clinical rating system. *Clin Orthop* 1989; 248:13–14.

perform normal activities of daily living, range of motion (ROM) of the knee, and teaching safe ambulation. In the initial stages (0 to 4 weeks) it is vital to maximize range of motion. Functional range of motion is considered to be between 110 and 120 degrees of flexion and full extension. Patients should be actively involved in home programs that focus upon the prevention of flexion or extension contractures of the knee.

In the period between 0 and 4 weeks after surgery, rehabilitation should focus upon strength gains in the quadriceps, hamstring, hip flexor, and hip extensor muscles. The patient may be allowed to progress to walking with full weight-bearing, as indicated by the physician. A patient who has undergone the cementless technique may be required to maintain limited weight-bearing for a period of 4 to 6 weeks or until sufficient new bone growth can be seen by the physician on an X-ray.

Desired Rehabilitation Outcomes for the TKR Patient

Patients who undergo TKR commonly require extensive outpatient physical therapy for a period of approximately 6 weeks in order to maximize ROM. Swelling may persist for several months until sufficient collateral circulation can develop. The use of home ROM programs as well as general conditioning exercises allow the patient to resume normal activities quickly. Strenuous exercise is to be avoided until approved of by the physician. A knee evaluation scale is shown in Box 24–1; it may be helpful in documenting postsurgical outcomes.

The patient may progress from using a walker to using a cane and then to ambulating with no assistive devices, as tolerated by the individual. Differences in leg length should be assessed and a shoe insert recommended if gait abnormalities persist. After several months, patients are often encouraged to resume in moderation physical activities such as golf, tennis, bicycle riding, and walking.

CONCLUSION

TKR is a surgical procedure commonly used in cases of advanced knee arthritis. There are many brand-name implants; they can be divided into three categories: linked prostheses, resurfacing implants, and conforming implants. The components of the knee replacement may be surgically fixed with bone cement, or a cementless technique can be used. Rehabilitation is similar after the use of both of these methods, but a patient who has had the cementless procedure may be limited in weight-bear-

ing for 4 to 6 weeks. Following discharge from the inpatient setting, continued rehabilitation should advance functional activities, restore normal ROM (110 to 120 degrees of flexion is desirable), and ensure safe walking. Normal physical activities can be resumed several months after the operation.

SUGGESTED READINGS

Falatyn S, Lachiewicz P, Wilson F. Survivorship analysis of cemented total condylar knee arthroplasty. *Clin Orthop* 1995; 317:208–215.

Malkani A, Rand J, Bryan R, Wallrichs S. Total knee arthroplasty with the kinematic condylar prosthesis: a ten-year follow-up study. *J Bone Joint Surg* 1995; 77A:423–431.

Vernereli P, Sutton D, Hearn S, Booth R, Hozack W, Rothman R. Continuous passive notion after total knee arthroplasty: analysis of cost and benefits. *Clin Orthop* 1995; 321:208–215.

Chapter 25

The Aging Bony Thorax
Jane K. Schroeder, M.A., P.T.

INTRODUCTION

The bony thorax has the primary function of protecting the organs of circulation and respiration. Some protection is also given to the liver and stomach. Secondarily, the muscles of respiration attach to the bony thorax and the ribs are mechanically involved in the mechanism of respiration. These elements are shown in Figure 25–1.

The thorax is composed of 12 thoracic vertebrae posteriorly, the sternum anteriorly, and 12 ribs, which encircle the thorax. The first 7 ribs are true ribs, with joints attaching them to the sternum and the thoracic vertebrae. Ribs 8 through 10 are false ribs, with joints connecting them to the thoracic vertebrae only. Anteriorly, there is no true attachment to the sternum, only a cartilaginous one. The last two ribs are floating ribs, with joints at the thoracic vertebrae and anterior ends that are unattached. These bony relationships are shown in Figures 25–2 and 25–3.

The sternum is composed of three parts—the manubrium, the body, and the xiphoid process—that are connected by fibrocartilage. The manubrium is the most superior and has notches for the clavicles. The body is a thin, flexible bone and is the part used for closed cardiac compression. The xiphoid process is attached to the distal part of the body.

Each rib has a small head at the posterior end

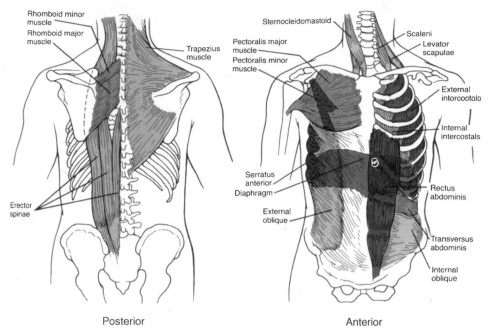

Figure 25-1 Muscles of ventilation, posterior and anterior views. (From Starr JA. Pulmonary system. In: Sgarlat-Myers R, ed. Saunders Manual of Physical Therapy Practice. Philadelphia: W.B. Saunders; 1995: 259.)

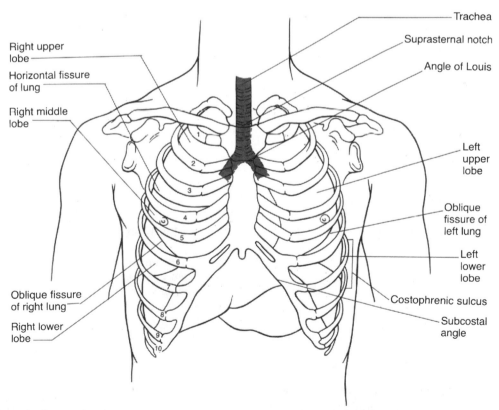

Figure 25-2 The bones of the thorax, anterior view. (From Starr JA. Pulmonary system. In: Sgarlat-Myers R, ed. Saunders Manual of Physical Therapy Practice. Philadelphia: W.B. Saunders; 1995: 254.)

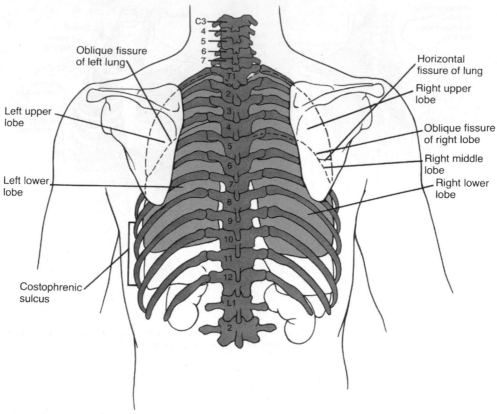

Figure 25–3 The bones of the thorax, posterior view. (From Starr JA. Pulmonary system. In: Sgarlat-Myers R, ed. Saunders Manual of Physical Therapy Practice. Philadelphia: W.B. Saunders; 1995: 254.)

that presents upper and lower facets divided by a crest. Each facet articulates with the adjacent vertebral body. The next part of the rib, the tubercle, articulates with the transverse process of the corresponding vertebra. The shaft of the rib curves gently from the neck to a sudden sharp bend called the angle of the rib. Each rib is separated from the others by an intercostal space that houses the intercostal muscles. On the lower border of each rib there is a costal groove. This groove provides protection for the costal nerve and blood vessels.

KINESIOLOGY

Mechanics of the Ribs

There are two kinds of rib movements. The pump-handle type is noted at the upper ribs, where movement is limited by joint articulations anteriorly and posteriorly. When these upper ribs move upward, because of the costosternal joints, the sternum is thrust forward and glides upward. This movement increases the anteroposterior diameter and depth of the thorax.

The lower ribs swing outward and upward during inspiration, each pushing against the rib above. This movement increases the transverse diameter of the thoracic cage. The movement is similar to a bucket-handle movement and is given this name. These two movements greatly increase the volume of the thorax, which creates the negative pressure responsible for air exchange.

Muscles of the Thorax

The primary muscle of respiration is the large dome-shaped diaphragm that separates the thoracic and abdominal cavities. It has two halves, each of which has attachments to the sternum at the posterior aspect of the xiphoid process.

The costal parts of the diaphragm arise from the inner surfaces of the four lower ribs and the lower six costal cartilages. These interdigitate and transverse the abdomen to insert into a central tendon. There is also a lumbar part that arises from the bodies of the upper lumber vertebrae and extends upward to the central tendon.

The intercostal muscles arise from the tubercles

Table 25–1 Muscles of Respiration: Their Innervations and Functions

Muscle (Innervation)	Functions
Inspiratory Muscles	
Diaphragm (C_{3-5})	Expands thorax vertically and horizontally; essential for normal vital capacity and effective cough
Intercostals (T_{1-12})	Anterior and lateral expansion of upper and lower chest
Sternocleidomastoid (cranial nerve XI and C_{1-4})	When head is fixed, elevates sternum to expand chest superiorly and anteriorly
Scalenes (C_{3-8})	When neck is fixed, elevate first two ribs to expand chest superiorly
Serratus anterior (C_{5-7})	When scapulae are fixed, elevates first 8–9 ribs to provide posterior expansion of thorax
Pectoralis major (C_5–T_1)	When arms are fixed, elevates true ribs to expand chest anteriorly
Pectoralis minor (C_{6-8})	When scapulae are fixed, elevates third, fourth, and fifth ribs to expand chest laterally
Trapezius (cranial nerve XI and C_{3-4})	Stabilizes scapulae to assist the serratus anterior and pectoralis minor in elevating the ribs
Erector spinae (C_1 down)	Extend the vertebral column to allow further rib elevation
Expiratory Muscles	
Abdominals (T_{5-12})	Help force diaphragm back to resting position and depress and compress lower thorax leading to higher intrathoracic pressure, which is essential for effective cough
Internal intercostals (T_{1-12})	Depress third, fourth, and fifth ribs to aid in forceful expiration

From Watchie J: *Cardiopulmonary Physical Therapy.* Philadelphia: W.B. Saunders Company; 1995.

of the ribs and travel above, down, and forward to the costochondral junction of the ribs below, where they become continuous with the anterior intercostal membrane. The membrane then extends forward to the sternum. These 11 external and 11 internal intercostals along with the erector spinae, rectus abdominus, internal oblique abdominals, and transverse abdominals also contribute to respiration. The specific muscles and their innervations and functions are listed in Table 25–1.

PATHOLOGIES INVOLVING THE BONY THORAX

Obstructive Lung Diseases

Obstructive lung diseases cause an overinflated state in the lungs. The thoracic cage tends to assume the inspiratory position and the diaphragm becomes low and flat. The anteroposterior (AP) and transverse diameters of the chest are increased and the ribs and sternum are always in a state of partial or complete expansion.

Restrictive Lung Diseases

In restrictive lung diseases, the lungs are prevented from fully expanding because of restrictions in the lung tissue, pleurae, muscles, ribs or sternum. The AP and transverse diameters of the chest should increase with inspiration but do not increase to normal levels in these conditions. Interstitial fibrosis, sarcoidosis, and pneumoconiosis are examples of disease processes that decrease elasticity (or compliance) of the lung tissue.

Tumors or abnormalities in the pleural tissue, such as pleurisy, pleuritis, and pleural effusion, cause compression of the lungs. Any condition that elevates the diaphragm and prevents full excursion of this muscle diminishes the ability of the chest to expand, for example, ascites, obesity, and abdominal tumors of any kind.

Numerous musculoskeletal conditions cause disturbed respiratory mechanics. The autoimmune (collagen) diseases can affect any joint in the body, including the costochondral and costovertebral joints. Additionally, these are systemic diseases and thus can also involve the pleural or lung tissue. Rheumatoid arthritis, systemic lupus erythematosus, and scleroderma are examples. Other, less severe forms of autoimmune disease such as fibromyalgia and dermatomyositis may affect the musculature and can cause pain and restriction of the myofascial structures and thereby limit chest expansion. Costochondritis (Tietze's syndrome) is an inflammatory condition of the costochondral tissue that can be viral or secondary to strain or can occur for unknown reasons. The symptom of chest pain can occur with this condition and be mistaken for a myocardial infarction. An effusion of the costosternal joint may be mistaken for a painful lump found during self-breast examination.

Orthopedic conditions such as kyphosis, scoliosis, and kyphoscoliosis affect primarily the vertebral segments and the costovertebral articulations. Even with mild changes of spine alignment, the mechanics of the ribs and sternum are altered. In severe cases, the lung tissue, heart, and major vessels may be compromised by the deformity and altered mechanics.

Ankylosing spondylitis can be considered in the autoimmune and orthopedic categories. It is considered separately here because of the severe consequences it can have on the thorax. In this condition, there is gradual fusion of spinal zygapophyseal joints, starting usually in the sacroiliac joints. As more and more of the spine becomes involved, x-rays demonstrate a bamboo-like image (bamboo spine). There is a calcification of the spinal segments as well as of the costovertebral joint, which causes severe restriction of chest expansion.

Trauma, accidental or surgical, can cause muscle splinting which may restrict chest expansion or relaxation. After thoracic and cardiovascular surgery there is a tendency for the patient to breathe in a shallow, rapid, and guarded manner, usually not using the diaphragm but, rather, accessory muscles such as the scalenes and sternocleidomastoid. Even after healing often the posture of such patients has changed and shows an increase in thoracic kyphosis, severe adduction of the shoulders, protraction of the entire shoulder girdle, and a marked forward-thrust head.

Another type of trauma to the thorax that is not often considered is injury that occurs in a motor vehicle accident. If the person is using a seat belt/shoulder strap type of restraint at the time of the accident, the shoulder strap may cause damage to the thoracic fascial structures, muscles, or sternum and ribs, as well as fractures. However, soft-tissue and joint injuries are often overlooked even though they may contribute to painful postural and respiratory dysfunction.

When muscular, fascial, spinal, rib, or sternal components are the cause of restriction of lung capacity, the patient may benefit from physical therapy which can improve the mechanics and lower the pain factor, thus improving quality of life in spite of the underlying disease process.

ASSESSMENT

History is very important. Understanding the underlying disease process or mechanism of trauma can help in defining the problem list and the goals for a particular patient. Histories of the present illness as well as of past medical and surgical problems are vital to proper examination and treatment. Laboratory and radiographic data, medication lists, particularly pulmonary and cardiac drugs, and psychosocial information should be gathered.

Examination can be broken down into many components, starting with general appearance (Box 25–1). This consists of assessing level of consciousness, which can indicate adequacy of oxygenation of brain tissues. Body type is evaluated as normal, obese, or cachectic. An obese person has higher energy demands, even for simple activities. General appearance can also indicate whether the person is deconditioned. Also, some respiratory conditions are caused by excessive weight which can cause restriction of the diaphragm. The cachectic patient may have had weight loss associated with a carcinoma, or eating may take too much energy, so caloric intake becomes insufficient.

In evaluating posture, the therapist should note any spinal malalignment or unusual postures. The extremities are observed for nicotine stains (which indicate a history of heavy smoking), clubbing of the fingers or toes (a sign of cardiopulmonary or small bowel disease), swollen joints, tremors, and edema. Any of these parameters may indicate respiratory system impairment.

The color of the skin and face should be noted. A patient might show evidence of a bluish tinge to the mucous membranes or nail beds, indicating severe arterial oxygen desaturation. A plethoric facial color (red or ruddy) may indicate hypertension, while a cherry-red coloring may be a sign of carbon monoxide poisoning.

Posture should be noted initially, especially sitting and standing patterns. In a patient with chronic obstructive pulmonary disease (COPD), usually there is a forward-thrust head, increased kyphosis in the thoracic area, and adduction and protraction of the shoulder girdles. There may be elevation of the shoulders as well, if the accessory muscles of breathing are the primary respiratory muscles. With spinal curvature, there are changes in posture from the sagittal and frontal views. When trauma is the mechanism of dysfunction, any or all of the above can be seen, as well as changes related to joint dysfunction and muscle involvement.

Vital signs, including blood pressure, heart rate and rhythm, and respiratory rate and rhythm should be noted. It may be pertinent to assess these at rest and with exertion. Pulmonary function volumes and disease are described in Chapters 7 and 49. Pulmonary function might have to be assessed by means of spirometry. Respiratory patterns include factors such as rate and rhythm and use of particular mus-

Box 25–1

Steps in Clinical Assessment of Patients with Breathing Dysfunction

General appearance
- Level of consciousness
- Body type
    - Obese
    - Cachectic

Posture

Skin and color
- Face
- Fingers

Vital signs

Respiratory pattern
- Rate
- Rhythm
- Accessory muscles

Chest wall movement
- Axilla
- Xiphoid tip
- Lower costal border
- Quiet and maximal inhalation and exhalation

Range of motion
- Neck
- Upper extremity
- Trunk
- Lower extremity

Auscultation

Strength
- Trunk posture

Functional abilities
- Activities of daily living
- Gait

Palpation
- Skin
- Fascia
- Muscles

Joint mobility
- Costosternal
- Costovertebral
- Spinal

Psychosocial factors
- Patient's goals
- Family's goals

Chest wall excursion can be recorded taking circumferential measurements with a tape measure at the floor of the axillae, at the tip of the xiphoid, and at the lower costal border at the midaxillary line of the 10th rib. These measurements should be taken during quiet breathing for inspiration and expiration, as well as with maximum inspiration and forced expiration. These landmarks (or others of the therapist's choice) should be consistent and reproducible.

Auscultation, or listening to the breath sounds, is another important aspect of assessment. When possible, the patient should sit forward for this part of the examination. The anterior and middle lobes can best be auscultated at the front of the patient, whereas the posterior lobes are best heard at the patient's back. The patient should breathe in and out through an open mouth. A comparison of breath sounds in each segment of each lung should assess the intensity, pitch, and quality.

There is a system of nomenclature and it is helpful to use these standard terms. Quality is defined as absent, decreased, normal, or bronchial. If abnormal sounds are heard, they can be further described as crackles, rales, wheezes, or rhonchi. During vocalization, sounds can be normal, increased, or decreased. All the above can help to define the area of the chest and lungs involved in the pathology. One can also hear rubs from the pleura or from the pericardium. Crunches may indicate air in the medialstinal space. See Figure 25–4 for auscultation sites.

Range of motion (ROM) assessment, formal or functional, should include the head, neck, upper extremities, lower extremities, and trunk. Emphasis on specific areas may change depending on the pathology. However, as the neck, upper back, and shoulder girdles are consistently involved to a large degree, these areas must be accurately assessed on an ongoing basis. Flexibility is an important parameter to consider, especially that of the anterior chest muscles. The pectoralis major and minor, sternocleidomastoid, and scalenes may all be shortened or overused. Unless a normal length can be regained in these muscles, normalization of posture cannot occur.

Strength may also be specifically or functionally tested. In most cases, testing of functional strength is all that is necessary. However, when working on postural correction, it may be important to test specifically the trapezius, rhomboids, and rotator cuff muscles as well as neck and back extensors. Coordination among muscle groups should be examined.

It is extremely important to note functional abilities, as it is these activities that most concern outcome measures. Basics such as bed mobility, trans-

cles for respiration. When accessory muscles are used, the upper chest and neck muscles are moving and strained. Bracing postures or any unusual postures taken to assist breathing increase the work of breathing. The depth of inspiration and whether expiration is passive (as is normally expected at rest) or forced should be observed.

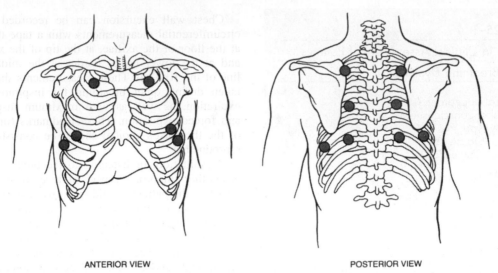

ANTERIOR VIEW   POSTERIOR VIEW

Figure 25–4 Anterior, lateral, and posterior auscultation sites. (From Starr JA. Pulmonary system. In: Sgarlat-Myers R, ed. Saunders Manual of Physical Therapy Practice. Philadelphia: W.B. Saunders; 1995: 270.)

fers, feeding, bathing, and toileting may be possible but higher-level activities such as housekeeping, food preparation, and shopping may be limited. Whatever the functional limitations, it is important to note them in measurable ways. Gait pattern, balance, endurance, and need of assistive devices should be evaluated. The ability to traverse a specific distance in a measured time clarifies functional mobility, which is so very important in persons who have to cross streets.

On palpation, skin, fascia, and muscles should be pliable and extensible, and each layer should be separate from the adjacent layers. With the absence of any of these qualities, movement at any or all layers or planes may be restricted and painful, thus creating guarding or spasm which may prevent normal joint kinematics and mobility.

Joint mobility can be restricted by surgical, traumatic, or soft-tissue conditions. The costosternal and costovertebral joints may be involved, which limits general mobility of the ribs in their upward and downward movements. The sternum can also be prevented from gliding by soft-tissue restriction or dysfunction of the sternoclavicular joints and acromioclavicular joints on one or both sides. To a lesser extent but still important are the spinal joints of the cervical and thoracic areas. The scapulothoracic joints may also affect the mobility of the ribs, and they certainly affect posture.

The joints can be assessed by passive mobility testing involving A–P, P–A springs at the costosternal, costovertebral, cervical, and thoracic segments. Monitoring the excursion of each rib anteriorly and/or laterally during inspiration and expiration demonstrates any dysfunctions. At the first rib, a distal

spring at the midpoint of the supraclavicular space and A–P and P–A springs can be used to assess mobility. Glides of the scapula in all planes detect disturbances of the scapulothoracic joints.

Psychosocial factors can affect a patient's condition, goals, treatment plan, and outcome measurements. The patient's family situation, the availability of a care-giver, and the type of dwelling should be recorded. The patient's and the family's reactions to the disease process may affect the pathology and the outcome, so it is important to allow the patient to discuss problems and concerns. It is to be hoped that the patient's and family's goals are congruent with those of the medical providers.

REHABILITATION INTERVENTION

Optimal breathing is performed by the diaphragm, with distal excursion on inspiration and return to baseline or elevation on expiration, normal or forced. This results in expansion of the lower chest and abdomen on inspiration and retraction in these areas on expiration. The person should be encouraged to inhale through the nose (to filter, warm, and moisturize the air) and to exhale through pursed lips to ensure the emptying of the alveoli.

Lateral costal expansion can also be promoted as this requires rib movement in a buckhandle fashion and may improve mobility. Use of tactile stimulation over the diaphragm or the lateral costal margins can facilitate the proper function. Resistance may also be performed by using weights on the diaphragm area or by resisting chest expansion with elastic exercise bands or tubing. When a specific area of the lungs is not expanding, segmental breathing exercises may be useful. Again, tactile stimulation may provide the sensory input that will promote increased expansion at the area.

In conjunction with proper breathing techniques, postural correction exercises can assist with more efficient breathing patterns. However, in the case of chronic cardiopulmonary diseases, postural changes may have occurred to assist air exchange and if so, those corrections can be detrimental to the patient's overall condition. Each case must be considered on an individual basis.

In order to improve posture, several factors must be considered. Some muscles will have shortened, whereas others will have overstretched and weakened. Joints may have lost passive mobility in one or several planes. Body awareness and proprioception may be impaired, so high patient motivation and a long-time commitment to exercise and awareness are necessary. ROM, strengthening, and flexibility exercises are vital for postural changes, functional improvements, and general well-being. All areas of the body should be considered, but practicality stresses exercises for the most severely involved areas. When pulmonary disease is present, the ability of the muscles to extract oxygen can be enhanced by strengthening exercises. This improved extraction of oxygen allows the patient better efficiency and endurance during routine activities.

Strengthening exercises may include any or all of the following: active ROM, progressive resistive exercises with gradually increasing weight and repetition, and use of exercise equipment, such as a bicycle ergometer, treadmill, rowing machine, or ski machine. Proprioceptive neuromuscular facilitation exercises and closed-chain activities or functional activities with increasing time and difficulty can enhance strength and fitness.

For patients with musculoskeletal conditions in the thoracic or rib area, physical therapy modalities including heat, cold, ultrasound, and electric stimulation may be indicated (see Chapters 68 and 69).

If, during the evaluation, restriction of skin, fascia, or muscle is identified, manual techniques may be used to regain tissue extensibility. Treatment techniques are identified by many different names, but the goals of all such techniques are the same—to improve the extensibility of tissues and to allow one layer to move separately from adjacent layers.

Mobilization of the joints may be necessary in order to recover full ROM, full flexibility, and correct posture. The first rib as well as the costosternal and costovertebral joints can be mobilized by A–P, P–A spring and distal glide mobilizations in grades I through IV, depending on the patient's condition

and tolerance. Mobilization techniques used on the ribs can encourage elevation or depression.

CONCLUSION

The bony thorax is often overlooked in caring for an aging patient unless there is frank pathology. In addition to overt pathologies of the thorax, insidious age-related declines contribute to changes in structure and function that necessitate thorough assessment. Breathing, posture, mobility, and strengthening exercises are important rehabilitation interventions.

SUGGESTED READINGS

Andreoli TE, Carpenter CC, Plum F, Smith LH Jr. *Cecil Essentials of Medicine.* Philadelphia: W.B. Saunders; 1986.

Atasoy E. Thoracic outlet compression syndrome. *Orthop Clin North Am* 1996; 27:265–303.

Donnelly LF et al. Airway compression in children with abnormal thoracic configuration. *Radiology* 1998; 206:323–326.

Frownfelter D, Dean E. *Principles and Practice of Pulmonary Physical Therapy,* 3rd ed. St. Louis: Mosby-Year Book; 1996.

Hollingshead WH. *Textbook of Anatomy,* 3rd ed. Hagerstown, Md.: Harper & Row; 1974.

Irwin S, Tecklin JS, eds. *Cardiopulmonary Physical Therapy,* I. St. Louis: C.V. Mosby; 1985.

Macklem PT. The mechanics of breathing. *Am J Respir Crit Care Med* 1998; 157:S88–S94.

Suga K et al. Ventilation abnormalities in obstructive airways disorder: detection with pulmonary dynamic densitometry by means of spiral CT versus dynamic Xe-133 SPECT. *Radiology* 1997; 202:855–862.

White AA III, Panjabi MM. *Clinical Biomechanics of the Spine.* Philadelphia: J.B. Lippincott; 1978.

Chapter **26**

Conditions of the Geriatric Cervical Spine

Jeff A. Martin, M.D.
Zoran Maric, M.D.
Robert R. Karpman, M.D.

INTRODUCTION

The aging process can be "a pain in the neck," literally as well as figuratively. Schmorl and Junghann reported that 90% of males over the age of 50 and 90% of females over the age of 60 have radiographic evidence of spinal degeneration. It is common for senior adults to experience neck symptoms, the majority of them related to cervical spondylosis or degenerative disease of the spine. These occur as a result of degeneration of the intervertebral disks, with loss of the water content within the disk, and subsequent disk collapse. The most common clinical syndromes associated with degenerative disk disease include cervical spondylosis, radiculopathy, and myelopathy.

COMMON CLINICAL SYNDROMES

Cervicalgia

Cervicalgia is defined as neck pain. The pain tends to be located posteriorly in the area of the paraspinous muscle. Patients often complain of occipital headaches as well as interscapular pain. The symptoms are exacerbated by neck motion and by abducting the arms in the over-the-shoulder position. Gore reported a 10-year follow-up of patients with cervicalgia and noted that 79% of the patients had decreasing neck pain, and 32% had only residual or moderate pain. The symptoms are relieved by various therapeutic modalities, including hot packs, ultrasound, electrical stimulation, traction, and soft-tissue techniques such as massage. Immobilization with a cervical orthosis along with neck-strengthening exercises may be helpful. It should be noted, however, that older patients have difficulty wearing a soft collar, as it tends to be too large and uncomfortable. Rigid supports should rarely be used.

Radiculopathy

Radiculopathy is defined as pain in a specific nerve root distribution. Radiculopathy is a result of herniation of a soft disk as opposed to constriction where the nerve root exits the spinal foramina due to the presence of osteophytes. Clinically, it is characterized by pain and paraesthesia both proximally and distally along the involved nerve root. It is not uncommon to find overlapping in multiple dermatomes. The interspace most commonly involved is the C5-6 interspace.

Myelopathy

Myelopathy is often missed but is commonly found in patients over 55 years of age. Typical neurological findings include lower motor neuron and reflex changes at the level of the lesion and upper motor neuron involvement below the level of the lesion. Gait abnormality is the most common clinical concern. The myelopathy tends to have an insidious onset and develops gradually over a long period of time.

HISTORY, PHYSICAL EXAMINATION, AND IMAGING

When taking a history, it is extremely important to specify the type of pain and its anatomical distribution. Complaints of deep aching pain and a burning sensation are suggestive of spinal cord involvement. Many patients lose hand dexterity. In patients who have been institutionalized for long periods, it may be difficult to assess an insidious myelopathy, as many patients already have bladder incontinence. In those instances, a more careful neurological examination is necessary to determine the cause of the incontinence.

On physical examination, most patients present with decreased range of motion of the neck and with paraspinous muscle spasm. There may or may not be tenderness directly over the spinous process. The pain is typically exacerbated by moving the shoulders and it is common for pain to radiate either within a specific nerve distribution down the arm or proximately into the occiput. Particularly in cases of cervical myelopathy, both upper and lower neurological examination should be performed. Imaging modalities are extremely useful in differentiating various types of cervical disease. Probably the most useful test is computerized tomography (CT) with intrathecal contrast. This technique provides an excellent differential between bone and soft-tissue lesions and can accurately demonstrate canal size and foraminal narrowing. Magnetic resonance imaging (MRI) is also useful as a noninvasive way of evaluating the spinal cord, soft tissues, and neural structures. Plain x-rays demonstrate bony changes and obvious foraminal narrowing but tend to be more generalized.

Differential Diagnosis

In generating a differential diagnosis when working with an older person, other diseases should be considered. Neoplasms, the most common being metastatic tumors from carcinoma of the breast, prostate, kidney, or thyroid, should be sought. Pain resulting from metastatic disease tends to be more intense at night and is often unremitting.

Sepsis of the skeleton occurs infrequently in the cervical spine but is commonly seen in the lumbosacral spine and can occur following urogenital procedures. Other inflammatory diseases can also lead to myelopathy; they include rheumatoid arthritis, ankylosing spondylitis, Reiter's syndrome, and diffuse idiopathic skeletal hypertrophy. However, most patients with such diseases present with other joint symptoms before the cervical spine becomes involved.

Cervical disc disease must be differentiated from primary shoulder disorders, too. Rotator cuff tendinitis, subacromial bursitis, and acromioclavicular joint problems can present with shoulder pain that radiates into the paraspinous muscle area. It is possible for a patient to have both primary shoulder disease and degenerative disk disease of the cervical spine. Selective injections, particularly into the subacromial space or the glenohumeral joint, can be helpful in differential diagnosis. Polymyalgia rheumatica should also be considered when an older patient presents specifically with significant proximal pain and stiffness in the morning.

This can develop into an acute emergency should the patient develop temporal arteritis and visual difficulties. The treatment of polymyalgia includes high-dose steroids. A patient who presents with these symptoms should be referred to a physician immediately for evaluation and treatment.

Other neurological findings that may be confused with cervical radiculopathies include compressive neuropathies such as entrapment of the suprascapular nerve, with pain in the upper scapular region and atrophy of the rotator cuff musculature. Median and ulnar nerve compression and thoracic outlet syndrome also present with shoulder pain, along with paraesthesia or weakness. Differentiation can be determined by nerve conduction studies or electromyelograms. (See chapters 35 and 36, which discuss neuropathies.)

TREATMENT

The majority of cervical symptoms in the geriatric patient can be treated by means of physical therapy and careful monitoring. Surgery is indicated primarily in a patient with myelopathy, progressive compression of the spinal cord, or significant nerve root encroachment that causes pain and progressive weakness in a specific nerve distribution. As mentioned previously, the remainder of musculoskeletal problems can be treated with heat, electrical stimulation, ultrasound, traction, soft-tissue massage, range-of-motion exercises, and muscle strengthening. Immobilization should be used only if necessary to prevent further stiffness and muscle atrophy.

Vigorous manipulation should not be used because of the risk of encroachment on the vertebral arteries and the possibility of stroke. Anti-inflammatory medications are a useful adjunct; however, many patients experience gastrointestinal irritation and bleeding as a result of such medication, and acetaminophen seems to provide similar symptomatic relief without the undesirable side effects. Generally speaking, a patient should not be restricted to bedrest for spinal abnormality unless it is absolutely necessary, and in those instances, careful monitoring is vital to avoid excessive pressure that could result in decubiti and to avoid pulmonary compromise and subsequent development of pneumonia.

CONCLUSION

Neck pain is common in persons over the age of 50. Degenerative changes, the cause of the majority of problems, may cause encroachment on the spinal cord or spinal nerves and present as myelopathy or radiculopathy. Differential diagnosis is crucial, as the other conditions mentioned above can cause the same or similar symptoms. Treatment with anti-inflammatory medications and physical therapy procedures and modalities may provide successful outcomes. Surgery is indicated for patients with myelopathy, progressive spinal cord compression, or significant nerve root encroachment. Bedrest is not a primary treatment.

SUGGESTED READINGS

Buszek MC et al. Hemidiaphragmatic paralysis: an unusual complication of cervical spondylosis. *Arch Phys Med Rehabil* 1983; 64:601–603.

Clark CR. Cervical spondylitic myelopathy: history and physical findings. *Spine* 1988; 13:847–489.

Gore DR et al. Neck pain: a long-term follow-up of 205 patients. *Spine* 1987; 12:1–5.

Harrington KD. Metastatic disease of the spine. *J Bone Joint Surg Am* 1986; 68:1110–1115.

Hawkins RJ. Cervical spine and the shoulder. *Instruct Course Lect* 1985; 34:191–195.

Modic MT et al. Imaging of degenerative disease of the cervical spine. *Clin Ortho* 1989; 239:109–120.

Simeone FA, Rothman RH. Cervical disc disease. In: Rothman RH, Simeone FA, eds. *The Spine*. Philadelphia: W.B. Saunders, 1992:440–476.

Schmorl G, Junghann S. Die gesunde und Kranke Wirbel Saule in Rontgenbild. Leipzig, Germany; 1932.

Wilberger JE Jr et al. Acute cervical spondylitic myelopathy. *Neurosurgery* 1988; 22:145–146.

Chapter **27**

Disorders of the Geriatric Thoracic and Lumbosacral Spine

Robert R. Karpman, M.D.

INTRODUCTION

Unlike the disorders typical of cervical and lumbosacral areas the disorder that most commonly affects geriatric patients in the thoracic spine is a result of metabolic diseases, particularly osteoporosis. As bone mass decreases in senior adults, the vertebral bodies are at particular risk for compression fracture. A patient with multiple compression fractures in the thoracic spine can develop a severe kyphosis, or "dowager's hump," and severe deformities. Minimal trauma or none at all is necessary to create compression fractures in a certain geriatric population. Patients complain of acute pain, often incapacitating, in the midthoracic region. Examination reveals significant tenderness with palpation of the spinous process and an obvious deformity when multiple vertebral bodies are involved. There is also significant paraspinous muscle spasm. The neurological examination generally remains intact. Plain radiographs demonstrate the abnormality as well as diffuse loss of bone mass in the adjacent vertebral bodies

Compression fractures, however, must be differentiated from malignancies. It is not uncommon for a patient with multiple myeloma or metastatic disease to present with a compression fracture. A bone scan, which may demonstrate lesions in other areas of the skeleton, is useful in differentiating a malignancy from a compression fracture as a result of osteoporosis.

Other spinal abnormalities include infections and degenerative disk disease. In addition, other visceral problems can present as acute back pain in older patients, particularly ruptured aneurysms, myocardial infarctions, mediastinal tumors, acute pneumonia, and peptic ulcer disease. A careful physical examination and laboratory and diagnostic studies can differentiate viscerogenic from spinal disorders.

TREATMENT OF COMPRESSION FRACTURES

The treatment of a compression fracture involves analgesics and bedrest for a short period of time, followed by gradual mobilization and weightbearing with assistive devices, if they are needed. Cau-

tion must be exercised because the biomechanics (long lever arm) of lifting a walker can actually provoke increased thoracic pain. A wheeled walker reduces biomechanical strain. Prolonged bedrest leads to further osteopenia caused by disuse and to other complications, including pneumonia and urinary incontinence. If analgesics are incapable of resolving these symptoms, or if polypharmacy is a concern a TENS unit may be helpful in relieving the paraspinous pain. External immobilization such as hyperextension braces are of little use for these patients as they are extremely uncomfortable and often cause chest compression and resultant difficulty in lung expansion and breathing. If necessary, a simple extended corset can be used for support. Once the symptoms have resolved, within a period of 1 to 2 weeks, extension exercises may be useful in preventing further deformity. Jewett extension braces or other rigid external supports are frequently found to have been placed in the drawer next to the patient rather than on the patient because of the discomfort involved in using the brace. Therefore, unless the deformity is severe, immobilization is not customary.

DISORDERS OF THE LUMBOSACRAL SPINE

As in the cervical spine, degenerative disorders of the lumbosacral spine are common in older individuals. These disorders include loss of the water content of and, thus, the pliability of the intervertebral disk, which leads to disk collapse and, occasionally, disk protrusion. As disks collapse, instability in the adjacent vertebrae develops, often causing mechanical low back problems. In addition, significant arthritic change can lead to stenosis of the central spinal canal or the nerve roots' foramina.

A patient with spinal stenosis tends to have a classic presentation. Typically, there is pain in the lower back or pain radiating down both legs, usually after walking for a brief time. The symptoms are relieved with rest or flexion of the spine. Once the patient resumes walking, the symptoms recur. This is similar to the experience of lower limb claudication as a result of vascular compromise. Examination of a patient with spinal stenosis often demonstrates a replication of the symptoms with hyperextension of the spine. Hyperextension leads to a narrowing of the spinal canal in the lumbosacral region and results in cord compression. The symptoms may also be aggravated by stenosis of the vertebral foramina, which often leads to radicular symptoms in addition to the claudication.

Treatment of spinal stenosis in severe cases is almost always surgical. A patient experiences acute relief of symptoms following decompression of the spinal canal. Often multiple vertebrae require decompression so fusion is necessary to prevent instability of the lumbosacral spine. This is often accompanied by spinal instrumentation to provide rigidity and stability of the spine until the vertebrae have fused. This also allows for earlier mobilization of the patient. In mild cases, nonsteroidal anti-inflammatories and occasionally epidural steroid blocks may be helpful in relieving the patient's symptoms. In addition to history and physical examination, the diagnosis of spinal stenosis can easily be made with the use of computerized tomography with or without intrathecal contrast.

As in the thoracic spine, lumbosacral supports and corsets are often uncomfortable and provide little if any relief of symptoms for a patient with low back problems. Abdominal exercises and stretching provide the most relief to a patient suffering from mechanical low back pain. Occasionally massage, hot packs, and ultrasound are also useful in resolving symptoms. Reduced weight-bearing walking exercises in an aquatic program or in a harness suspension on land may reduce symptoms and improve exercise tolerance.

When a patient experiences an acute onset of low back pain, a compression fracture or neoplasm must be considered. Plain radiographs and laboratory tests should differentiate the two abnormalities.

CONCLUSION

Common disorders of the thoracic and lumbosacral spine are the result of osteoporosis and degenerative changes. However, the cause of the patient's complaints must be investigated with appropriate laboratory and radiographic studies because metastatic disease and visceral problems may present as acute back pain.

In most cases, it is extremely important that patients with any kind of spinal disorder be mobilized as quickly as possible, in order to prevent further osteopenia due to disuse. All attempts should be made to provide appropriate assistive devices, so that patients can be ambulatory as soon as possible.

SUGGESTED READINGS

Grasland A, Pouchot J, Mathieu A, et al. Sacral insufficiency fractures. *Arch Intern Med* 1996; 156:668–674.
Harrison KD. Metastatic disease of the spine. *J Bone Joint Surg Am* 1986; 68:1110–1115.
Hulkins D, Nelson M, eds. *The Aging Spine.* Manchester, England: Manchester University Press, 1987.
Lane JM. Osteoporosis: Medical prevention and treatment. *Spine* 1997; 22(24S):325–375.

Chapter 28

Orthopedic Trauma
E. Frederick Barrick, M.D.

INTRODUCTION

Although some special consideration must be given to the geriatric population, the basic principles of rehabilitation after orthopedic trauma described in this chapter apply to all ages. Here, attention has been directed to the rehabilitation of the geriatric patient because of the aging population and the influence of Medicare. It is recognized that the elderly can lead productive and interesting lives.

Orthopedic trauma in this context covers everything from the fractured wrist that occurs because of a trip and a fall to the multiple injuries sustained in a motor vehicle accident. The more severe the injury, the more intensely the basic principles have to be applied.

It has been demonstrated that accelerated rehabilitation after proximal femur fracture in elderly patients significantly reduces cost at a savings of up to 38% per patient.[1]

BASIC PRINCIPLES FOR REHABILITATION

The goals of rehabilitation are, in sequence, (1) mobility, (2) motion, (3) motor control and coordination, (4) strengthening, and (5) adaptation. These objectives are taken up in order but are overlapped as shown on the time line in Figure 28 1. One begins by mobilizing the patient out of bed, into a chair, and up on crutches or a walker, but at the same time, motion of the joints is necessary. As the patient is gaining functional mobility, more attention can be given to regaining full motion of the involved joint or joints. Emphasis may have to be placed on regaining motor control and coordination, especially if pain and muscle splinting are factors.

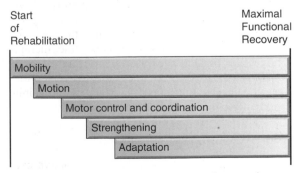

Figure 28–1 Rehabilitation time line.

When reasonably comfortable motion and motor control are being obtained, strengthening should be started. As rehabilitation progresses and it becomes apparent that preinjury status may not be attainable, then adaptations with prosthetics, orthotics, or lifestyle may be necessary.

The first objective is to get the patient out of bed. Depending on the patient's condition, mobilization can begin immediately or days or even weeks may pass before it can be started. The latter may be especially true of patients with spine injuries.

If an upper extremity is injured, then the necessary instruction may be only to keep the arm elevated or to learn how to get out of bed without using that arm. With a lower extremity injury, the patient must learn how to get out of bed while keeping the leg elevated. Assistance in lifting is often needed as there is sometimes not enough strength in the extremity so the patient can lift it without help.

Learning to walk using crutches or a walker with reduced or no weight-bearing is a challenge to most people. The amount of energy required is 30 to 50% greater than is required by normal walking.[2] This extra requirement can be especially taxing on the elderly because of their decreased cardiopulmonary reserves.

Of course, the more extremities injured, the greater the obstacle to mobilization. Attention may have to be concentrated on transfers. Forearm supports may be needed on ambulatory assistive devices.

The geriatric patient may already have impairment of mobility that has to be taken into account. The goal is to get the patient back to preinjury status.

Motion

The therapist's job is to instruct and assist the patient in regaining range of motion after injury. Any precautions or contraindications should be noted by the physician who may need to provide direct supervision. Active exercise is done by the patient. Active assistive exercise is performed with help from the therapist who makes sure, with gentle persuasion, that the motion is taken to the maximum range possible. In passive exercise, the therapist moves the patient; it is used in resistant cases, in unconscious patients, or for paralyzed extremities. It has been shown that age is no barrier to regaining or even increasing strength.

Motor Control and Coordination

Motor control is necessary before any active exercise can begin or progress. Sometimes electrical stimulation is needed to activate muscles with atrophy or painful splinting.

Coordination is crucial to motor control. It involves smooth, accurate movement of the joints in the kinematic chain. The timing and sequencing of the movement of ipsilateral and contralateral joints requires neural control and musculoskeletal integrity. For example, a humeral fracture disrupts the coordinated movement of the involved arm, but it can also reduce the contralateral arm swing during normal reciprocal gait. Coordination is facilitated by proper breathing, decreased splinting, and reduced abnormal flexor and adductor tone.

Strengthening

When some degree of comfortable motion and some muscle control are obtained, strengthening can be started. Increased strength often results in better motion.

An effective method of strengthening is progressive resistance exercises. One technique exercises each muscle group with enough weight (resistance) to allow 20 to 30 repetitions. Once 30 repetitions can be done, the resistance is increased. Other popular methods include 3 sets of 10 to 15 repetitions with decreasing weights for each set or 3 sets using the same weight with decreasing repetitions (20–15–10).

Adaptation

At some point during rehabilitation, it may become evident that there will be some permanent impairment. These changes in anatomy and consequently in function may force changes in the patient's life. In order to adapt to physical changes some aspect of training or equipment may be needed. This stage may come early if, for instance, there has been a major amputation. In other cases, it may become evident later in the course of rehabilitation that permanent loss of joint motion or strength is inevitable and that compensation during work or play is needed.

The ability to return to some form of useful activity is one of the major goals of rehabilitation—although it is not always achievable. It may mean the patient must get used to a more sedentary lifestyle or pursue an activity in which remaining physical abilities may be used. It can mean learning to adapt to new limitations in order to regain a meaningful life.

REHABILITATION AFTER SPECIFIC INJURIES

Colles' Fracture

The most common musculoskeletal injury in the geriatric population is a displaced fracture of the distal radius, which accounts for about one quarter of all fractures in the population over 65 years of age. The classic Colles' fracture is displaced dorsally (apex volar). Variations of distal radius fractures have similar rehabilitation demands.

Mobility. Screen for balance and mobility defects that may have caused the fall that resulted in the fracture.

Motion. Range of motion and strengthening of the part of the upper extremity that is not immobilized is helpful during the initial healing period to try to prevent stiffness of the shoulder and fingers. Motion of the elbow usually returns after immobilization is discontinued without the need for more than active exercises. Once wrist motion can begin, active and active assistive exercises are encouraged in all six directions—flexion, extension, radial and ulnar deviation, pronation, and supination. Modalities such as hydrotherapy, electrical stimulation, heat, cold, or ultrasound may be helpful. The end goal should be to match the range of motion of the uninjured hand and wrist. Some degree of permanent loss of range may occur, especially in supination and extension.

Motor Control and Coordination. The initiation of muscle function may be difficult when all motion is painful. Postural changes in the head, neck, and trunk may need attention.

Strengthening. After some reasonable range has been obtained, strengthening with motion against resistance can commence.

Adaptation. One complication of a distal radius fracture, especially in the elderly, can be some degree of malunion. As a result, there may be prominence of the distal ulna which causes a mild degree of deformity. The patient may have to adapt to this cosmetic change.

Hip Fracture

Fractures of the proximal femur, both intertrochanteric and intracapsular, are common in people over the age of 60 and even more common in persons over 80.[3] Less common in the geriatric patient is fracture of the acetabulum. A hip fracture is likely to cause significant disruption in the patient's life. This injury requires a considerable amount of rehabilitation if the patient is to return to a life of independence. The cause of most hip fractures is impaired mobility, rather than osteoporosis. Impaired mobility is commonly associated with parkinsonism and Alzheimer's disease. Nocturia can precipitate a fall in those with impaired mobility. Proximal femur fractures make up about 10% of fractures in the elderly. Fracture of the acetabulum is seen in the more active patient and results from a higher-energy injury, such as a motor vehicle accident or a fall from a ladder or roof.

Surgery is universally recommended to permit mobilization that can prevent complications and even death. Rehabilitation depends on the type of surgery required. For intertrochanteric fractures and nondisplaced intracapsular neck fractures, internal fixation is performed. For displaced neck fractures, a hemiarthroplasty is generally done, although a few surgeons still do closed reductions of fractures inside the hip joint and fix the fracture with lag screws.

Internal Fixation for Fracture of the Proximal Femur

Mobility. A major goal of rehabilitation after a hip fracture is to enable the patient to walk, especially if mobility is already impaired. Mobilization is begun immediately after surgery. With an intertrochanteric fracture, protected weight-bearing is usually necessary. An alert patient can understand the necessity and accommodate accordingly. A patient who is not strong enough to manage "weight-of-the-leg" weight-bearing or not coherent enough to understand the therapist's instructions must be limited to a wheelchair or to pregait activities, such as sit-to-stand and static stance with weight shift, until stronger or until the fracture has healed sufficiently to permit unrestricted weight-bearing. Early assisted swing (slide) phase of gait with the involved leg may be helpful to facilitate proper weight-bearing and return to functional gait in the future. This is achieved with the patient standing in the parallel bars or with a walker, and simply sliding the involved foot forward and backward, or lifting it over a low obstacle (cane) that is placed on the floor in front of the foot. This type of patient should be expected to perform safe ambulation and transfers at home or on the nursing floor where proper guidance and assistance are not likely to be available.

Motion. Range-of-motion exercises are encouraged soon after the initial pain subsides and the patient can cooperate. Motion in all directions is advised, especially abduction and extension, which are the most difficult and the least likely to be worked on by the patient when alone. These motions are especially important to prevent the common flexion and adduction contractures that can make walking difficult.

Motor Control and Coordination. Work to control the involved limb is essential to permit adequate mobility in bed and prevent decubiti and to allow transfer out of bed. Balance and coordination instructions are given concurrently with all phases of ambulation.

Strengthening. Strengthening abduction gradually reduces the lurching (Trendelenburg) limp seen after a hip injury. Progressive resistance exercises are used, starting with abduction while standing or supine on a powder board. As strength increases, the patient is instructed in the exercise while lying on the contralateral side, abducting against gravity. Coexisting musculoskeletal and cardiovascular conditions may necessitate modification of these positions. Once 20 to 30 repetitions can be performed, progressively greater weight is added. Strengthening is encouraged for flexors, extensors, and adductors as well.

Adaptation. The patient may have to adapt to even more limited mobility. The patient may have to accept the permanent need for a cane, or even a walker, for aid in balance and to reduce the Trendelenberg lurch associated with weak abductors. There may be a necessity for placement in an assisted living facility or a full-care nursing home.

Hemiarthroplasty for Proximal Femur Fracture

Mobility. If a posterior surgical approach is used in performing hip replacement, precautions against dislocation must be taken for the first month. Dislocation can occur with the combination of flexion and adduction and internal rotation, and there is a natural tendency for the hip to go into this position after injury. Some people must be warned not to put on their shoes and stockings in this position and these precautions also apply when the patient is lying in bed and particularly when sitting. Sitting in a lean-back chair so that the hip is flexed no more than 60 degrees is advised. The abduction pillow is useful when in bed. A knee immobilizer should prevent dislocation, as the hip cannot be flexed enough to dislocate unless the knee can bend also.

If an anterior approach is used, these precautions are not needed. The hip will dislocate only in extension which is not a natural position for the hip after injury.

Motion. Same as with internal fixation with the precautions taken.

Motor Control and Coordination. Same as with internal fixation.

Strengthening. Same as with internal fixation with the precautions taken.

Adaptation. Same as with internal fixation.

Internal Fixation for Displaced Fracture of the Acetabulum

This procedure is indicated if there is disruption of the weight-bearing dome of the acetabulum and if the patient's general condition permits it. It is a much more extensive procedure than either of the above hip operations. Blood transfusion is more likely to be required, and the patient is likely to be more depleted.

Mobility. Usually weight-bearing will have to be restricted for a longer time—8 to 12 weeks—using a partial weight-bearing (weight-of-the-leg) gait.

Motion. Same as with internal fixation of the proximal femur; a longer period of rehabilitation is to be anticipated.

Motor Control and Coordination. These aptitudes may be more seriously impaired because of the severity of the injury and the intensity of the surgical treatment. Much more attention must be given to regaining initial muscle control at the hip and the rest of the leg.

Strengthening. Same as with internal fixation.

Adaptation. Same as with internal fixation.

Fracture of the Proximal Humerus

Fracture of the proximal humerus is an injury that is also common to members of the geriatric population. The treatment is essentially the same, whether or not operative treatment is needed. Open reduction and internal fixation are occasionally required. A hemiarthroplasty is indicated if there is extensive comminution.

Mobility. It is important for the patient to avoid using the affected arm when getting out of a bed or chair. There is a natural tendency to do so, but such assistance can displace the fracture even after surgery. It is especially likely to be done if there are multiple injuries and if the patient has some mental impairment. If this seems to be the situation, the orthopedic surgeon often does not perform such an operation, knowing that it is doomed to failure without the patient's cooperation.

Motion. Balance must be observed. The fracture must be kept immobilized long enough for the bone to heal to the point at which the patient can move the shoulder but not too long, or the shoulder will become incapable of movement. As early as 10 to 14 days after surgery, stooping exercises (pendulum exercises), as first described by Codman[4] early in this century, can begin. Passive range of motion is started even earlier (2 to 3 days) after hemiarthroplasty. It is also used later, after other methods of treatment. Active and passive ROM exercises are carried out for months until maximum improvement has been obtained. The hand, wrist, and elbow should be exercised with active and resistive motion as well. Motion of the neck, scapula, and trunk should not be ignored either.

Motor Control and Coordination. In most cases active muscle control of the shoulder is discouraged, the emphasis being placed on passive pendulum exercises. However, muscle control education for the rest of the upper extremity and the trunk is encouraged.

Strengthening. After 3 to 4 weeks, active exercise involving the deltoid and shoulder rotators can be added.

Adaptation. Although some loss of motion results in most cases, it does not seem to impair function enough to cause concern. The patient should be informed of the prognosis.

Compression Fracture of the Spine

Osteoporosis is a major factor in compression fracture of the vertebral body. This type of fracture occurs more commonly in women. It is often associated with a fall on the buttocks, but can take place spontaneously. Treatment consists of initial rest and analgesics.

Mobility. In most cases, mobilization is begun as early as pain permits. It is rare that surgery is needed. Instruction in the performance of transfers, activities of daily living, deep breathing, and ambulation is the primary rehabilitation.

Motion. Flexion of the spine is to be avoided, as it duplicates the mechanism of injury. Extension exercises of the trunk and hips are useful. Ranging of the shoulders and scapular retraction exercises are helpful also.

Motor Control and Coordination. Recovery of trunk control and coordination is to be started immediately, as soon as the initial pain has subsided sufficiently.

Strengthening. Strengthening in extension should be continued. General fitness exercises have proven to be helpful, especially to prevent recurrence of osteoporotic fractures.

Adaptation. The patient may have to accommodate herself or himself to repeat fractures. Treatment of osteoporosis has been shown to reduce the incidence of refracture. (See Chapter 19, "Osteoporosis.")

Multiple Trauma

The basic principles of treatment of multiple orthopedic trauma apply to the aged. Immediate internal fixation or external immobilization of all long-bone fractures is known to increase survival and improve long-term function. Early mobilization of the patient is extremely important if it is at all possible. Resuscitation may be hampered by a patient's preexisting medical condition. If the patient is unresponsive because of head injury, passive range-of-motion exercises and splinting in the position of function are important to prevent disabling contractures.

CONCLUSION

After fractures or dislocations in the aged, rehabilitation is applied as in younger patients but with its intensity tempered by the restrictions imposed by the patient's underlying general physical condition. The injured elderly will respond if consideration is given to their limitations.

REFERENCES

1. Cameron ID, Lyle DM, Quine S. Cost-effectiveness of accelerated rehabilitation after proximal femur fracture. *J Clin Epidemiol* 1994; 47:1307–1313.
2. Waters RL, Campbell J, Perry J. Energy cost of three-point ambulation in fracture patients. *J Orthop Trauma* 1987; 1:170–173.
3. Jarnlo GB. Hip fracture patients. *Scand J Rehab Med* 1991; 24 [suppl]:1–31.
4. Codman EA. *The Shoulder: Rupture of the Supraspinatis Tendon and Other Lesions in or About the Subacromial Bursa.* Brooklyn: G. Miller; 1941:202.

SUGGESTED READINGS

Goldstein FC, Strasser DC, Woodard JL, Roberts VJ. Functional outcome of cognitively impaired hip-fracture patients on a geriatric rehabilitation unit. *J Am Geriatr Soc* 1997; 45:35–42.
Randell A, Sambrook PN, Nguyen TV, et al. Direct clinical and welfare costs of osteoporotic fractures in elderly men and women. *Osteoporos Int* 1995; 5:427–432.
Stravrou ZP, Erginousakis DA, Loizides AA, Tzevelekos SA, Papagiannakos KJ. Morality and rehabilitation following hip fracture: a study of 202 elderly patients. *Acta Orthop Scand Suppl* 1997; 275:89–91.

2

NEUROMUSCULAR AND NEUROLOGIC INVOLVEMENT

Chapter 29

Rehabilitation After Stroke

Robert C. Wagenaar, Ph.D.
Gert Kwakkel, Ph.D., P.T.

INTRODUCTION

A patient suffering from a cerebrovascular accident (CVA, or stroke) commonly has severe and complex deficits of both action and perception. An inability to move the side of the body contralateral to the cerebral infarct (hemiplegia) is the most typically observed consequence of a stroke. Immediately after a stroke, one side of the body is often completely flaccid. In industrialized countries 10% of all deaths are caused by strokes.[1] If recovery takes place, pathological movement patterns emerge, and they will not, in most cases, be replaced by normal movement coordination.[2] The largest amount of recovery occurs within approximately the first 6 months after the stroke. Perceptual deficits such as hemi-neglect are often part of the hemiplegic syndrome, and they tend to hamper recovery of the ability to perform activities of daily living. In addition, speech deficits, depression, and neuropsychological disorders such as apraxia are typically observed in stroke patients, leaving rehabilitation specialists—physical therapists, occupational therapists, speech therapists, and physicians—with a bewildering complexity of impairments and disabilities to deal with.[3]

EPIDEMIOLOGY OF STROKE

A stroke is usually understood to be the sudden onset of neurological deficits due to local disturbances in the blood supply to the brain, that is, a vascular occlusion (ischemic infarct) or a vascular disruption (hemorrhage). In the Netherlands, about 26,000 cases of stroke (approximately 173 per 100,000 inhabitants) are reported each year.[4] The risk increases considerably with age, with males having a significantly higher incidence than females for all age groups below 75 years. About 30% of

the stroke patients died within 21 days. Of those who survived the acute phase (defined as the first 3 weeks poststroke), 42% remained dependent upon other persons for their activities of daily living (ADL), 24% were hospitalized or sent to a nursing home, 11% were unable to walk, and 66% were unable to return to work.

Comparison among members of the international community is difficult because of inconsistencies in reporting and study design, but stroke mortality rate per 100,000 persons varies across political and geographical borders. As can be seen in Figure 29–1, the mortality varies among the Russian Federation, the United Kingdom, and the United States, but the clear age-related trend is obvious. Genetics may be an influence, but modifiable lifestyles (diet, blood pressure, obesity, cigarette smoking, and physical activity) and improved medical care may explain the decrease in stroke mortality rate in many but not all countries between 1960–64 and 1985–89, which is shown in Figure 29–2. Although the incidence of stroke mortality is decreasing, the prevalence of stroke is stable or increasing, thereby placing high demands on rehabilitation services.

Early and adequate prediction of functional recov-

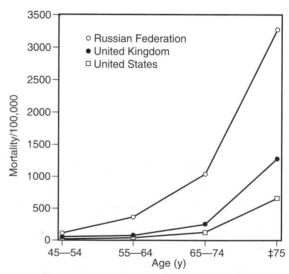

Figure 29–1 Stroke mortality rates per 100,00 by age for men in three countries. (Redrawn with permission from Khaw KT. Epidemiology of stroke. *J Neurol Neurosurg Psychiatry* 1996; 61:333–338.)

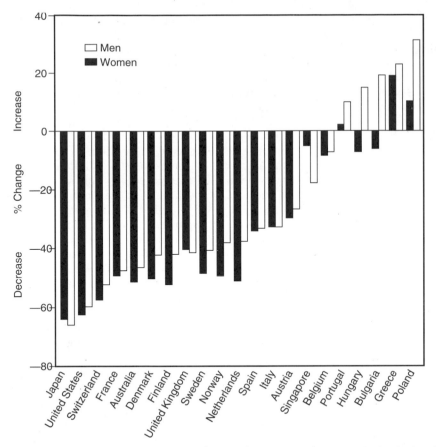

Figure 29–2 Changes in age-standardized mortality rates from stroke in men and women 1960–1964 and 1985–1989 in selected countries. (Redrawn with permission from Khaw KT. Epidemiology of stroke. *J Neurol Neurosurg Psychiatry* 1996; 61:333–338.)

ery after stroke is important in order to facilitate proper discharge planning, anticipate the need for home adjustments and community support, and set realistic and attainable goals for treatment.[5] In several reviews, a number of predictors for functional recovery after stroke have been suggested: disability on admission, sitting balance, severity of paralysis, urinary incontinence, level of consciousness within 48 hours poststroke, disorientation in time and place, prior stroke, age, level of social support, and metabolic rate of glucose outside the infarct area.[5] Predictive models formulated for functional recovery after stroke appear to have limited predictive validity because of methodological shortcomings in prognostic studies and a lack of information about functional recovery patterns dependent on patient characteristics.[6]

REHABILITATION AFTER STROKE

Special stroke rehabilitation wards based on a multidisciplinary approach have been in existence since the 1950s.[7] It has been suggested that such wards provide the opportunity to raise the standard of care, improve the level of therapy, and coordinate resources, while at the same time constituting a focus for staff training and instruction of caregivers in the precise management of individual patients and opportunities for study and research.[8] In addition, a large number of different methods of physical and occupational therapy have been developed during the past 4 decades. These methods range from neurological exercise therapies [9] to cognitive remediation programs for perceptual deficits.[10] The frequently applied neurological exercise therapies are Neuro-Developmental Treatment (NDT, derived from the Bobath method), the motor relearning program, Brunnstrom, Proprioceptive Neuromuscular Facilitation (PNF), and electromyography (EMG) feedback therapy. Major controversies exist among proponents of the various neurological exercise therapies (e.g., Bobath or NDT versus Brunnstrom).

One of the basic principles of the Bobath method is the treatment of the pathological muscle tone with the aid of reflex inhibiting patterns (RIPs) in order to facilitate normal movement coordination.

An example is the reduction of flexor activity in the trunk and arm, achieved by extending the neck and spine while externally rotating the paretic arm at the shoulder with an extended elbow.[11] Intensive exercises involving the hemiplegic side of the body (the "healthy" side) are discouraged as long as they provoke pathological muscle tone in the paretic arm and leg. The method prescribes exercising both sides of the body as symmetrically as possible. The patient has to learn to exert conscious control over his or her muscle tone when performing the activities of daily living. Davies has extended the ideas of Bobath to training in functional tasks such as grasping, standing up, climbing stairs, bouncing a ball, getting dressed, preparing meals, washing, brushing teeth, and having a bath or shower.[12] Because of these changes, the Bobath method was renamed NDT. The motor relearning program formulated by Carr and Shepherd offers another approach to functional training; in it, an attempt is made to incorporate ideas that stem from theories about motor control and learning.[13]

According to Brunnstrom, six phases can be distinguished during successful recovery by the stroke patient: (1) no movements can be carried out (flaccidity); (2) flexion synergy in the upper extremity and extension synergy in the lower extremity become apparent as associated reactions and spasticity begin to develop; (3) spasticity increases, and the patient is able to control basic synergy patterns; (4) the patient is able to break through synergy patterns; (5) as spasticity decreases the patient is able to make selective movements, more difficult movement combinations can be learned, and basic synergies disappear; and (6) a normal coordination of movements is reestablished.[14] According to the Brunnstrom method the therapist should facilitate this "natural and lawful" process from no movement through basic synergy patterns to dissociated motor behavior. For example, the stimulation of associate reactions in the paretic extremities by applying resistive exercises on the healthy side of the body is advocated when synergy patterns have not yet developed. As soon as dissociation of basic synergy patterns becomes possible, the training of selective movements should be initiated. With the exception of the training of basic functional activities such as grasping, sitting, and walking, training for ADL is hardly discussed by Brunnstrom.

Effects of Stroke Rehabilitation

In a published meta-analysis of 10 studies, Langhorne et al. have shown that recovering in a stroke rehabilitation ward significantly reduces the rate of mortality in comparison to the rate that exists in traditional wards.[15] Wagenaar and Meijer found in their critical review that expert care, as compared to traditional care, has a significant positive effect on recovery of function.[16] At this time, it is still unclear which part of the expert care causes the effect—team care, active family participation, special staff education, early start of treatment, or intensity of treatment. The results of a few studies suggest that intensive rehabilitation has a positive influence on functional recovery after stroke, reducing impairment and disability.[17]

Optimal forms of physical and occupational therapy have, however, not yet been discovered, and all of the available approaches appear to promote improvement in functional ability.[18] Most studies reveal differential treatment effects, but these effects are often limited to the activity in which the patient was trained. Facilitation techniques, inhibition techniques, functional electrostimulation, and EMG feedback therapy have resulted in differential effects on parameters defined on the neuromuscular level, but showed hardly any transfer effects to ADLs. The exception appears to be visual perception training, for which some transfer effects have been demonstrated within the neuropsychological domain; transfer effects are found for tasks such as reading and writing, but not for gross motor tasks such as wheelchair navigation and driving performance.

Only a small number of studies have found specific effects on functional tasks; for example, Cozean et al.[19] noted the effect of the combination of functional electrostimulation and EMG feedback therapy applied during sitting and walking on ankle and knee angles during gait; Shumway Cook et al.[20] and Winstein et al.[21] noted the effect of postural sway feedback therapy on postural lateral sway; and Webster et al.[22] noted the effect of visual scanning training on wheelchair navigation. Such studies appear to indicate that ADLs must be specifically taught if the functional recovery of stroke patients is to be improved.[19-22] The findings of studies of the effects of forced use in the treatment of hand dexterity and walking corroborate this finding. Applying a sling to the healthy arm[23] and walking on a treadmill,[24] have produced impressive positive findings in terms of usage of the paretic arm in ADLs and independent walking, respectively. It should be noted, however, that in general, spontaneous recovery appears to account for much of the improvement in functional ability.

Relearning Dynamics after Stroke

The rehabilitation of the stroke patient has often been described as a relearning process. The necessity of providing specific training in ADLs, however, implies that we need to know more about the nature of the coordination deficits that prevent the performance of functional tasks and, thus, more about the natural laws of coordination and control required for the performance of such tasks. Only when we know precisely what is being relearned can we really begin to come to terms with questions about how relearning takes place. A better theoretical understanding of the deficits in motor coordination and perception may turn out to be a prerequisite for designing new and more effective rehabilitation methods.

For example, a number of gait studies done from a dynamic systems perspective have shown that walking velocity is an important independent (or control) parameter in the evaluation of healthy and hemiplegic gait.[25] In human walking, a transition in the coordination of the transverse pelvic and thoracic rotation, as well as in the arm and leg movements, occurs in the velocity range of 0.75 to 1.0 m/s, which, perhaps, could be summarized as a transition from controlling step frequency to controlling stride frequency. An important aspect of this change in gait pattern is that from 0.75 m/s onward, the pelvic rotation starts contributing to a lengthening of the stride, which in itself demands a changeover from an in-phase relation between pelvic and thoracic rotations and the movement of both arms toward a counterrotation, or a more or less out-of-phase relationship. Within the velocity range of 0.25 to 0.75 m/s the frequency of arm movement is dominantly synchronized with the step frequency, whereas from 0.75 m/s onward, the frequency of arm movements is locked into the stride frequency.

In hemiplegic gait, disordered frequency, or phase relationship, between pelvic and thoracic rotation and arm and leg movements has been observed; it can be summarized as a lack of timing within coordination patterns and a general inability to switch between coordination patterns. Results from intervention studies on hemiplegia after stroke suggest that walking velocity as well as auditory rhythms can have a positive impact on the disordered coordination patterns in trunk rotation and arm and leg movements.[25]

CONCLUSION

An important aspect of the efficacy of expert care for stroke patients appears to be the early start of intensive rehabilitation after the stroke. Facilitation and inhibition techniques have resulted in differential effects on parameters defined on a neuromuscular level; the transfer to ADLs appears to be minimal. The findings of studies of the effects of postural sway feedback therapy, visual perception training, and forced use in the treatment of hand dexterity and walking strongly suggest that stroke patients must be trained specifically to perform the activities necessary for daily life.

A large gap exists between theories of motor control and learning and the practice of rehabilitation. Future research should establish the expediency of using dynamic systems theory in the evaluation and treatment of movement disorders. Tweaking the perception-action coupling by means of external rhythms or oscillators can offer an interesting theoretical paradigm that has promising practical consequences for exercise therapy.

It should be noted, however, that return of function appears to be determined to a large extent by spontaneous recovery which, itself, is found to be constrained by characteristics unique to the patient, such as the severity of the stroke, a history of prior stroke, and older age. Future research should define the natural history of recovery of relevant functional tasks and classify its various patterns according to patient characteristics over time. This classification can then be used as a framework to evaluate the contribution of rehabilitation strategies to the relearning process.

REFERENCES

1. Khaw KT. Epidemiology of stroke. *J Neurol Neurosurg Psychiatry* 1996; 61:333–338.
2. Twitchell TE. The restoration of motor function following hemiplegia in man. *Brain,* 1951; 75:443–480.
3. Wade DT, Langton-Hewer R. Rehabilitation after stroke. In: Toole JF, ed. *Handbook of Clinical Neurology 11, Vascular Diseases III.* North Holland, the Netherlands: Elsevier Science; 1989:233–254.
4. Herman B, Leyten ACM, van Luijk JH, Frenken CWGM, Op de Coul AAW, Schulte BPM. Epidemiology of stroke in Tilburg, The Netherlands. *Stroke* 1982; 13:629–634.
5. Kwakkel G, Wagenaar RC, Kollen B, Lankhorst GH. Prognosis of functional recovery after stroke: a critical review of literature. *Age Ageing,* 1996: 25:479–489.
6. Gladman JRF, Harwood DMJ, Barer DH. Predicting the outcome of acute stroke: prospective evaluation of five multivariate models and comparison with single methods. *J Neurol Neurosurg Psychiatry* 1992; 55:347–351.
7. Garraway M. Stroke rehabilitation units: concepts, evaluation and unresolved issues. *Stroke* 1985; 16:178–181.
8. Stevens RS, Ambler NR, Warren MD. A randomized controlled trial of a stroke rehabilitation ward. *Age Ageing* 1984; 13:65–75.
9. Wagenaar RC. *Functional Recovery after Stroke.* Amsterdam: VU University Press; 1990.
10. Diller L, Weinberg J. Hemi-inattention in rehabilitation: the evolution of a rational remediation program. In: Weinstein EA, Friedland RP, eds. *Hemi-Inattention and Hemisphere Specialization.* New York: Raven Press; 1977:63–82.
11. Bobath B. *Adult Hemiplegia: Evaluation and Treatment.* London: William Heinemann Medical Books; 1978.
12. Davies PM. *Steps to Follow: A Guide to the Treatment of Adult Hemiplegia,* Berlin: Springer-Verlag; 1985.

13. Carr JH, Sheperd RB. *A Motor Relearning Programme for Stroke.* London: William Heinemann Medical Books; 1982.

14. Brunnstrom S. *Movement Therapy in Hemiplegia: A neuro-physiological approach.* Hagerstown, Md.: Harper & Row; 1970.

15. Langhorne P, Williams BO, Gilchrist W, Howle K. Do stroke units save lives? *Lancet* 1993; 342:395–398.

16. Wagenaar RG, Meijer OG. Effects of stroke rehabilitation 1, 2: A critical review of the literature. *J Rehabil Sci* 1991; 4:61–73, 96–108.

17. Langhorne P, Wagenaar RC, Partridge C. Physiotherapy after stroke: more is better? *Physiother Res Int* 1996; 1:75–88.

18. Ernst E. A review of stroke rehabilitation and physiotherapy. *Stroke* 1990; 21:1081–1085.

19. Cozean CD, Pease WS, Hubbell SL. Biofeedback and functional electric stimulation in stroke rehabilitation. *Arch Phys Med Rehabil* 1988; 69:401–405.

20. Shumway-Cook A, Anson D, Haller S. Postural sway biofeedback: its effect on reestablishing stance stability in hemiplegic patients. *Arch Phys Med Rehabil* 1988; 69:395–400.

21. Winstein CJ, Gardner ER, McNeal DR, Barto PS, Nicholson D. Standing balance training: effect on balance and locomotion in hemiparetic adults. *Arch Phys Med Rehabil* 1989; 70:755–762.

22. Webster JS, Jones S, Blanton P, Gross R, Beissel GF, Wofford J. Visual scanning training with stroke patients. *Behav Ther* 1984; 15:129–143.

23. Hesse S, Bertelt C, Jahnke MT, et al. Treadmill training with partial body weight support compared with physiotherapy in nonambulatory hemiparetic patients. *Stroke* 1995; 26:976–981.

24. Taub E, Miller NE, Novack TA, et al. Technique to improve chronic motor deficit after stroke. *Arch Phys Med Rehabil* 1993; 74:347–354.

25. Wagenaar RC, van Emmerik REA. Dynamics of pathological gait. *Hum Movement Sci* 1994; 13:441–471.

Chapter **30**

Neurological Trauma

Nancy M. Prickett, M.A. M.P.T., N.C.S., G.C.S.

INTRODUCTION

Trauma to the central and peripheral nervous systems is often misdiagnosed or initially missed because of the subtle and varied signs and symptoms, especially in the elderly patient. Trauma experienced by an older person is often not associated with symptoms that are expressed or noted a week or so after a relatively minor incident. Also, inaccurate reporting of events due to cognitive deficits compounds the challenge to the medical practitioner to determine the accurate diagnosis. Physical therapists often receive orders for treatment of a condition that has been misdiagnosed. Examinations to ascertain accurate physical and mental status help to determine the proper diagnosis and management for the elderly person experiencing trauma to the neurological system.

CLOSED HEAD TRAUMA

Falls, assaults, and motor vehicle accidents are the primary causes of traumatic brain injury in the elderly. Concussions, contusions, and hemorrhage of the brain tissues and fractures of the skull result. The symptoms of a concussion, the most minor head injury, can be loss of consciousness for a short period of time, a degree of amnesia, vomiting, headaches, sleepiness, and difficulty in focusing. Close observation of the individual presenting with these symptoms is indicated. In addition, x-rays are helpful to screen for skull and cervical fractures and intracranial hematomas.

A person who experiences an epidural hematoma, which is usually arterial in origin, may initially be unconscious, have a period of lucidity, and then lapse into a state of unconsciousness as the hematoma enlarges. Other symptoms that may follow the unconsciousness include hemiparesis, headache, personality changes, dysmetria, ataxia, anisocoria (difference in pupil size), and cranial nerve deficit.

A subdural hematoma is often the result of an acute venous hemorrhage. An acute hematoma develops within a week after injury and a subacute subdural hematoma shows signs and symptoms within 7 to 10 days after injury. Both acute and subacute subdural hematomas cause similar symptoms and can best be confirmed by a computed tomography scan or angiography.

Medical team members who work with the elderly must be aware that chronic subdural hematomas are most common in the aged patient on anticoagulant therapy. A seemingly minor trauma with no immediate effects can be the cause of a chronic subdural hematoma. The patient may present with a chronic headache and have tenderness over the lesion when the skull is percussed. Often the signs and symptoms presented by a person with a chronic subdural hematoma are taken to indicate a cerebral vascular accident, encephalitis, metabolic encephalopathy, or psychosis. Progressive dementia with generalized rigidity is another possible symptom. Only when it has been appropriately diagnosed can proper management for a patient with severe neurological impairment be provided. The Glasgow Coma Scale rates the level of consciousness (see Box 30–1). Posturing and motor responses are noted. If a patient obeys commands, localizes painful stimuli, or withdraws from pain, all descending motor pathways are intact.

Box 30-1

Glasgow Coma Scale

EYES	SCORE
OPEN:	
Spontaneously	4
To verbal command	3
To pain	2
No response	1
BEST MOTOR RESPONSE	
TO VERBAL COMMAND:	
Obeys	6
TO PAINFUL STIMULUS:	
Localizes pain	5
Flexion-withdrawal	4
Flexion-abnormal	3
Extension	2
No response	1
BEST VERBAL RESPONSE	
Oriented and converses	5
Disoriented and converses	4
Inappropriate words	3
Incomprehensible sounds	2
No response	1
Glasgow Coma Scale Total	3-15
(Eyes + Motor + Verbal)	

Rehabilitation

Rehabilitation of a person with head injuries includes orientation to time, place, and person and treatment strategies designed to decrease confusion, which may be best achieved in a closed room rather than an open treatment area. Complaints of diplopia and dizziness must be taken into consideration when gross and fine motor tasks are performed. When doing mobility training, balance strategies must be considered, as they may be compromised as a result of the head injury. A stepping strategy for balance may be employed initially to maintain balance when agitated. More advanced balance strategies (using muscles crossing the hip and ankle joints) may follow as recovery occurs. Motor weakness and tonal changes may affect efforts to walk. Inappropriate behavior, apathy, restlessness, and fearfulness affect the treatment sessions and set limits on short-term treatment outcomes.

Patience, understanding, and encouragement are necessary elements for all therapuetic interventions. The therapist must be mindful not to frustrate or overwhelm the elderly patient with tasks beyond his or her current abilities. A comfortable and organized atmosphere helps a patient with a head injury to achieve his or her physical and mental potentials, if given appropriate time.

SPINAL CORD TRAUMA

Falls and other accidents can also lead to spinal cord and peripheral nerve injuries. For the elderly person with a spinal cord injury, whether it be complete or incomplete, the chances that medical complications will develop are higher than they are for the younger patient. The elderly are at greater risk for developing pneumonia, gastrointestinal hemorrhage, pulmonary emboli, and renal stones. Premorbid conditions, such as arthritis and congestive heart failure, may complicate the rehabilitation process. For instance, the wearing of halo traction may limit ambulation secondary to balance difficulties for the elderly individual with kyphosis and a flexed hip and knee posture. The halo traction may also lead to disorientation and depression, both of which directly affect rehabilitation outcomes. The ultimate function achieved by the elderly spinal cord patient is directly related to the motor strength present. Regaining strength is possible if the cord is intact, but it may be slowed because of aging and comorbid conditions. Attaining the ability to perform the activities of daily living requires greater assistance for the elderly than for the younger patient with a spinal cord injury.

PLEXUS AND PERIPHERAL INJURY

Conditions of aging such as spinal stenosis and spinal deformities may predispose the elderly individual to plexus and peripheral nerve injuries with relatively minor exertion or trauma. Overextending an upper extremity reach accompanied by force may result in a brachial plexus stretch injury in an individual with kyphoscoliosis and a narrowed spinal canal. If the nerve root is evulsed there will be a flail motor response and no chance for the return of motor strength. Motor function can be regained after stretch injuries; appropriate positioning (with a brace or sling) of the involved limb is necessary if deformity is to be minimized and recovery maximized. Graded therapeutic exercises performed in positions of the limb where the effect of gravity is lessened or eliminated, along with the use of electrical simulation will retard further deleterious effects on the musculotendinous unit and may thus promote return of motor function. Motor and sensory tests assist the therapist in determining the extent of injury and provide a baseline against which to monitor recovery.

Fractures and other injuries to the limbs can result in peripheral nerve damage that leads to motor and sensory involvement. The radial, medial, ulnar, and peroneal nerves are most commonly affected. The extent of nerve damage is classified into three categories: (1) neurapraxia, a brief interruption of physiological function; (2) axonotmesis, Wallerian degeneration of axons with intact Schwann sheaths; and (3) neurotmesis, complete nerve severance. Nerve conduction studies and electromyography assist in determining the extent of nerve damage. See Chapters 35 and 36 for further information on generalized and localized peripheral neuropathies.

Instructing the patient in skin protection, the use of splints, strengthening exercises, joint range of motion, and sensory reeducation is the recommended therapeutic regimen. Functional electrical stimulation is useful in the recovery process. Periodic sensory examinations using Semmes-Weinstein filaments and manual muscle tests assists both the physical therapist and the patient in noting changes in the peripheral nerve's innervated tissues and in directing case management.

CONCLUSION

Trauma in the aging patient may not present clinically in the same fashion as it does in a younger person. In addition, preexisting conditions such as spinal stenosis and arthritis may complicate the physical findings. Therefore, the skilled clinician must be vigilant during evaluation and treatment in looking for signs and symptoms that vary from the diagnosis or change over time.

SUGGESTED READINGS

Jennett B, Teasdale G. *Management of Head Injuries.* Philadelphia: F.A. Davis; 1981:78.
Netter FH, Jones HR Jr, eds. *Nervous System, Part II: Neurologic and Neuromuscular Disorders, The Ciba Collection of Medical Illustrations.* West Caldwell, N.J.: CIBA Pharmaceutical; 1986.
Rosenthal M, Griffith E, Bond M, Miller JD. *Rehabilitation of the Head-Injured Adult.* Philadelphia: F.A. Davis; 1984.

Chapter 31

Senile Dementia and Cognitive Impairment
Osa Jackson, Ph.D., P.T.

INTRODUCTION

The rehabilitation goal for every patient with temporary or permanent cognitive impairment is to promote maximal involvement in self-care and meaningful life activities. Each individual defines the things that constitute meaningful life activities in a unique and personal way. The physical therapists who work with a patient with temporary or permanent cognitive impairment face the challenge of helping the patient, significant others (family and friends), and care-givers to support the individuality and self-determination of each patient and to enhance his or her sense of safety. The physical therapy intervention can include, but is not limited to, consultation and training for care-givers and hands-on treatment for specific patient problems. Examples include ergonomics (such as wheelchair fit to maximize safe mobility), functional evaluation and training in the performance of the activities of daily living (ADLs) (such as helping care-givers with rolling the patient over and with mobility in bed), neurological rehabilitation focusing on kinesthetic cuing to enhance participation in ADLs through modified communication (such as showing care-givers how sitting to one side and using light touch can enhance self-feeding), and environmental adaptation (such as setting up key environmental cues that enhance safety, for example, curbs painted bright yellow for contrast).

DEFINITION OF TERMS

The patient with cognitive limitations presents a unique set of needs because hands-on care and touch, rather than speech, eventually become the key tools for communication. The entire medical team is involved in making the diagnosis of dementia or cognitive impairment. Accuracy of diagnosis is a key factor as some temporary cognitive impairments can be reversed. Common examples of conditions in which impairment may be temporary include medication toxicity, depression, nutritional deficiency, anesthesia, and allergic reaction.[1]

When working with dementia and cognitive impairment, definitions of terms are helpful.

1. Delirium: a decline in the level of cognitive function combined with drowsiness or agitation.
2. Dementia: a global decline in cognitive abilities in a person who is awake and aware of surroundings. The decline from previous status affects several kinds of cognitive tasks.
3. Alzheimer's disease: a degenerative disease of the brain of unknown cause.

Alzheimer's Disease

The most common symptoms of Alzheimer's disease include the following (some of these symptoms may also apply to other dementing illnesses):

- recent memory loss affecting skills in performing job or tasks,
- difficulty performing familiar tasks,
- problems with language,
- disorientation in terms of time and place,
- poor or decreased judgment,
- problems with abstract thinking,
- misplacing things,
- changes in mood or behavior,
- changes in personality, and
- loss of initiative[2]

At this time, Alzheimer's disease is a diagnosis that is made after ruling out the other major causes of cognitive impairment such as depression, cerebral infarct, thyroid dysfunction, normal-pressure hydrocephalus, tuberculosis, metal poisoning, and Parkinson's disease.[3]

Progressive Phases of Alzheimer's Disease

In dementia/Alzheimer's, the behavior of the patient often progresses through three distinct phases, although each patient presents with unique minor variations in the progression of the disease. The common aspects of the three stages can be described as follows.

1. Between 2 and 4 years leading up to and including diagnosis: Common symptoms include low energy, emotional lability, slow reactions, picking up new information more slowly, showing less initiative and greater reluctance to try new things, sticking to familiar and predictable activities, taking longer to do routine chores, being unable to think of words, especially names of things, losing one's way to familiar places, having trouble with finances, and experiencing heightened anxiety.

2. Between 2 and 10 years after diagnosis: Common symptoms include having trouble recognizing familiar people, finding it difficult to make decisions, making up stories to fill empty memory spaces, little speech with content or meaning noticeably impoverished, having trouble comprehending what is read, writing illegibly, becoming more self-absorbed, experiencing late afternoon restlessness (sundown syndrome), having difficulty with perceptual motor coordination, showing lability, acting impulsively, losing ADL skills, monitoring physical appearance inappropriately, repeating physical movements, experiencing delusions or hallucinations, overreacting to minor events, and needing gradually increasing supervision as the severity of symptoms increases.

3. Between 1 and 3 years (terminal phase): Commons symptoms include becoming apathetic and remote, being unable to recognize self or family, having poor short-term and long-term memory, losing orientation in familiar environments, becoming incontinent, losing the ability to communicate with words, gradually becoming unable to walk or get around, and possibly experiencing seizures or weight loss or the urge to put objects to the mouth. Note: In the third phase, the person can still understand emotion and tone and can still be responsive in small ways to physical care.[4]

REHABILITATION: EMPOWERING THE PATIENT

Contributions can be made by physical therapy intervention at any phase of the cognitive decline in order to enhance patient participation in ADLs and communication and minimize care-giver burnout. The key strategy is to build on the patient's intact skills, to explore new possibilities for communication, and to create a sense of safety and enjoyment that includes modified ADL tasks for the patient. The clearest means of communication is to relate in ways that allow the person to feel emotionally safe and to build from an emotional tone that is perceived by the patient as being nurturing and positive.

Empowering the patient during interaction with care-givers and family means that individuality and a sense of safety and self-determination are the most important outcomes for each interaction. For staff and family this means that there is a need to become aware of what works for the patient, and what the patient can emotionally sense if the intention of the care-giver is to support his or her determination and self-esteem.

The physical therapy intervention that is provided for a person with dementia or cognitive impairment requires that the therapist be trained beyond the entry level. When a therapist or assistant is interested in working with older persons with cognitive impairment, advanced training in kinesthetic contact, communication, neurological rehabilitation, and handling skills is necessary. Emphasis on mastering neurological rehabilitation techniques to empower the patient through functional training and kinesthetic cuing is critical. The physical therapist works closely with care-givers to enhance the effectiveness of daily tasks that are important to the patient. The patient should always be seen for treatment in his or her own environment if possible, and any new therapists should be introduced by someone who has a history of months of nurturing contact with the patient.

Training of Care-Givers and Significant Others

As a therapist, assistant, care-giver, or health-care team member begins work with a person with cognitive impairment, it is critical that training include an inventory of personal communication habits plus refinement so that communication with hands-on cuing is clearly reinforced by communication through posture, facial expression, breathing rate, and so forth. The primary approach to communicating with a person with cognitive impairment is to start with a single clear intention and then reinforce it with touch, gestures, and body language that are perceived by the patient as helpful.

Hands-on contact and touch can be a key strategy for communication that will enhance the life of a person with cognitive impairment. It is helpful to get input from family and care-givers about historical information and special cultural or social significance of touch that are unique to the individual. A first step in a consultation is to help the family and care-givers to explore their awareness of their own quality of touch, of the cultural history related to touch, and of their own body language. When words are not the main tool of communication, it becomes even more important to clarify the intention of each communication before initiating that communication. A place to start may be for the staff and family to develop a statement of philosophy concerning interaction with the patient (e.g., agree that the most important thing to get across to the patient is that everyone supports that patient's having the highest quality of life possible, as defined by the patient). The detailed definition of a philosophy provides the rationale for ongoing problem-solving and consultation such as what behavioral cues are needed to support the philosophy and still get the patient out of another patient's room.

Key Questions

Another way of empowering the patient is to use the patient's own perceptions as the guiding factors in all communication. As the consultant, the therapist guides staff members in identifying key questions for each individual patient. These can include but are not limited to the following:

1. What are the habits for nurturing or comforting at the present time?
2. Under what conditions does the patient enjoy being with other people?
3. What rituals appear to be important to the patient?
4. What are some of the patient's favorite activities?

5. How does this patient communicate enjoyment and displeasure?
6. What is the preferred rest/activity and eating/toileting cycle?
7. What activities, objects, or persons appear to anchor the patient into cognitive reality in the present?
8. What activities are known to produce agitation or discomfort?

It is hoped that this type of information can be collected by care-givers and family and incorporated into the care plan.

Enhancing Self-Care

It is critical that all care-givers (family and health-care personnel at all levels) have up-to-date information about the desires and abilities of each patient they are caring for on a particular shift. Other specific issues for the elderly with dementia or cognitive impairment that can enhance self-care abilities include the following:

1. Establish a staffing pattern that allows the patient and the care-givers to gain familiarity with and be comfortable with each other. A person with cognitive impairment does poorly in a constantly changing environment and develops better self-care habits in an environment in which there is a small, familiar team of care-givers. It is important for the supervision of patients and the detection of new problems that the care-givers be familiar with the habits, likes, and dislikes of each particular patient.[5]
2. Modify the pace of activity to the pace and abilities of each individual.
3. Provide options for one-to-one pleasant, nurturing contact several times each day.
4. Change the position of the nonambulatory patient every hour as desired and allow rest for half an hour in bed, as needed; as a patient's abilities decline, it is important to allow the patient to rest in bed and to get up from bed as often as is desired.
5. Provide stable furniture in the environment so that patient can use it for balance and support during ambulation.
6. Encourage early introduction of rolling carts or walkers so that patients can remain safely mobile as long as possible.
7. Encourage care-givers to walk and talk with patients and provide nurturing contact such as holding the patient's hand or arm.
8. Eat with patients in a normal social manner (one staff member joins two or three clients at a table and eats along with them, family style. When a client is unable to participate in this way, the staff member may eat with one client at a time; when the client no longer wishes to eat, the staff member

should simply sit and read, sing, or talk to the patient in order to provide socially nurturing contact.

9. Encourage the patient to make choices as part of care-giving as long as the patient can be empowered by doing so. When this is not nurturing for the patient, then a predictable structure of events can help.

10. Help to perform ADLs so that the patient enjoys living. This could mean changing the style of clothing to avoid pulling clothing over the head which may be irritating; a shirt with an opening in the front and a velcro closure would avoid this.

11. Perform functional cognitive assessments of the patient as part of daily care-giving. This means that the care-giver must be trained as appropriate to his or her educational background in order to moni-

tor gross changes in the cognitive function of the patient.

Mini Mental-State Examination

The Mini Mental-State Examination can be a valuable resource and can be introduced to the majority of family members and care-givers.[3] (See Box 31–1.) It is critical that persons providing day-to-day care in the home or institutional setting be able to verify that cognitive abilities are present and unchanged from the previous day. The rationale is that the staff member or care-taker is the person who must modify the communication strategy if there are changes in the patient's abilities. The rationale for daily review of cognitive status is that it forms the basis for clear and reasonable communi-

---

Box 31–1

The Folstein Mini-Mental State Examination

Maximum Score	
	Orientation
5	What is the (year) (season) (date) (day) (month)?
5	Where are we (state) (county) (town) (hospital) (floor)?
	Registration
3	Name three objects: one second to say each. Then ask the patient all three after you have said them. Give one point for each correct answer. Repeat them until he learns all three. Count trials and record number.
	Attention and Calculation
5	Begin with 100 and count backward by 7 (stop after five answers). Alternatively, spell "world" backward.
	Recall
3	Ask for the three objects repeated above.
	Language
2	Show a pencil and a watch and ask the patient to name them.
1	Repeat the following: "No ifs, ands, or buts."
3	A three-stage command: "Take a paper in your right hand, fold it in half, and put it on the floor."
1	Read and obey the following: (show written item) CLOSE YOUR EYES
1	Write a sentence.
1	Copy a design (complex polygon).
30	Total score possible.

Source: Adapted with permission from *Journal of Psychiatric Research* (1975;12:196–197), Copyright © 1975, Pergamon Journals Ltd.

cation with the patient at the highest and most accurate level.

Supporting Quality of Life

The interventions necessary to support a good quality of life for each patient fall into the categories of treating excess disability, reducing patient stress, and creating a supportive environment. Physical therapy consultation can be used by the health-care team to maximize participation in ADLs in many areas of problem-solving. The ergonomic aspect involves creating a fit between the patient and the environment that encourages normalization of lifestyle. Common problems that are addressed include selection, fitting, and training to use canes, walkers, wheelchairs, and beds. (Note: bed height should be at chair height—approximately 16 to 18 inches from seat surface to floor—if an assistive device such as a sliding board is to be used to help with transfers. It is critical to understand the importance of sliding boards in the third phase of cognitive impairment in which the patient becomes less and less able to get in and out of bed without help. A patient and a care-giver trained in the use of a sliding board can easily get up during the night to go to the toilet. The idea is that the patient is slid onto the board so that the care-giver may need to use only 40 pounds of effort to help a 160-pound patient. Both the patient and care-giver benefit because the transfer takes less effort and is more pleasant. If beds are too high they appear to promote fear and falls in some patients, and two or more nurse's[2] aides are required to help a 160-pound patient out of bed and into the bathroom. Several ready resources are available for teaching sliding-board transfers from bed, chair, toilet, and car.[6]

The physical therapist can provide consultation for the care-giver when ADLs are no longer easy to perform. There are many functional profiles that can be used but it is important that a measure of how long tasks take to perform be included along with the amount of help (physical assistance) and the assistive devices required. It is critical that the actual care-givers be present during physical therapy so that they can then demonstrate solutions to the care-givers on the other shifts. It is important that written instructions be left with care-givers after training is complete and the care-givers are able to perform independently. The physical therapy goals will be written in a way that trains care-givers to assist a patient to perform a particular task within a specific environment and time and with specific assistive devices. Functional evaluation for ADL problem-solving can be very helpful during the third phase of cognitive decline when the patient

will tend to want to spend an increasing amount of time in bed. For example, if there is only one care-giver and the patient needs to roll over but is "dead" weight, the care-giver who knows basic handling skills can involve the patient to whatever degree possible and thus use less energy.

The physical therapist who has mastered a particular technique of neurofacilitation (such as the Bobath, Brunstromm, or Feldenkrais method) has available a series of strategies that a nontrained person does not have access to when it comes to helping a person to move or to perform a specific task such as sitting up, standing up, and walking. It is important to acknowledge that evaluation and treatment have been going on from moment t moment and that this is not a strategy that can be taught in 5 minutes to someone else. However, it is possible to teach a person how to reinforce the patient in using a mastered technique by employing a specific kinesthetic cue.

Spaced repetition creates mastery of and strength in a new pattern of action so care-givers can provide valuable practice of new skills that the patient has mastered during a therapy session. An example can help to clarify the teamwork that can exist between the care-giver and the physical therapist: The patient, when resting supine, becomes rigid in the legs and then is very hard to roll and help to a sitting position. The therapist explores and finds that placing a small towel roll ($3'' \times 6''$) below the knees relaxes the hips and legs slightly. The therapist tries lightly stroking the feet one at a time for 3 to 4 minutes, and this appears to desensitize the feet. The therapist then explores various possibilities and finally finds that tapping the forefoot one at a time, allows the legs to relax enough that support under the knees combined with rolling the leg out (externally rotating and abducting the hip) allows the knees to be bent; thus, rolling the patient over becomes possible. The next step is to demonstrate this procedure on the care-giver so that the person can feel the contact and points of pressure that create the response. Lastly, the care-giver explores and practices the process under the tutoring of the therapist until the procedure has been mastered.

Environmental adaptation to enhance independence is well described by Karlquist.[7] Organizing the furniture and rituals of care-giving to build on the patient's strengths is critical to enhance the sense of safety and enjoyment for the patient through each phase of the decline in cognitive function. It is often likely to be necessary to continue to solve environmental concerns at regular intervals. The patient may find an extra blanket comforting at one time, but in 6 months that same extra blanket on the bed may be irritating. As a patient experiences cognitive changes, there will be periods when he or she will favor physical contact such as holding hands or walking arm in arm. Some patients may literally need someone to sit at the bedside for 5 minutes and sing in order to feel safe and be able to go to sleep.

The physical therapy consultation can involve a variety of detailed refinements. Sometimes it is as simple as the fact that if you sit on a patient's hemiplegic side, the patient becomes agitated, but if you sit on the unaffected side, the patient is calmed by your presence and goes to sleep. The key is to be available to support staff and care-givers so they can accept the patient as he or she is and accept a show of affection even if it is not how we would expect an adult to act.

The family commonly needs referral to a family support group or to formal counseling so they can work through their emotional reactions (i.e., grief and anger). Counseling is often helpful to answer questions of grandchildren who may not have been present to see the gradual decline and then are introduced to a person who looks like grandmother but does not even recognize them. Children are often fine at accepting the limited abilities of a relative if they are given the right tools and support so they can be comfortable and feel safe in the situation.

Physical Therapy: Hands-On Treatment and Teaching Care-givers

For a therapist or assistant trained in neurorehabilitation handling techniques, guided touch or hands-on facilitation can be a strategy to enhance communication, relaxation, balance, coordination, and self-determination. When the therapist meets the patient, it is common to find him or her sitting in a primitive posture, such as with feet unsupported and hips flexed, head forward, hands resting unnaturally, and showing overall tension and shallow breathing. Commonly, a therapist has been called in because bathing or some other basic task has become a source of great stress to the patient and has resulted in conflict between the care-giver and the patient. The first step is to create a sense of safety and comfort. It is helpful to know what has been comforting to the patient in the recent past. A negotiation between the therapist and the care-givers should occur so that there can be agreement from the beginning about the desired goals and the willingness of the care-giver to make minor but possibly key changes in the way a desired task is performed. There is an old statement that says, "To keep doing the same thing and then being surprised that the results are the same is common when we are too stressed to see the obvious." When the therapist meets the patient, a bond of trust must be established. This can involve any number of stimuli—a hot pack in the lap, a heating pad, a doll, some music to listen to, or simply a hand to hold—and the ability to just sit and smile and wait for acceptance of the contact. The goals of therapy will vary but the component skills that create a positive therapeutic outcome are often the same.

Key Physical Changes

Key physical changes that may facilitate relaxation and thus the patient's involvement in assisted ADLs may include the following:

1. Evaluate the patient's breathing pattern for 1 minute and take corrective actions if appropriate. Gentle tapping and touching procedures as described by Speads[8] may enhance the ease of ventilation.

2. Place the patient in a supine position so that the legs can roll out slightly and the ankles are at or near neutral, not plantar-flexed.

3. Allow active assistive and passive range of motion in each leg as needed to assist with dressing. This can be achieved by comfortably abducting each lower extremity one at a time to approximately 30 degrees.

4. Position the patient in a seated posture with the feet relaxed, foot-flat, placed hip-width apart, and covered with comfortable footwear for skin protection.

5. Use a correctly fitted, ergonomically appropriate firm seat, especially for a wheelchair or a chair that is used frequently. This will enhance the sit-to-stand pattern of action.[9]

6. Place the patient's hands on arm rests or in the lap, with the wrists at a neutral position; avoid flexion of the wrists.

7. Use a functional lumbar support as needed for comfort, especially if the patient will be sitting for more than 15 minutes.

The Importance of Touch

During the therapist's process of exploration to discover what will enhance self-determination for the patient and minimize stress for the care-giver, touch can have many effects. Touch can be used simply to relax and to comfort, as in light massage, and the relaxation response will occur if that is what the patient needs. Touch can also be used to create awareness, as in helping a person prepare to stand by having him or her touch one foot to the top of the other or by rubbing the person's feet against each other in a gentle fashion. Touch can also be used to suggest change, to create a distraction and help a person to redirect. If a patient is focused on getting something that the care-giver cannot provide and then a new stimulus is offered, the first object is forgotten. Touch can also be used to actually initiate change, as in a directional movement to assist in communicating the need to stand up or sit down. In this application, the touch is usually clearly visible to the patient and the care-giver and involves more pressure than the others. The techniques of neurofacilitation use a repetitive or gradually increasing or decreasing touch to stimulate or to erase a reflex response which can then be used to reinforce improvement in functional activities.

For a person with cognitive impairment, the use of touch to enhance functional abilities and participation in ADLs starts at the point of the patient's awareness of his or her habitual response to what the care-giver is doing. In hands-on treatment, the habitual response of the patient to a particular input can often be changed from an undesirable response to a desirable response simply by making very minor changes in the stimulus—slowing down, using an ounce more or less pressure, using two fingers of contact rather than one, or using a flat hand rather than the fingertips. The patient with cognitive impairment has the ability to know clearly what he or she needs and can make precise distinctions in methods of handling that to the outsider watching are not at all obvious. The patient with cognitive impairment is often sensitive to contact and touch and can respond to physical therapy by showing improved participation in life. The big question is whether the care-giver and the therapist are willing to acknowledge the tiny distinctions (such as flat-hand versus fingertip pressure) desired by the patient and modify input so the patient can comfortably participate in life on his or her own terms and feel empowered rather than having to submit to others' terms.

CONCLUSION

Recognizing the possibility of reversing cognitive impairments due to temporary conditions is important. In Alzheimer's disease, the stage to which it has progressed affects the intervention. The involvement of the family and care-givers is crucial, so educating them is a priority. Every change that enhances the treatment and facilitates the patient's participation in self-care is of great value. Working with cognitively impaired patients can be deeply rewarding, but it requires a willingness to explore the fine distinctions that can appear meaningless but that make the difference between creating a pleasant environment for the patient or a living hell.

REFERENCES

1. Jackson-Wyatt O. Aging, the brain and dementia. In: Umphred D, ed. *Neurological Rehabilitation* 3rd ed. St. Louis: C.V. Mosby; 1995.
2. *Is it Alzheimer's? Ten Warning Signs.* Alzeimer's Association, Detroit Area Chapter; 1997.
3. Mace N, Hardy SR, Rabins P. Alzheimer's disease and the confused patient. In: Jackson-Wyatt O, ed. *Physical Therapy of the Geriatric Patient,* 2nd ed. New York: Churchill Livingstone; 1989.
4. Ronch J. *Alzheimer's Disease: A Practical Guide for Families and Other Caregivers.* Alzheimer's Association, Detroit Area Chapter, 1997.
5. Murray R, Huelskotnner M. *Psychiatric Mental Health Nursing: Giving Emotional Care.* Englewood Cliffs, N.J.: Prentice-Hall; 1983.
6. Buchwald LE. *Activities of Daily Living: A New Form.* New York: New York University Medical Center, Institute of Rehabilitation Medicine; 1979.
7. Karlquist L. Environmental assessment: adaptations for maximal independence. In: Jackson-Wyatt O, ed. *Therapeutic Considerations for the Elderly.* New York: Churchill Livingstone; 1987.
8. Speads C. *Ways to Better Breathing,* 2nd ed. Great Neck, N.Y.: Felix Morrow; 1986.
9. Jackson-Wyatt O. *Natural Ease for Daily Living: Can You Move to Get the Job Done?* Rochester, Mich.: Physical Therapy Center; 1994.
10. Umphred D. *Neurological Rehabilitation,* St. Louis: C.V. Mosby, 1995.

Chapter 32

Multiple Sclerosis
Deborah L. Cooke, Ph.D., P.T.

INTRODUCTION

Multiple sclerosis (MS) affects an estimated 250,000 to 500,000 people in the United States alone. Onset of MS usually occurs between the ages of 20 and 60. Although rare, it is not impossible for the onset of disease to occur in childhood or after the age of 60. Twice as many women as men have the disease. It has long been thought that people living in temperate zones are at greater risk of developing the disease than those living in subtropical areas. However, ethnic background, family history, and diet may also be noteworthy factors influencing disease risk.

COURSE AND PROGNOSIS

Many MS patients can expect a normal lifespan. Mean survival after being diagnosed with MS has been reported to be between 25 and 38 years, although in very serious cases, the mortality rate is more than four times that of the general population. Death due directly to the disease is uncommon, but cases of herniation of the brainstem or primary respiratory failure have been reported to be caused by the disease and to result in death. Secondary complications such as those arising from upper respiratory or urinary tract infection are uncommon today because of the modern antibiotic treatments available. The rate of suicide in persons with MS has been reported to be as much as seven times higher than that of the general population, but social, religious, and ethnic factors no doubt affect the probability of death by suicide in any individual.

Classification of MS

Classification of MS is based on the course of clinical symptoms (Box 32–1). Relapsing-remitting is the most common type, occurring in approximately 70% of people with MS. The rate of clinically relevant MS exacerbations varies widely and tends to decrease with advancing disease. Although one might assume that the patient with more frequent clinical relapses would have more severe disability, there is, in fact, only a weak association between the rate of MS relapses and disability outcome. It may be that the accumulation of subclinically active MS lesions is more important in determining long-term severity of disability. A frustration for the clinician and the patient may be the difficulty in distinguishing the temporary effects

of viral infections, fever, or fatigue from true symptoms associated with the disease processes. As the disease progresses this distinction may become more difficult. No definite clinical criteria exist for identifying an active disease state, but one rule of thumb may be that MS symptoms last longer than 24 hours and can be documented clinically by the presence of sensory or motor changes. Patients with relapsing-remitting MS are at greatest risk for poor clinical outcome (1) if they suffer frequent exacerbations involving motor systems that result in residual deficits 6 months following relapse, (2) if they are older at the time of the onset of symptoms, or (3) if they have moderate disability within 5 years of diagnosis (Box 32–2).[1]

Relapsing-remitting MS may later develop into a secondary, progressive phase in which disability progresses more rapidly. Of significance to those working with a geriatric population is a Dutch study that followed 214 patients with relapsing-remitting disease and found that disability accrues more rapidly in older women, who experienced frequent relapses that ultimately converted to progressive MS.[2] There tends to be a great deal of variability within and between patients in the transition from relapsing-remitting to secondary progressive MS. The transition is difficult to identify clinically or pathologically at the time it is occurring, although in retrospect the patient may be able to identify an extended period of time in which remission of active symptoms did not occur.

Persons with primary progressive MS make up less than 10% of the MS population and are thought to have a later age of onset and a higher morbidity. Symptoms tend to progress more slowly in primary progressive than in secondary progressive, but the ultimate level of disability may be as severe.[2] It is more common for primary progressive MS to present as a progressive paraparesis or with progressive cerebellar involvement. Rather than representing a variety of MS in clinical course, primary progressive may be a distinct pathological form with a poorer response to traditional immune-directed treatments.[1] For those working with the geriatric patient, it is significant to note that older age at onset of MS symptoms is related to poorer outcome for both primary and secondary progressive MS.

The term "benign multiple sclerosis" is ambiguous and poorly defined in the MS literature. It is generally used to describe patients with little disability after 10 years, who make up 20 to 40% of the population with MS, and therefore the classification can be used reliably only in retrospect. The term "benign" is misleading in that some persons with this slow course may eventually develop severe disability.

Box 32–1

Classification of MS

Based on Clinical Course

Relapsing-remitting	Fluctuating course characterized by sudden onset of new or reappearance of previous symptoms followed by partial or total remission of symptoms
Secondary progressive	Absence of remission phases with more rapid progression of symptoms and disability; develops from relapsing-remitting course
Primary progressive	Slow progression of symptoms from onset of disease with no remission of symptoms

Box 32–2

Kurtzke Expanded Disability Status Scale

0	Normal neurological exam (all grade 0 in FS; mental grade 1 accepted)
1.0	No disability, minimal signs in one FS other than mental
1.5	No disability, more than one grade 1 in FS other than mental
2.0	Minimal disability, one FS grade 2, other 0 or 1
2.5	Minimal disability in two FS with grade 2, others 0 or 1
3.0	Moderate disability in one FS with grade 3, others 0 or 1; or three/four FS with grade 2, others 0 or 1; fully ambulatory
3.5	Fully ambulatory but with moderate disability in one FS with grade 3 and one/two FS grade 2; or two FS grade 3; or five FS grade 2
4.0	Fully ambulatory without aid or rest at least 500 meters, self-sufficient, up and about some 12 hours a day despite relatively severe disability of FS grade 4 (others 0 or 1), or combinations of lesser grades beyond limits of preceding step
4.5	Fully ambulatory without aid or rest at least 300 meters, up and about much of day, able to work full day, may have some limits of full activity or require minimal assistance; relatively severe disability consisting of one FS grade 4 (others 0 or 1) or combinations of lesser grades beyond limits of preceding step
5.0	Ambulatory without aid or rest for 200 meters; impaired ability to carry out full daily activities; FS of one grade 5 or combination of lesser grades beyond preceding step
5.5	Ambulatory without aid or rest for about 100 meters; unable to carry out full daily activities; FS of one grade 5 or combination of lesser grades beyond preceding step
6.0	Intermittent or unilateral constant assistance to walk 100 meters with or without rest; more than 2 FS grades 3+ and combinations of lesser grades
6.5	Constant bilateral assistance required to walk 20 meters without resting; two FS grade 3+ with combinations of lesser grades
7.0	Unable to walk beyond 5 meters even with aid; wheels self in standard wheelchair and transfers independently; up in w/c approximately 12 hours a day; FS scores are combinations with more than one grade 4+
7.5	Unable to take more than a few steps; may need aid in transfer, cannot be up in chair full day, but wheels self, may require motorized w/c, FS as in 7.0
8.0	Restricted to bed or chair, may be up in chair most of day; able to perform self-care functions with effective use of arms; FS as in 7.0
8.5	Restricted to bed much of day; some use of arms; some self-care functions; FS as in 7.0
9.0	Unable to help in bed; can communicate and eat; FS grades mostly 4+
9.5	Totally helpless bed patient; unable to communicate or eat/swallow; almost all FS grade 4+
10	Death due to MS

FS, Functional systems.

Kurtzke JF. Rating neurologic impairment in multiple sclerosis: an expanded disability status scale (EDSS). *Neurology* 1983; 33:1444.

PATHOLOGY AND CAUSES

Multiple sclerosis is a disease characterized by demyelination of the central nervous system, with relative axon sparing. In chronic stages of the disease, loss of axons does occur. Although rare, peripheral nervous system involvement in MS has also been reported and may represent a subset of MS with immune responses to antigens present in both the central nervous system (CNS) and peripheral nervous system (PNS). The disease process is a dynamic one, with inflammation and edema occurring in the early stages, followed by scarring and plaque formation. A disruption of the blood-brain barrier is involved in early stages of lesion formation. Demyelination produces characteristic MS plaques, which are grossly visible on magnetic resonance imaging (MRI), and result in the slowing of axon conduction, leading to the primary clinical symptoms associated with the disease. Although remyelination can occur in the early stages of the disease process, it rarely leads to clinical improvements. MS lesions may occur at various sites throughout the CNS, producing a wide variety of clinical pictures. However, in North America and Europe there seems to be a prevalence of involvement of the optic nerve, periventricular white matter, brain stem, and spinal cord.

Although much is still misunderstood about the cause of MS, current thinking is that it involves a genetic predisposition modified by environmental factors. A disturbance of immunological function is the primary pathogenesis. There are currently two competing theories that attempt to explain the cause of multiple sclerosis. Briefly summarized, they are (1) an infection, probably of the viral type, that may attack the oligodendroglia of the central nervous system or (2) an autoimmune process that may begin with an infection of the peripheral lymphatic immune system, producing antibodies that cross the blood-brain barrier and cause destruction of myelin.

DIAGNOSTIC CRITERIA

The standard clinical criterion for the diagnosis of MS is the occurrence of symptoms reflecting involvement of at least two areas of the central nervous system separated in time and in anatomical space, for example, double vision at one time followed by tingling in the legs 6 months later. MRI is rapidly becoming the standard tool for both diagnosis and monitoring of disease progression. Using the Poser criteria, for plain MRIs to be diagnostic there must be two or more lesions with a diameter of more than 2 mm.[3] There is poor correlation between site and size of the lesions on plain MRI and clinical manifestations of MS, and it may be that the accumulation of plaques in the CNS, as much as location, is the more significant aspect of the clinical picture. Godalinium-enhanced MRI and proton MR spectroscopy are newer techniques that may detect subclinical disease processes and more accurately reflect the clinical picture.

Visual evoked potential tests can be sensitive measures of abnormalities in the early stage of MS, as optic tract involvement is common as an early sign. Abnormal cerebral spinal fluid is found in 80 to 90% of persons with MS at some time during the disease, although the features of an abnormal spinal tap are not specific to MS.

IMPAIRMENTS AND DISABILITIES

Primary impairments are those symptoms that are a direct result of the disease process. Primary impairments in MS may involve a single nervous system function but more often involve multiple CNS systems (Box 32–3). Secondary impairments result from restrictions imposed on the individual by the primary problem and are often preventable with timely interventions. Disability, or limitations in daily living skills, does not always reflect the level of impairment in MS, as many patients develop adaptations over time and remain remarkably functional despite profound physical impairment.

Sensory System Impairments

Visual impairments due to demyelination of the optic nerve are often an early symptom of MS and are characterized by painful visual acuity loss, scotoma, diplopia, and loss of sensitivity to color and contrast. Partial recovery often occurs.[4] In terms of the motor aspect of the visual system, defects in eye movement control are common, particularly internuclear ophthalmoplegias and nystagmus. Hearing loss occurs in 10% of persons with MS, with onset acutely or up to 10 years after onset of the disease. Partial or complete remissions are common.[4] Vestibular involvement may include central and peripheral vestibular components, as the most proximal portion of the PNS is myelinated by oligodentrocytes. Only about 20% of patients with MS have symptoms of true vertigo, which is a sense that oneself or the environment is moving.[5] More commonly patients report dizziness and unsteadiness. The majority of patients with MS experience problems with balance at some time in their disease, but this may be secondary to multisensory deficits. Somatosensory system impairments in proprioception, light touch, and temperature may be caused by spinal sensory tract involvement. Permanent or transient paresthesias may occur. Bandlike sensations around the trunk and tingling or numbness in the limbs or face are sometimes reported. Lhermitte's sign is a transient sensation radiating down the spine following neck flexion. Although they have been reported, peripheral neuropathies are uncommon and are usually associated with secondary effects in advanced disease, such as malnutrition or cytotoxic drug effects. The reported incidence of pain in MS patients varies widely in the literature, ranging from 10 or 20%[6] to 80%.[7] Burning or searing pain may be caused by nerve root or spinal cord involvement and may follow a dermatomal pattern. Radicular-type pain originating from the lumbar spinal roots may be experienced, as well as

Box 32–3

Summary of Common Impairments

Sensory systems	Visual
	• Diminished acuity
	• Scotoma
	• Double vision
	• Color and contrast sensitivity loss
	• Ocular pain
	Vestibular
	• Dizziness
	• Unsteadiness
	• Vertigo
	Somatosensory
	• Numbness
	• Pain
	• Distorted sensations
Motor systems	Spasticity
	Weakness
	Ataxia
	Intention tremors
	Difficulty with speech and swallowing
	Disequilibrium
	Fatigue
Bowel and bladder	Urgency
	Frequency
	Urinary retention
	Incontinence
	Constipation
Sexual	Impotence
	Diminished sensitivity
	Diminished lubrication
Cognitive/ emotional	Deficits in
	• Short-term memory
	• Attention
	• Word-finding
	• Problem-solving
	• Conceptual thinking
	Depression
	Emotional lability
	Euphoria

misalignment resulting from muscle weakness or spasticity. Of course, a patient with MS may also experience pain from concurrent pathologies not related to MS, such as fibromyalgia or osteoarthritis.

Motor System Impairments

Spasticity is a common impairment in MS and may be mild or severe, limiting basic hygiene functions. The most common pattern of spasticity is in the hip flexors and adductors, the knee flexors, and the ankle plantar flexors. Upper extremity spasticity is less common but may occur in flexor muscles in advanced MS. Contractures may occur secondary to severe spasticity and prolonged immobility, and are most common in hip and knee flexors, hip adductors, and ankle plantarflexors (see Chapter 17, "Contractures"). Edema may be a problem in lower limbs secondary to prolonged dependent immobility and lack of muscle-pumping actions. Other secondary, and often preventable, effects of immobility and confinement to bed may include decubital ulcers, upper respiratory tract infections, bronchitis and bronchopneumonia, deep-vein thrombosis, and subsequent pulmonary infarction.

Muscle weakness is most evident upon repeated testing. In other words, a muscle may appear strong in an isolated muscle test, but as the duration of an activity such as ambulation increases, selective muscle weakness may appear. Ankle dorsiflexors, knee flexors and extensors, hip abductors, and trunk muscles, including upper back muscles, most often show such weakness. Cerebellar involvement may be exhibited as ataxia, postural and intention tremors, and dysmetria. These symptoms may be seen in the extremities, trunk and head, and ocular and oral musculature. Bulbar difficulties are more common in advanced disease. Involvement of tracts innervating cranial nerves V, VII, IX, and X may contribute to difficulties in eating, swallowing, and speaking. In addition, spasticity, weakness, or poor timing of respiratory and cervical muscles play a role.

Fatigue may be a factor in speech production. In fact, fatigue is a characteristic and early symptom of the disease. It is most notable in the early afternoon and evening and may worsen all MS symptoms. Different types of fatigue have been described: (1) fatigue from activity or exercise may be experienced more quickly in persons with MS; (2) "nerve fatigue," thought to be caused by the short-circuiting of demyelinated nerves, may be experienced as muscle weakness or fatigue; (3) fatigue associated with depression may go unrecognized; and (4) lassitude or an overwhelming sense of fa-

episodes of trigeminal neuralgia. Pain may also be experienced secondary to spasticity, most commonly taking the form of painful extensor spasms of the legs. Joint pain may occur secondary to tigue out of proportion to activity level is described by some persons with MS.

Postural instability is a common problem in MS, even in the early stages of the disease. Difficulties with static and dynamic balance control may be caused by impaired processing and integration of multisensory information relevant to the body's placement in the environment. Delayed timing of antagonistic muscle responses during dynamic activities may also be a source of postural instability. In addition, instability may be secondary to spasticity, muscle weakness, or ataxia.

Bowel and Bladder Involvement

Bowel and bladder problems are commonly reported by patients with MS. An estimated 50 to 80% of persons with MS develop bladder dysfunction at some time in the disease.[8] A neurogenic bladder is the most common cause of bladder problems in MS. Urinary frequency and urgency may occur in an uninhibited neurogenic bladder (cortical and subcortical involvement). Urinary retention and incontinence may be symptoms of a reflex neurogenic bladder (spinal cord above conus medullaris). Urinary tract infections may be secondary symptoms of a neurogenic bladder. Approaches to management of bladder dysfunction include timed voiding programs and intermittent self-catheterization. Foley catheters may be used in some patients who are ataxic and cannot self-catheterize. Constipation and bowel incontinence may occur in more advanced cases of MS. Bowel irregularity can be controlled with timing after meals, bulk-formers, suppositories, or enema, if needed. A rectal bag may be necessary for the more severely involved patient.

Neuropsychological Impairments

Although severe dementia from MS is rare, prevalence rates of some form of cognitive deficit range from 13 to 64%.[9] In some instances, neuropsychological impairment may be the initial or primary symptom. Deficits in attention, short-term memory, word-finding, conceptual thinking, and problem-solving are the most typical findings. Cognitive impairments may affect employment and social interactions. Frequency and rate of progression of neuropsychological impairments are not known.

Behavioral Changes

Depression, emotional lability, and euphoria, a persistent feeling of well-being and optimism that is inappropriate to the situation are possible emotional changes that may be seen in patients with MS, although the degree of prevalence of these emotions is not known. Debate exists as to whether these emotional responses are caused by brain dysfunction resulting from the disorder or are secondary to the stress placed on the patient and family by the uncertainty of the disease course. As with physical symptoms, behavioral responses may vary considerably from one patient to another and certainly within an individual over time.

Sexual Dysfunction

MS has no effect on fertility, fetal viability, or delivery. Relapses decrease during pregnancy and increase during the first 3 months following delivery. Sexual dysfunction is common in both men and women with MS and includes difficulty in achieving and maintaining erection, diminished sensitivity, problems with vaginal lubrication, and difficulty in achieving orgasm. In some patients, corticosteroid treatment, often given for other symptoms, can improve sexual functioning.

CLINICAL ASSESSMENT IN MS

The Kurtzke Expanded Disability Status Scale (EDSS) is an impairment/disability-level scale that is the gold standard for MS clinical drug trials (see Box 32–2). It is also used widely in other MS research and by clinicians to classify the extent and impact of the disease and to document change over an extended time. The scale has been criticized for not describing neuropsychological or upper extremity function well, for being biased toward ambulation, and for lack of sensitivity to short-term change. There is also little correlation between change in EDSS scores and lesion burden when viewed on MRI. The Minimal Record of Disability (MRD)[10] is a tool used to standardize assessment of the disability and handicap associated specifically with MS. This internationally approved scale is meant to be used in conjunction with the EDSS. Other scales, which are not exclusive to MS but have been used to classify disability and handicap, include the PULSES Profile,[11] the Barthel Index,[12] and the Functional Independence Measure (FIM).[13] The FIM, included in this text in Figure 79–1, has been shown to be useful in predicting the burden of care and in identifying MS patients' satisfaction with their lives.

REHABILITATION

General Principles

Rehabilitation for persons with multiple sclerosis may occur in many settings, including the acute hospital, rehabilitation center, outpatient clinic, nursing home, and client's own home. Ideally, rehabilitation involves an interdisciplinary team, with the patient and family members working as active participants in the team. The goals of rehabilitation should focus on maximizing the quality of life and independence of the patient within the constraints imposed by physical and psychological impairments. The dynamic interactions of the patient within his or her family and community as well as available resources should be considered when planning the goals of functional outcomes. Rather than being seen as a last resort, early team rehabilitation can provide patients with the basic skills and knowledge needed to assume responsibility for managing areas of life and health that can be controlled. Rehabilitation can offer education, emotional support, guidance as to realistic vocational and avocational choices, exercise recommendations, instruction in energy conservation and work-simplification techniques, and choices in selection of assistive and adaptive equipment. An emphasis on wellness and patient responsibility can help to develop a positive sense of control over what can be a very unpredictable disease.

Interventions

Motor system symptoms of MS may be treated with many of the same techniques used with other neurological problems. Spasticity may respond to daily range-of-motion and stretching exercises, especially in rotational and diagonal patterns, to slow rolling from supine to side-lying, to positions of side-lying with muscle elongation, to inhibitive splinting, and to cool baths or towels. Proper wheelchair positioning and seating devices may be helpful in controlling tone as well as preventing skin breakdown. These measures also help prevent contracture. Surgical release may be necessary in severe cases of contracture that interfere with hygiene or positioning. Limb edema may be treated with elevation and massage or with compression garments.

Muscle strengthening may be performed with light weights or rubber tubing, using exercises directed toward specific muscle weaknesses. Isokinetic equipment has been used to improve muscle endurance using high-speed, high-repetition protocols. Ataxia may be decreased with lightweight cuffs or vests, weight-bearing exercises in developmental patterns, and functional strengthening directed toward proximal muscle groups. Balance training may be task-specific and have little carryover from one situation to another; therefore, repetitive practice of a variety of functional activities is recommended. Assistive devices such as canes and walkers may be necessary to compensate for balance deficits. Weighting the device at the distal end with light cuff weights may help to improve control when ataxia is severe. Braces such as ankle-foot-orthotics (AFOs) may be necessary when the patient has weakness at the ankle, poor endurance in walking, impaired sensation, or poor knee control resulting in hyperextension. Severe foot edema, severe spasticity in the lower limb, or extreme muscle weakness at the hip are likely to be contraindications to the use of an AFO. It is important that braces be lightweight to avoid the compounding problems of proximal weakness and poor endurance. Customized fit, which requires the skills of a trained orthotist, is usually required.

Naps and rest periods are helpful in reducing fatigue. Cool environments, clothing, and baths may help. Exercise may actually reduce fatigue when done properly. Endurance exercises are performed at low intensity with repetition. In persons who are sedentary or who have chronic diseases, 10 minutes of continuous activity three times a day may provide the same aerobic training effect as 30 minutes of continuous exercise. Exercise should be done in a cool environment, and intensity can be kept at a level at which the person can still talk comfortably. For geriatric patients or others limited to wheelchairs, continuous range-of-motion exercises in a seated position, alternating arms and legs and done for 10 minutes twice a day may provide aerobic benefits. Exercise can also be incorporated into everyday activities like shopping, walking in the yard, or putting away dishes. However, household activities that involve continuous use of the same body parts in static positions for even short periods of time, such as folding laundry or washing dishes, may be more fatiguing. Recent research has shown that persons with mild to moderately severe MS may tolerate and actually benefit from aerobic training at intensities between 70 and 80% of HR_{Max} for 30-minute sessions on an exercise bike that incorporates arm and leg work.[14] Water activities are also excellent exercise for some patients with MS. To reduce fatigue and spasticity, water temperature should be 25° to 27.5°C (77° to 81.5° F). Free swimming, calisthenics, or water aerobics can be beneficial, depending on the client's skills and interests.

Problems in swallowing (dysphagia) and speech production (dysarthria) may occur in the patient with more advanced disease and are particularly important to address in the geriatric client. Difficulty in swallowing presents safety concerns because of the potential for aspiration. In addition, fatigue or difficulty eating may contribute to nutritional deficiencies, placing the geriatric patient at further risk for secondary complications. Treatment of dysphagia includes a focus on body positioning, swallowing techniques, and selection of food textures. The patient should sit upright to eat, with the neck elongated and the head flexed slightly forward to prevent aspiration. If automatic swallowing is impaired, the patient can focus on a conscious swallow. Light pressure on the thyroid notch timed with the attempt to swallow may facilitate the action. Thick fluids and semisoft foods are easier to swallow than thin fluids or coarse foods. The patient should be discouraged from talking during eating and encouraged to eat small meals frequently during the day or to take large meals early in the day. In the severely involved patient, a nasogastric feeding tube or percutaneous gastrostomy is an option, depending on the patient's wishes for long-term care.

Maintaining communication is critical for the geriatric patient in order to reduce the perception of isolation. The focus of treatment for dysarthria is generally to compensate for the dysfunction. The patient may be encouraged to slow down and pause between phrases or to exaggerate word formation. Good upright postural alignment, even if external positioning support is needed, can help to increase voice volume. Exercises to increase oral ROM and strength may help some patients. If production is severely limited, communication devices such as simple alphabet, word, or picture communication boards that may be accessed by pointing may be an option. More sophisticated computer-driven devices are used less frequently by the geriatric population.

Pharmacological Treatment

Although long-term corticosteroid treatment is not indicated, short-term courses of methylprednisolone have long been the standard of treatment during relapses. Options for pharmacological management of MS are changing rapidly as new drugs to delay the course of the autoimmune response come on the market. Interferon beta-1b, released in 1993 for treatment of relapsing-remitting MS, is reported to delay the rate of relapse and decrease overall lesion burden as seen on MRI. Other new autoimmune system drugs include inteferon beta-a and copolymer 1. Clinical trials are under way to determine the efficacy of these new treatments in relapsing-remitting and progressive forms of MS. Another approach to treatment is the use of potassium-channel-blockers called aminopyridines. These agents have been found to reduce symptoms in some patients with MS, presumably by improving nerve conduction in partially demyelinated nerves.

Other medications are also used to treat the symptoms of MS.[7] The most frequently used antispasticity drugs include baclofen (Lioresal), dantrolene sodium (Dantrium), and diazepam (Valium). Clonazepam may be useful for night spasms, and carbamazepine (Tegretol) may help with flexor and extensor spasms. Botulinum toxin (Botox) injections have been used to decrease severe, unmanageable tone. Intrathecal baclofen pumps have also been used for severe spasticity. Tremor from cerebellar involvement is difficult to treat but may respond to propranolol (Inderal). Fatigue has been treated with amantidine (Symmetrel), pemeline (Cylert), and fluoxetine (Prozac). Painful dysesthesias may respond to treatment with carbamazepine (Tegretol), phenytoin (Dilantin), or amitriptyline (Elavil). Dizziness is sometimes treated with meclizine (Antivert), which is a vestibular suppressant.

CONCLUSIONS

Life expectancy approaches that of the general population for persons with multiple sclerosis, so they are faced with the same social, psychological, and physical issues related to normal and pathological aging as others are. The effects of coexistent disease processes associated with aging, such as osteoarthritis, diabetes, peripheral vascular disease, or osteoporosis may be compounded with MS-related symptoms. In addition, patients with MS may be diagnosed with other autoimmune diseases, such as rheumatoid arthritis and fibromyalgia syndrome. With increasing age and duration of disease, a greater proportion of persons with MS need the assistance of wheelchairs, ambulatory aids, or another person.[15] Rehabilitation may become more complex and the demands on social services and families may increase. The rehabilitation specialist should consider the special needs of the geriatric client with MS within a wholistic context of client, family, and community.

REFERENCES

1. Winshenker BG. The natural history of multiple sclerosis. *Neurol Clin* 1995; 13:119.
2. Minderhound JM, Van Der Hoeven JH, Prange AJA. Course and prognosis of chronic progressive multiple sclerosis: results of an epidemiological study. *Acta Neurol Scand* 1988; 78:10.
3. Poster CM, Paty DW, Scheinberg L, et al. New diagnostic criteria for multiple sclerosis: guidelines for research protocols. *Ann Neurol* 1983; 13:227.

4. Baloh RW, Honrubia V. Other neurologic disorders. In: Baloh RW, ed. *Clinical Neurophysiology of the Vestibular System,* 2nd ed. Philadelphia: F.A. Davis; 1990: 274.

5. Herrera WG. Vestibular and other balance disorders in multiple sclerosis. *Neuro Clin* 1990; 8:407.

6. Franklin GM, Burks JS. Diagnosis and medical management of multiple sclerosis. In: Maloney FP, Burks JS, Ringel SP, eds. *Interdisciplinary Rehabilitation of Multiple Sclerosis and Neuromuscular Disorders.* Philadelphia: J.B. Lippincott; 1985: 32.

7. Schapiro RT. Symptom management in multiple sclerosis. *Ann Neurol* 1994; 36: S123.

8. Augspurger RR. Bladder dysfunction in multiple sclerosis. In: Maloney FP, Burks JS, Ringel SO, eds. *Interdisciplinary Rehabilitation of Multiple Sclerosis and Neuromuscular Disorders* Philadelphia: J.B. Lippincott; 1985: 48.

9. Prosiegel M, Mertin J, Michael C. Neuropsychology and MS: diagnostic and therapeutic approaches. In: Wietholter H, Dichgans J, Mertin J, eds. *Current Concepts in Multiple Sclerosis.* Amsterdam, Netherlands: Elsevier; 1991: 165.

10. International Federation of Multiple Sclerosis Societies. *M.R.D.: Minimal Record of Disability for Multiple Sclerosis.* New York: National Multiple Sclerosis Society; 1985.

11. Moskowitz E, McCann CB. Classification of disability in the chronically ill and aging. *J Chron Dis* 1957; 5:342.

12. Mahoney FI, Barthel DW. Functional evaluation: Barthel Index. *Md State Med J* 1965; 14:61.

13. Granger CV, Cotter AC, Hamilton BB, et al Functional assessment scales: a study of persons with multiple sclerosis. *Arch Phys Med Rehabil* 1990; 71:870.

14. Gappmaier E, White AT, Mino L, et al. Aerobic exercise in multiple sclerosis. *Neurology* 1995; 19:41.

15. Baum HM, Rothschild BA. Multiple sclerosis and mobility restriction. *Arch Phys Med Rehabil* 1993; 64:591.

Chapter **33**

Parkinson's Disease
Michael Moran, Sc.D., P.T.

INTRODUCTION

Parkinson's disease (PD), also known as paralysis agitans, is a progressive neurodegenerative disease that affects approximately 1% of those over the age of 60 years. Men and women are equally affected. PD results from a loss of pigmented neurons in the substantia nigra which leads to a reduction in the production of the neurotransmitter dopamine. The resulting movement disorders are characterized by tremor, rigidity, bradykinesia and postural instability. (See Figure 33–1 for a sample evaluation.) Diagnosis is usually by observation of signs and symptoms although magnetic resonance imaging (MRI) and computerized tomography (CT) can be useful in differentiating PD from other disorders. A clinical presentation that mimics but is different from PD is called Parkinson's syndrome or parkinsonism.

SIGNS AND SYMPTOMS

The signs and symptoms of PD vary, depending on the stage of the disease. The early stage may include tremor (often unilateral) and a sense of fatigue. The middle stage usually includes tremors, varying degrees of rigidity and bradykinesia, and postural changes and instability, and the patient may begin to require assistance from care-givers. The final stage of PD includes extensive motor disorders, requiring that the patient be assisted in performing activities of daily living and moving. Cognitive changes (depression, dementia) commonly accompany PD.

Tremors are present at rest and usually disappear as a patient attempts to move and during sleep. The term given to the commonly observed repetitive finger movements is "pill-rolling." Clinically, it has been observed that PD patients move slowly, and with inconsistent acceleration, and this bradykinesia is often noticeable when the patient progresses from the early stages of the disease. A complete lack of movement (akinesia) may occur. PD patients can "freeze" in a certain position (including standing) and then spontaneously begin to move again. Rigidity has been linked to the development of contractures, fixed kyphosis, and loss of pelvic mobility. Postural instability most likely reflects central nervous system pathology as well as the musculoskeletal changes mentioned above.

INTERVENTIONS

The management of PD usually combines nonpharmacological and pharmacological treatments. The former should include a multidisciplinary approach involving various therapies (physical, occupational, and speech) emphasizing the patient's independence and training of the care-giver. Musculoskeletal changes associated with aging should not be confused with the changes typically seen in PD—a forward-thrust head, increased thoracic kyphosis, posterior pelvic tilt, and a slow, shuffling gait. Instead, a PD patient should be objectively evaluated using an appropriate device such as the Unified Parkinson's Disease Rating Scale (Box 33–1). The clinical assessment can be videotaped, which allows changes in movement disorders to be more easily tracked.

Nonpharmacological Management

Therapeutic intervention should begin as early in the disease state as possible. Avoiding soft-tissue contracture, loss of joint range of motion, reduction

---

PARKINSON'S DISEASE EVALUATION FORM   (Circle Appropriate Score)

Bradykinesia of hands
0   No involvement
1   Detectable slowing of supination/pronation rate evidenced by beginning difficulty in handling tools;
     buttoning clothes; and with handwriting
2   Moderate slowing of supination/pronation rate, one or both sides, evidenced by moderate impairment
     of hand function. Handwriting is greatly impaired, micrographia
3   Severe slowing of supination/pronation rate. Unable to write or button clothes. Marked difficulty in
     handling utensils

Rigidity
0   Undetectable
1   Detectable rigidity in neck and shoulders. Activation phenomenon is present. One or both arms show
     mild, negative, resting rigidity
2   Moderate rigidity in neck and shoulders. Resting rigidity is positive when patient not on meds.
3   Severe rigidity in neck and shoulders. Resting rigidity cannot be reversed by meds.

Posture
0   Normal posture. Head forward flexed less than 4 inches
1   Beginning poker spine. Head flexed forward up to 5 inches
2   Beginning arm flexion. Head flexed forward up to 6 inches. One or both arms flexed but still below waist
3   Onset of Simian posture. Head flexed forward more than 6 inches. Sharp flexion of hand, beginning
     interphalangeal extension. Beginning flexion of knees

Upper Extremity Swing
0   Swings both arms well
1   One arm decreased in amount of swing
2   One arm fails to swing
3   Both arms fail to swing

Gait
0   Step length is between 18–30 inches. Turns effortlessly
1   Step length shortened to 12–18 inches. Foot/floor contact abnormalities in one side. Turns around
     slowing and takes several steps
2   Step length 6–12 inches. Foot/floor contact abnormalities on both sides
3   Onset of shuffling gait. Occasional stuttering gait with feet sticking to floor. Walks on toes. Turns very
     slowly

Tremor
0   No tremor
1   Less than 1 inch amplitude tremor observed in limbs or head at rest or in either hand while walking
2   Maximum tremor envelope fails to exceed 4 inches. Tremor is severe but not constant. Patient still has
     some control of hands
3   Tremor envelope exceeds 4 inches. Tremor is constant and severe. Writing and feeding are impossible

Face
0   Normal. Full animation. No stare
1   Detectable immobility. Mouth remains closed. Beginning features of anxiety or depression
2   Moderate immobility. Emotion shows at markedly increased threshold. Lips parted some of the time
     Moderate features of anxiety or depression. Drooling may occur
3   Frozen face. Mouth slightly open. Severe drooling may be present

Speech
0   Clear, loud, resonant, easily understood
1   Beginning of hoarseness with loss of inflection and resonance. Good volume. Still easily understood
2   Moderate hoarseness and weakness. Constant monotone, unvaried pitch, early dysarthria, hesitancy,
     stuttering, difficult to understand
3   Marked hoarseness and weakness. very difficult to hear and understand

Self-care
0   No impairment
1   Still provides full self-care but rate of dressing definitely slowed. Able to live alone and still employable
2   Requires help in certain critical areas such as turning in bed, rising from chairs etc. Very slow in
     performing most activities but manages by taking time
3   Continuously disabled. Unable to dress, feed self or walk alone

Overall Disability (Sum of the scores from all categories)

1 – 9 Early stage   **10 – 18 Moderate disability**   **19 – 27 Severe or advanced stage**

Figure 33–1 Parkinson's Disease Evaluation Form. (Modified with permission from Turnbull GI. *Physical Therapy Management of Parkinson's Disease.* New York: Churchill-Livingstone; 1992.)

Box 33–1

Unified Parkinson's Rating Scale
(Hohn and Yahr Scale)

Stage 0 = No signs of disease
Stage 1 = Unilateral disease
Stage 2 = Bilateral disease, without impairment of balance
Stage 3 = Mild to moderate bilateral disease; some postural instability; physically independent
Stage 4 = Severe disability; still able to walk or stand unassisted
Stage 5 = Wheelchair-bound or bedridden unless aided

in vital capacity, depression, and dependence on others enhances the quality of life of the PD patient. It is important to include the care-givers and others significant to the patient in goal setting and treatment planning.

A treatment plan should be goal oriented (restoring or maintaining function is the desired outcome) and individually tailored, based on the stage the patient is in. Relaxation exercises may be useful to reduce rigidity and there is some support for the idea that strengthening exercises may help to prevent falling. Stretching and active range-of-motion (ROM) exercises are vital, and the patient should be provided with a home program to facilitate improvement in functional postural alignment. Breathing and endurance exercises can help to maintain vital and aerobic capacities. They are important, as PD patients have a high incidence of pulmonary complications such as pneumonia. Balance, transfer, and gait activities (including weight shifting) are also recommended.

Balance training should include practice at varied speeds as well as self-induced and external displacements. Self-induced displacements are necessary to help the patient in tasks such as leaning, reaching, and dressing. Displacements of an external origin may be expected if a patient is walking in crowds or attempting to negotiate uneven or unfamiliar terrain. External displacements may be simulated by the use of gradual resistance via rhythmic stabilization.

Transfer training should focus on those activities reasonably expected of the patient. At a minimum,

bed mobility and transfers and chair and commode transfers should be considered. Limitations in active trunk and pelvic rotation may impair a PD patient's mobility in bed. Satin sheets or a bed cradle may reduce resistance to movement from friction. An electric mattress warmer may ease mobility by reducing the need for and thus the weight of covers. If the PD patient cannot be taught to perform a transfer independently, accommodations should be considered. Examples include bed rails or a trapeze, a lift chain, and a commode with arms. It is possible that the PD patient may require the assistance of another to perform transfers. Careful instruction and guided practice will help to ensure effective carryover of the learning experience.

Gait training should focus on musculoskeletal limitations that can be quantified. PD patients tend to have limitations in ankle dorsiflexion, knee flexion/extension, stride length, hip extension, and hip rotations. Joint mobilization and soft-tissue stretching can be effective to increase ROM and improve gait. It is important to include trunk mobility (rotation) and upper extremity ROM (large, reciprocal arm swings) in a comprehensive gait training program for PD patients. Rhythm or music may facilitate movement, but the use of assistive devices such as canes and walkers is not always appropriate for PD patients. At times, the use of an assistive device increases a festinant gait or aggravates problems with balance or coordination. Care should be taken to avoid excessive musculoskeletal stress and falls. Conditions such as osteoporosis may predispose a patient to injury.

For PD patients, a primary problem is difficulty in motor planning. Complex tasks such as transferring out of bed and walking to the bathroom have to be broken down into simple components. It is important for patients and care-givers to remember that verbal and physical cuing (and other forms of assistance) should be oriented toward completion of a number of simple tasks in order to accomplish the overall goals of maintaining function and mobility. Further, it has been noted that stress, fatigue, anxiety, or need to hurry imposed by the care-giver may exacerbate the freezing associated with PD.

When evaluating or treating a PD patient, common age-related changes must be considered. For instance, older individuals are more sensitive to glare and benefit from contrasting colors when determining depth. These facts are especially evident when working in some environments during activities such as gait training on steps. Further, some signs and symptoms of PD have been confused with changes associated with aging. PD patients may present with a reduced or lost sense of smell, handwriting that is difficult or impossible to read, and changes in sleep patterns.

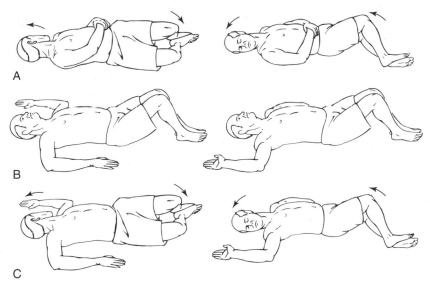

Figure 33–2 A sequence of exercises that can be used in the supine position to increase the range of motion of the neck and trunk. Any combination of motions can be used. (A) Head is slowly rotated side to side within the available range of motion while lower extremities are rotated side to side in the opposite direction. (B) Upper extremities are positioned in 45 degrees of shoulder abduction within 90 degrees of elbow flexion. One shoulder is externally rotated; the opposite shoulder is internally rotated. From this initial position the shoulders are slowly rotated back and forth from an internally to an externally rotated position. (C) In an advanced exercise, the head, shoulders, and lower extremities are simultaneously rotated from one position to the other. (Used with permission from Turnbull GI. *Physical Therapy Management of Parkinson's Disease.* New York: Churchill-Livingstone; 1992.)

Specific nonpharmacological treatment approaches for relaxation include biofeedback, proprioceptive neuromuscular facilitation, and Feldenkrais work. Stretching, active ROM, and strengthening exercises should emphasize safety: patients should be placed in a fully supported position initially and progressed to unsupported positions. In addition, spinal mobility must be oriented toward complete rotation, including elongation of trunk musculature. A loss of pelvic motion occurs and can be addressed by means of lateral and anterior/posterior tilts; for instance, the functional task of standing from a seated position can incorporate anterior pelvic tilts. Mobility in bed such as rolling over can include trunk rotation. To improve

postural (i.e., balance) responses, repetition of balance activities has been recommended. It is noted however, that a variety of tasks should be practiced, as skills tend to be task-specific. Examples of some of the mobility skills are shown in Figures 33–2, 33–3, and 33–4.

The PD patient may experience frustration because of a loss of independence in performing normal activities. That frustration may lead to social withdrawal as symptoms worsen. Social withdrawal can be related to facial involvement—the "mask" face typical of PD patients, which includes prolonged eyelid closure, slurred speech, and drooling. Drooling may be reduced by correcting forward head posture and using speech therapy to address

Figure 33–3 In a side-lying position; the thorax is slowly rotated forward and backwards relative to the pelvis while the upper extremity is protracted and retracted relative to the thorax. (Used with permission from Turnbull GI. *Physical Therapy Management of Parkinson's Disease.* New York: Churchill-Livingstone; 1992.)

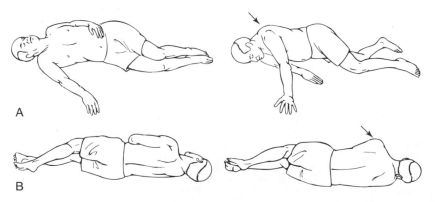

tongue and swallowing dysfunctions. Speech therapy may also assist in improving voice volume and inspiratory muscle strength. Sucking ice chips 20 to 30 minutes before a meal may help swallowing and decrease coughing and choking. See Chapter 58 for additional information about dysphagia.

Pharmacological Management

Pharmacological management of PD includes dopamine replacement (Sinemet, a combination of carbidopa and levodopa), dopaminergic drugs that act at the postsynaptic site such as pergolide (Permax) and bromocriptine (Parlodel), anticholinergic drugs like trihexyphenidyl (Artane), and neuroprotective medications, including selegiline (Eldepryl). A drug that can be used to test for suspected PD is amantadine (Symmetrel), as it is believed to have dopaminergic and anticholinergic properties.

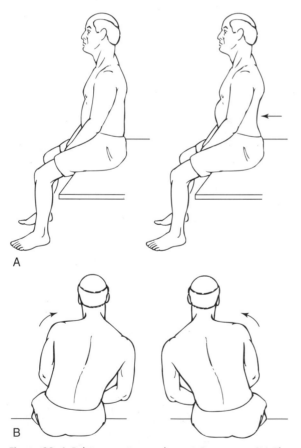

Figure 33–4 Pelvic exercises in the sitting position. (A) The pelvis is anteriorly and posteriorly tilted while the shoulders remain at midline. (B) The pelvis is laterally tilted (by lumbar lateral flexion) while the shoulders remain at midline. (Used with permission from Turnbull GI. *Physical Therapy Management of Parkinson's Disease*. New York: Churchill-Livingstone; 1992.)

Medications used for PD have a great number of side effects that can hamper rehabilitation. Nausea, vomiting, confusion, lightheadedness, and dyskinesia are only a few clinical signs that may be evident. Some clinical problems may be medication-related; Sinemet and Parlodel can cause hallucinations, vivid dreams, leg cramps, and daytime drowsiness. In addition, levodopa is associated with the "on-off" syndrome in which the PD patient demonstrates periods of time when motor control is intact (on) or not (off). As dosages increase, a wearing-off effect may be noted. This is a deterioration of motor performance as the time nears for the next dose of medication. Because of these limitations of levodopa, some physicians delay using it, preferring to start with selegiline. Generally, as the disease progresses, finding the right dose of medication becomes difficult and patients may be over- or undermedicated.

Surgical Treatment

Surgical treatments are varied as are the reported outcomes. Specific techniques include thalamotomy, a surgical lesion of the thalamus (which is reported to reduce tremor), and pallidotomy, a surgical lesion of the globus pallidus (which is reported to alleviate bradykinesia more than tremor). Patients apparently demonstrate reduced dyskinesia associated with anti-Parkinson medications following both procedures. Fetal tissue transplant procedures have been done in some countries but are banned in others. Clinical results are varied, with some sources claiming a higher success rate with pallidotomy.

Cognitive and Social Issues

Cognitive deficits that have been associated with PD are dementia and depression (mood disorders). These deficits are demonstrated by changes in cognitive abilities such as memory impairments, spatial abilities, word finding, and dealing with new or complex tasks. Cognitive deficits should be considered when planning a treatment program for PD patients, as modifications may be required to accommodate specific patient limitations. Varying the style of interaction and reducing the pace of communication may be helpful. Therapists should use caution when deciding a PD patient is being uncooperative or stubborn, as cognitive deficits may not have been adequately addressed. Possibly, cognitive changes from an earlier injury such as a cerebrovascular accident may already exist. It is important to educate care-givers regarding a patient's cognitive deficits and find strategies to reduce frustration for both.

CONCLUSION

Parkinson's disease is a neurodegenerative disease that results from a loss of pigmented neurons in the substantia nigra and leads to movement disorders characterized by tremors, rigidity, bradykinesia, and postural instability. Therapeutic interventions should begin in the early stages of the disease in order to enhance mobility and quality of life. Pharmacological intervention is a mainstay in the treatment of Parkinson's disease, but therapists must be cognizant that the potential side effects of medicines and the on-off syndrome may hamper rehabilitation. Surgical treatment such as thalamotomy and pallidotomy have shown varied results.

SUGGESTED READINGS

Ciccone CD. *Pharmacology in Rehabilitation,* 2nd ed. Philadelphia: F.A. Davis; 1996.

Cutson TM, Cotter-Laub K, Schenkman M. Pharmacological and nonpharmacological interventions in the treatment of Parkinson's disease. *Phys Ther* 1995; 75:363.

The Parkinson's Web. http://neuro-chief-e.mgh.harvard.edu/parkinsonsweb/Main/PDmain.html

Protas EJ, Stanley RK, Jankovic J, MacNeil B. Cardovascular and metabolic responses to upper- and lower-extremity exercise in men with idiopathic Parkinson's disease. *Phys Ther* 1996; 76:34–40.

Schenkman M, Custon TM, Kuchibhatla M, Chandler J, Pieper C. Reliability of impairment and physical performance measures for persons with Parkinson's disease. *Phys Ther* 1997; 77:19–27.

Turnbull GI. *Physical Therapy Management of Parkinson's Disease.* New York: Churchill Livingstone; 1992.

Chapter **34**

Tremors, Chorea, and Other Involuntary Movements

Michelle Lusardi, Ph.D., P.T.

INTRODUCTION

Health professionals in geriatric rehabilitation often observe extraneous or involuntary movements that interfere with the older person's ability to accomplish his or her functional goals. There is great variation in cause, presentation, characteristics, and management of the numerous types of involuntary movement and dyskinesias. This can create a chal-

lenge in setting goals and assessing the efficacy of rehabilitation.

DEFINITION OF TERMS

Tremor

Tremor is an involuntary movement characterized by a rhythmic oscillation around a fixed axis, often congruent with a joint axis. The frequency (period) and wave form (timing and sequence of muscle activity) of any one type of tremor is markedly consistent over time, even though the amplitude varies with intra- and extraindividual factors. Tremor occurs because of the alternating contraction of striatal muscle on both sides of a joint. The underlying central nervous system (CNS) mechanisms of tremor are not well understood. Four systems may contribute to the motor expression of tremor: the oscillating tendencies of the mechanical systems of the joints and muscle, short- and long-loop spinal cord and brainstem reflexes, and closed-loop feedback systems of the higher motor centers, including the cerebellum. Tremor can occur during movement, at rest, or while maintaining a relatively fixed posture. Physiological tremor is a normal phenomenon that becomes more obvious under conditions of stress or fatigue. Most other types of tremors indicate CNS pathology. The amplitude of most types of tremor increases in times of stress, anxiety, or fatigue and often decreases or disappears during sleep. Tremor is the most commonly occurring form of dyskinesia.

Chorea

Chorea is a random and rapid contraction of muscle groups that usually involves the muscles of the extremities or of the face. The movement of chorea is often described as graceful or dance-like. Both proximal and distal muscle groups of the extremities may be affected. Persons with chorea often learn to blend their involuntary movement with a purposeful movement in an effort to mask or minimize the unwanted movement; for example, a choreic movement of the arm over the head might be turned into a smoothing of the hair. As a rule, axial muscles are minimally involved, so static postural control is usually uncompromised. Choreiform movements are usually bilateral and somewhat symmetrical. Chorea is often associated with hypotonia. Frequency and amplitude of choreic movements increase during periods of stress and usually decrease during sleep. Chorea occurs when there is damage in the corpus striatum, especially in the caudate nucleus, either because of a hereditary disorder such as Huntington's disease or as consequence of other physiological diseases. Choreic movements also occur in tardive dyskinesia, a complication that results from long-term use of neuroleptic drugs or dopamine therapy. Although the underlying mechanism of chorea has not been established, several have been proposed. Heightened sensitivity to the neurotransmitter dopamine among surviving striatal neurons in the damaged caudate nucleus may randomly trigger fragments of motor patterns. Alternatively, abnormal striatal activity may "release" long-latency reflexes that would otherwise suppress unwanted movement.

Ballismus

Ballismus (hemiballismus) is an involuntary, often wild and forceful flailing or throwing motion that commonly affects the proximal joints of one or more extremities. Trunk and facial muscles are usually not involved, so that posture and bulbar function (speech, swallowing, respiration) are uncompromised. The movements of hemiballism are usually much more stereotypical and often more severe and disruptive than those seen in chorea. Hemiballism also differs from other dyskinesias during periods of sleep; with it, there is no decrease in frequency or amplitude of the ballistic movements, so that all phases of the sleep cycle can be disrupted. Hemiballism is much less prevalent than other dyskinesias. It is the result of damage to the contralateral subthalamus, typically caused by a lacunar stroke. Damage to the subthalamus is thought to "release" activity of the globus pallidus nucleus, which triggers the stereotypical forceful limb movements. Hemiballistic moments typically diminish in amplitude in the weeks following stroke. Haloperidol (Haldol) is often used early in recovery to minimize involuntary movements and allow effective sleep.

Athetosis

Athetosis is described as a continuous, slow, sinuous, somewhat irregular, writhing movement. It is the result of continuous and unpredictable variation in underlying muscle tone, which can range from hypotonia (low tone) to hypertonia (spasticity). Athetosis tends to be more obviously expressed in distal musculature but also affects axial and postural muscles, including those of the face and mouth. It usually involves both sides of the body in a fairly symmetrical pattern, and it is often accompanied by chorea or spasticity or both. Persons with athetosis

have difficulty sustaining positions at rest, which compromises their postural stability. They also have difficulty sustaining tone during volitional movement, which interferes with functional activity. Athetosis occurs when there has been damage to the corpus striatum (the caudate and putamen nuclei) in the forebrain. It has been associated with perinatal ischemia and hypoxia or bilirubin toxicity; premature infants are especially at risk. It is often diagnosed as cerebral palsy during the first or second year of life. Although the severity of athetosis does not change with maturity, function may become more challenging with the accumulation of age-related musculoskeletal and neuromuscular changes and unrelated pathologies.

Dystonia

Dystonia is a movement disorder characterized by a sustained positioning or a slowly changing movement. Dystonia is much slower and more severe than athetosis. It can affect one or several parts of the body and is seen clinically as tonic posturing. Dystonic positions are frequently described as "unnatural" or "bizarre," they are abnormal movement patterns that cannot be recreated volitionally. Some idiopathic dystonias, such as spastic torticollis, may have a familial distribution. Certain dystonias, such as writer's cramp or laryngeal dystonia, occur only during a particular type of motor activity. An idiopathic torsion dystonia with onset of symptoms in later life typically affects axial (torticollis), facial, or arm musculature, and although it interferes with functional activities, it is usually nonprogressive. Symptomatic dystonias are also associated with damage to the putamen nucleus of the basal ganglia in the forebrain, which can result from tumor, ischemia or infarct, or head trauma. Dystonias can occur in progressive degenerative diseases such as progressive supranuclear palsy, Huntington's chorea, Wilson's disease, or Parkinson's disease. Persons with long histories of spasticity associated with cerebral palsy, stroke, or multiple sclerosis may exhibit dystonic posturing of the hands (hyperextension of the fingers) or feet (equinovaus). Dystonic posturing may also evolve, along with reappearance of tonic hindbrain-moderated reflexes (for example, the tonic labyrinthine supine and prone reflexes, the assymetrical tonic neck reflex, or the positive supporting reaction), in the end stages of Alzheimer's disease. Medications used to manage severe dystonia include anticholinergics, diazepam, haloperidol, baclofen, and carbamazepine. Severe dystonia may be treated with injection of botulism toxin.

Myoclonus

Myoclonus is a rhythmic, involuntary movement that can resemble tremor. It can occur through three mechanisms: (1) as the expression of a hyperactive, spinal-cord-level stretch reflex, (2) during a partial or generalized seizure of the cerebral cortex, or (3) as a familial, idiopathic, or physiologically induced movement disorder.

Myoclonus associated with hyperactive stretch reflex can be either transient (lasting for several beats) or sustained (appearing to be tremor-like) over a period of time. It is triggered by a quick passive stretching or elongation of muscle fibers as occurs in deep-tendon reflex testing or passive range-of-motion exercises. Annulospiral sensory receptors wrapped around the centers of the muscle spindles' intrafusal fibers are stimulated by the deformation of the muscle during a rapid stretch. Information about muscle length is carried to the spinal cord via 1a sensory neurons. These afferent neurons directly facilitate alpha motor neurons, triggering contraction of the elongated extrafusal muscle fibers. The resulting contraction elongates antagonistic muscles on the opposite side of the joint, often triggering the stretch reflex in the antagonists as well. Hyperactive stretch reflex myoclonus occurs when there has been upper motor neuron damage to the pyramidal motor system, such as that which occurs in stroke or spinal cord injury. Myoclonus can also occur in people without pathology who are extremly anxious, stressed, or fatigued. On testing deep-tendon reflexes, persons with myoclonus are often graded as 4+ (several beats of clonus) or 5+ (sustained clonus). Most people with myoclonus due to pyramidal system dysfunction also exhibit a positive Babinski response (an upward-pointing great toe with fanning of the second through fifth toes).

Myoclonus that occurs during CNS seizure may involve a single limb segment (in a partial seizure of the motor cortex) or may involve rhythmic jerking of all extremities (during a generalized seizure involving the entire cerebral cortex). The combination of loss of consciousness and myoclonus during a generalized seizure differentiates this involuntary movement from tremor. During a partial seizure, consciousness is unaltered, and the involuntary myoclonus may be confused with tremor. An electroencephalogram recorded while the abnormal movement is occurring would indicate focal abnormality of the motor cortex during partial seizure, whereas patterns during tremor would be likely to be "normal."

Hiccups and "sleep starts" (nocturnal myoclonus) are examples of physiologically triggered myoclonus. A movement-triggered myoclonus has been reported during recovery from severe cerebral hypoxia or ischemia following myocardial infarction or near drowning, and it may significantly interfere with functional activity and gait. Myoclonus may occur as a component of uremic or hepatic encephalopathy or infectious encephalopathy. Occasionally myoclonus presents as a symptom of toxicity to drugs such as penicillin, tricyclic antidepressants, or L-dopa or to other toxins such as strychnine. A familial form of myoclonus, benign essential myoclonus, is a relatively rare movement disorder.

Fasciculation

Fasciculation (pseudotremor) is a spontaneous asynchronous contraction of motor units that is often mistaken for tremor. On careful observation, fasciculation presents as a random twitching rather than a rhythmic, oscillating contraction of muscle fibers as is seen in tremor. Fasciculation may be a result of side effects or an overdose of certain drugs (e.g., excessive caffeine), electrolyte imbalance or sodium deficiency, muscle denervation, nerve root irritation (herniated disk or spondylosis), diseases of the anterior horn cell (polio, amyotrophic lateral sclerosis), periods of extreme fatigue or stress, or strenuous exercise.

Tics

Tics (also called mimic spasms) are stereotypical, often complex movements that sometimes resemble tremor or chorea. They may be expressed as repetitive eye blinking, throat clearing, shoulder shrugging, arm gesturing, or skipping while walking. Patients often report a sense of increasing muscle tension that can be relieved only when the stereotypical movement occurs. Tics differ from other types of involuntary movement in that they are somewhat under volitional control and can be suppressed for a length of time. Idiopathic tics may occur for short periods, especially during childhood, and are often associated with anxiety or other psychological stress factors. The tics observed in Tourette's syndrome persist over the lifespan and may include vocalizations (barking, grunting, echolalia, and swearing) in addition to the stereotypical repetitive motions.

Asterixis

Asterixis is a brief but recurring loss of muscle tone in postural, antigravity muscles, usually extensors.

It is often seen clinically as a "flapping" of the hands when the arms are held horizontally with wrists extended against gravity during neurological testing. It commonly occurs because of physiological consequences of hepatic and renal encephalopathy, pulmonary failure, and malabsorption syndromes and when there is drug toxicity. It has also been reported as a consequence of anticonvulsant therapy and when there is a CNS lesion between the brain stem and the thalamus.

Akathisia

Akathisia is a subjective sense of restlessness or discomfort of the limbs, typically accompanied by agitation, which may or may not be relieved by movement. Patients report great difficulty sitting or lying still and a powerful urge to move. They may begin to pace or rock, and they often have difficulty sleeping. Akathisia can occur when individuals are at rest or during movement. It is one of a group of extrapyramidal side effects of antipsychotic medication and may be the presenting symptom of an episode of tardive dyskinesia.

CLASSIFICATION STRATEGIES AND DIFFERENTIAL DIAGNOSIS OF TREMORS

There is much variation in the presentations and causes of tremors, and no single classification system can fully capture the nature of all tremors. Tremors have been categorized according to how and when they occur, their wave forms, the body segments involved, whether there is a family history of tremor or other movement disorders, their responsiveness to medication, and their conjunction with other CNS-oriented signs or symptoms. A brief discussion of classification strategies may help to distinguish among the various tremors commonly seen in geriatric rehabilitation. These classification systems are summarized in Table 34–1.

A behavior classification scheme considers when the tremors are most likely to be observed. Those that occur in an otherwise relaxed or inactive extremity are described as resting tremors. Resting tremors are a characteristic symptom of Parkinson's disease. It has also been reported in cases of Wilson's disease (a hereditary disorder involving the metabolism of copper), normal-pressure hydrocephalus, heavy-metal poisoning, neurosyphilis and as a side effect of neuroleptic medication. Tremors that occur when a body segment is held in a sustained position, usually against gravity, are called postural tremors. Essential tremors are the most common postural tremors, but they also occur in other conditions, including senile tremor, Parkinson's disease, Wilson's disease, Charcot Marie Tooth disease (hereditary motor and sensory neuropathy), and spastic torticollis. Tremors that occur during volitional movement are classified as kinetic, or action, tremors. Some action tremors are relatively constant in amplitude from the beginning to the end of purposeful movement, as is seen in many cases of essential tremor. Action tremors that worsen as a voluntary movement moves toward completion are called intention tremors. The amplitude of intention tremors (which occur perpendicular to the line of the intended volitional movement) increases as the movement's goal is approached. Clinically, this is evaluated using a finger-to-nose or heel-along-shin movement task. Intention tremors are a classic sign of damage of the cerebellum or its interconnections or of brain-stem dysfunction or damage. Tremor-like movements that occur during passive movement are called myoclonus.

Tremors have also been characterized by the frequency (period) at which they occur. Tremor frequency is measured by EMG recording or by accelerometer, it cannot be reliably estimated by observation alone. The frequencies of most pathological tremors are relatively stable within and across individuals. For example, the resting tremor of Parkinson's disease most typically falls within the range of 4 to 6 cycles per second (cps) (Hz), whereas essential tremor has a frequency of 8 to 10 cps, and physiological tremor falls between 11 and 13 cps. Amplitude is not typically a reliable indicator of the severity of tremor because it varies within the individual over time, usually becoming more pronounced at times of stress or fatigue and decreasing during sleep.

An attempt has also been made to classify tremors according to the part of the body affected. For example, the resting tremors of Parkinson's disease are expressed in the distal upper extremity as a "pill-rolling" motion. Most postural tremors affect the head, neck, or trunk and are most obvious when sustaining a position against gravity. Action tremors tend to impact on the proximal limb girdles, the connections between extremity and trunk. Physiological tremors affect all muscle groups and may be seen at rest, in posture, during movement, or all three.

Neurologists often clarify a clinical diagnosis of movement disorder by assessing the impact of medication on the amplitude of tremors. Anticholinergic agents are used to reduce the resting tremors of Parkinson's disease, and essential tremors diminish with ingestion of alcohol or administration of β-antagonists (β-blockers) such as propranolol. Cerebellar intention tremors are often unresponsive to pharmaceutical intervention.

Table 34-1 Comparison of Classification Strategies for Tremor

Type of Tremor	Frequency (cps)	Behavior	Mechanism/Site of Pathology	Response of Tremors to Medication
Normal physiological	11–13	At rest	Cardioballistic, passive resonance of limb	Increase with sympathetic activity
"Enhanced" physiological	8–12	Postural	Unknown	Increase with epinephrine, isoprenaline, neuroleptics, and L-dopa; decrease with alcohol, β-blockers, benzodiazepines
	7–11	Action	Occurs with stress, anxiety, altered metabolic function	
Essential	8–10	Postural, action	Possible interconnections among Inferior olivary nucleus, cerebellum, and/ or red nucleus	Decrease with alcohol, β-blockers, primidone, phenobarbitone, benzodiazepines; increase with isoprenaline, epinephrine, neuroleptics, L-dopa
Muscle fatigue	6	Action	Unknown	
Parkinsonian antagonists	5–7	Postural	Unknown	Decrease with L-dopa, dopamine
	4–5	At rest	Imbalance in long latency reflex of BG circuit and VL nucleus	Decrease with anticholinergics, amantadine, alcohol; increase with physostigmine, isoprenaline, epinephrine, or neuroleptics
Intention	3–5	Action, postural	Cerebellar disease, damage to dentate nucleus, superior cerebellar peduncle, or red nucleus	May decrease with choline or isoniazid; often increase with alcohol or epinephrine

BG, basal ganglia; VL, ventrolateral nucleus of the thalamus.

Alternatively, the type of tremors observed during the clinical evaluation can suggest the location of the dysfunction within the CNS. Resting tremors associated with the rigidity and bradykinesia of Parkinson's disease are a hallmark of degeneration of the substantia nigra in the midbrain. Intention tremors in goal-directed, volitional movement suggest damage to the cerebellar peduncles, deep cerebellar nuclei, or cerebellar cortex. Choreiform movement and athetosis indicate damage to or dysfunction in the corpus striatum (caudate and putamen nuclei), and ballistic movement is evidence of subthalamic damage.

Types of Tremor
Physiological Tremor

Physiological tremor is a normal oscillation of the extremities or trunk that has a frequency of between 11 and 13 cps. Typically, the amplitude of physio-logical tremor is very small and difficult to observe. Physiological tremor occurs as both a postural and an action tremor. It is thought to result from the combination of the resonant properties of the musculoskeletal system, the synchronization of agonist/antagonist motor neuron activity and muscle spindle feedback, and the distal expression of the force generated by the heartbeat (cardioballistic force). It is important to note that physiological tremor usually affects all muscle groups (axial, limb girdle, and distal) simultaneously, whereas pathological tremors tend to affect selected areas or segments.

Physiological tremor is enhanced by any mechanism that triggers activity in the sympathetic nervous system (β-adrenergic activity and catecholamine release)—stress, anxiety, fright, sleep deprivation, alcohol ingestion, cardiac medications, CNS stimulants, exercise, and also fatigue. Physiological tremor has been observed in metabolic disorders such as hypoglycemia and thyrotoxicosis, in withdrawal from sedatives or alcohol, and in carbon monoxide or heavy-metal poisoning. Toxic levels of certain medications (lithium, bronchodilators, and tricyclic antidepressants) may also lead to tremor. Physiological tremor diminishes with administration of the β-blocker propranolol. Amplitude of physiological tremor often begins to diminish in midlife and is often difficult to observe in later life.

Essential Tremor

Essential tremor is an action or postural tremor that commonly affects neck and axial musculature and may be expressed as head-nodding or an oscillating flexion/extension movement of the trunk. Essential tremors are also evident when the upper extremities must sustain a relatively fixed position during functional activity. Involvement of the pharynx and larynx may compromise speech and swallowing. As an action tremor, essential tremor often interferes with the efficiency of fine motor tasks, such as writing, grooming, or bringing full feeding utensils to the mouth. It is the most commonly occurring of the involuntary movements, affecting between 1 and 7% of the U.S. population over age 40. The exact mechanism of essential tremor is unclear, although a disruption in the connections among the cerebellum, the red nucleus in the midbrain, and the inferior olivary nucleus in the hindbrain has been implicated. Essential tremor is considered "benign" because it is not associated with significant or progressive neuropathology; however, it can significantly interfere with independent function in later life. The temporary reduction in amplitude of essential tremor following ingestion of alcohol (lasting less than 30 minutes) is often used to support clinical diagnosis. Medications such as propranolol and other β-blockers reduce tremor over longer periods (several hours) and are very useful in the long-term management of the disorder (except in the presence of congestive heart failure, A-V heart block, asthma, insulin-dependent diabetes, and other diseases in which β-blockers may be harmful). Sedatives, tranquilizers, and anti-Parkinson's medications are not effective in reducing essential tremor. While essential tremor tends to be familial, no clear pattern of heredity has been identified.

An action tremor similar to essential tremor affects approximately 10 to 15% of persons with Parkinson's disease and occurs most commonly in cases of onset of Parkinson's symptoms prior to age 60. Although often considered essential tremor, it does not typically diminish with alcohol ingestion, and although it does respond to propranolol, it is somewhat unresponsive to other β-blockers such as primidone and clonazepam.

Intention Tremor

An intention tremor (also called a rubral or cerebellar tremor) is an oscillation around the intended path of a voluntary movement that typically increases in amplitude as the movement draws to its conclusion. This characteristic, coupled with its relatively low frequency (3 to 5 cps) has led to the description of intention tremor as "coarse." Intention tremor occurs when there has been damage to the cerebellar cortex or dentate nucleus (in tumor or stroke), to the superior cerebellar peduncle (in multiple sclerosis, traumatic head injury, or brain-stem stroke), or to structures of the midbrain, especially the red nucleus and its efferent fibers. Damage to these structures interferes with the delivery of ongoing feedback to the motor system about the accuracy of movement as it occurs and is especially evident when fine control is necessary. Intention tremor has also been observed in patients with severe Parkinson's disease or essential tremor, in alcohol, barbiturate, or sedative intoxication, and in hypothyroidism. It may also be a result of high serum levels of the anticonvulsants phenytoin or carbamazepine.

Intention tremor typically compromises function of the shoulder and hip girdles as well as of muscles at each joint of an extremity. In severe cases, there may be tremor at rest and in posture, as well as the classic disruption of goal-oriented movement. It is often accompanied by nystagmus, hypotonia and weakness, dysmetria, ataxia in gait, and an overall decomposition of movement associated with cerebellar dysfunction. Interestingly, the amplitude of cerebellar tremor often decreases when the eyes are closed; perhaps less visual feedback to the cerebellum reduces the tendency toward dysmetria.

Resting Tremor

Resting tremor is one of the most common symptoms of Parkinson's disease, but it can also occur in progressive supranuclear palsy, normal-pressure hydrocephalus, exposure to toxic levels of heavy metals, and in the traumatic encephalopathy associated with boxing or repeated head injury. It is most commonly expressed in the distal upper extremities as alternating supination and pronation of the forearm and lumbrical flexion and extension of the fingers and thumb. Resting tremor in idiopathic Parkinson's disease has historically been described as "pill-rolling" because the movement of the fingers and thumb resembles that used by early pharmacists to form tablets of medication by hand. The cycle of a resting tremor is relatively slow at 4 to 6 cps (Hz). This tremor, which typically lessens or disappears with onset of volitional movement, may result from the release of inhibition of the long-latency reflexes associated with the reduction of nigral-striatal function. Anticholinergic medications such as trihexyphenidyl (Artane) and benztropine (Cogentin) are more successful in minimizing resting tremor than are dopamine agonists and L-dopa therapy. Selective surgical ablation of the contralateral ventrolateral nucleus of the thalamus has also been used to reduce the amplitude of severe resting tremor.

Neuropathic Tremor

Neuropathic tremor has been reported in many diseases involving dysfunction of sensory or motor peripheral nerves. The presentation of neuropathic tremors is quite variable; tremor may occur at rest or during voluntary movement or even as a postural tremor. How and why tremor occurs in the presence of neuropathy is not well understood. Tremor has been observed in acquired neuropathies (for example, in diabetic polyneuropathy, in patients with end-stage renal disease, and in patients with chronic alcoholism), in hereditary neuropathies (for example, in Charcot Marie Tooth disease/hereditary motor sensory neuropathy), and in infectious or inflammatory neuropathy (for example, in Guillain-Barré polyneuritis). Management of these tremors can be challenging; many medications that are successful in controlling other types of tremor are often not as effective in the presence of neuropathy.

Posttraumatic Tremor

Two types of posttraumatic tremor have been associated with head injury. An action tremor similar to essential tremor sometimes occurs following mild head injury. Usually, this type of tremor begins within 1 to 4 weeks after injury. In most instances, no structural damage can be identified on computed tomography or magnetic resonance imaging scan. This tremor is usually unresponsive to propranolol and primidone. Although signs of this mild tremor may diminish over time, it sometimes persists and is bothersome. A delayed-onset posttraumatic action tremor has also been reported after head injury. It usually evolves in the 12 to 18 months following injury and often persists, although symptoms may diminish in amplitude and intensity over a period of several years.

Orthostatic Tremor

An orthostatic tremor is a relatively rare action tremor that occurs only during unsupported standing and preparation for it. The frequency of this tremor (14 to 18 cps) is somewhat faster, and its amplitude somewhat smaller than those of essential tremor. It does not respond to alcohol or propanalol, the medications used to manage essential tremor. Instead, clonazepam, a mediation that typically has no effect on essential tremor, has been found to be useful. Patients with orthostatic tremor report a sense of unsteadiness when upright and frequently are reluctant to stand for fear of falling. Orthostatic tremor greatly reduces quality of life and significantly interferes with functional ability.

Senile Tremor

Senile tremor is the term used to describe a mild movement disorder that develops in the seventh decade of life or later. It is chronic in nature, is very slowly progressive, and is diagnosed only when there is no familial history of essential tremor. Usually, a senile tremor affects the head (titubation), mouth, and lips but has little significant impact on functional status. Whether it is a distinct movement disorder or a variation of essential tremor is open to debate.

Hysterical Tremor

A diagnosis of hysterical tremor (conversion disorder) is made when apparently involuntary movements differ in appearance from the "classic" patterns of resting, postural, or intention tremors, especially if they move from one area of the body to another within the same individual. Onset of hysterical tremor is typically abrupt, whereas most other tremors develop slowly. The frequency and amplitude of hysterical tremor are typically variable over time. In most other types of tremor, there is often an increase in amplitude of the involuntary movement when patients are given a competitive, anxiety-producing cognitive task such as subtracting 7 serially from 100. In hysteria, however, the tremor is often reduced or may disappear when attention is focused on competitive tasks.

CHOREA AND OTHER TYPES OF INVOLUNTARY MOVEMENT

Huntington's Chorea

Huntington's chorea is an autosomal dominant hereditary disorder characterized by progressive degeneration of the corpus striatum. The gene for Huntington's disease is located on the short arm of chromosome 4. Huntington's disease has a progressively deteriorating course that lasts 10 to 25 years after diagnosis. The first signs and symptoms of the disease typically appear in midlife and may include restlessness, emotional lability, neurosis, or personality disorder. Over time, cognitive function declines and involuntary movement appears. As choreiform movements become more pronounced, there is marked impairment of gait, speech production, and swallowing. Late in the disease, rigidity and dystonia develop. Typically, there is reduction in the neurotransmitter γ-aminobutyric acid (GABA) and its associated enzymes in the corpus striatum (caudate and putamen nuclei), while dopamine levels are close to normal. On CT or MRI scan there is marked degeneration of the caudate nucleus, enlargement of the anterior horn of the lateral ventricles, and cerebral atrophy. Treatment of Huntington's disease is symptomatic; choreiform movements can sometimes be controlled by dopamine-blocking agents, such as haloperidol, reserpine, or tetrabenzanine.

Sydenham's Chorea

Sydenham's chorea appears insidiously several weeks after recovery from childhood rheumatic fever. Characterized by facial grimacing and rapid twitching of the trunk and proximal extremities, this type of chorea is often accompanied by emotional lability, uncharacteristic listlessness, and hypotonia. It typically affects one extremity or one side of the body. Whether persons with a history of Sydenham's chorea are more likely to develop movement disorders in later life is being investigated.

Wilson's Disease

Wilson's disease is a disorder involving metabolism of copper. It is inherited in an autosomal recessive pattern of transmission of a gene on chromosome 13. If untreated, Wilson's disease is fatal. Neurological symptoms of the poorly managed disease include resting or postural tremor, chorea of the extremities, Parkinson-like symptoms, dystonia, pseudobulbar palsy, and cognitive dysfunction. In addition, patients with Wilson's disease have marked hepatic dysfunction that eventually develops into chronic cirrhosis. Ongoing treatment with penicillamine, which effectively binds copper, and restriction of dietary copper often halts progression of the disease, although neurological symptoms may persist. Onset of the disease usually occurs in adolescence or young adulthood, but there have been reports of initial symptoms occurring as late as 60 years of age.

Paroxysmal Choreoathetosis

Paroxysmal choreoathetosis (also described as striatal epilepsy) presents as jerking, writhing movements of limbs and trunk that are associated with being startled. It is seen in the presence of other CNS pathologies such as multiple sclerosis.

Familial Choreoathetosis

Familial choreoathetosis is a rare and relatively benign hereditary movement disorder that is inherited in an autosomal recessive pattern. The intermittent "attacks" of jerking and writhing choreoathetoid movements of this disorder are associated with physical exertion and caffeine and alcohol ingestion.

Senile Chorea

Senile chorea is a term used to describe involuntary movements, especially of the mouth, tongue, and trunk, when there is no apparent history of psychotropic or dopamine therapy, Huntington's disease, or other types of dementia or familial movement disorders. It is sometimes called oral-facial-lingual dyskinesia. Senile chorea affects less than 1% of people between the ages of 50 and 59 but may be present in as many as 7% of people over the age of 70. The lip movements seen in senile chorea are similar to—and should be differentiated from—the facial movements of tardive dyskinesia and to the lip and jaw movements observed in older persons who have lost all of their teeth and no longer are able to wear dentures.

Other Causes of Chorea

Damage to the basal ganglia caused by infarction, calcification, and a relatively rare seizure disorder of the basal ganglia, may result in choreiform movement. Chorea may also be one of a constellation of symptoms of other disease states. It occasionally occurs in thyrotoxicosis, systemic lupus erythematosus, polycythemia rubra, hypoparathyroidism, neurosyphilis, estrogen or contraceptive use, hypocalcemia, hepatic cirrhosis, and Wilson's disease.

Tourette's Syndrome

Tourette's syndrome is an idiopathic movement and behavioral disorder that is characterized by multiple motor and vocal tics. The behavior of persons with Tourette's syndrome has been described as bizarre and peculiar, and patients may be misdiagnosed with a psychiatric illness. Onset of the tics often occurs in childhood or adolescence and persists over the lifespan, with some variation in the intensity of symptoms over time. Initial symptoms are commonly motor tics of the face that progress over time to involve vocal manifestations (grunts, barks, throat-clearing, cursing, or echolalia) and involuntary, sometimes self-damaging, movements of the extremities. These motor tics are often similar to the stereotypical involuntary movements of chorea. Although the pathomechanics of the syndrome are not fully understood, it appears to be a disorder of the basal ganglia involving excessive levels of the neurotransmitter dopamine. Symptoms can often be controlled by dopamine-blocking agents, clonidine, haloperidol, or pimozide.

Drug-Induced Movement Disorders

Extrapyramidal dysfunction may be caused not by direct damage or pathology of the basal ganglia or their interconnections but as an undesired side effect of psychotropic therapy or certain other medications. The tendency to have less efficient metabolism and excretion of medications in later life makes older adults on these types of medications more susceptible to drug-related movement disorders. Medications that have been associated with extrapyramidal side effects are listed in Table 34–2.

There are several classes of psychotropic drugs that may cause iatrogenic extrapyramidal dysfunction:

- phenothiazines
- reserpine
- benzodiazepines
- thioxanthenes
- butyrophenones

Tricyclic antidepressants have been reported to have similar side effects in some patients. The underlying mechanism may be a supersensitivity to dopamine that is related to the blocking of postsynaptic dopamine receptors by neuroleptic medication. The incidence of drug-induced movement problems among psychiatric patients treated by long-term use of neuroleptic medications has been estimated to be as high as 25%. Akathisia may be an early sign of extrapyramidal side effects, especially in patients being treated with a medication in the phenothiazine group. Patients may develop a movement disorder that mimics Parkinson's disease, including hypokinesia, rigidity, stooped or flexed upright posture, shuffling gait, and impairment of balance reactions. An acute dyskinetic reaction may occur within days of initiation of drug therapy with phenothiazines, butyrophenones, tricyclic antidepressants, and sometimes phenytoin, carbamazepine, propranolol, and certain calcium-channel-blockers. This reaction is more common in young women but it has been reported in those in later life as well. Such a sudden onset of choreiform movements of the face, head and neck, or limbs can be frightening, but is usually reversible if the offending medication is withdrawn.

Tardive dyskinesia, the most severe of the extrapyramidal side effects, occurs in long-term drug therapy (3 to 12 months after initiation of treatment) with dopamine antagonists. It is characterized by rapid onset of involuntary rhythmic choreoathetoid movement of the face, mouth, and tongue that can include repeated thrusting of the tongue, lip smacking, sucking, pouting, grimacing, and blinking. Patients with tardive dyskinesia may also experience chorea of the extremities and dystonias, including torticollis of the neck, oculogyric crisis of the eyes, and opisthotonos of the trunk. Symptoms of extrapyramidal dysfunction appear and progressively worsen until the precipitating medication dose is reduced or discontinued, but sometimes they persist for extended periods after medication has been withdrawn. If the offending medication cannot be changed, mild extrapyramidal symptoms may be treated by certain anti-Parkinson medications or benzodiazepines. Severe cases of tardive dyskinesia may be managed by dopamine-blocking agents such as reserpine or tetrabenazine, but unwanted side effects, including orthostatic hypotension and depression, are likely to occur. A variation of tardive dyskinesia has also been reported in patients without previous symptoms when neuroleptic medication is suddenly withdrawn.

Choreiform movement and other abnormal involuntary movement have been reported with long-term use of medications other than neuroleptics. A common side effect of long-term L-dopa therapy in Parkinson's disease is the development of choreic moments of the face, tongue, and sometimes the lower extremities. The severity of the unwanted movements is dose-related, fluctuating with levels of circulating L-dopa. Frequent administration of smaller doses, which reduces or stabilizes L-dopa levels, may reduce extraneous movements, but then the disabling symptoms of Parkinson's often intensify. Chorea is also an infrequent side effect of anticonvulsant medications such as phenytoin and carbamazepine. In managing seizures, medications should be withdrawn when chorea becomes apparent, even if blood levels fall within therapeutic range. Onset of choreic movement is one of many signs of lithium toxicity. Certain CNS stimulants, including amphetamine, methylphenidate, and pemoline, may induce oral-facial choreiform movements.

Table 34–2 Medications Associated with Extrapyramidal Side Effects

Type of Medication	Symptoms	Examples
Psychotropic/Neuroleptic	Akathisia, pseudo-Parkinson's, chorea, tardive dyskinesia, acute dyskinetic reaction	Phenothiazines (chlorpromazine, triflupromaxine, fluphenazine, perphenazine, trifluoperazine, pericyazine, promazine, mesoridazine) Thioxanthines (thiothizene, chlorprothixene) Butyrophenones (droperidol, haloperidol) Dibenzapines (loxapine) Diphenylbutylpiperidines Indolones (molindone) Many sleeping medications
Antidepressants	Chorea, athetosis, akathisia	Tricyclic antidepressants, mono-oxide inhibitors
	Tremor, myoclonus, pseudo-Parkinson's	Lithium carbonate, amoxapine
Stimulants	Postural tremor, chorea	Amphetamines, methadone, methylphenidate, fenfluramine Caffeine, cocaine
CNS Depressants/Sedatives	Physiological, intention tremor; chorea, dystonia	Alcohol Diazepam
Anticonvulsants	Intention tremor, chorea, asterixis	Phenytoin, valproic acid, carbamazepine Phenobarbital, clonazepam
Anti-Parkinson medications	Akathisia, chorea, dystonia	Amantadine, bromocriptine, L-dopa
Other types of medication	Tremor	Bronchodilators (theophylline, doxapram) Hypoglycemics Corticosteroids
	Chorea, tremor	GI meds (cimetadine, terfenadine)
	Chorea dystonia, tremor	Antiarrhythmic (propranolol, tocainide)
	Tardive dyskinesia	Antiemetic (prochlorperazine, thiethylperazine, promethazine)
	Intention tremor, ataxia	Cyclosporin A
	Chorea	Estrogen/oral contraceptives

NONPHARMACOLOGICAL INTERVENTIONS

Nonpharmacological intervention in the treatment of tremors is not well validated in the research literature, so the following ideas will be mentioned only briefly. These possible treatments are specific to movement dysfunction only and should not be considered to have residual effects on the tremors themselves. Individual practitioners should apply these techniques with sound clinical reasoning on an individual basis.

Passive range of motion, stretching, joint approximation, splinting, and postural inhibiting positions have been used to decrease tone, provide stability, and improve movement. Various neurodevelopmental techniques or aquatic therapy may provide individual patients with some increase in motor control. Strengthening exercises or functional electrical stimulation may be helpful to overcome weakness, especially in functional ranges. Balance and gait training with or without devices may help mobility and increase safety. Ankle or cuff weights may improve mobility in gait. Heat, cold, or neutral warmth are suggested as potential adjuncts to therapeutic exercise. Usually, these techniques are more effective if applied in conjunction with medications.

CONCLUSION

When providing rehabilitative services to elderly patients, therapists commonly see various extraneous or involuntary movements. Definitions and classification strategies enable the clinician to differentiate these tremors, choreas, and dyskinesias. Pharmacological treatments should be specific to the particular movement disorder. The efficacy of physical intervention techniques has yet to be validated.

SUGGESTED READINGS

Aminoff MJ. *Neurology and General Medicine,* 2nd ed. New York: Churchill Livingstone; 1995.

Ciccone CD. *Pharmacology in Rehabilitation* Philadelphia: F.A. Davis; 1990.

Findley LJ, Capildeo R. *Movement Disorders: tremor.* New York: Oxford University Press; 1984.

Guberman A. *An Introduction to Clinical Neurology.* Boston: Little Brown; 1994.

Jankovic J, Tolosa E. *Parkinson's Disease and Movement Disorders,* 2nd ed. Baltimore: Williams & Wilkins; 1993.

Lohr JB, Wisniewski AA. *Movement Disorders: A Neuropsychological Approach.* New York: Guilford Press; 1987.

Marsden CD, Fahn S. *Movement Disorders 3.* Oxford: Butterworth Hienman; 1994.

Malone T. *Physical and Occupational Therapy: Drug Implications for Practice.* Philadelphia: J.B. Lippincott; 1989.

Simon RP, Aminoff MJ, Greenberg DA. *Clinical Neurology.* Norwalk, Conn.: Appleton & Lange; 1989.

Chapter 35

Generalized Peripheral Neuropathy

James K. Richardson, M.D.

INTRODUCTION

Disorders of the peripheral nerves are common in the elderly, and they are likely to have a significant impact on the rehabilitation plan. Generalized peripheral polyneuropathies are regularly encountered in the elderly. It is estimated that 18% of Caucasian Americans and 26% of African-Americans older than 60 have diabetes mellitus; half of these people have peripheral neuropathy (PN). Therefore, approximately 10% of Americans over 60 have PN due to diabetes, and another 10% have PN due to other causes, which reveals a prevalence of about 20% in the older American population.[1] The prevalence of PN in older Americans requiring rehabilitation is undoubtedly much higher. Recognizing a generalized peripheral polyneuropathy and the functional limitations associated with it is important and necessary if a patient is to be successfully rehabilitated. This chapter provides the rehabilitation clinician with knowledge that will allow the recognition and treatment of a functionally significant generalized peripheral neuropathy.

RECOGNIZING A GENERALIZED PERIPHERAL NEUROPATHY

If it is understood that the longer the peripheral nerve, the more greatly it is affected by neuropathic processes, then the signs and symptoms of PN will make intuitive sense. Because lower extremities are longer than upper extremities and because sensory nerves are longer than motor nerves (as a result of the former's intraspinal dendritic processes), it follows that in PN, distal lower extremity sensory function is the first and most severely affected, followed in order by distal lower extremity motor function, distal upper extremity sensory function, and distal upper extremity motor function.

Patients are extremely variable with regard to their insight into PN, so historical features are variable as well. Many patients are acutely aware of their numbness and pain whereas others simply note that they must be more careful in performing activities requiring balance. When pain or numbness is apparent to the patient, the symptoms are most marked in the forefoot and then lessen proximally. In the upper extremity, symptoms may not occur or may occur in the fingertips only or may involve the hand and distal forearm, depending upon the severity of disease. A typical distribution of nerve dysfunction is demonstrated in Figure 35–1. Motor symptoms are usually not noted but with severe disease, foot-drop and lessening of hand dexterity may develop. Balance problems consistent with PN include difficulty standing on one foot while turning, problems with lower extremity dressing, and difficulty climbing stairs without a railing. Patients often note the insidious onset of the need to be touching something while walking, particularly if the floor surface is irregular or the lighting is low.

On examination, there is loss of sensory function in a distal-to-proximal gradient. This is best noted with a 128-Hz tuning fork maximally struck and placed at the base of the great toe, malleolus, and then tibial tubcrosity. The examiner should record the number of seconds the patient feels the buzz at each level. This can be done similarly in the upper extremity at the base of the second finger, distal radius, and olecranon. In the presence of PN, the number of seconds the patient feels the vibration

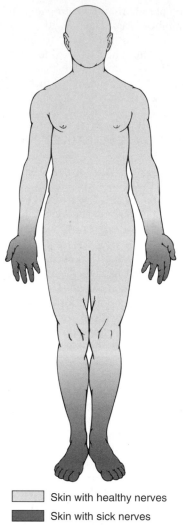

☐ Skin with healthy nerves

■ Skin with sick nerves

Figure 35–1 The typical distribution of sensory loss and, to a lesser extent, weakness in a patient with mild to moderate peripheral neuropathy. (Redrawn with permission from Richardson JK, Ashton-Miller JA. Peripheral nerve dysfunction and falls in the elderly. *Postgrad Med* 1996; 99:161–172.)

increases proximally in the extremities affected by PN. If the older patient is able to perceive the maximally struck tuning fork for 10 seconds or more at the base of the great toe, then PN is absent; if a similar patient perceives the same vibration for less than 10 seconds at the malleolus, then PN is likely to be present. Light touch and pinprick sensation can be used also and they produce similar findings but are less reliable than vibratory sense.

Muscle-stretching reflexes are also lost in a distal-to-proximal gradient. Loss of Achilles tendon reflexes is almost uniform in PN; patellar tendon and internal hamstring reflexes are progressively less affected. The intrinsic musculature of the foot is commonly atrophied, which causes changes in

foot architecture such that the metatarsophalangeal joints are extended and the interphalangeal joints are flexed ("hammer toes"). Toes move minimally or only in a stiff, gross manner. In more advanced or severe PN, anterior compartment muscles and, less commonly, posterior calf muscles can atrophy. Usually by the time the lower extremity changes have occurred, the intrinsic muscles of the hand have begun to weaken and atrophy. The sense of position of the great toe is also affected in functionally significant PN. The inability to correctly identify at least 8 out of 10 small (approximately 1 cm) great toe movements by a noncuing examiner has been correlated with decreased ankle inversion/eversion proprioception.[2]

Gross motor function is affected too. The patient may have a positive Romberg's sign in that he or she is stable standing with feet together and with the eyes open, but is not stable if the eyes are closed, which suggests a deficit in somatosensory input and excessive reliance upon vision for balance. A positive Romberg's sign suggests that the PN is relatively severe; however, many patients with functionally significant PN demonstrate a negative Romberg's sign. A more sensitive test of balance impairment secondary to PN is the assessment of unipedal stance time. If the patient can balance on one foot for 10 or more seconds (the best of three tries on the foot of choice), then functionally significant PN is likely not present. If the patient can balance on one foot for only 3 to 4 seconds or less, then the PN is functionally significant. It should be noted that the unipedal stance test is not used to identify PN but, rather, to determine the extent of loss of balance caused by the PN once it has been identified by the other elements of the clinical examination. In the upper extremity, a patient with functionally significant PN can be identified by the inability to fasten buttons without seeing them (the "upper extremity Romberg's sign"). Table 35–1 lists the clinical characteristics of a patient with functionally significant PN.

Few other diseases mimic PN. Lumbar stenosis, which is common in older populations, can present in a similar fashion, with gradual-onset numbness and weakness in the distal lower extremities. However, symptoms of lumbar stenosis increase with prolonged standing and walking and improve with sitting or lying down. There is usually some accompanying back pain as well. This contrasts with painful PN in which the pain is similar at all times or worse at night. On examination, the patient with lumbar stenosis does not usually demonstrate the symmetrical gradient of sensory loss that is found in the PN patient. If there is motor involvement, the patient with lumbar stenosis is likely to have asymmetrical weakness, and weakness that com-

Table 35–1 Clinical Detection of Functionally Significant Peripheral Neuropathy

Test or Condition	With Peripheral Neuropathy	Without Peripheral Neuropathy
Vibratory sense (128-Hz tuning fork)	Obvious gradient	Minimal or no gradient
	Vibration felt at malleolus for < 5–10 seconds	Vibration felt at metatarsophalangeal joint for > 10 seconds
Foot deformities, calluses	Present	Absent
Heel jerk	Absent	Present
Position sense at great toe	< 8 of 10 correct responses	≥ 8 of 10 correct responses
Unipedal stance (3 attempts on foot of choice)	≤ 5 seconds in each attempt	≥ 10 seconds in 1 of 3 attempts

From Richardson JK, Ashton-Miller JA. Peripheral nerve dysfunction and falls in the elderly. *Postgrad Med* 1996;99:169.

monly involves the gluteal as well as the distal musculature. In contrast, the patient with PN has symmetrical weakness that is always most severe distally and improves proximally.

THE FUNCTIONAL RAMIFICATIONS OF PN

Peripheral neuropathy has a clear impact on the functioning of the older patient in rehabilitation. Two studies have demonstrated that patients with isolated PN are about 20 times more likely to fall than are patients without PN.[3, 4] The subjects in these studies had PN and no other functionally relevant diagnoses and were all community ambulators without assistive devices. PN will undoubtedly have an equal or greater impact on the functioning of rehabilitation patients who have accompanying diagnoses and worse baseline functioning.

Other studies comparing matched older patients with and without PN have demonstrated that PN subjects have impaired ankle proprioception[2] and decreased ability to maintain unipedal stance.[5] The difficulty PN subjects had with unipedal stance was present whether or not the subjects were performing that task with preparation time or immediately upon command, with no preparation. This somewhat surprising finding suggests that patients with PN simply cannot do tasks requiring reliable unipedal stance, even if they take their time and are prepared. Therefore, climbing stairs without a support or dressing while standing will always be a challenge, even if done in a calm, leisurely fashion. The other study demonstrated that ankle inversion/eversion

proprioceptive thresholds in subjects with PN were about 1.5 degrees but only 0.3 degrees in age- and sex-matched controls without PN. The 1.5 degrees of motion at the ankle allows the body's center of mass to travel to the edge of the patient's base of support during unipedal stance without the patient's perceiving the change. As a result, the ability to maintain unipedal stance reliably is impaired.

In the older rehabilitation patient, PN is rarely isolated, as in the research subjects described above; therefore, PN exacerbates the clinically obvious impairments already present. If, for example, a patient with PN has hemiparesis or an above-knee amputation as the primary rehabilitation diagnosis, then the patient's ability to use the "good" lower extremity is impaired also. If the PN is not recognized, unrealistic expectations or care-giver confusion over difficulty with progression to certain goals develop. Patients with disruption of the other systems that help to maintain balance—the visual and the vestibular—have even greater difficulty staying upright if PN is present. Patients with ataxia from cerebellar or vestibular dysfunction and patients with visual or visual-spatial dysfunction have even worse problems when PN complicates their clinical situations. The early recognition of PN in such patients allows the formulation of reasonable goals and an early start in the learning process that enables patients to compensate for PN.

TREATING THE PATIENT WITH PN

If a PN is identified or suspected clinically, should it be further investigated? The answer depends on the circumstances. Some of the more common causes are shown in Box 35–1. A number of them, such as alcohol abuse, diabetes mellitus, chronic obstructive pulmonary disease (COPD), and critical-care illness, are quite common in the older population. The identification of PN, particularly if it has had a gradual onset, in a patient with any of these disorders does not necessarily mean further investigation is necessary. On the other hand, if PN develops in a patient with no risk factors or if it develops in any patient and exhibits relatively rapid progression, the case deserves further investigation. PN can be the presenting manifestation of many treatable systemic diseases. Electrodiagnostic studies are the best place to start as they will be helpful in characterizing the PN as primarily axonal or demyelinating. Making that distinction on clinical grounds is challenging; clues to a demyelinating PN are early loss of all reflexes, with relative preservation of muscle mass, whereas clues to an axonal PN are maintenance of proximal reflexes and relatively greater muscle atrophy distally. In general, axonal PN is associated with metabolic disorders or toxins, and demyelinating PN is associated with immune processes that are, at times, related to malignancy.

The most important aspect of treatment, in terms of the functional impact of PN, is education. The

patient and the patient's family must understand the nature of the disorder—that the patient has lost a special sense in the distal lower (and sometimes upper) extremities. They must further understand that as a result of this lost special sense, the patient's balance is impaired and compensatory techniques will be necessary to avoid an increased risk for falls.

Visual input must be maximized to compensate for the impaired somatosensory input. Vision should be tested and if it is impaired, referral to the appropriate health professional is indicated. Equally important, the patient must be taught to use proper lighting. This is particularly important at night during trips to the bathroom; the temptation to avoid putting on glasses and to leave the lights off so as not to disturb other household members as they sleep must be avoided.

A patient with PN should use proper footwear. The shoes that are best for balance have a wide base of support and thin soles. Thick crepe soles or the heavily cushioned soles of athletic shoes should be avoided. If significant foot deformity exists, custom orthotics, possibly in association with extra-depth shoes to accommodate the foot deformities, should be prescribed. Sometimes a patient with poor balance finds custom-molded, plastic ankle-foot orthoses to be of benefit; however, care must be taken in fitting them to avoid the initiation of a foot wound.

A patient with balance impairment due to PN should use support when walking. This support may be a cane, a walker, or furniture placed strategically around the house; such furniture should be steady and without sharp edges or corners. The use of a cane for stabilization of patients with PN has been studied.[6] Subjects were asked to transfer onto an unsteady surface that tilted during midtransfer and maintain 3 seconds of unipedal balance (Fig. 35–2). Under such circumstances the PN subjects failed to maintain their balance without a cane about half the time but succeeded 96% of the time with a cane. It has been further demonstrated that to obtain maximal benefit from a cane in preventing a fall, a patient must be able to support approximately 25% of his or her body weight with the cane. The patient should be instructed to place the cane down with each contralateral footstep so as to assist in preventing falls away from the cane as well as toward it. Patient and family are often reluctant to accept the use of a cane. Acceptance and compliance may be greater if they are told that the cane is a substitute, like glasses or a hearing aid, for a special sense that has been lost and is a way to prevent falls, not a sign of infirmity. The patient also complies better if the cane is used as needed and not all the time. A patient can usually be free of the

---

Box 35–1

Common Causes of a Generalized Peripheral Polyneuropathy in Older Persons

Alcohol abuse

Chronic obstructive pulmonary disease

Diabetes mellitus

Monoclonal gammopathy (benign or malignant)

Neoplasm (especially leukemia, lymphoma)

Past or long-term use of certain drugs, including nitrofurantoin macrocrystals (Macrodantin), phenytoin (Dilantin), lithium, gold compounds, vincristine sulfate (Oncovin, Vincasar PFS), isoniazid, ethambutol HCl (Myambutol), disulfiram (Antabuse)

Renal disease

Thyroid disease

Use of antiarrhythmic drugs (amiodarone HCl [Cordarone])

Vitamin B_{12} deficiency

cane when the lighting is good and the walking surface is firm, flat, and familiar.

There is no evidence that physical training improves balance in cases of PN, but if a patient is interested and motivated, the practice of unipedal stance (with eyes open) is recommended. It should focus on one foot at a time as the patient stands in front of a sink, counter, or other flat, supportive surface. First, the patient is to balance with two hands on the supportive surface, then with one hand, and finally with no hands touching the surface. This exercise strengthens ankle musculature and theoretically sharpens residual distal sensory input or input interpretation. A patient with inadequate upper extremity strength should work with grip, shoulder depression, and elbow extension so as to be able to support 25% of his or her body weight with a cane if necessary.

Pain can be a significant problem for a patient with PN, particularly at night. A trial of the medication capsaicin is indicated if the patient has the intellectual capacity and manual dexterity to apply it correctly. Although it is cumbersome to use, as it must be applied 3 to 4 times per day, and it can make symptoms worse at first, capsaicin has the distinct advantage of causing no systemic side effects, a particularly important point in a debilitated older patient. Other options include one of the tricyclic antidepressants with low anticholinergic effects in a low dosage, for example, nortriptyline 10 to 50 mg before bed. Other agents include anticonvulsants such as carbamazepine (Tegretol), phenytoin (Dilantin), and gabapentin (Neurontin), but the side effects of these drugs limit their use in an older population. Transcutaneous electric nerve stimulation (TENS) can be helpful and, like capsaicin, it has the advantage of producing no systemic side effects.

CONCLUSION

Approximately 20% of older Americans have PN, which is likely to have an impact on rehabilitation. Sensory impairment is usually more prominent than motor impairment, and distal lower extremities are affected more than distal upper extremities. These changes usually impair balance control and often lead to falls. Generalized PN usually compounds existing clinical impairments. The patient and the patient's family must be educated about the loss and advised of potential risk for further injury and what can be done to mitigate risks. The use of assistive devices for mobility, therapeutic exercises for functional activities, and medication or TENS for pain is encouraged.

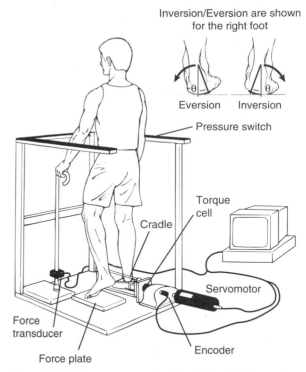

Figure 35–2 The apparatus developed (by Dr. James A. Ashton-Miller) to assess the ability of subjects to transfer onto an unstable surface and maintain balance on one foot with and without vision and/or a cane. This apparatus also helped determine ankle inversion/eversion proprioceptive thresholds in subjects with and without PN. (Modified with permission from Vanden Bosch CG, Bilsing M, Lee SG, Richardson JK, Ashton-Miller JA. Effect of peripheral neuropathy on ankle inversion and eversion detection thresholds. *Arch Phys Med Rehabil* 1995; 76:850–856.)

REFERENCES

1. Richardson JK, Ashton-Miller JA. Peripheral nerve dysfunction and falls in the elderly. *Postgrad Med* 1996;99:161–172.
2. Vanden Bosch CG, Gilsing M, Lee SG, Richardson JK, Ashton-Miller JA. Effect of peripheral neuropathy on ankle inversion and eversion detection thresholds. *Arch Phys Med Rehabil* 1995;76:850–856.
3. Richardson JK, Ching C, Hurvitz EA. The relationship between electromyographically documented peripheral neuropathy and falls. *J Am Geriatr Soc* 1992;40:1008–1012.
4. Richardson JK, Hurvitz EA. Peripheral neuropathy: a true risk factor for falls. *J Gerontol A Biol Sci Med Sci* 1995;50A:211–215.
5. Richardson JK, Ashton-Miller JA, Lee SG, Jacob K. Moderate peripheral neuropathy impairs weight transfer and unipedal balance in the elderly. *Arch Phys Med Rehabil* 1996;77:1152–1156.
6. Ashton-Miller JA, Yeh MW, Richardson JK, Galloway T. A cane lowers the risk of patients with peripheral neuropathy losing their balance: results from a challenging unipedal balance test. *Arch Phys Med Rehabil* 1996;77:446–452.

Chapter 36

Localized Peripheral Neuropathies

James K. Richardson, M.D.

INTRODUCTION

Localized peripheral neuropathies are even more common than generalized neuropathies, and the two often coincide. Because a diffusely diseased peripheral nervous system is less able to recover from a mechanical insult than is a healthy peripheral nervous system, it is a clinical rule that a patient with generalized peripheral neuropathy is at increased risk for specific, discrete neuropathies. In addition, mechanical insults are particularly common in the rehabilitation setting as patients learn alternative strategies for self-care and mobility. Such strategies often involve stressing intact musculoskeletal regions to compensate for regions that are impaired, which increases the risk for nerve trauma in the intact regions. For example, more than 50% of wheelchair users have carpal tunnel syndrome. Obviously, early recognition, prevention and, when necessary, treatment of these specific neuropathies are critical to the prevention of further impairment and disability in older patients.

Unfortunately, localized, or regional, neuropathies are often a particular challenge for the health-care practitioner. The difficulty in diagnosing such problems stems from the fact that even the most articulate patient often has trouble describing the onset, location, quality, and aggravating and alleviating factors of neuropathic pain. Such patients commonly have severe pain but few motor signs to help localize the lesions. Conversely, a patient who has significant weakness due to a peripheral nerve disorder often has few sensory complaints, which can also obscure the diagnosis. However, the proper diagnosis and treatment of these local or regional peripheral neuropathies are often critical to the patient's rehabilitation. Furthermore, some rehabilitative strategies such as assistive devices and orthotics are often the cause of peripheral neurological disorders or delayed healing. Finally, peripheral neurological disorders, even when benign, can cause patients and families significant anxiety, for they worry that the symptoms represent the progression of a previously existing neurological disease or a new, potentially malignant entity. Therefore, although it may be challenging at times to obtain, a clear understanding of a patient's peripheral neurological status is of great benefit to the patient and the health-care practitioner.

In organizing this chapter, the author considered simply enumerating peripheral neurological disorders by anatomical region. The difficulty with this approach is that a patient does not tell a health-care practitioner about an "ulnar mononeuropathy at the elbow" or "an L-5 radiculopathy on the left." Rather, a patient mentions a numb hand or a foot that drops. Therefore, this chapter will be organized around typical (and nonspecific) symptoms and complaints. The potentially responsible focal neuropathy will be identified for each symptom. The details of clinical presentation and approach to each potentially responsible focal neuropathy will be discussed as well.

NUMB HAND

Hand numbness and pain are extremely common complaints. Usually, one of the three nerves that serves the hand distally—the median, radial, or ulnar—is at fault. Hand numbness is also a possible presentation of a more proximal process such as a radiculopathy or plexopathy.

Median Nerve Compression

Although classical median nerve compression at the wrist (carpal tunnel syndrome, CTS) involves the second and third digits (the palmar cutaneous branch to the thenar eminence often branches off proximal to the carpal tunnel), the patient often senses that the "whole hand is numb." Examination should focus on sensation in the median distribution (avoiding the thumb). Pinprick sensitivity should be determined by first pricking a noninvolved area and then comparing the differences between sides. Ask, "If this (the normal side) is 100 cents, how much is this (the affected side)?" Do not just request perception of sharp or dull, as that is often maintained, even in the presence of a clinically significant localized or generalized neuropathy. An additional clue is the presence of Tinel's sign, tingling that radiates from the percussed median nerve at the site of entrapment. The site of entrapment is more distal than is often perceived, approximately 1 to 2 cm beyond the distal wrist crease. This is the area that should be percussed (Fig. 36–1). Phalen's sign, in which the wrists are held in flexed positions for 30 to 60 seconds by pushing the dorsa of the hands together in front of the chest, is often used; however, it is overly sensitive, in that pain of a nature other than due to carpal tunnel syndrome is often elicited. A particularly misleading "positive" Phalen's test occurs when the hands turn numb because of the stretching of compressed ulnar

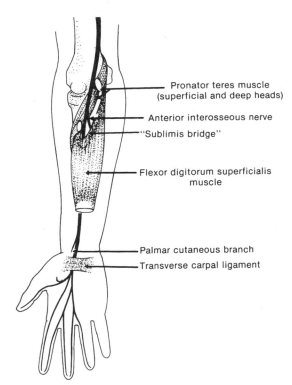

Figure 36–1 The site of compression of the median nerve at the wrist. Note the palmar cutaneous branch taking off proximal to the site of compression. (From Stewart JD. *Focal Peripheral Neuropathies,* 2nd ed. New York: Raven Press; 1993:158.)

Pronator teres muscle (superficial and deep heads)

Anterior interosseous nerve

"Sublimis bridge"

Flexor digitorum superficialis muscle

Palmar cutaneous branch

Transverse carpal ligament

nerves across the flexed elbows rather than because of median nerve compression at the wrist. Attention should also be paid to the muscles in the hand that are served by the median nerve, those of the thenar eminence. An obvious difference in bulk and strength suggests significant axonal damage to the median nerve and a prolonged, often incomplete recovery, even with surgical decompression. It is important for the examiner to test the strength of the patient's thumb abductors by opposing them with his or her own.

Treatment

Treatment requires decreasing the pressure within the carpal tunnel. The pressure in the canal is increased in positions of hyperflexion or hyperextension. Avoidance of wrist extension and gripping is particularly difficult for those who use assistive devices such as walkers and canes. The temporary use of forearm platforms rather than hand grips on assistive devices lessens the pressure on the median nerve without compromising mobility and safety. The use of a splint, which prevents flexion and extension, particularly at night when a patient's

tendency is to sleep with the wrists flexed or extended, is recommended. A patient who routinely uses a sliding board is also at risk. Using splints during transfers may allow continued function without repetitively compressing the median nerve. Injections of steroids into the carpal tunnel may provide temporary symptomatic relief but there is no evidence of a lasting benefit. Surgical decompression may be helpful as a last resort, but compression may recur in those who routinely use the upper extremities for weight-bearing.

Ulnar Nerve Compression

The second most common cause of hand numbness is ulnar nerve compression. This occurs most commonly at the elbow. Decreased pinprick response in the ulnar distribution (the fourth and fifth digits), hand-intrinsic muscle wasting, and a positive Tinel's sign over the ulnar nerve at the elbow are common findings. When severe, hand-intrinsic wasting leads to a characteristic hand position of hyperextension at the metacarpophalangeal joints and flexion at the interphalangeal joints. As was true with testing the thumb abductors for carpal tunnel syndrome, the hand's interossei should be tested against the examiner's hands interossei so that a true estimation of strength is possible.

Cause and Treatment

The cause of an ulnar neuropathy in an older patient is usually compression at the elbow within the groove between the olecranon and the medial epicondyle, or the stretching of the nerve from a prolonged, hyperflexed elbow position (Fig. 36–2). The latter often occurs while a patient sleeps holding the hand against the neck and chest when lying on one side. Compression commonly occurs in wheelchair users as forearms and elbows rest on wheelchair arms. This problem is particularly common in thin and cachectic patients. Treatment is best accomplished by protecting the elbow with an elastic pad such as is often used in athletics. The pad can be maintained posteriorly during the day to prevent compression and anteriorly during sleep to prevent hyperflexion. If these measures are not successful, ulnar transposition surgery can be performed to remove the nerve from its usual position over a bony prominence.

Radial Nerve Involvement

One of the pitfalls in the treatment of CTS is the development of a radial sensory neuropathy of the

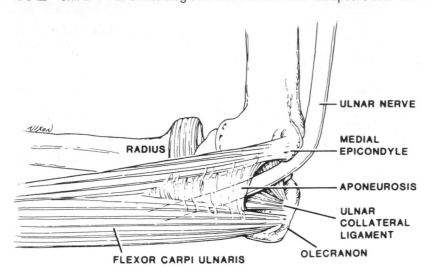

Figure 36–2 The vulnerability of the ulnar nerve to compressive or stretching forces at the elbow is obvious. (From Kincaid JC. *Minimonograph #31: The Electrodiagnosis of Ulnar Neuropathy at the Elbow*. Rochester, Minn.: American Association of Electrodiagnostic Medicine; 1983.)

distal forearm (Fig. 36–3). In this situation, the splint compresses the superficial radial nerve over the distal and radial aspects of the forearm. The only clinical consequence is sensory loss, as there is no radial motor function in the hand-intrinsic musculature. The numbness that was initially attributed to CTS persists in the second and third digits of the hand despite the splint. At this point, however, the numbness involves the dorsum of the hand rather than the palmar aspect, but the patient may not recognize or report this subtle change. Decreased pinprick and light-touch sensation in the radial nerve distribution is noted on examination, and usually a Tinel's sign can be noted with gentle percussion over the superficial radial nerve in the distal forearm. The CTS signs may coexist or may

have resolved. Treatment should relieve the compression of the nerve by discontinuing the splint (if the CTS is resolved) or by modifying the splint.

The radial nerve can be affected proximally, as well. This occurs most commonly following a humeral fracture due to a fall by an osteoporotic patient, but it can also occur after a prolonged compression of the posterolateral humerus (see Fig. 36–3). When the radial nerve is injured proximally, the hand numbness in the radial distribution is accompanied by weakness of the brachioradialis muscle and the wrist and digit extensors. At times, the nerve is not injured acutely at the time of fracture but becomes compressed by bony callus as the fracture heals. This pattern of injury would be most evident to the patient's rehabilitation team. Dy-

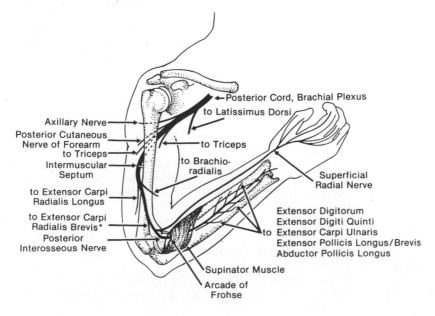

Figure 36–3 The superficial radial nerve in the forearm and the radial nerve as it wraps around the humerus are vulnerable to compressive forces. (With permission from Lotem M, Fried A, Levy M. Radial palsy following muscular effort: a nerve compression syndrome possibly related to a fibrous arch of the lateral head of the triceps. *J Bone Joint Surg Br* 1971; 53B:500–506.)

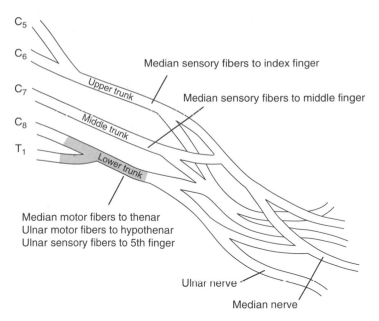

Figure 36–4 The lower trunk of the brachial plexus supplies the hand intrinsic musculature and supplies sensation to the medial (ulnar) aspect of the forearm and hand; the upper trunk supplies the shoulder musculature and elbow flexors, giving sensation to the lateral aspect of the forearm and hand. (From Wilbourn A. *Case Report #7: True Neurogenic Thoracic Outlet Syndrome.* Rochester, Minn.: American Association of Electrodiagnostic Medicine; 1982.)

namic orthotics can substitute for some of the digit extensors' functions while awaiting return of neurological function.

Brachial Plexopathy

Another cause of hand numbness that is seen in the older population is an injury to the brachial plexus. Common causes include trauma, tumor, and remote effect from radiation, most commonly to the chest and axilla during treatment for breast or lung cancer. Motor vehicle accidents typically affect the upper trunk, when the patient's head has been laterally flexed and the shoulder depressed. Such patients experience weakness in the humeral rotators and abductors and the elbow flexors, with numbness involving the lateral aspect of the arm and the first and second digits of the hand more than the fifth. Trauma after surgery usually results from the upper extremity's being abducted and externally rotated, which leads to excessive stretching of the lower trunk of the plexus. This results in weakness of the hand-intrinsic musculature and to numbness in the fourth and fifth digits (Fig. 36–4).

Tumor—metastatic, recurrent, or primary—can cause plexopathy. The two most common tumors to affect the plexus are those of the lung and breast. Classically, these tumors cause shoulder pain and a predominantly lower trunk plexopathy with numbness along the medial aspect of the forearm and hand weakness. It is rare for the brachial plexopathy to be the first manifestation of the tumor, except for Pancoast's syndrome, a carcinoma involving the apex of the lung. Finally, radiation to the upper chest or shoulder, such as occurs with lymphoma, breast or lung cancer, can lead to plexopathy. Plexopathy does not occur in every patient who has received radiation to the area, but the likelihood increases with higher doses of radiation. Symptoms and signs of plexopathy can occur anywhere from a few months to several years after the completion of radiation therapy. Although it has been suggested that pain and lower trunk involvement are more commonly due to recurrence of tumor, and that upper trunk involvement is more likely to be due to radiation effects, it is not possible to distinguish the two based on clinical grounds, and more extensive investigation is indicated.

Regardless of cause, brachial plexopathies that are primarily demyelinating in nature can improve rapidly and leave a fully functional limb. Plexopathies that are associated with significant axon loss typically improve slowly, and the patient is usually left with some residual weakness and sensory loss. Atrophy is an important clinical clue to significant axon loss; electrodiagnostic studies can much more precisely determine the degree and distribution of axon loss, thus assisting the rehabilitation clinician with prognosis.

Cervical Radiculopathy

Radiculopathy can be a cause of hand numbness in the older patient. Although C-7 is the most common level to be affected by acute disk herniations, C-5 and C-6 are the levels most commonly affected by chronic degenerative changes and are therefore the most commonly affected in the older population.

With a cervical radiculopathy at this level, the patient experiences numbness over the lateral aspect of the forearm and the first and second digits. Weakness occurs predominantly in the humeral rotators and elbow flexors. In a C-7 radiculopathy, the third digit feels numb and the elbow extensors and shoulder depressors are weak. With lower cervical radiculopathies (C-8 and T-1), the fourth and fifth digits are numb and weakness is most prominent in the hand-intrinsic musculature. Atrophy, weakness, and decreased reflexes in the proper distribution are clues to the presence of a radiculopathy. In addition, if compression of the nerve roots by simultaneously extending, laterally flexing, and rotating the head to the symptomatic side increases upper extremity symptoms and pain (Spurling's sign), radiculopathy is likely. Extension of the neck should be undertaken cautiously in the older patient with vascular or degenerative disease. The addition of axial compression of the head to the above maneuvers, as is often advocated for Spurling's test, should be avoided in the older patient undergoing rehabilitation. Electrodiagnostic studies should be obtained to assist with specific diagnosis, prognostication, and treatment.

Radiculopathies and plexopathies have functional ramifications. Upper plexopathies and high cervical radiculopathies lead to shoulder weakness; this weakness, in turn, predisposes the patient to rotator cuff tendinopathies and impingement. This is particularly true if the extremity is used regularly or is overused, for example, during ambulation with a cane or walker. If possible, the extremity should not be used to assist with mobility skills. If that is not possible, the use of a platform rather than a standard cane or walker may be helpful, as these allow the shoulder to bear weight with less internal rotation. C-7 radiculopathies cause weakness of shoulder depressors and elbow extensors. As a result, the extremity is much less effective during transfers. It can still assist with ambulation but less effectively; the patient may benefit from a shortening of the cane so that the elbow can lock when the cane is placed on the ground. Lower trunk plexopathies and C-8/T-1 radiculopathies result in hand and finger weakness. Assistive devices can still be used effectively but compensation for the weakened grip may have to be made. Activities of daily living (ADLs) that require fine motor function become very difficult, and adaptive techniques are usually necessary.

Stenosis and Myelopathy

It should be noted that the same cervical degenerative processes that cause upper extremity radiculo-pathies in older patients can cause cervical stenosis and resultant myelopathy; this is particularly true following a fall or motor vehicle accident when the spinal cord is "shaken" against a narrowed, irregular cervical spinal canal. Such patients have weak, atrophied upper extremities and minimally atrophied, often spastic lower extremities; these changes are sometimes associated with bowel or bladder dysfunction. Muscle stretching reflexes give the best clinical clues. Depressed reflexes in the upper extremities associated with hyperactive reflexes and extensor plantar (Babinski) responses in the lower extremities suggest a cervical myelopathy. If this syndrome is suspected, then appropriate imaging studies and neurosurgical consultation are indicated.

FOOT-DROP

Foot-drop, or dorsiflexor weakness, is a common observation or complaint in the older population. Both upper motor neuron dysfunction leading to equinovarus posturing and lower motor neuron dysfunction can cause functionally significant foot-drop. This section focuses on the latter. The common areas of peripheral nerve compression that lead to foot-drop are demonstrated in Figure 36–5.

Common Peroneal Neuropathy

Probably the most frequent cause of foot-drop is a common peroneal neuropathy at the fibular head. Older patients in rehabilitation have many risk factors for such a lesion. Common peroneal neuropathy typically occurs in patients with prolonged hospitalization, weight loss, knee replacement surgery, plaster casts, and fractures of the fibular head or neck. Weakness occurs in the ankle dorsiflexors and evertors. Numbness and decreased sensation are present along the anterolateral calf and dorsum of the foot. At times, Tinel's sign can be found over the peroneal nerve just inferior and posterior to the fibular head. Significant wasting of the musculature of the anterior and lateral compartments suggests significant axon loss and a prolonged or incomplete recovery. Electrodiagnostic studies can further clarify both diagnosis and prognosis. Treatment should protect the peroneal nerve from further mechanical trauma. Weight gain and careful positioning in bed to prevent knee hyperflexion and pressure over the area are helpful. As the patient becomes ambulatory, it is imperative that the ankle-foot orthosis prescribed to compensate for the foot-drop does not prolong it by putting pressure on the peroneal nerve adjacent to the fibular head.

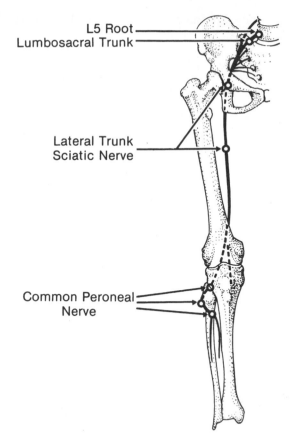

L5 Root

Lumbosacral Trunk

Lateral Trunk
Sciatic Nerve

Common Peroneal
Nerve

Figure 36–5 The common sites of compression or trauma that lead to foot-drop. (From Stewart JD. *Focal Peripheral Neuropathies,* 2nd ed. New York: Raven Press; 1993:355.)

Deep Peroneal Neuropathy

Less commonly, foot-drop can be caused by a deep peroneal neuropathy. The common peroneal nerve divides into the superficial and deep branches just distal to the fibular head. The deep branch provides innervation of the anterior compartment muscles, which are ankle dorsiflexors and toe extensors, plus sensation to a small space between the dorsal aspects of the first and second toes. Lesions to the deep peroneal nerve are commonly caused by anterior compartment syndromes which result from high pressure within the anterior compartment due to tissue trauma, tibial fracture, or hemorrhage. Compartment syndromes are usually handled surgically in the acute care setting. The deep peroneal nerve is not influenced by external compression forces or positioning so that little can be done in the rehabilitation setting to influence the course of recovery either positively or negatively. Certainly, following the guidelines mentioned above for the common peroneal nerve makes sense so that a lesion more proximal to the peroneal nerve does not develop.

L-5 Radiculopathy

Another cause of foot-drop is a low lumbar (usually L-5) radiculopathy. This can develop as the result of an acute disk herniation, which is uncommon in older populations, or it can develop more gradually as the result of degenerative changes. Such patients usually have a years-long history of low back pain with or without leg pain. It should be kept in mind that tumor can be a cause of back pain and radiculopathy, especially in patients over 50. Clinical clues that suggest a malignant cause of back pain and radiculopathy include age greater than 50, insidious onset, pain for more than 1 month, and a history of any kind of cancer. Worsening pain at night is almost universal in patients with a malignant cause of back pain, but it occurs commonly in benign causes of back pain as well. As a result, the absence of night pain is reassuring and suggests that the source of pain is not malignant, but the presence of night pain is less diagnostically helpful. L-5 radiculopathy can be differentiated clinically from a lesion at the fibular head by a variety of clinical findings.

A patient with an L-5 radiculopathy, as compared to one with peroneal neuropathy, usually has the following: weakness in the hip abductors and knee flexors; loss of an internal hamstring reflex on the affected side; a positive straight-leg-raising sign (straight-leg-raising causes pain or dysesthesia in the anterolateral calf and dorsum of the foot); and absence of Tinel's sign at the fibular head. If the cause of the radiculopathy is not known, appropriate imaging studies should be performed. If the cause is benign, electrodiagnostic studies can provide prognostic information. As the patient begins to ambulate, it is important to accommodate for the foot-drop with an orthosis and also to support the weakened gluteal musculature by using a cane in the opposite hand. Doing so helps to avoid a trochanteric bursitis on the affected side and difficulty during the swing phase of gait on the contralateral side.

Sciatic Neuropathy

Despite the fact that the sciatic nerve contains fibers that give rise to both the tibial and peroneal nerves, a sciatic neuropathy can cause foot-drop. The reason for this is that the peroneal division of the sciatic nerve lies in a more lateral and superficial position as it travels through the buttock and proximal posterior thigh and is thus more vulnerable to external forces. Although in such instances foot-drop, or dorsiflexion weakness, is the predominant finding, close examination usually suggests that there is some degree of tibial division involvement as demonstrated by decreased ankle muscle stretching reflex or plantar flexor weakness or both. In addition, sensation commonly decreases in both the peroneal and tibial distributions. Risk factors for sciatic neuropathies in older patients include hip surgery, repeated intramuscular injections in the hip, cachexia, and malpositioning (hips flexed for too long, lying supine on an operating-room table), and a history of trauma to the hip or pelvis. Avoiding pressure over the posterior thigh and buttock, such as that caused by sitting on a ledge, and avoiding prolonged time either supine or with hips flexed are important to allow healing. Ankle-foot orthotics are important functionally but must be carefully fitted to prevent the development of a more distal peroneal neuropathy at the fibular head or a foot wound.

Lumbosacral Plexopathy

Several disorders common among older patients could affect the lumbosacral plexus which, in turn, can cause foot-drop. These include radiation, proximal diabetic neuropathy, and retroperitoneal disorders such as hematomas, aortic aneurysms, malignancies, and abscesses. Radiation plexopathy does not occur in the lumbar region as frequently as it does in the cervical region. When it does occur, symptoms develop a few months to several years after the radiation and are associated with relatively painless weakness. Proximal diabetic neuropathy typically causes symptoms in the thigh and hip, although more distal involvement is possible and will be discussed in a later section. Retroperitoneal hematomas can occur in any anticoagulated patient; resultant neurological compromise is usually related to hemorrhage into the psoas muscle. Usually the thigh muscles are more affected than the distal muscles. Postural lightheadedness or weakness is often associated with retroperitoneal hemorrhages, as large amounts of blood can be lost from the intravascular space into such lesions.

Several tumors that are common among older populations occur in the retroperitoneal area and lead to plexopathy. These include lymphoma and carcinomas of the prostate, bladder, kidney, cervix, and colon. The initial manifestation of retroperitoneal tumors is lumbosacral plexopathy in 15% of cases. Sensory and motor symptoms develop, as does pain.

All of these diagnoses have serious ramifications. If foot-drop develops and there are proximal signs or symptoms as well (weakness of the knee extensors, hip flexors and abductors, and numbness proximal to the knee) suggestive of a plexopathy, then proper diagnostic studies should carried out as soon as possible. Imaging the area with MRI or CT and electrodiagnostic studies are typical ways to start.

THIGH NUMBNESS OR WEAKNESS

Thigh numbness or weakness is a common problem in the older patient involved in rehabilitation. Obviously, if there is no numbness and the complaints are bilateral, a muscular cause such as disuse or a metabolic myopathy is the likely underlying cause. This section focuses on the patients who have associated numbness or unilateral symptoms.

Meralgia Paresthetica

One of the most benign and common causes of thigh numbness is entrapment of the lateral femoral cutaneous nerve, often referred to as meralgia paresthetica. This nerve is purely sensory and often gets entrapped between an external force and the inguinal ligament or anterior superior iliac spine (Fig. 36–6). The nerve then travels distally, supplying the anterior and lateral thigh. Entrapment can occur because of belts or restraints and commonly occurs because of thoracolumbosacral orthoses (TLSOs). Anxiety often develops in patients with TLSOs as well as in their families and health-care providers when meralgia paresthetica develops, as there is a natural concern that spinal instability is developing along with progressive neurological compromise. Patients can be reassured if the numbness is just over the anterior and lateral aspects of the thigh, and the knee muscle stretching reflex and quadriceps muscle bulk are maintained. Further confirmatory evidence is sometimes available if Tinel's sign is found where the skin just medial and inferior to the anterior superior iliac spine is percussed. If the diagnosis is clear, no further studies are needed; although electrodiagnostic evaluation can rule out other diagnoses, it is surprisingly ineffective in confirming the presence of meralgia paresthetica and is generally not indicated.

The natural history of meralgia paresthetica is spontaneous resolution. Tightness of the rectus femoris and iliotibial band muscle tendon complexes, if present, should be corrected and this correction can help to hasten improvement. Avoiding compression medial to the anterior superior iliac spine will prevent prolonging the syndrome. If symptoms become severe or long-lasting, injection with local anesthetic and corticosteroid may be helpful; surgical treatment is efficacious as well.

Upper Lumbar Radiculopathy

Thigh numbness and weakness due to an upper lumbar radiculopathy are more common among

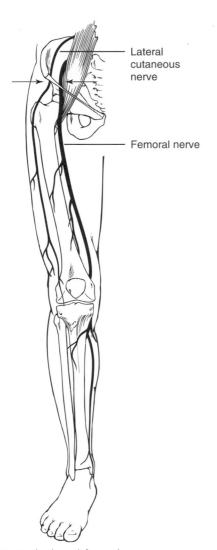

Figure 36–6 The lateral femoral cutaneous nerve is at risk for compression medial to the anterior iliac spine, whereas the femoral nerve is vulnerable to compression by hematoma and other retroperitoneal processes. (Redrawn from Smorto MP, Basmajian JV. *Clinical Electroneurography: An Introduction to Conduction Testing,* 2nd ed. Baltimore: Williams & Wilkins; 1979:59.)

older patients than among the young. One of the reasons is that as patients age, the L-4/L-5 and L-5/S-1 disks degenerate, decreasing movement at these interspaces. As motion and stress increase in the upper lumbar segments, disk displacement, injury, and degenerative changes become more likely. An upper level (L-2, L-3, or L-4) radiculopathy may result. The patient experiences unilateral knee weakness and numbness of the anterior and medial thigh. On examination there is evidence of muscle wasting, which can be subtle and is best found by looking for side-to-side differences in vastus medialis oblique mass or measuring circumferences

10 cm above the superior pole of the patellae. Other findings include decreased sensation over the anterior and medial thigh and a reverse straight-leg-raising sign. This occurs when the patient experiences dysesthetic pain into the anterior thigh while lying prone and having the thigh passively extended by the examiner while maintaining knee flexion of about 90 degrees. The side-lying position can be used as well, if care is taken that lumbosacral motion is not substituted for true hip extension. Imaging studies are indicated in older patients to rule out malignant causes of radiculopathy. Electrodiagnostic studies are indicated to provide information concerning location and severity of the lesion if the patient does not improve.

Retroperitoneal and Femoral Neuropathy

Thigh numbness and weakness can result from any of the retroperitoneal processes described earlier, in the section on foot-drop. As was true for foot-drop, a careful examination usually demonstrates abnormalities of reflex, sensation, or strength in the gluteals or leg muscles as well as in the thigh, which would lead the examiner to suspect a plexopathy. In anticoagulated patients, however, an isolated femoral neuropathy can develop because of a hematoma in the iliacus muscle. (The close relationship between the iliopsoas musculature and the femoral nerve can be seen in Figure 36–6.) The patient keeps the lower extremity flexed at the hip and bruising may be seen in the proximal thigh. Loss of patellar reflex and knee extension strength on the affected side is usually present; sensory loss may be less remarkable and occurs over the anterior or lateral thigh and medial knee and leg.

Diabetic Neuropathy

The major clinical manifestation of proximal diabetic neuropathy (which is also known by other terms, including diabetic amyotrophy, diabetic polyradiculopathy, diabetic radiculoplexopathy) often involves the thigh, so the entity is included in this section. However, it should be recognized that proximal diabetic neuropathy may involve multiple roots or multiple lesions at the level of the lumbosacral plexus. Commonly, the patient experiences the abrupt or subacute onset of pain in the hip and thigh. Lower extremity weakness soon develops and has a predilection for the anterior thigh musculature. The pain usually diminishes as the weakness develops. The weakness is often accompanied by dramatic weight loss. Many times, the pain and weight loss lead to a search for neoplasm. Most patients have evidence of a generalized polyneuropathy at the onset of the proximal diabetic neuropathy. Similarly, most patients are known to have diabetes when proximal diabetic neuropathy develops, but it can be the presenting manifestation of diabetes. Symptoms are usually bilateral but often so asymmetric that the less affected side is not functionally impaired.

Although it is not clear that there is any way to influence the recovery of the nerves from the presumed metabolic or vascular insult associated with proximal diabetic neuropathy, it makes good clinical sense to maximize the patient's neuromuscular anabolism by optimizing glycemic control and instituting a graded therapeutic exercise regimen. Joint protection with orthotics, particularly to stabilize the knee, is often indicated. Careful education of patient and family to prevent falls is critical, as the majority of these patients have peripheral neuropathy as well as marked proximal weakness. Pain control can be difficult. Tricyclic antidepressants, preferably with low anticholinergic side effects, anticonvulsants, capsaicin, and transcutaneous electrical nerve stimulation (TENS) units may be helpful. Pain lessens after the first few weeks or months. Strength returns slowly over a period of 6 to 18 months. A full recovery occurs in slightly fewer than half of all patients, but most have sufficient recovery to develop functional mobility skills.

When the patient walks again it is important to avoid superimposed compression neuropathies as described above; the median, ulnar, and peroneal nerves are at particular risk.

CONCLUSION

Localized peripheral neuropathies are common complaints; they manifest as numbness, weakness, and radicular pain. The common causes of these clinical problems have been discussed for upper and lower extremities. Accurate diagnosis is crucial for prognosis and effective treatment, which is aimed at reducing compression or entrapment; educating the patient and family; teaching proper use of protective equipment, orthotics, or assistive devices; preventing further injury; controlling pain; and restoring function.

SELECTED READINGS

Brown MJ, Asbury AK. Diabetic neuropathy. *Ann Neurol* 1984;15:2–12.

Davidoff G, Werner R, Waring W. Compressive mononeuropathies of the upper extremity in chronic paraplegia. *Paraplegia* 1991;29:17–24.

Steward JD. *Focal Peripheral Neuropathies,* 2nd ed. New York: Raven Press; 1993.

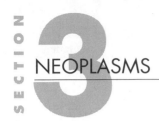

Chapter 37

Neoplasms of the Brain

Stephen A. Gudas, Ph.D., P.T.

INTRODUCTION

Primary tumors of the central nervous system (CNS) have an annual incidence rate of between 4.8 and 19.6 per 100,000 of the total U.S. population, which means an average of 18,000 new cases occur annually in the United States.[1] The actual age-related incidence is bimodal, with an early peak in infancy and childhood and another, more sustained peak in the fifth through the eighth decades. In the adult, primary brain cancer ranks 13th in frequency of all adult cancers. Throughout history, brain tumors have evoked some very special emotional and psychosocial sentiments, for they affect the organ of our intellect, function, and humanity. Contemporary neuro-oncology, however, stresses some of the more hopeful clinical features of these tumors, while remaining aware of the realities of tumor progression and symptom production. Approximately 50% of patients with primary brain tumors are now treated successfully, and many have excellent long-term prognoses.[2]

PRESENTATION AND DISTINGUISHING FACTORS

Some unique therapeutic considerations govern the diagnosis and management of tumors in the central nervous system. They are different from tumors arising elsewhere. For one thing, the distinction between benign and malignant histology in tumors in the central nervous system is not an absolute concept, as a benign tumor in a vital area of the brain is just as lethal as a frankly malignant one if it is surgically inaccessible or ineradicable. Unlike the rest of the body, the brain lacks a defined lymphatic drainage system; this, in conjunction with the fact that brain neoplasms rarely, if ever, metastasize hematogenously outside of the central nervous system, gives these tumors special significance. Tumors can be locally progressive and invasive, compressing structures with their own substance and also with the cerebral edema that commonly occurs, especially in metastatic lesions.

The exact cause and pathophysiology of most brain tumors remain obscure despite the fact that in small, discrete groups of subpatients, definite genetic predisposition to brain tumor involvement has been identified. Most commonly observed is an increased incidence of patients with neurofibromatosis; interestingly enough, these patients are also prone to soft-tissue sarcoma as a complication of the disease process.[3] Other genetic syndromes that carry an increased incidence of nervous system tumors are uncommon, leaving the vast majority of brain tumors in the category of being spontaneous, or apparently so. The fact that as many as 7% of primary brain tumor patients with gliomas have a blood relative with a positive history of brain tumor is intriguing and demands further study.[2] Although there is currently little evidence to support a viral basis for most brain tumors, this concept cannot be ignored completely, especially considering the relationship between primary cerebral lymphomas and the Epstein-Barr virus.[4]

Results of studies seeking to blame environmental carcinogens in brain tumor etiology and development have been conflicting; some questionably positive statistical associations between brain tumor occurrence and work in the rubber, petrochemical, and farming industries have been suggested, but none have been proven definitively. Much work has to be done in brain tumor etiology and pathogenesis. This chapter focuses on primary and secondary tumors of the brain; tumors of the spine and pituitary gland are excluded, as space does not permit their discussion. They are much less common than primary or secondary brain tumors, even though they are just as important clinically to the patients who develop them.

CLINICAL RELEVANCE

Gliomas

Brain tumors are classified on the basis of both cellular origin and histological grade. Tumor location, independent of tumor pathology, can be a critical factor that governs therapy and prognosis. Although neurons have an extreme tissue density in the CNS, they have no reproductive capabilities and are therefore rarely the cause of CNS tumors. The glial cells, on the other hand, have tremendous replicative ability and are the cells most likely to be the origin of central nervous system tumors, the gliomas, accounting for more than 50% of all primary brain tumors. Other, less common cells of origin are the meninges, choroid plexus, blood vessels, and primitive embryonal cells. Primary lymphomas of the brain, once uncommon and accounting for only 1 to 2% of brain tumors, have risen dramatically in incidence during the past decade, partly because they tend to occur in AIDS patients and transplant recipients and also in other individuals with significant immunoincompetence.[5]

Gliomas of various types make up the majority of brain tumors. The astrocytomas, graded 1 through 4, depending on their differentiation and degree of malignancy, are the most common and most frequently seen by health-care practitioners. The glioblastoma multiforme is a grade 4 astrocytoma characterized by cellular atypia, high mitotic activity, exuberant endothelial proliferation, and necrosis. These latter tumors are the classical type that used to kill the elderly patient in 6 months or less. Oligodendrogliomas make up 30% of brain tumors and are characterized by a somewhat earlier age of occurrence, slow growth, calcification, and indolent course. Meningiomas make up approximately 20% of brain tumors, have a 3:1 female/male ratio, occur most commonly in elderly individuals, and carry a very good prognosis with surgical removal. Regardless of tumor type, tumor recurrence after surgical removal is common, and the tumors typically recur with a higher-grade pathology, rendering treatment decisions difficult.

The brain, at least initially, has a surprisingly high tolerance for the compressive and infiltrative effects of an expanding cranial lesion, but in time all tumors produce symptoms by several mechanisms: increased intracranial pressure, compression or destruction of brain tissue or cranial nerves, and local electrochemical instability which results in seizures.[2] Headache occurs in 30% of patients at diagnosis and is a symptom in 70% during the course of the disease. Papilledema, increased intraoptic nerve pressure, occurs in 50 to 70% of patients and is often detected early. Seizures are the presenting symptom in one third of patients and occur in 50 to 70% of patients during the disease course.

Tumors in subcortical areas tend to be less epileptogenic. Altered mental status occurs in approximately 15 to 20% of cases; tumors of the frontal lobe more commonly cause this sign. Focal neurological signs are characterized by a gradual and progressive loss of neurological function, especially when the frontoparietal lobe is involved; hemiparesis and loss of sensation are of particular interest to rehabilitation clinicians. Tumors of the temporal lobe typically cause seizure activity; tumors of the occipital lobe, uncommon in comparison to tumors in other brain areas, cause homonymous hemianopsia. However, there may be false localizing signs. Tumors of the cerebellum cause headaches, vertigo, ataxia, akinesia, and nausea and vomiting, all symptoms that affect function.

Diagnosis is now made by CT scan and MRI; the former detects 90% or more of tumors, but the latter provides much greater anatomical detail and resolution in multiple planes, and is particularly useful in visualizing skull base, brain stem, and posterior fossa tumors. Cerebral angiography is now indicated only when excessive vascularity is anticipated. Outlining the blood supply of a brain tumor preoperatively by angiography can do much to assist the surgeon in planning approach and technique.

Metastases

Metastatic complications of cancer are an escalating clinical problem; brain metastases occur in 20% of patients with cancer, with lung and breast being the most common primary tumors, and renal cell carcinoma and melanoma following.[6] Although usually occurring late in the clinical course of a malignancy, brain metastases are being seen earlier with some cancers, particularly lung carcinoma, and it is not uncommon for a silent lung primary to present with brain metastases as the first symptom of cancer. The frontal and parietal lobes are favored, owing to the vascular territory of the middle cerebral artery. Multiple metastatic lesions are present in over one half of cases, many of them subclinical. The evolution of symptoms in brain metastases is rapid, often measurable in days to weeks. This is partially due to cerebral edema, which is disproportionate in comparison to the edema effected by primary brain tumors. Solitary brain lesions may present a diagnostic problem in the face of an unknown primary; histological confirmation may be necessary. The symptoms caused by brain metastases are in other ways similar in frequency and type in comparison to primary tumors.

THERAPEUTIC INTERVENTION

The treatment of malignant brain tumors is guided by the principle that it is worthwhile to prolong the survival of patients, as most of this additional time is good; functional decompensation tends to occur late in the clinical course. For virtually all types of brain tumors, surgical resection is the most important form of initial therapy. Surgery establishes the tissue diagnosis, quickly relieves intracranial pressure and mass effect, and achieves the oncological cytoreduction that will facilitate later chemotherapy, if done. Collectively, many advances in neurosurgical techniques, including lasers, intraoperative ultrasound, and computer-based stereotaxic resection procedures have given new dimensions to neurosurgical procedures and strategies. Even if not curative, tumor resection is a reasonable surgical goal provided a neurological deficit is not imposed. Corticosteroids are a mainstay, as they relieve cerebral edema, which is so common in brain tumors. Also, these medications can sometimes produce dramatic improvements in clinical function and neurological status.

Radiation Therapy

Radiation therapy is a proven and effective method of treatment for most brain tumors. There is at least a short-term survival advantage to be obtained from radiation therapy, so it is often used in conjunction with surgery for tumor treatment.[7] Older and younger individuals do not differ significantly in their response to radiation therapy; age alone should not be a factor in making decisions concerning the employability of radiation therapy as a treatment modality. Effects of radiation therapy can be divided into acute and chronic; the acute brain syndromes that occur as a result of swelling and irritation of the brain microvasculature are self-limited and respond to steroids. Long-term chronic effects are fortunately uncommon, and they include brain necrosis, endocrine disturbances, and neuro-oncogenesis. The newer techniques of interstitial brachytherapy and stereotaxic radiotherapy employ different radiation physics but are designed to deliver a highly concentrated, discrete, and well-controlled dose of radiation directly to the tumor, sparing uninvolved brain tissue. The availability and popularity of these procedures are increasing, and favorable clinical results are now being reported.

Chemotherapy

Although chemotherapy has not made major breakthroughs in brain tumor treatment, except in some brain neoplasms in children, it can provide modest extensions of survival for some patients, but these gains may be overshadowed by other variables, such as age, performance status, and neurological deficit. Immunotherapy has some clinical appeal, as brain tumors cause a marked reduction in immunocompetence. The potential role of biological response modifiers and the use of active and passive immunotherapy are increasing.

Rehabilitation

In terms of rehabilitation, clinical problems arise that are amenable to therapeutic intervention. Any patient with a hemiparesis or other motor syndrome secondary to the tumor or its treatment will respond to therapeutic strategies designed to return and enhance motor function. All neurophysiological approaches are applicable and may be tried sequentially or concurrently. The efficacy of many of the standard exercise and facilitative approaches is empirical, and choice of treatment is sometimes made by trial and error. Postural and balance control exercises may be necessary, even in the absence of frank hemiparesis. Pain management and proper breathing exercises are useful in many patients with brain tumors. Because so many of the patients have symptoms attributable to brain edema, relief of this complication through corticosteroids will assist the health-care practitioner in returning improved function to the patient.

Wheelchair prescription and management, evaluation for assistive devices, and education in performing the activities of daily living and related activities are tantamount to a good functional outcome. The various therapeutic disciplines should combine their efforts in a team approach to the patient, with each field contributing its expertise. Nutritional intake should be monitored to prevent malnourishment, dehydration, and weight loss. Nursing staff must attend to skin integrity and bowel and bladder function as well as to infection control. Social interaction with other patients is crucial to success. Family involvement and teaching are also integral; psychosocial support and intervention are very helpful, especially when the family is confronted with an individual with altered mental status and severe motor and sensory deficit. Formal rehabilitation in an inpatient setting is sometimes indicated, and the health-care professional should be available to assist in this transition in care when it occurs.

CONCLUSION

In summary, the treatment of primary and metastatic tumors of the central nervous system offers unique and challenging clinical opportunities to the health-care practitioner. The clinical course may be long and at times slow to progress, so, the rehabilitation professional should be on hand to provide the services necessary to bring the patient to his or her highest level of function. New and exciting treatment techniques, particularly in the delivery of radiation therapy, are allowing longer survival and thus creating extended periods during which the trained health-care professional is needed to respond to the clinical syndromes and rehabilitative problems that arise.

REFERENCES

1. Landis SH, Murray T, Bolden S, Wingo PA. Cancer statistics, 1997. *CA Cancer J Clin* 1998; 48:6–30.
2. Tjhaper K, Laws E. Tumors of the central nervous system. In: Murphy GP, Lawrence L, Lenmhard RE, eds. *American Cancer Society Textbook of Clinical Oncology,* 2nd ed. Atlanta: American Cancer Society; 378:1995.
3. Blatt J, Jaffe R, Deutsch M, Adkins JC. Neurofibromatosis and childhood cancers. *Cancer* 1986; 57:1225.
4. O'Neil BP, Illig JJ. Primary central nervous system lymphoma. *Mayo Clin Proc* 1989; 64:1005.
5. Deangelis LM. Primary central nervous system lymphoma: a new clinical challenge. *Neurology* 1991; 41:619.
6. Patchel RA. Brain metastases. *Neurol Clin* 1991; 9:817.
7. Leibel SA, Sheline GE. Radiation therapy for neoplasms of the brain. *J Neurosurg* 1987; 66:1.

Chapter **38**

Neoplasms of the Breast
Stephen A. Gudas, Ph.D., P.T.

INTRODUCTION

Breast carcinoma remains one of the most challenging diseases for health-care practitioners and their patients. Its extensive metastatic capability combined with intriguing responses to treatment make breast carcinoma a compelling enigma for all involved in oncology. Until just a few years ago, breast cancer was the number one cause of cancer death in females, now it is surpassed by cancer of the lung (Box 38–1). An estimated 44,000 women died of breast cancer in 1998.[1] It is curious that breast cancer mortality has been stable for almost 50 years. During that time there has been a 15% increase in its occurrence in women 55 years of age or older and a concomitant decrease in women younger than 55.[2] Breast cancer, like many other cancers, is getting "older." People are living longer; people are living longer with cancer; people with breast carcinoma are living considerably longer.

Box 38–1

The Leading Causes of Cancer Death in the United States, 1997

Male
1. Lung carcinoma
2. Prostate carcinoma
3. Colon and rectal carcinoma

Female
1. Lung carcinoma
2. Breast carcinoma
3. Colon and rectal carcinoma

Other leading causes of cancer death include pancreas, stomach, and esophagus in males and ovary, pancreas, and stomach in females.

The recognition that breast cancer is a treatable disease has set the stage for numerous clinical trials utilizing various forms of treatment.

PRESENTATION AND DISTINGUISHING FACTORS

The median survival of patients with metastatic breast cancer is more than 2 years.[3] As many as 10% of those who have metastatic disease live more than a decade. During this long interval, symptoms arise that result in functional disability. Thus, many geriatric individuals with breast cancer have problems related both to the disease process and to its treatment.

Breast cancer in the geriatric patient does not differ greatly from that found in younger individuals. It is common for clinicians to encounter patients with long-standing, indolent disease. There is not much difference, for example, in the detection and patterns of spread of breast cancer when older and younger groups are compared. Women 70 years of age or older who were enrolled in clinical trials were similar to their younger counterparts in terms of response rates, time interval to disease progression, survival, and effects of chemotherapy.[4]

The fact is that many elderly patients with breast cancer suffer from intercurrent diseases that not only significantly reduce their life expectancy but also increase their operative risk. Despite a high percentage of deaths from concomitant diseases, long-term survival of elderly breast cancer patients is possible and is comparable to the rate of survival found in the general population of those with breast cancer.[5]

CLINICAL RELEVANCE

The clinical relevance of breast cancer to the rehabilitation professional stretches across the disease process from detection and primary treatment and through a long period of metastatic disease, culminating in involvement with terminal patient care. Although some forms of breast cancer may be treated with simple lumpectomy followed by radiation therapy, the modified radical mastectomy is the mainstay of breast cancer surgery today, and for more than two decades has replaced the standard Halstead radical technique. In the former, the breast and axillary lymphatics are removed, but the pectoralis major and minor are preserved. Surgical drains are present after the procedure for a day or two, and aggressive movement is not indicated during this time. Even with the less extensive pectoral-sparing procedure, loss of glenohumeral flexion and abduction are the usual temporary sequalae.

More extensive disease, such as attachment to the chest wall muscles will, of necessity, require a more extensive surgical procedure to manifest a definitive cure. At times, the pectoralis major and minor, although not surgically removed, are displaced and mobilized to obtain a good surgical field, and the resultant postoperative soreness inhibits movement for varying lengths of time after surgery. Much attention was paid in the past to limitation of internal rotation, which interfered with activities such as bathing and hooking a bra behind the back. This appears to be less of a problem than formerly thought; actually, limitation of external rotation is seen more often but typically resolves before glenohumeral flexion and abduction return to normal. This observation tends to be true for both older and younger patients.

The functional disabilities following mastectomy are usually transient and respond favorably to physical therapy intervention. Elderly patients who do not gain their full range of motion within 6 to 8 weeks after surgery are not likely to do so. The reasons for this are not entirely clear; a sedentary patient combined with a nonaggressive therapist may be contributory. The window of opportunity to avoid loss of range and function is not a large one, and an aggressive approach with these patients during the second month after surgery is warranted in otherwise healthy individuals.

Edema of the ipsilateral arm occurs in a significant percentage of postmastectomy cases.[6] The incidence of this complication of mastectomy has declined considerably over the past two decades, owing to early detection, improved radiation therapy and surgical techniques, and early and comprehensive management to effect control. In some cases, edema can be severe and can result in a grossly enlarged upper extremity with resultant loss of range and function. This is usually largely preventable with active rehabilitation intervention.

Metastases

Few cancers can match carcinoma of the breast regarding metastatic patterns; the disease spreads both lymphatically and hematogenously, the latter process actually occurring long before the primary is detected and the surgery performed. The skeleton is the most common site of blood-borne spread, and lesions favor the axial skeleton because of Batson's vertebral plexus of veins. The pelvis, spine, rib, upper femora, upper humeri, and scapulae are most commonly involved; lesions are usually lytic, but blastic-predominating and mixed patterns may occur. Large lytic lesions carry the great risk of pathological fracture. Unfortunately, these usually happen over weight-bearing areas such as the proximal femur. In bone metastases, pain typically heralds positive radiographs, but occasionally pain may be severe in the absence of both radiographic evidence of the disease and scan negativity.

Occasionally axillary metastases and local recurrence in the chest wall produce troubling edema and complex wound-care problems. More common are metastases to other organs, following or concomitant with the bony lesions that are most often the first sign of metastatic carcinoma. The liver, pleura, lungs, central nervous system, and intra-abdominal area can all be involved, each area producing its particular family of symptoms. Liver metastases produce fatigue, early caffeine intolerance, anorexia, metabolic disturbances, and weakness, most of which are rehabilitative problems. Pleural effusions are painful, debilitating, and require frequent thoracentesis and, at times, chest tubes, which limit mobility and function. Lung metastases are of several types. Parenchymal rounded areas that eventually coalesce occur but do not affect symptomatology until a sufficient amount of lung tissue has been compromised. Lymphangitic metastases, on the other hand, in which the tumors are within the lymphatics of the lung, cause an early and distressing pulmonary syndrome of cough, dyspnea, and intense sputum production. Metastases to the brain cause symptoms and signs comparable to primary brain tumors, which are addressed in Chapter 37.

Metastatic breast carcinoma, after lung carcinoma, is the second leading cause of epidural spinal cord compression, a medical emergency. Sudden or subacute onset of sensory disturbances and motor weakness of the lower extremities in a metastatic breast cancer patient with known spinal disease warrants prompt attention. The pattern and degree of weakness may well fluctuate with treatment and may improve, unlike traumatic spinal cord injury. This presents a dynamic and changing clinical picture to the health-care practitioner. Metastasis of any type debilitates the patient; pain may be one of the major limiting factors in any rehabilitative efforts. Adequate pain control is tantamount to successful rehabilitative intervention.

From the foregoing, it can be seen that breast cancer is a complex disease process that raises a multiplicity of rehabilitative issues for the clinician. Because patients are living longer with treatable metastatic disease, these issues will continue to pose unique and challenging clinical problems to the clinicians who confront them.

THERAPEUTIC INTERVENTION

The therapeutic treatment and rehabilitative intervention for breast cancer is comprehensive and ongoing throughout the disease process. Preoperative physical therapy screening is a sound clinical practice, as the information imparted can do much to allay fears and establish a good clinical rapport with the patient; the common existence of a premorbid functional loss of range of motion in the shoulder on the operated side underscores the value of preoperative intervention. If the patient cannot be seen preoperatively, a physical therapy visit the day after surgery is desirable. After a modified radical mastectomy procedure, often accompanied by an axillary node dissection, glenohumeral flexion and abduction should be limited to 90 degrees until the surgical drains have been removed. One should proceed gently with other shoulder movements such as extension and external rotation. Because the hospital stay of these patients, even of the elderly without complications, is very short, early and consistent intervention ensures optimal functional and physical return.

Rehabilitation

A scoliotic curvature is common in elderly women and thus should be a consideration when treating a postmastectomy patient. Positioning, range of motion and strengthening exercise of the trunk chest wall movement, and breathing exercises may offset the potential effects of the curvature that result from both the surgery and the weight imbalance after mastectomy.

Various exercises are used to regain range of motion and function in the shoulder; no single program has proven superior to another in terms of functional result. Most regimens call for gradual stretching of the pectoralis major muscle; pulley exercises and wall climbing are often used. Emphasis on external rotation, slowly bringing the clasped hands behind the head, is another standard approach. Early monitoring for lymphedema is important, and the fitting of elastic compression garments has become a large part of the care of these individuals. If intermittent compression with a pneumatic device is necessary, a sequential pump should be entertained, as graded application of the pneumatic pressure is more efficacious. Manual lymph drainage performed by specially trained therapists and followed by wrapping with a specific-pressure elastic material has gained favor in clinical practice as an approach to lymphedema management. It is to be hoped that research comparing manual techniques with pneumatic compression is forthcoming; it should shed light on treatment decision-making. Perhaps even more important is lymphedema prevention through patient and family education.

Older breast cancer patients tend to have more bony and soft-tissue disease than younger counterparts, and sometimes an indolent clinical course occurs in which bony metastases predominate.[7] Even in an elderly woman with extensive bony lesions, the lesions may be asymptomatic. Pain may be worsened by activity, particularly weight-bearing. If a patient experiences a pathological fracture and is treated surgically or has the procedure performed prophylactically, aggressive rehabilitative therapy is warranted as soon as the patient can tolerate it. Internal fixation of the femur facilitates nursing care, potentiates ambulatory ability, and makes transportation of the patient easier; ease in handling the patient facilitates radiotherapy treatments. The health-care providers and surgeons should realize that early mobilization, cautious early weight-bearing, and graduated exercises should be employed to ensure maximal functional outcome. Strength and range of motion can be restored, and the complications of being bedridden can be avoided.

Orthotic devices to relieve weight-bearing may be tried, but extensive bracing should be avoided in a moribund patient except when used for pain control. Thoracolumbar stabilization with an orthotic device may be required if the spine is heavily involved with tumor. Patients with liver metastases have poor exercise tolerance and this must be respected, weighing the pitfalls faced with immobility. Pleural effusions and lung metastases respond to physical therapy techniques when pulmonary symptoms require intervention. Epidural spinal cord compression is approached assertively, with all rehabilitation techniques pertinent to traumatic spinal cord injury being applicable. The often changing weakness picture and the common and sometimes dramatic motor return that can take place merit intense rehabilitation efforts. Finally, supportive and palliative care for terminally ill geriatric breast cancer patients is integral to total patient care and is most appreciated by those patients who need it.

CONCLUSION

Breast cancer rehabilitation in the elderly patient begins at diagnosis, continues through the early postsurgical phase, and is both reactive and active. As metastases spread and cause specific symptoms and disabilities, rehabilitation again plays a major role in preventing immobility. Palliative and comfort care round out the intervention, and with patients living for an appreciably longer time, the period of rehabilitative care may span decades. Breast cancer is a treatable disease, and rehabilitation is an integral part of this treatment.

REFERENCES

1. Landis SH, Murray T, Bolden S, Wingo P. Cancer Statistics, 1998. *CA Cancer J Clin* 1998; 48:6–30.
2. Harris JR, Lippman ME, Veronsesi U, Willet W. Breast cancer. *N Engl J Med* 1992; 327:319.
3. Clark GM, Sledge GW, Osborne CK, McGuire WL. Survival from first recurrence: relative importance of prognostic factors in 1015 breast cancer patients. *J Clin Oncol* 1987; 5:55.
4. Christman K, Muss HB, Case LD, Stanely V. Chemotherapy of metastatic breast cancer in the elderly. The Piedmont Oncology Association experience. *JAMA* 1992; 268:96.
5. Hunt EL, Fry DE, Bland KL. Breast carcinoma in the elderly patient: an assessment of operative risk, morbidity, and mortality. *Am J Surg* 1980; 140:339.
6. Dietz JH. Rehabilitation of the cancer patient. *Med Clin North Am* 1969; 53:607.
7. Ratner LH. Management of cancer in the elderly. *Mt Sanai J Med* 1980; 47:224.

Chapter 39

Gastric and Colon Neoplasms

Stephen A. Gudas, Ph.D., P.T.

INTRODUCTION

Gastric carcinoma was the number one cause of cancer mortality up until about 1940. Despite the fact that the treatment and overall survival of patients with gastric cancer has not changed appreciably in the past 50 years, mortality from stomach cancer has been decreasing during the same period.[1] These figures are from the United States; in other areas of the world, stomach cancer is the most common form of the disease. Ongoing studies are attempting to delineate the purported dietary factors that are believed to play a major role in the geographic differences in incidence. Changes in the methods of food preparation and the increased use of vitamin C are believed to be partly responsible. In 1998, there were an estimated 23,000 new cases of stomach cancer in the United States, with approximately 14,000 deaths.[2] Stomach cancer is the third most common gastrointestinal neoplasm, after colorectal cancer and pancreatic cancer. There is a male: female ratio of 1.7:1, so it is a disease of men rather than of women—actually, of older men, as the peak incidence is in people between 50 and 70 years of age.

PRESENTATION AND DISTINGUISHING FACTORS

Atrophic gastritis seems to be more common in countries that have a high incidence of gastric cancer, an association explained only in part by the natural progression of a dysplasia or inflammatory process to frank cancer. Similarly, there is a slight increase in incidence in those who have undergone a partial gastric resection for peptic ulcer disease. The stimulus for this pathological chain of events has not been clearly defined. Nitrosamines can produce carcinoma in the stomach, at least in the experimental animal, but the synthesis of these compounds is blocked by normal stomach acid. This, however, may explain the increased incidence of gastric carcinoma in those individuals with pernicious anemia and the accompanying achlorhydria.

Colon Cancer

Colon cancer is the third leading cause of cancer death for both men and women in the United States, with approximately 130,000 new cases per year, resulting in 60,000 deaths[2] (see Box 38–1). This number is surpassed only by lung cancer and breast cancer in females and by lung cancer and prostate cancer in males. The average age at diagnosis is between 60 and 70 years.[3] The 5-year survival rate for colorectal cancer is about 45%, and that figure has remained stable for the past 3 decades. There has been a trend toward finding more proximal bowel tumors that is only partly the result of increased access to the proximal bowel by means of colonoscopy procedures.

Several known predisposing conditions for colon cancer exist, the most common of which are ulcerative colitis and familial polyposis. In the former, duration of disease is as important a factor as severity of symptoms. Fortunately for patients with a predisposition to colon cancer, the removal of the colon and rectal mucosa while preserving sphincter function has been a rather remarkable clinical advance of recent years. Prevention has advanced, too. Likewise, in familial polyposis, which is inherited as an autosomal dominant gene, patients who do not have the large intestine mucosa removed will more or less uniformly undergo malignant transformation of one of their multiple polyps. Notwithstanding the benefit of prophylactic surgery for these select patients, the vast majority of colon cancer patients are "sporadic."[4] However, in the future, partly because of major breakthroughs in the molecular biology of colon adenocarcinoma (the most common histological type), medical genetics will perhaps define an additional population of individuals with premalignant colon phenotypes to whom model systems of genetics and screening can be applied, thus finding at an earlier stage the polyps that are believed to be precursors of colon cancer.

CLINICAL RELEVANCE

Gastric Cancer

Gastric cancer usually arises from the distal portions of the lesser curvature of the stomach, but there seems to be an increasing trend toward more proximal origin.[5] Gastric cancer originates in the mucosa or submucosa of the stomach, but by the time of diagnosis, in the United States, it has penetrated the muscular layers of the gastric wall and can commonly be seen on the outer serosal surface of the stomach when the patient is in surgery. It is common for the tumor to invade anatomical structures contiguous to the stomach, which results in involvement of the pancreas and the transverse mesocolon in particular. Gastric cancers also spread across the peritoneal surface of the abdominal cavity, making survival less certain, as ascites, peritoneal implanting, or "caking," as well as frank abdominal carcinomatosis all portend serious prognoses. In almost two thirds of patients, gastric cancer will have spread to the abdominal lymphatics by the time it is surgically explored, with the lymph nodes adjacent to the primary tumor usually involved first. The rich mixture of lymphatic, nerve, and vascular tissues in the abdominal area affords the tumor abundant opportunity to spread. After the regional lymphatics on the greater and lesser curvature are involved, then the lymphatics along the hepatic and splenic vessels become infiltrated.

Hematogenous dissemination of gastric cancer occurs late in the course of the disease, usually to the liver via the portal vein, but other distant sites may be involved. Spread may be asymptomatic; whereas 25% of patients at autopsy show lung metastases, they are uncommonly detected clinically prior to death. This is because of the silent nature of parenchymal lung metastases and because the late clinical course is marked by other, more pressing issues.

Clinically, gastric carcinoma commonly presents with vague epigastric discomfort, postprandial pain, or early satiety in eating. Because these somewhat nonspecific symptoms may be attributed to simple gastritis or dietary indiscretion, the patient may delay seeking medical attention. Anemia, weakness, and weight loss may all occur, alerting the patient to a more serious source of the abdominal discomfort. Physical examination of the patient is often unrevealing, except when advanced disease is present. A palpable tumor in the upper abdomen is not a common presentation, but when it does occur it is usually a poor prognostic sign. A thorough workup is indicated for any individual who exhibits persistent symptomatology. An upper GI endoscopy accompanied by biopsy of the suspected lesion will provide the diagnosis in over 95% of cases. Endoscopic ultrasound evaluation is a relatively new technique that shows some promise because it enables the clinician to visualize all walls of the stomach.

Colon Cancer

Colon cancer spreads through the bowel wall, and the TNM classification (tumor, node, metastases, each graded as to size and number) has begun to replace the old Duke's ABC terminology (related to size and depth of bowel invasion). In classic colon or rectal carcinoma, spread occurs sequentially from the bowel wall into pericolonic or rectal mesentery and its nodes, then into regional nodes, and then into venous channels where blood-borne dissemination occurs. The route of distant metastasis is usually the liver, because of the portal vein, but the lungs, the bone, and even the brain may be involved. Direct extension of a rectal or low colonic tumor into the sacral area and eventual involvement of the lumbosacral plexus sometimes occurs, causing varying syndromes of plexopathy or nerve compression. Tumor compression neuropathies are usually a late event in the progression of colon cancer. Recently, it has become apparent that, in addition to the carcinoembryonic antigen (CEA) that is commonly followed in these patients, there may be other markers present in the marrow that determine metastatic proclivity to certain distant sites. With this knowledge, selected patients may be followed more closely for distant spread.

Diagnosis of colon cancer is difficult despite more widespread use of the digital exam and sigmoidoscopy. One of the reasons is that the presenting symptoms depend on the site of the tumor. Circumferential tumors ("apple-core lesions") of the lower colon are usually the cause of changes in bowel habits, whereas almost complete obstruction may effect a paradoxical diarrhea. More proximal lesions may cause weakness because of the anemia that occurs as a result of the slow bleeding. Melena (blood in the stool) is a common and sometimes presenting symptom of colon cancer, and the nature of the blood is specific for different regions in the bowel. Frank obstruction is most common in the left colon, where colicky pain is often experienced. In rectal carcinoma, for example, the pain is constant and gnawing in character, and the melena is bright red; there may be tenesmus (painful stool passage). Distant metastases are often to the liver, where hepatic function may be compromised, making the patient weak and moribund. Other sites of metastases produce symptomatology specific to their locations and, sometimes, function.

THERAPEUTIC INTERVENTION IN GASTRIC CANCER

Surgery

In gastric carcinoma, surgery is the only effective method of treatment when cure is a goal, and this approach is utilized for palliation as well. Survival rates remain low for all except those with early carcinoma, which is not commonly diagnosed.[6] All patients except those with obvious distant spread should have exploratory celiotomy in order to find selectively curable patients and those who would benefit from a palliative procedure. Unfortunately, fewer than 40% of patients can be considered potentially curable and of these, many experience recurrence and early, cancer-related death. Distal, proximal, or total gastrectomy may be performed, using various methods and pouches to restore or ensure continuity of the alimentary tract. Resection of adjacent organs may be performed, but that makes cure less likely. Careful abdominal exploration at the time of surgery is necessary not only to avoid unnecessarily radical procedures but also to confirm the diagnosis histologically. For the 60% or so of patients who are not curable, some type of palliative

resection is usually done to relieve symptoms and prolong survival.

Since the usual reason for palliation is anatomical unresectability, radiation therapy is not often employed when surgery has failed. Some surgeons are trying intraoperative radiation therapy, but the results are inconclusive, and trials are pending. External beam radiation therapy postsurgery may be used in selected cases to relieve obstruction or control bleeding, but it is not commonly employed. Many chemotherapeutic trials of various drugs have been tried over the years; most regimens include 5-fluorouracil (5-FU). Because surgery alone is a disappointing method of treatment, there is interest in aggressive clinical trials employing adjuvant combination chemotherapy. The overall survival rate is only 10 to 15% when all gastric adenocarcinomas are included, so further trials are clearly indicated.

Rehabilitation

The gastric cancer patient needs rehabilitation postsurgically, when assistance in mobilization and ambulation is mandatory to avoid complications and to get the alimentary tract functioning again. Older patients should be moved out of bed gently but firmly on the first postoperative day, barring serious complications. Mild exercise programs are helpful in restoring muscle strength and functional mobility.

After recovery from gastrectomy, long-term sequelae are more important that short-term ones. The former include the "dumping syndrome" in which gastric transit is greatly accelerated owing to the loss of the normal pyloric function of adjusting food entry into the duodenum. This can usually be controlled by diet and the common employment of gastric reservoirs during surgery. Anemia and its accompanying weakness may occur if there is impairment of iron absorption or loss of the intrinsic factor when large portions of the stomach have been removed. Metastatic disease is managed in the same ways as metastatic disease arising from other tumors.

THERAPEUTIC INTERVENTION IN COLON CANCER

Surgery

Colon cancer is usually treated surgically, with the creation of a colostomy after the distal colon and rectum are resected. More proximal tumors may allow end-to-end colonic anastomosis, a less radical procedure that causes much less dysfunction. During surgery, the entire tumor is removed; the analysis of depth of invasion through the bowel wall is made; analysis of the lymphatic drainage is performed; and surgical evaluation, often now through intraoperative ultrasonography, of the adjacent and noncontiguous abdominal organs is made. The amount of bowel removed depends on the tumor but also on its location, as blood vessels must be respected, and definitive procedures for various areas have been outlined for some time. The major limiting factor in utilizing procedures less extensive than an abdominal peritoneal resection for low rectal cancer is the lack of adequate preoperative staging techniques. The ability to define microscopic lymphatic spread prior to or even during surgery is negligible and contributes to the overall failure rate of surgical intervention. Approaches to sphincter preservation, in particular, should not sacrifice curative surgical principles. All in all, elderly patients seem to tolerate the necessary surgery well, and chronological age alone is not a deterrent to surgery.[7]

Rehabilitation

The creation of a temporary or permanent colostomy or ileostomy engenders loss of voluntary control of bowel function. Ostomy rehabilitation is a specialty now, and enterostomal therapists, nurses with formal training, are used to handle the many problems that ensue. The diversification of collection devices, skin adhesives, and related appliances has been remarkable over the past few decades. A regular elimination schedule, skin protection, and edor control are a few of the many issues addressed in the postoperative care of these patients. Like gastric cancer patients, the postop colon cancer patient needs gentle but persuasive out-of-bed mobilization, and exercise when necessary. Health-care practitioners also must keep in mind special problems of the elderly patient. Liver metastases are so common in colon cancer that the health-care worker involved with these patients must be alert to the decreased exercise tolerance, generalized weakness, and cachexia that may occur. Even the patient with widespread metastases from colon cancer could benefit from a therapeutic program that emphasizes exercise, ambulation, and pain control.

Radiation Therapy and Chemotherapy

The use of radiation therapy and chemotherapy in colon cancer has seen many clinical trials. It has been shown that concurrent or subsequent radiation therapy and chemotherapy have afforded a survival advantage, and additional trials are under way. The drug 5-FU and folic acid have been used and have consistently elicited improvement, so they warrant further attention. A multidisciplinary team approach is the best method of supporting and rehabilitating the patient. It is of interest that fewer than 10% of cases are unresectable at surgery, and nearly 50% of patients will be alive and free of disease 5 years after therapy. These results are encouraging, and the rate continues to improve.

CONCLUSION

Gastric cancer is no longer the number one cause of cancer mortality in the United States, but it remains a predominant cause of death in other areas of the world. Colon cancer is the third leading cause of death in the United States, and the 5-year survival rate is approximately 45%, a rate that has remained unchanged for the past 30 years. Both gastric and colon cancer are treated surgically. Rehabilitation is important in order to regain functional mobility and ambulation. Gentle therapeutic exercise is needed to restore muscle strength. Both gastric and colon cancer may metastasize to the liver, which may contribute to weakness, fatigue, and cachexia.

REFERENCES

1. Correa P. A human model of gastric carcinogenesis. *Cancer Res* 1988; 48:3554.
2. Parker SL, Long T, Bolden S, Wingo PA. Cancer statistics, 1997. *CA Cancer J Clin* 1997; 65:5.
3. Bader JF. colorectal cancer in patients older than 75 years of age. *Dis Colon Rectum* 1986; 29:728.
4. Vogelstein B, Fearon ER, Hamilton SR, et al. Genetic alterations during colo-rectal tumor development. *N Engl J Med* 1988; 319:525.
5. Meyers WC, Damiano RJ, Postlethwait RW, Rotlo F. Adenocarcinoma of the stomach: changing patterns over the last four decades. *Ann Surg* 1987; 205:1.
6. Itoh H, Oohata Y, Nakamura K. Complete 10-year postgastrectomy follow-up of early gastric cancer. *Am J Surg* 1989; 158:14.
7. Gingold BS. Local treatment for carcinoma of the rectum in the elderly. *J Am Geriatr Soc* 1981; 29:10.

Chapter **40**

Neoplasms of the Skin
Stephen A. Gudas, Ph.D., P.T.

INTRODUCTION

Skin cancer is one of the most common forms of cancer in human beings.[1] It accounts for almost one quarter of all cancers diagnosed in the United States.[2] The most common forms of skin cancer are basal cell carcinoma, squamous cell carcinoma, and malignant melanoma. Other, rarer types also occur, and the skin can be the site of metastatic tumors, as well. Each of the three most common types are discussed in turn regarding incidence, clinical relevance, and therapeutic intervention.

PRESENTATION AND DISTINGUISHING FACTORS

Basal Cell Carcinoma

Basal cell carcinoma (BCC), the most commonly occurring of the three main types of skin cancer, occurs primarily on sun-exposed skin surfaces, specifically on areas of skin exposed to ultraviolet (UV) light. Although historically this disease affected more men than women, there is currently only a slight preponderance of males affected by it. Traditionally a disease of older persons, it is becoming more common in younger individuals; some cases occur during the third decade of life. Increased sun exposure, as culturally defined, and a depletion of the protective ozone layer in the Earth's atmosphere are both believed to play a role in the etiology of this disease. Cumulative exposure to UV light over many years is necessary for the development of this tumor. Those with outdoor professions or extensive outdoor recreation are at the greatest risk. Ionizing radiation can also be implicated; the resultant basal cell carcinoma occurs after a long latency period and is usually in the area of previous irradiation. The immune system may play a role, but this is less well appreciated in basal cell carcinoma than in squamous cell carcinoma.

Basal cell carcinomas are locally destructive, but they rarely if ever metastasize.[3] Metastases usually occur in head and neck basal cell tumors of long standing. The tumor follows the path of least resistance, so bone, cartilage, and muscle are invaded late in the course of the disease. The primary lesion may vary in size and appearance, but usually is nodular-ulcerative in nature. The margin of the lesion demonstrates a pearly, raised, or rolled border, with reactive telangiectasis and central necrosis. A superficial multicentric variant can occur, more commonly on the trunk and extremities than on the head and neck, the latter being the most frequent sites of BCC.

Squamous Cell Carcinoma

Squamous cell carcinoma (SCC) of the skin is a tumor of the keratinizing cells of the epidermis, and its behavior is like that of squamous cell carcinoma arising elsewhere in the body. Unlike BCC, SCC has a propensity to metastasize to regional lymph nodes and distant sites. It is second in occurrence only to BCC, and the risk of occurrence increases dramatically with increasing age.[4] The mean ages for SCC are 68.1 and 72.7 years for men and women, respectively, and very few cases occur before the age of 40. The factors that initiate and promote SCC are the same as those for BCC; both are related to sun exposure, and light-skinned, poorly tanning individuals are at the greatest risk. Other predisposing factors are chemical carcinogens and exposure to ionizing radiation; the list of the former is increasing in length.

The metastatic potential of SCC is determined by tumor size and location, the extent of cellular differentiation, whether it is mucocutaneous or purely cutaneous, and a host of other factors. SCC tumors may present in a variety of ways, usually as a plaque-like lesion that is raised and erythematous. SCC lacks the pearly raised border and telangiectasia of BCC.

Malignant Melanoma

Malignant melanoma develops from the malignant transformation of the melanocyte, a cell of neural crest origin that produces melanin pigment. It is surprising that the disease is not more common, considering that most individuals have numerous pigmented moles or other lesions. Melanoma accounts for 3% of all cancers and is increasing, mainly as a result of increased sun exposure. In the past 30 years, survival has increased from 60 to 84% partly because of new methods of treatment but, more importantly, because of new methods of detection.[4] Melanoma appears as a change in an existing mole, with rapid growth, bleeding, or change in color noted. However, the lesion can arise de novo; the increased incidence has caused some public concern for all pigmented nevi.

Four patterns of melanoma are seen: superficial spreading melanoma, nodular melanoma, lentigo melanoma, and acral lentigo melanoma. The nodular type has the worst prognosis, owing to great depth of invasion. Pathological staging of melanoma is based on microscopic assessment of thickness and level of invasion, the latter evaluated as Clark's level I to IV.[5] Melanoma does not kill by local extension but by distant metastases. No other human tumor possesses the metastatic potential and virulence of an aggressive melanoma. Virtually any organ of the body can be involved, but the regional lymph nodes are usually involved first. Distant sites are the brain, lung, and bone. Prognostic factors are multiple and variable and depend on stage of the disease. Tumor thickness is the most important and dominant variable; other factors include site, sex, age of patient, ulceration, number of nodes involved, and length of disease. Melanomas can metastasize years after the primary lesion has been treated, a fact not often appreciated among health-care practitioners.

THERAPEUTIC INTERVENTION

Surgery and Radiation Therapy

Basal cell carcinomas and squamous cell carcinomas are treated primarily by surgery or radiotherapy. Curretage and electrodissection are commonly used for small tumors, with total surgical excision saved for the larger lesions. Mohs micrographic technique, a method employed for large and stubborn BCCs, has enjoyed some popularity as it allows maximum conservation of normal tissues. Wide surgical margins are necessary; the fact that BCC and SCC can spread deeply into tissue must be respected and recognized in surgical treatment procedures. Alternative removal methods include lasers, cryosurgery, and radiation therapy, the latter paradoxical as a method of treatment as it can also induce the development of cancer. Radiation therapy is best used for small lesions or in patients that cannot or will not tolerate a surgical procedure.

Both SCC and BCC can be treated with these methods, but the propensity for SCC to metastasize must be considered. All therapies are designed to effect total tumor removal, always the primary goal in treating these cancers. Recurrence rates are high in certain areas and with certain histological variants, and may call for more extensive surgery or an alternative technique. Many older individuals can be freed from tumors with the procedures described above. Follow-up visits are essential to promptly diagnose recurrence or new primaries, for which the patient is at risk.

Malignant melanoma demands some special considerations regarding treatment, as regional lymph node involvement may be high and subclinical, and the high metastatic potential of these tumors must be taken into account in treatment planning. A therapeutic node dissection is employed in stage III carcinomas (large and/or deep primary lesions), whether or not the nodes are involved clinically. Specific guidelines have been established for the accepted surgical margin, depending on the thickness and size of the lesion. Patients with enlarged regional nodes have a greater than 85% chance of having distant hematogenous metastases, and their survival rate at 10 years is less than 10%. This does not mean that palliative surgery cannot be used for stage IV patients (distant spread already present at diagnosis), as it is common practiced to remove surgically accessible lesions and it may palliate the patient significantly.

Chemotherapy

The response rates of metastatic melanoma patients to combination chemotherapy is encouraging, and many trials are under way. Immunotherapy and gene therapy have been studied and tried more often in malignant melanoma than in other tumors, with varying degrees of response and success. All of these approaches are still experimental in that they provide palliation and relief of distressing symptoms, but cures are few once the disease has metastasized to distant areas. That principle drives the intense research that is currently being performed.

Basal cell and squamous cell carcinomas are treated with chemotherapy and other methods when disease is unresectable, or there are local or distant metastases. Health-care practitioners can do much to assist the patient in planning treatment and in decision-making. It is important to note that because of the lesions' common location on the head and neck, and the sometimes cosmetically disfiguring surgery that is required, psychosocial intervention is important to total patient care.

Rehabilitation

Noncomplicated surgical removal rarely requires rehabilitation intervention except when function is involved or the surgery is extensive and normal function is compromised. However, caution should be used when applying heat or electrical modalities to areas of previous surgery or to areas where extensive pigmented or raised nevi are present. Exercise and manual techniques should be applied judiciously also. The surgical site should be examined carefully.

CONCLUSION

Like lung cancer, skin cancer is largely preventable. Health-care practitioners should assist in efforts to educate the public to limit sun exposure and reduce exposure to chemical carcinogens that can cause skin tumors.

REFERENCES

1. Betchel MA, Cullen JP, Owen LG. Etiological agents in the development of skin cancer. *Clin Plast Surg* 1980; 7:265.
2. Miller SJ. Biology of basal cell carcinoma. *J Am Acad Dermatol* 1991; 24:1.
3. Von Domarus H, Stevens PJ. Metastatic basal cell carcinoma: report of five cases, and review of 170 cases in the literature. *J Am Acad Dermatol* 1984; 10:1043.
4. Koh HK. Cutaneous melanoma. *N Engl J Med* 1991; 325:171.
5. Clark WH, From L, Bernerdino EA, Mihm MC. The histogenesis and behavior of primary human malignant melanomas of the skin. *Cancer Res* 1969; 29:705.

Chapter **41**

Neoplasms of the Prostate

Stephen A. Gudas, Ph.D., P.T.

INTRODUCTION

Prostate cancer is the most common male cancer that occurs in the United States, accounting for approximately 32% of all cancers newly diagnosed in males. It is also the second leading cause of cancer death in men, accounting for 13% of all male cancer deaths. The median age of onset is 70, making it a geriatric problem; the incidence increases each decade after the age of 50. It is estimated that in 1998 there were 335,000 new cases of prostate carcinoma diagnosed in the United States, and 42,000 deaths.[1] It is a curious fact that the incidence of histological prostate cancer at autopsy increases with advancing age, from 5 to 14% in the fifth decade to 40 to 80% in the ninth decade.[2] This is quite constant across cultures and countries, but the incidence of frank prostatic cancer is low in Japan, for example. With the aging of the U.S. population, it is expected that the incidence of prostate cancer will continue to increase.

Although the exact etiology of prostate cancer is unknown, there appears to be a hormonal relationship, as many tumors respond to orchiectomy, implying that testosterone augments cancer growth in males. The precise factors that facilitate or enhance the gradual, if not multistep, transition of a benign epithelial cell to adenocarcinoma are unknown. Cancer of the prostate has been found to occur at a disproportionately higher rate in certain industrial workers—tire and rubber manufacturing workers, sheet metal workers, and those who work with cadmium.[3] The exact reasons for the increased incidence of and mortality from prostate cancer in these individuals is unknown. Familial factors may also play a role, although these too are not fully explained.

PRESENTATION AND DISTINGUISHING FACTORS

Almost 60% of prostate cancer patients have clinically localized cancer at diagnosis, making cure a real possibility. The ones with resectable tumors are usually asymptomatic or have few symptoms of urinary tract obstruction. In the absence of infection, marked bladder symptoms should warrant a search for prostate cancer. If the clinical presentation is advanced, there are symptoms of bladder outlet obstruction and anuria, uremia, anemia, and anorexia will ensue. Patients are very ill at that point and most will have sought medical attention.

The digital rectal exam still finds most primary prostate cancerous tumors; approximately 50% of palpable nodules in the prostate are proven to be carcinoma. The PSA, or prostate-specific antigen, is a prostate marker that is useful in the early detection of prostate cancer. If the level is above 10 ng/mL, there is a 66% chance that the biopsy will be positive.[4] However, the use of the PSA as a screening tool for the general geriatric male population is still in question; PSA levels are determined after a nodule is palpated on digital examination. A baseline PSA should be taken in males after age 50 and repeated at intervals. Because early detection of prostate cancer is just now becoming a reality, it will be many years before the impact of this detection ability upon the natural history of and survival with prostate cancer is known. Further investigation is required to determine the true value of screening and of clinical staging procedures. Prostatic acid phosphatase (PAP) is used to detect metastatic disease, as elevated levels signify spread at least as far as the lymph nodes.

Metastases

Prostate carcinoma, like breast and lung cancer, spreads both lymphatically and hematogenously. The regional lymphatics are involved in over 60% of cases. Most patients with prostate carcinoma who die of their disease do so with relatively successful local tumor control. Metastatic disease develops in the vast majority of fatal cases, and the favored site is the skeletal system. Like tumors of the chest or chest wall, Batson's vertebral plexus of veins is causative, and the axial skeleton is preferred. Fully 70% of men with prostate cancer develop bony metastases, commonly to the sacrum, pelvis, lumbar spine, and femurs.[5] The osseous lesions may portend considerable pain and disability, making management of these patients a challenging clinical problem. For reasons not entirely clear, the bony metastases tend to be osteoblastic rather than osteolytic and, occasionally, mixed patterns are seen. For this reason, pathological fracture because of metastatic lesions is seen much less frequently in prostate carcinoma than in women with metastatic breast cancer. Bony pain, however, may be severe and out of proportion to the extent of bone involvement or the number of bones involved.

Other distant organs may be involved, and spinal involvement may lead to epidural spinal cord compression. As in breast and lung cancer, this complication has increased markedly, partly because people with metastatic disease are living longer—long enough with spinal disease to develop the complication. Epidural spinal cord compression is treated the same as compression arising from other tumors (see Chapter 38, "Neoplasms of the Breast"). Patients with widespread metastatic disease from prostate cancer are quite debilitated and appear older than their stated age. The lungs, liver, pleura, and other organs may be involved via the blood stream, but it is the bony metastases that cause the most pain, distress, and dysfunction in these patients. Occasionally, prostate carcinoma can spread beyond the regional pelvic lymph nodes to distant lymphatics, such as lumbar, paraortic, and even higher lymph nodes. Large tumors here can compress organs in close contiguity, effecting symptoms referable to that organ.

THERAPEUTIC CONSIDERATIONS

Although at present there is no cure for patients with extensive bone or visceral metastases, surgery, radiation therapy, hormonal therapy, and chemotherapy have all been used to combat this disease, with varying degrees of success.[6] A radical prostatectomy through the retropubic route is the surgical method of choice; here, the prostate gland, seminal vesicles, and a part of the bladder neck are all removed. At the time of this procedure, pelvic lymph nodes are resected and sampled for tumor. A pelvic lymphadenectomy is not therapeutically curative, but it allows for precise staging, as the pelvic lymph nodes are the first site of metastatic spread in the vast majority of cases. A laparoscopic approach to the pelvic node dissection can be employed in those with suspected node involvement but for whom radical prostatectomy is not an option. A nerve-sparing procedure has been designed in which the capsular and periprostatic nerves are spared, and it has preserved potency in most patients. Impotence was an operative sequela for most patients until the advent of this surgical procedure.[7]

Highly focused modern radiotherapeutic techniques enable a large dose—60 to 70 Gray (one Gy is equal to 100 rads)—to be delivered to the tumor with relatively little morbidity to the patient. Pelvic lymph nodes can be irradiated as well. The major role of radiotherapy, however, is to control bone pain from metastatic disease, and radiation therapy is an extremely effective modality for this purpose. Patients can also undergo a surgical or chemical orchiectomy, with good local and systemic control of disease for varying periods of time. Ambulatory patients survive 1 to 3 years, with good symptom control. A wide variety of chemotherapeutic agents, singly and in combination, have been employed in metastatic prostate carcinoma, but no standard effective chemotherapy regimen exists that is uniformly efficacious.

It appears that both radiation therapy and surgery are equally effective, especially in early disease, but there is no randomized study that compares the two in early-stage adenocarcinoma of the prostate. In cases of large tumors with expected spread, biological recurrences occur in over 90% of patients by the end of 3 years. On occasion, the course is indolent and carries slow decline in function and mobility. Extensive bony lesions eventually lead to general debilitation.

Rehabilitation

In terms of rehabilitation, it is good to remember that patients with prostate carcinoma survive longer than a year or two, and therapeutic intervention designed to maximize function and mobility are standard in patient management. For patients who undergo surgical treatment, it is important to begin gentle exercises and the erect bipedal posture as soon as possible, as postoperative pain encourages hip and trunk flexion that can develop into contractures. Severe spinal involvement may lead to restricted motion and a bedfast condition in which even turning and positioning may require assistance. Most patients are elderly and have concomitant diseases which themselves influence function. Light range-of-motion exercises, ambulation with appropriate assistive devices, usually a walker, can be used and should be encouraged in all patients.

Although bony lesions are usually osteoblastic, lytic lesions and fractures can occur and are treated accordingly. Orthotic devices to stabilize the spine tend not to be tolerated well in the elderly, and the weight and pressure of a brace may actually aggravate symptoms and bone pain. Degenerative joint disease of the spine may complicate the clinical picture. Transcutaneal electric nerve stimulation (TENS) may be used on occasion for pain control, lessening the amount of narcotics needed for effective pain relief.

CONCLUSION

Prostate carcinoma ranks number one in incidence and number two in deaths for males in the United States. With the possibility of diagnosing this illness in its early stages, when confined to the prostate itself and therefore curable by surgery and radiation, many more individuals will be living free of cancer in the future. Prostate carcinoma is one cancer site that should demonstrate an increase in survival rates and length of survival. Health-care practitioners should respond with appropriate intervention to ensure that this trend continues.

REFERENCES

1. Landis SH, Murray T, Bolden S, Wingo PA. Cancer Statistics, 1998. *CA Cancer J Clin* 1998; 48:6–30.
2. Sheldon CA, Williams RD, Fraley EE. Incidental carcinoma of the prostate: review of the literature and reappraisal of classification. *J Urol* 1980; 124:626.
3. Carter BS. Epidemiologic evidence regarding predisposing factors to prostate cancer. *Prostate* 1989; 16:187.
4. Catalona WJ, Smith DS, Ratliff TL, et al. Measurement of prostate-specific antigen in serum as a screening test for prostate cancer. *N Eng J Med* 1991; 324:1156.
5. Forman JD, Order SE, Zinreich ES. Carcinoma of the prostate in the elderly: the therapeutic ratio of definitive radiotherapy. *J Urol* 1986; 136:1238.
6. Barnes RW. Endocrine therapy of prostate carcinoma. *Cancer Detect Prev* 1979; 2:761.
7. Walsh PC, Lepor H. The role of radical prostatectomy in the management of prostatic cancer. *Cancer* 1987; 60[suppl]:526.

Chapter 42

Exercise Considerations for Cardiopulmonary Disease

Pamela Reynolds, M.S., P.T., G.C.S.

INTRODUCTION

The age-related cardiopulmonary changes are described in Chapters 6 and 7. This Chapter presents an overview of exercise considerations for the typical age-related degradations and cardiopulmonary pathologies. These specific conditions and diseases and the appropriate treatments are discussed in Chapters 43 through 49.

When applying therapeutic exercises and mobility techniques to patients with known or unrecognized cardiopulmonary diseases, the availability and easy use of oxygen by the body is a fundamental factor. This is addressed in the Fick equation: $\dot{V}O_2$ = CO $\times$ a-vO_2 difference; $\dot{V}O_2$ represents functional capacity, or the amount of oxygen available for utilization. This can also be described as a person's physical fitness level or functional capacity. The amount of oxygen ($\dot{V}O_2$) the body can obtain and effectively utilize is dependent on two factors: (1) the delivery system, or cardiac output (HR [heart rate] $\times$ SV [stroke volume]), which is also called the central component, and (2) the peripheral factor, or the body's ability to extract and utilize the delivered oxygen (a-vO_2 difference), especially in muscles. Cardiopulmonary dysfunctions are usually the result of impairments in the delivery system. However, the benefits of increased peripheral utilization of oxygen by metabolically active tissues, particularly the muscles, should not be underestimated in rehabilitation considerations. A person with very limited cardiac function, especially left ventricular dysfunction, can make small improvements of 1 to 2 metabolic equivalents (METs) in his or her physical fitness level, or $\dot{V}O_2$. Current research indicates that this improvement is usually due to more efficient utilization of oxygen by the muscles, not improvements in the delivery systems and function of the left ventricle.

EXERCISE CONSIDERATIONS

When developing an exercise program or prescription, it is important to consider the following:

- medical screening or clearance,
- baseline functional capacity,
- mode, intensity, frequency, and duration,
- gradual progression,
- safety,
- motivation, and
- regular reevaluation

Screening

Aging does have some immutable factors that increase a person's risk for exercise. Many disorders do not demonstrate significant clinical signs during regular daily activities, but they may become evident during exercise. Experts at the American College of Sports Medicine (ACSM) state, "Virtually all sedentary individuals can begin a moderate exercise program safely." They define "moderate" in the elderly as 40 to 60% of the person's functional capacity. They also recognize the "potential negative impact of physical activity participation . . . by insisting that all sedentary persons receive medical clearance prior to becoming more active." ACSM recommends medical clearance if a person has one or more major signs or symptoms suggestive of cardiopulmonary disease, or two or more risk factors (see Box 42–1). It is also important to identify the medications a patient is taking. Regular use of cardiovascular drugs, tranquilizers, diuretics, and sedatives can effect physiological response to exercise.

Baseline Functional Capacity

Establishing a baseline functional capacity is an essential beginning for those participating in an exercise program. As the person progresses through an exercise program, comparison of the initial exercise test with subsequent tests provides feedback regarding the individual's success in the program. The test protocol should be chosen based on the

Box 42–1

Symptoms and Signs and Risk Factors of Cardiovascular Disease

SYMPTOMS OR SIGNS SUGGESTIVE OF CARDIOPULMONARY DISEASE

1. Pain, discomfort (or other anginal equivalent) in chest neck, jaw, arm, or other areas that may be ischemic in nature
2. Shortness of breath at rest or with mild exertion
3. Dizziness or syncope
4. Orthopnea or paroxysmal nocturnal dyspnea
5. Ankle edema
6. Palpitations or tachycardia
7. Intermittent claudication
8. Known heart murmur
9. Unusual fatigue or shortness of breath with usual activities

POSITIVE RISK FACTORS FOR CORONARY ARTERY DISEASE

1. Age: Men > 45 and women > 55 years old
2. Family history: myocardial infarction or sudden death in first-degree relative; male before age 55, female before age 65
3. Current cigarette smoking
4. Hypertension: $\geq 140/90$ mmHg
5. Hypercholesterolemia: total serum cholesterol > 200 mg/dL or HDL < 35 mg/dL
6. Diabetes mellitus: IDDM > age 30 or IDDM > 15 years
7. Sedentary lifestyle, physical inactivity: sedentary jobs involving sitting for a large part of the day and no regular exercise

American College of Sports Medicine. *Major Symptoms or Signs Suggestive of Cardiopulmonary Disease and Coronary Artery Disease Risk Factors.* Baltimore: Williams & Wilkins; 1995:17, 18.

person's expected capabilities. Such assessments have been shown to play a significant role in decreasing attrition rates in exercise programs.

Regardless of the specific test, the following protocols are recommended for establishing a baseline functional capacity in deconditioned individuals or patients with cardiovascular or respiratory disease. At a minimum, heart rate, blood pressure, respiratory rate, and, if possible, ECG responses should be recorded at rest, immediately upon completion of test, and until the person regains his or her pretest or resting measures. It is also highly recommended that vital signs be monitored during the stages of the test. The following tests and protocols are suggested:

1. A 6- or 12-minute walk; in addition to exercise response, record distance walked and note any other physical signs and symptoms such as fatigue, sweating, leg cramps, shortness of breath, and so forth.
2. Naughton-Balke or Modified Balke Protocol (Table 42–1).
3. University of Minnesota Cardiopulmonary Fitness Step Test developed by Amundsen et al.; this is another simple test that requires only a bench 8" or 12" in height, a metronome, and a timer. MET level is given for each stage (Table 42–2).

Consideration of Mode, Intensity, Frequency, and Duration

When developing an exercise prescription or training program, careful consideration must be given to mode or type of activity, duration, frequency, and intensity. The information in the following figures and tables may be helpful: metabolic costs of selected treadmill tests (Fig. 42–1) and the Bruce and STEEP treadmill protocols (Fig. 42–2 and Tables 42–3 and 42–4).

Activities can be classified into two groups—continuous or sustained activities and discontinuous or intermittent exercise. Any activity that requires work from large muscle masses for a prolonged period of time elicits an exercise training response from the cardiovascular system. Discontinuous or intermittent exercise activities are often required for those with low functional capacities or any condition that limits performance, such as chronic obstructive lung disease, intermittent claudication, moderate cardiovascular disease, or orthopedic limitations. Cahalin has enumerated criteria necessary prior to initiation of an exercise program for patients with congestive heart failure (Fig. 42–3). Examples of continuous and intermittent walking or exercise protocols are illustrated in Tables 42–5 and 42–6.

Table 42-1 Naughton-Balke and Modified Balke Treadmill Protocols

	Naughton-Balke Treadmill Protocol		
MPH	**% Grade**	**Minutes**	**METs**
3.0	2.5	2	4.3
(constant)	5.0	2	5.4
	7.5	2	6.4
	10.0	2	7.4
	12.5	2	8.4
	15.0	2	9.5
	17.5	2	10.5
	20.0	2	11.6
	22.5	2	12.6

	Modified Balke Treadmill Protocol		
MPH	**% Grade**	**Minutes**	**METs**
2.0	0	3	2.5
2.0	3.5	3	3.5
2.0	7.0	3	4.5
2.0	10.5	3	5.4
2.0	14.0	3	6.4
2.0	17.5	3	7.4
3.0	12.5	3	8.5
3.0	15.0	3	9.5
3.0	17.5	3	10.5
3.0	20.0	3	11.6
3.0	22.5	3	12.6

(*Guidelines for Exercise Testing and Prescription.* American College of Sports Medicine. Philadelphia: Lea & Fabiger; 1991:62)

Table 42-2 University of Minnesota Cardiopulmonary Fitness Step Test

Stage[a]	0 Resting	1	2	3	4	5	Recovery
Resting heart rate							
Resting B/P							
Respiratory rate						Final:	
2 minute heart rate						Final:	
2 minute B/P						Final:	
Other signs and symptoms							
CPM[b] (8″ bench/step)		52	40	60	80	104	
MET level		2	3	4	5	6	
CPM[b] (12″ bench/step)		52	44	72	104	136	
MET level		2	4	6	8	10	

a Each stage is 3 minutes in duration
[b] CPM = counts per minute and is divided by 4 to account for a step up and down with each foot, thus yielding the mounts per minute, for example, 52 counts yield 13 complete mounts per minute.
(Compiled by P. Reynolds, based on Amundsen L, et al., University of Minnesota Step Test.)

METS	1.6	2	3	4	5	6	7	8	9	10	11	12	13	14	15	16
Balke				3.4 miles/hr												
				2	4	6	8	10	12	14	16	18	20	22	24	26
Balke			3.0 miles/hr													
			0	2.5	5	7.5	10	12.5	15	17.5	20	22.5				
Naughton	1.0	2.0 miles/hr														
	0	0	3.5	7	10.5	14	17.5									
METS	1.6	2	3	4	5	6	7	8	9	10	11	12	13	14	15	16
O₂,mL/kg/min	5.6	7		14		21		28		35		42		49		56
Clinical Status	Symptomatic patients / Diseased, recovered / Sedentary healthy / Physically active subjects															
Functional Class	IV	III			II			I and normal								

Figure 42-1 Metabolic cost of selected treadmill test protocols. One metabolic equivalent (MET) signifies resting energy expenditure, equivalent to approximately 3.5 mL of oxygen uptake per kg of body weight per min (mL/kg/min). Unlabeled numbers refer to treadmill speed (top) and percentage grade (bottom). (With permission from Wenger NK, Hellerstein HK. *Rehabilitation of the Coronary Patient*, 3rd ed. New York: Churchill-Livingstone; 1992:150.)

Table 42-3 STEEP Treadmill Protocol

Workload (stage [min])	1	2	3	4	5	6	7	8	9	10	11	12	13	14	15
Speed (mph)	1.5	2.0	2.0	2.0	2.5	2.5	2.5	3.0	3.0	3.0	3.5	3.5	3.5	4.2	5.0
Elevation (%)	0	0	1.5	3	3	5	7	7	9	11	11	13	16	16	16

(From Wenger NK, Hellerstein HK. *Rehabilitation of the Coronary Patient*, 3rd ed. New York: Churchill Livingston; 1992.)

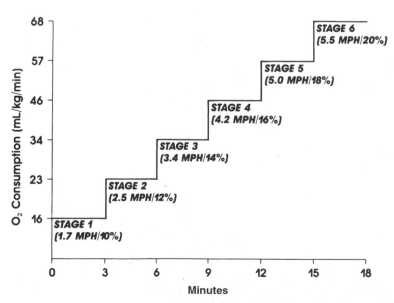

Figure 42-2 The standard Bruce treadmill protocol showing progressive stages (speed, percent grade) and the corresponding aerobic requirement, expressed as mL/kg/min. (With permission from Wenger NK, Hellerstein HK. *Rehabilitation of the Coronary Patient*, 3rd ed. New York: Churchill-Livingstone; 1992:150.)

Table 42–4 STEEP Bicycle Protocol Showing the Workload for Each of the 15 Stages of the Protocol as Determined by the Subject's Body Weight

| Weight | | Work Load (W)[a] at Stage (min) | | | | | | | | | | | | | | |
kg	lb	1	2	3	4	5	6	7	8	9	10	11	12	13	14	15
50	110	15	20	25	30	40	50	60	70	85	95	110	125	145	170	185
55	121	15	20	30	35	45	55	65	80	95	105	125	140	160	185	205
60	132	15	25	30	40	45	60	70	85	100	115	135	150	175	200	225
65	143	20	25	35	40	50	65	80	90	110	125	145	165	190	220	240
70	154	20	25	35	45	55	70	85	100	120	135	155	175	205	235	260
75	165	20	30	40	45	60	75	90	105	125	145	170	190	220	250	280
80	176	25	30	40	50	65	80	95	115	135	155	180	200	235	270	295
85	187	25	35	45	55	65	85	100	120	145	165	190	215	250	285	315
90	198	25	35	45	55	70	90	105	130	150	175	200	225	265	300	335
95	209	25	35	50	60	75	95	115	135	160	180	215	240	280	320	350
100	220	30	40	50	65	80	100	120	140	170	190	225	250	295	335	370

[a] For conversion of watts to kilogram·meters per minute, 1 W = 6.12 kg·m/min.
(From Wenger NK, Hellerstein HK. *Rehabilitation of the Coronary Patient,* 3rd ed. New York: Churchill-Livingstone; 1992.)

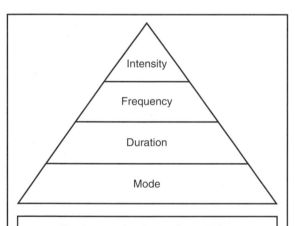

Figure 42–3 The pyramidal structure of exercise training. (From Cahalin LP. Exercise tolerance and training for healthy persons and patients with cardiovascular disease. In: Hasson SM, ed. *Clinical Exercise Physiology.* St. Louis: Mosby-Year Book; 1994:148.)

Table 42–5 Seniors' Walking Exercise Program

Continuous Walking Protocol

1. At the start of the walking program, do not allow the client to walk longer than the time indicated on the test results.
2. To increase the client's motivation and sense of control, have the client choose how often (frequency) he/she will exercise per week.

3. Have the client determine how long he/she would like to walk, and set that as the time goal.
4. Expect progress at a rate of 2 to 5 minutes per week until the time goal has been achieved.

	Time	Frequency (times/week)
Walk	45 to 50 minutes	3
Walk	34 to 38 minutes	4
Walk	27 to 30 minutes	5
Walk	23 to 25 minutes	6
Walk	17 to 19 minutes	8 (or twice a day 4 times week)

Intermittent Walking Protocol

Repeat each walk/rest cycle 3 times. DO NOT progress to the next stage until 3 cycles can comfortably be completed within set exercise tolerance parameters.

Stage	Exercise (minutes)	Rest (minutes)	Total Exercise (minutes)
1	2	1	6
2	3	1	9
3	4	1	12
4	5	1	15
5	6	1	18
6	7	1	21

Recommended frequency: 5 to 7 times per week

(Reynolds P. Seniors' Walking Exercise Program. *Focus on Geriatric Care and Rehabilitation.* 1991; 4:8.)

Duration is inversely proportional to intensity. The lower the intensity, the longer the duration should be. The frequency of exercise for those with low functional capacity should be daily. Individuals with very low endurance may need multiple short sessions per day. Cahalin succinctly summarizes the safe, effective fundamentals of exercise training in his pyramid structure (see Fig. 43–3).

Prescribing the appropriate exercise intensity is the most difficult challenge in designing an exercise program. Because a linear relationship exists between functional capacity ($\dot{V}O_2$) and heart rate, the intensity of exercise is usually prescribed based on a target heart-rate range, which is a percentage of the patient's cardiac reserve. The Karvonen method is recommended for this calculation (see Box 42–2).

Because persons with cardiovascular disease are commonly taking medications such as digoxin or beta-blockers, which blunt the heartrate response to exercise, Borg's Rating of Perceived Exertion (RPE) (Table 42–7) can be used to prescribe intensity. Rating of perceived exertion is a widely used measure that quantifies the subjective sensation of physical exertion. The RPE correlates closely with several measurable variables such as peak $\dot{V}O_2$ and percent of heart-rate reserve, so it can be used to prescribe intensity, especially when a person is taking a medication that alters the cardiopulmonary response to exercise.

The original RPE scale is numbered from 6 to 20. Although the numbering system may appear unusual, it correlates heart rate with a specific number. For instance, the number 11, described as "fairly light" exertion, generally corresponds to a heart rate of 110. An RPE of 11 to 16 associates closely with exercise intensities of 50 to 75% of functional capacity. Numerous studies have demonstrated reproducible results among a wide variety of individuals using this scale. The newer scale, with numbers from 0 to 10, was designed on the premise

Table 42–6 Example of Exercise Progression Using Intermittent Exercise

			A. Functional Capacity (FC) > 3 METs		
Week	**% FC**	**Total Minutes @ % FC**	**Minutes Exercised**	**Minutes Rest**	**Repetitions**
1	50–60	15–20	3–5	3–5	3–4
2	50–60	15–20	7–10	2–3	3
3	60–70	20–30	10–15	Optional	3
4	60–70	30–40	15–20	Optional	2
			B. Functional Capacity (FC) < 3 METs		
Week	**% FC**	**Total Minutes @ % FC**	**Minutes Exercised**	**Minutes Rest**	**Repetitions**
1	40–50	10–15	3–5	3–5	3–4
2	40–50	12–20	5–7	3–5	3
3	50–60	15–25	7–10	3–5	3
4	50–60	20–30	10–15	2–3	2
5	60–70	25–40	12–20	2	2
6	Continue with two repetitions of continuous exercise with one rest period or progress to a single continuous bout				

Note: Functional capacity is determined by Vo_2.
(American College of Sports Medicine. *Guidelines for Exercise Testing and Prescription.* Baltimore: Williams & Wilkins; 1995:186.)

Box 42–2

Calculating Target Heart-Rate Range Utilizing the Karvonen Method

Maximal heart rate	220		
Age	−70		
	150		
Subtract resting heart rate	−60		
Equals heart-rate reserve	90		90
Multiply by % intensity	× .40		× .60
	36.0		54.0
Add back resting heart rate	60		+ 60
Target heart-rate range for 40 to 60%	96 bpm	to	114 bpm

Table 42–7 Borg's Original and Revised Perceived Exertion Scales

Original Scale Category RPE Scale		Revised Scale Category-Ratio Scale	
Value	Description	Value	Description
6		0	Nothing at all
7	Very, very light	0.5	Very, very weak
8		1	Very weak
9	Very light	2	Weak
10		3	Moderate
11	Fairly light	4	Somewhat strong
12		5	Strong
13	Somewhat hard	6	
14		7	Very strong
15	Hard	8	
16		9	
17	Very Hard	10	Very, very strong
18		•	Maximal
19	Very, very hard		
20			

(Borg GA, Psychophysical basis of perceived exertion. *Med Sci Sports Exerc* 1982; 14:377–381. Scales © American College of Sports Medicine.)

Box 42–3

Guidelines for Termination

of an Exercise Session

These signs and symptoms are general indicators of exercise intolerance:

1. Severe breathlessness: able to speak only in two- to three-word sentences

2. Drop in heart rate with an increase in or continuous steady workload: > 10 beats per minute

3. Drop in systolic blood pressure (SBP) while exercising: > 20 mmHg

4. Light-headedness, dizziness, pallor, cyanosis, confusion, ataxia

5. Loss of muscle control or fatigue

6. Onset of angina, tightness, or severe pain in chest, arms, or legs

7. Nausea or vomiting

8. Excessive rise in blood pressure: SBP ≥ 220 mmHg or DBP ≥ 110 mmHg

9. Excessively large rise in heart rate: > 50 bpm increase with low-level activity

10. Severe leg claudication: 8/10 on a 10/10 pain scale

11. ECG abnormalities: ST-segment changes and multifocal PVCs > 30% of complexes

12. Failure of any monitoring equipment

that exercise intensity appears to increase as a power function rather than as a linear progression. It allows for more fine-tuning through subjective responses to small increases in objective exercise intensity. Whatever method is used, it is critical that all involved individuals be educated in its application to ensure that ratings are reliable and consistent.

Progression, Safety, and Reevaluation

Each participant in an exercise program should be taught to monitor himself or herself and should be strongly encouraged to do so. At the least, an individual should know how to monitor pulse and breathing and should also be aware of the signs of exercise intolerance, as enumerated in Box 42–3. The Activity Log provides useful feedback to both the participant and the health professional (Fig. 42–4).

Exercise training requires systematic, progressive increases in exercise activity. As a person progresses in an exercise program, he or she experiences a conditioning, or training, response such as a decrease in heart rate or blood pressure when it is

Activity Log					
Name					
Date					
Time of day					
Heart rate before exercise					
Heart rate after exercise					
Heart rate 5 min after exercise					
Blood pressure before exercise					
Blood pressure after exercise					
Blood pressure 5 min after exercise					
Exercise activity and minutes of activity					
Pain (Y = yes; N = no) If yes, where?					
Fatigue, tiredness					
Weakness					
Sweating (amount?)					
Shortness of breath? How long?					
RPE: Rating of perceived exertion after exercise					
Other comments					

Figure 42–4 Prototype activity log to be used by patients with cardiovascular disease in order to record specific exercise considerations before and after exercising.

measured immediately upon cessation of exercise at the same work level as the previous measurement. When this occurs, the individual is able to increase his or her workload. Currently, a symptom limited approach (see Box 42–3) is used in exercise training and progression for most populations. A decrease in heart rate or blood pressure or both and improved endurance that is observed between preexercise testing and retesting clearly indicates a favorable conditioning response to exercise.

CONCLUSION

Motivating and maintaining exercise participation is difficult. Research has demonstrated a 50% drop-out rate after 6 months from most supervised exercise programs. Exercise approaches that highlight organization and safety but focus primarily on individuals' personal goals have better program compliance. This approach assumes that a participant feels a personal commitment to exercise and considers it an opportunity for self-expression. The goal is to encourage safe progression of exercise activity to the point where it can be performed in an unsupervised environment because it is based on education and enjoyment.

Generally, a person is ready to progress if:

1. Signs of overexertion are not exhibited (see Guidelines for Termination of an Exercise Session (Box 42–3).
2. Pulse rate returns to within 5 beats of resting level within 5 minutes.
3. Breathing returns to preexercise rate and comfort within 10 minutes.

SUGGESTED READINGS

Amundsen L, Ellingham C, Shore S. Cardiopulmonary fitness test. *Cardiopulmon Rec* 1987; 2:13.
Cahalin LP. Heart failure. *Phys Ther* 1996; 76:516–533.
Cronqvist A, Faager G, Larsen F, Schenck-Gustafsson K. Stepwise versus symptom-limited in-hospital mobilisation after acute myocardial infarction. *Physiotherapy Theory and Practice* 1996; 12:67–75.
Francis K. Physical activity in prevention of cardiovascular disease. *Phys Ther* 1996; 76:456–468.
Hillegass E, Sadowsky S. *Essentials of Cardiopulmonary Physical Therapy.* Philadelphia W.B. Saunders; 1994.
McArdle WD, Katch FI, Katch VL. *Essentials of Exercise Physiology.* Philadelphia: Lea & Febiger; 1996.

Chapter 43

Atherosclerosis and Coronary Artery Disease
Joanne Dalgleish, M.D.
Pamela Reynolds, M.S., P.T., G.C.S.

INTRODUCTION

Cardiovascular disease is the leading single cause of death in the United States, accounting for 43% of all deaths. Coronary artery disease (CAD) is atherosclerosis, or the thickening and hardening of the arterial walls, specifically in the cardiac vessels. The general term for this is arteriosclerosis. The underlying pathology in coronary artery disease, aortic aneurysms, and arterial disease in the vessels of the lower limbs and brain is atherosclerosis.

The normal aging process affects the arterial walls in a slow but continuous fashion. The most common feature is symmetrical thickening of the innermost wall (intima), which manifests as increased smooth muscle and connective tissue. The lipid content, which is an accumulation of phospholipids and cholesterol, in the arterial wall also increases with age. These normal age-related intimal changes are diffuse, whereas atherosclerotic disease causes focal raised lesions in addition to the aging process. The normal changes that occur with aging result in a gradually increasing rigidity of the vessel walls. Larger arteries can become dilated, elongated, and tortuous, which lead to the development of aneurysms, especially at areas of bifurcation, at vessel curvatures and at points with little external support. (See Chapter 8 for further information about age-related changes in blood vessels.)

ATHEROSCLEROSIS

Atherosclerosis is a patchy, nodular form of arteriosclerosis. The lesions are distributed irregularly, with the aorta usually becoming involved early and often being the area most severely affected. Lesions are more common in the legs than the arms, the majority of atherosclerotic plaques are found in the larger proximal vessels used such as the femoral and iliac arteries.

Atherosclerosis of the coronary arteries is commonly widespread. The most usual site of plaques is within the main part of each vessel just after it arises from the proximal ascending aorta. However, lesions can be distributed through the branch vessels as well. The degree of lumen narrowing is variable. The saphenous vein and internal mammary artery are common vessels for coronary artery bypass grafts (CABG). A process similar to atherosclerosis can subsequently develop in them, too, making CABG necessary again.

Patchy changes occur in the cerebral vessels as well especially in the carotid, basilar, and vertebral arteries. The proximal portion of the internal carotid artery is a common site, with a concentration of lesions located near the bifurcation.

Angiographic visualization of deformity to a vessel lumen is still the best evidence of silent atherosclerosis. Doppler probes to measure blood flow, used in conjunction with ultrasound, are excellent techniques for determining the location of atherosclerotic plaques and narrowing of lumens in carotid and femoral vessels but not for coronary or other, more deeply set blood vessels.

The development of atherosclerosis has been linked to the presence of certain factors and conditions. The presence of these risk factors can dramatically accelerate the progression of atherosclerosis. When multiple risk factors are present, the possibility of atherosclerosis escalates even further. The most significant risk factors in the causation and acceleration of atherosclerotic disease are generally hypercholesterolemia, hypertension, and cigarette smoking. Other factors that play an important role include, age, gender, and heredity. Some influence is also exerted by body habitus (obesity), diet, hyperglycemia and diabetes mellitus, sedentary lifestyle, stress, and personality type. The last two of these factors are difficult to measure and are subject to differing expert opinions regarding their contribution to atherosclerosis and ischemic heart disease.

The clinical outcomes of atherosclerosis can be reduced by removing or reversing a single risk factor or group of risk factors. In particular, alteration of diet, reduction of blood cholesterol levels, treatment of hypertension, and cessation of smoking are the major targets to prevent the progression of atherosclerotic disease. Physical activity has been shown to reduce the negative effects of some of these factors. Exercise lets a person attain or maintain a higher metabolic rate which allows better caloric intake tolerance—one can enjoy a few more calories without gaining weight. Reduction of blood cholesterol and blood pressure along with successive reductions or elimination of reliance on blood-pressure-lowering medicine are other benefits of exercise. The general rehabilitation exercise considerations presented in Chapter 42 are all applicable to persons with atherosclerosis.

CORONARY ARTERY DISEASE

The most common cause of death in elderly persons is coronary artery disease (CAD). By the age of 70, its occurrence peaks, affecting both men and women similarly. Elderly patients with acute myocardial infarction (MI) account for over 50% of hospital admissions due to ischemic heart disease. Recognizing the presenting symptoms of CAD or MI becomes more challenging with the advancing age of the patient. Despite the high incidence of coronary artery disease, only about 10% of the elderly population have angina pectoris. Beyond the age of 80, less than 50% experience chest pain, and less than 20% experience diaphoresis, whereas the incidence of weakness, dizziness, and vomiting remains similar to that of younger groups. The presenting symptoms of myocardial infarction in the elderly that become increasingly common with advancing age are syncope, acute confusion, and stroke.

Generally, the risk factors for myocardial infarction and mortality due to coronary heart disease are similar to those for younger adults, although their relative importance changes. With advancing age, the relative risk of hypertension dramatically increases. Although the significance of high-density lipoproteins remains the same, an overall decline in the risk of elevated total cholesterol levels is seen. Smoking still remains a significant risk factor, even in the elderly, and it is associated with a 50% increase in mortality as a result of coronary artery disease. Diabetes mellitus also remains a major risk factor, especially in older women. Obesity continues to be a powerful risk factor in both elderly men and, to a lesser extent, women. Physical activity, even a moderate amount, has a definite protective effect, as does estrogen therapy in elderly women. Daily low-dose aspirin therapy is believed to reduce the risk of myocardial infarction as well as stroke in the elderly.

Older people have a higher frequency of complications of CAD, including arrhythmias, heart failure, and cardiac rupture. Increasing age is also associated with higher rates of complications in surgical treatments for myocardial infarction and coronary artery disease, but age alone should not be a basis for exclusion from invasive intervention. One-year mortality rates after infarction are four times higher in the elderly than in younger patients. The annual mortality after 3 years is 12% in those with non-Q-wave infarcts.

Treatment regimens for the elderly with chronic artery disease are similar to those for younger patients. Drug doses usually have to be reduced by one third to one half when treating patients older than 65 years of age because of their increased drug sensitivity and the prolongation of the drug's half-life. Polled analysis of data suggests that the elderly do derive significant benefit from thrombolytic therapy, even though initial studies showed no change in mortality in the elderly and an increase in hemorrhagic complications with this treatment.

Although the indications for surgical intervention in the elderly remain the same as for younger patients, the number of contraindications increases; thus, the risks of complication may exceed the risks of help. Perioperative mortality shows a progressive increase with increasing age: in those under 65 years it is 1.9%, in those between 65 and 69 years it is 4.6%, in those between 70 and 74 years it is 6.6%, and in those 75 and over it is 9.5%. The 5-year survival is 87% in all elderly patients who survive surgery, but it is slightly lower in persons 75 and over—about a 77% survival rate. Angioplasty has equally favorable survival rates and has shown benefit for persons over the age of 75 years. As it is a less invasive procedure, angioplasty has the advantage of involving fewer postoperative complications. It is interesting to note that the recurrence of angina among older people is less frequent than among younger people; this rate may reflect their less demanding lifestyle.

Rehabilitation considerations for a person with coronary artery disease and angina pectoris are discussed in Chapter 44, "Ischemic Heart Disease and Myocardial Infarction"; treatment considerations for a person after angioplasty are addressed in the medical and surgical Chapter 48, "Invasive Cardiac Procedures."

CONCLUSION

Atherosclerosis is a major health problem that necessitates medical and surgical intervention and contributes to death. Risk factors have been identified, hypercholesterolemia, hypertension, and smoking are the most significant. Reducing or eliminating these risks and adding an appropriate program of physical activity mitigates the unfavorable clinical outcomes of atherosclerosis.

Coronary artery disease is atherosclerosis of the arterial walls of the myocardium, and it leads to myocardial infarction, a significant cause of death in elderly persons. Risk factors include hypertension, elevated cholesterol levels, smoking, diabetes mellitus, and obesity. Appropriate physical exercise (see Chapter 42) and estrogen therapy for females (see Chapter 61) help to reduce the chance of its occurrence.

SUGGESTED READINGS

Bayer AJ, Chadha JS, Faray RR, et al. Changing presentation of myocardial infarction with increasing old age. *J Am Geriatr Soc* 1986; 34:263.

Blessey RL, Irwin S. Atherosclerosis: overview of the basic mechanism of atherogenesis, pathophysiology, and natural history. In: Irwin S, Tecklin JS, eds. *Cardiopulmonary Physical Therapy,* 3rd ed. St. Louis: Mosby-Year Book; 1996:6–21.

Braunwald E, Sobol BE. Coronary blood flow and myocardial ischemia. In: Braunwald E, ed. *Braunwald's Heart Disease.* Philadelphia: W.B. Saunders; 1988.

Cahalin LP. Heart failure. *Phys Ther* 1996; 76:516–533.

Fleg JL. Alterations in cardiovascular structure and function with advancing age. *Am J Cardiol* 1988; 51:33C.

Francis K. Physical actvity in prevention of cardiovascular disease. *Phys Ther* 1996; 76:456–468.

Fuster V, Badimon L, Badimon JJ, et al. The pathogenesis of coronary artery disease and the acute coronary syndromes. *N Engl J Med* 1992; 326:242, 310.

Hazzard WR. Aging and atherosclerosis. In: *Principles of Geriatric Medicine and Gerontology,* 3rd ed. New York: McGraw-Hill; 1993.

Hillegass E, Sadowsky S. *Essentials of Cardiopulmonary Physical Therapy.* Philadelphia: W.B. Saunders; 1994.

Chapter **44**

Ischemic Heart Disease and Myocardial Infarction

Joanne Dalgleish, M.D.
Pamela Reynolds, M.S., P.T., G.C.S.

INTRODUCTION

In the United States, approximately 1.5 million myocardial infarctions occur each year. Mortality with acute infarction is approximately 35%, with slightly more than half the deaths occurring before the patient reaches a hospital. Overall, an additional 15 to 20% of survivors die in the first year following a myocardial infarction; however, in the elderly, this number increases fourfold. Angina is a symptom of myocardial ischemia or anoxia of an area of the myocardium. Infarction is often a sequela of this ischemia which leads to necrosis, or death, of that part of the heart muscle. Complex ventricular arrhythmias that occur during ischemia and infarction are significant but independent factors in early mortality and are, unfortunately, much less predictable than other risk factors.

Ischemic heart disease and its complications cause the greatest number of deaths in the United States—about 700,000 each year; over 50% result from arriving at a hospital too late. Many processes produce the imbalance between myocardial oxygen supply and demand that develops into ischemia, but by far the most common cause is atherosclerosis of the coronary arteries, or coronary artery disease (CAD). CAD is a multifactorial disorder with seven major risk factors for its development: age, male gender, family history, cigarette smoking, hypertension, hypercholesterolemia, and diabetes mellitus.

The natural history of CAD is determined primarily by two pathophysiological factors—the extent of arterial obstruction (how many vessels are obstructed) and the function of the left ventricle. Consideration of these two factors can help to explain the relationship among the symptoms, the clinical signs, and the course of CAD. Significant CAD can exist without clinically evident symptoms and can occur in 2.5 to 10% of the general population. A coronary artery can be 70% occluded before a person experiences any symptoms. Over the past 30 years, mortality from CAD declined by 40% in the United States as a result of better education, modification of risk factors in the general population, and improvement in the medical care of symptomatic CAD.

MYOCARDIAL ISCHEMIA

Myocardial ischemia results from a deficient blood supply to the heart muscle because of either obstruction or constriction of the coronary vessels. Underlying this deficiency is an imbalance between the oxygen supply to the myocardial muscle cells and the oxygen demand of the myocardial cells. Abnormalities in one or both of these factors—that is, supply or demand—may be the cause of the ischemia. The overwhelming majority of diseased coronary arteries have fixed obstructions in the form of atherosclerotic lesions, but the incidence of coronary artery spasm, otherwise known as Prinzmetal's angina which includes pain when at rest, is greater than was previously appreciated. It is equally capable of reducing the supply of blood and therefore of oxygen to the myocardial muscle cells.

Ischemia produces major changes in two of the important functions of a myocardial cell, electrical activity and contractility. Alteration in electrical activity generates many of the arrhythmias seen with angina and acute myocardial infarction (AMI). Impairment of myocardial contractility affects the function of the left ventricle and results in a reduced ejection fraction (the amount of blood pumped out with each heartbeat) and decreased cardiac output, which further worsens the problem of supply to the coronary arteries.

Angina Pectoris

The term "angina pectoris" describes paroxysmal or spasmodic chest pain that is usually caused by myocardial cell anoxia and is usually precipitated by exertion or excitement. Stable angina is characterized by episodic chest pain that usually lasts 5 to 15 minutes, is provoked by exertion or stress, and is relieved by rest or sublingual nitroglycerin. The pain almost always has a retrosternal component and commonly radiates to the neck, jaw, shoulders, down the left or the left and right arms. Radiation to the back is also possible. Additional symptoms, such as lightheadedness, palpitations, diaphoresis, dyspnea, nausea, or vomiting, may accompany the pain. An ECG shows specific changes of ischemia, usually ST segment depression of more than 1 mm, in about 50% of cases during an acute attack.

Unstable angina represents a clinical state between stable angina and AMI. It is also referred to as crescendo or preinfarction angina. The clinical definition of unstable angina includes any of the following subgroups: (1) exertional angina of recent onset, usually within past 4 to 8 weeks (which means that all newly diagnosed angina is essentially unstable); (2) angina of worsening character, either with increasing severity of pain, increasing duration of pain, increasing frequency of pain, or increasing requirement for nitroglycerin; and, (3) angina at rest. Also included within this group of unstable anginas is postinfarction angina which, as its name suggests, occurs after an AMI. It is important to remember that it can occur within days or weeks after an acute infarction, or even months to years later (occurring after an angina-free period dating from the AMI). Those who experience angina after successful coronary artery bypass surgery are yet another group of individuals who are considered unstable. Once again, the onset of pain may occur several months or years after surgery.

Unstable angina is thought to be caused by a progression in the severity and extent of coronary atherosclerosis, coronary artery spasm, or bleeding into nonocclusive plaques in the coronary artery. It eventually results in complete occlusion of the artery. Studies have shown that those with unstable angina have a 40% incidence of acute infarction and a 1% incidence of death within a 3-month period. With intensive education, treatment, and avoidance of coronary risk factors, the risk of infarction dips to 8% and of early death to 3%. Therefore, it is vital to recognize, hospitalize, and treat patients with unstable angina.

Another form of angina is variant, or Prinzmetal's, angina. It occurs primarily at rest and without any precipitants. Unlike the other types of angina, the exercise capacity in those with variant angina is preserved. There is also a tendency for the pain to occur at about the same time each day. Arrhythmias, or conduction disturbances, may accompany episodes of variant angina. Considering that up to one third of variant angina sufferers have no atheroscle-

Table 44-1 Differentiation of Nonanginal Discomforts from Angina

Stable Angina	Nonanginal Discomfort (chest wall pain)
1. Relieved by nitroglycerin (30 sec to 1 min)	1. Nitroglycerin generally has no effect
2. Comes on at the same heart rate and blood pressure and is relieved by rest (lasts only a few minutes)	2. Occurs any time; last hours
	3. Muscle soreness, joint soreness, evoked by palpation or deep breaths
3. Not palpable	4. Minimal additional symptoms
4. Associated with feelings of doom, cold sweats, shortness of breath	5. No ST-segment depression
5. Often seen with ST-segment depression	

(From Irwin S, Blessey RL. Patient evaluation. In: Irwin S, Tecklin JS, eds. *Cardiopulmonary Physical Therapy*, 3rd ed. St. Louis: Mosby-Year Book; 1996.)

rotic disease of the coronary vessels, the current theory of pathogenesis is that variant angina is caused by the spasm of one or more of the coronary arteries. Spasm is not isolated to variant angina; it is also seen in people with typical angina and AMI. Unlike other forms of angina, history alone is not adequate to diagnose variant angina. Also unlike other forms of angina, an episode of variant angina actually causes ST segment elevation on an ECG.

Rehabilitation Considerations for the Person with Angina

Differentiating angina pain from nonangina pain and musculoskeletal pain is challenging. The person experiencing the angina initially denies it and passes it off as a musculoskeletal pain. It is commonly described as pressure, squeezing, or tightness in the substernal area. However, there are other individuals whose angina presents in atypical areas such as the jaw, neck, epigastric area, or back. Table 44-1 suggests some guidelines for differential diagnosis guidelines.

Angina can be quantified for evaluation purposes in two ways. First, the rate pressure product (RPP), also called the double product, is closely correlated with the myocardial oxygen requirement. A person with stable angina usually develops symptoms at a consistent level of RPP. Exercise training programs can therefore be designed to keep the person from reaching the anginal threshold by closely monitoring heart and systolic blood pressure.

Rate pressure product (RPP) = Systolic blood pressure (SBP) × Heart rate (HR)

Angina threshold = SBP × HR at onset of angina pain or ECG instability (ST segment depression <1mm)

Second, the subjective experience of the intensity of angina can be graded on a scale such as the one developed at Ranchos Los Amigos Medical Center (see Table 44-2).

An individual known to have angina should always carry nitroglycerin. The two most common forms are sprays and sublingual tablets. When an

Table 44-2 Angina Levels: An Individual's Subjective Response to Discomfort

Level 1	1. First perception of discomfort or pain in the chest area; this does not require one to stop physical activity
Level 2	2. Discomfort that increases in intensity, extends in distribution, or both, but is tolerable; patient slows activity in an attempt to decrease angina level
Level 3	3. Severe chest pain that increases to intolerable levels; patient must stop activity, take nitroglycerin, or both
Level 4	4. The most severe pain imaginable (infarction-like pain)

(From Temes WC. Cardiac rehabilitation. In: Hillegass E, Sadowsky HS, eds. *Essentials of Cardiopulmonary Physical Therapy*. Philadelphia: W.B. Saunders; 1994:643.)

individual begins to experience angina, he or she should begin taking one tablet of nitroglycerin every 5 minutes. If the angina pain is not relieved after 3 tablets or 15 minutes, the person should seek emergency care immediately.

ACUTE MYOCARDIAL INFARCTION

The vast majority of people with AMI have CAD, but there is no universal agreement about exactly what precipitates the acute event. Current concepts concerning the immediate cause of AMI include the interaction of multiple trigger factors: progression of the atherosclerotic process to the point of complete occlusion; hemorrhage at the site of an existing, narrowing coronary artery embolism; coronary artery spasm; and thrombosis at the site of an atherosclerotic plaque. Previous approaches to the treatment of AMI, such as resting the cardiovascular system while monitoring and treating only the complications, if they develop, is being replaced by interventions that are aimed at reversing the precipitating causes of the infarction.

Like ischemia, infarction produces changes in the electrical depolarization and the contractility of myocardial cells. These functions are important, and derangement in one or both of them can cause the common complications of AMI. During the first few hours after the onset of pain, there are areas of infarction interspersed with or surrounded by areas of ischemia, so in the early phases, infarction is not a completed process. These ischemic areas can be saved by the early application of medical and surgical therapy. The overall amount of infarcted myocardium remains one of the most critical factors in determining the prognosis, especially future morbidity and mortality.

Arrhythmias such as tachycardias, ventricular ectopy, bradycardias, and atrioventricular blocks, are commonly seen in AMIs and are the major manifestations of the disruption of the electrical depolarization of the myocardial cells and the specialized conducting system. The major result of impaired contractility is the failure of the left ventricular pump. Heart failure usually develops if 25% of the left ventricular myocardium is damaged. Cardiogenic shock is also common and involves more than a 40% impairment of left ventricular function. If the papillary muscles of the mitral valve are involved, acute mitral valve regurgitation may develop and cause acute pulmonary edema and hypotension. Rupture of the myocardial wall or ventricular septum, resulting from autolysis in the infarcted area, can also occur and cause cardiac tamponade or an acutely acquired ventricular septal defect.

Both of these conditions can present as sudden death after AMI.

Clinical Aspects of AMI

The classic symptom of AMI is retrosternal chest pain, which is usually the same as angina pain but lasts for more than 15 to 30 minutes. Individual variation in the site and radiation of the pain and also in the nature and severity of the pain is very common. Associated features such as dyspnea, diaphoresis, palpitations, nausea, and vomiting are common accompaniments, but not all are present all of the time. The degree of heart muscle damage and extent of infarction is usually independent of the presence of associated features or the severity of the pain. A long duration of pain often indicates more damage. AMIs in elderly patients, as opposed to those in younger people, are likely to present with no pain or with a noncardiac type of pain. Longitudinal studies indicate that up to 25% of myocardial infarctions are not recognized clinically but are diagnosed later in routine ECGs performed for unrelated conditions. Also, the person with diabetes is more susceptible to silent (painless) myocardial infarction.

The physical examination can be quite normal. Mild to moderate increases in pulse rate are common despite the fact that inferior infarcts are usually associated with bradycardia. The pain and the activation of the sympathetic nervous system can cause elevation of blood pressure. However, if left ventricle function is impaired by the pain, hypotension is more likely. Alteration in the heart sounds can occur too, particularly additional sounds that may be referred to as third (S_3) and fourth (S_4) heart sounds. New systolic murmurs are also of great concern as they may indicate that muscle damage has affected the cardiac valves, causing regurgitation, or that rupture of the septum has occurred.

AMIs may involve the full thickness of the myocardial wall (transmural) or only part of it (subendocardial or nontransmural). In the clinical setting they are referred to respectively as Q-wave and non-Q-wave infarctions, depending on the presence or absence of pathological Q waves on the ECG. Non-Q-wave infarction accounts for 30 to 40% of AMIs. A history of frequent angina and the added risk of its extending to a transmural infarct are also features of non-Q-wave AMIs. Occlusion of a coronary artery occurs in about 80% of Q-wave and 20% of non-Q-wave infarctions. Mortality and complications depend on the extent of myocardial damage rather than on the presence of Q waves; however, Q-wave AMIs do tend to be larger and produce more myocardial necrotic tissue. Non-Q-wave infarctions on the whole result in lower in-hospital mortality but also result in a far greater number of complications, especially recurrent infarction and postinfarct angina. Taking all these factors into account, the long-term morbidity for each type of infarction equal out after about 3 years.

Diagnostic Tests

The ECG is an important diagnostic test for an AMI. However, only 50% of AMIs show diagnostic changes on the initial ECG. Normal readings or evidence of nonspecific changes on the ECG do not mean that hospitalization is unnecessary, as such a decision should be based on clinical assessment and risk. The classical AMI produces ECG changes that include ST segment elevation, T-wave inversion, and Q waves. Both the pain and the ECG changes resolve with relief of the ischemia and infarction. In differentiating ischemia from infarction, it is to be noted that infarction eventually creates an electrically dead area of myocardial muscle that produces Q wave in an overlying electrode. In an acute AMI, the ST segment changes occur rapidly, T-wave inversion is variable, and Q waves usually require several hours to become apparent. The area of infarction can be localized on the ECG by using lead sites of the ST segment elevation and Q waves. Localization of the AMI is important for prognosis, as the type and incidence of complications vary with the site and size of infarction.

Damage to cardiac muscle cells results in the release of enzymes into the bloodstream. Creatine kinase (CK) is an enzyme found in skeletal muscle, myocardial muscle, and brain tissue. A specific iso-enzyme of CK, CK-MB, is found primarily in myocardial cells, and elevation of its level in the bloodstream is specific for myocardial injury. Serial blood-testing for cardiac enzyme levels in the setting of suspected AMI is now routine and is especially useful when ECG changes are nonspecific or absent. If the CK-MB is not elevated within 3 to 4 hours of the onset of symptoms, the probability of a myocardial infarction is extremely small. CK-MB may also be elevated after cardiac surgery and cardiopulmonary resuscitation.

Echocardiography is a form of ultrasound that is used to look at the cardiac muscles' contraction and motion and also to observe the function of the cardiac valves. Its primary use is in the detection of complications of AMIs that may need surgical intervention, such as rupture of the myocardial wall or valve damage. It is also used after AMIs to determine the extent of impairment to cardiac function.

Radionuclide scans are also used to detect both ischemia and infarction. Two radionuclides, thallium, which is taken up by normal myocardial cells, and technetium, which is deposited in infarcted myocardial tissue, are commonly used to determine the amount of cardiac tissue involved.

Complications of AMIs

Lethal arrhythmias are most common during the prehospital phase of an AMI. The site of infarction does not usually influence the incidence of arrhythmias, but it does play an important role in the type of arrhythmias that occur. For example, sinus tachycardia is more common with anterior AMIs, whereas sinus bradycardia frequently accompanies inferior AMIs. Atrial fibrillation usually occurs within the first 48 hours after an AMI and is often associated with heart failure. Nearly all people with acute AMIs have premature ventricular contractions (PVCs), and their significance in heralding more serious arrhythmias is still an issue of debate. Ventricular tachycardia always requires intervention, and in a hemodynamically unstable patient, immediate cardioversion is essential.

Ventricular fibrillation (VF) is divided into two forms, primary VF, which occurs suddenly, in the absence of left ventricular failure or cardiogenic shock, and secondary VF, which follows progressive left ventricular pump failure. Primary VF is seen in 5 to 10% of AMIs and occurs early in the presentation—in about 60% of cases, in the first 4 hours, and in 80% of cases, in the first 12 hours after AMI. It is nearly always successfully managed with defibrillation. In contrast, secondary VF treatment rarely has long-term success.

AMIs can damage the conducting system, which leads to complete, or third-degree, heart block. The risk of developing complete heart block is dependent on the site of infarction and the presence of preexisting conduction disturbances such as first- or second-degree conduction disturbances in conjunction with bundle branch or fascicular blocks.

AMIs nearly always produce an impairment of left ventricle pumping ability. The greater the area of damage, the more likely it is that symptoms are clinically apparent. Clinical findings ranging from no cardiac failure, through mild failure and worsening pulmonary edema, to cardiogenic shock correlate with increasing likelihood of mortality, from 5% with no cardiac failure to 80% with cardiogenic shock.

Cardiac wall rupture at the site of infarction occurs more often in those with persisting postinfarction hypertension, in the elderly, and in those having a first AMI. Mortality from cardiac wall rupture is about 95%, with half of the cases occurring in the first 5 days after AMI and 90% in the first 14 days postinfarction. Immediate surgical intervention and repair are essential for survival. The risk of both venous thrombosis and pulmonary embolism is higher after an AMI because of the prolonged bedrest required after AMI. Atrial fibrillation, obesity, and old age also contribute to this risk.

The Return to Physical Activity

Early ambulation and commencement of a symptom-limited rehabilitation program is very important for anyone in the postinfarction period. In the acute setting, the physician should determine the upper limits of exercise while considering the deconditioning effects of bedrest and lack of exercise. For persons who are asymptomatic and do not show signs of ischemia, tolerance of exercise is more important than exercising at a specific heart-rate intensity. The American College of Sports Medicine (ACSM) offers general criteria for exercising after an acute cardiac event (see Box 44–1). In addition, "Guidelines for Termination of an Exercise Session" in Box 42–4, should be followed.

CONCLUSION

Ischemic heart disease, which leads to myocardial infarctions, is a significant cause of death. Angina pectoris with its retrosternal symptoms and other complaints of pain to the neck, jaw, shoulders and upper extremities result from myocardial anoxia usually precipitated by exertion or excitement. Angina is commonly denied and dismissed as a musculoskeletal complaint. Appropriate therapeutic exercise training programs must be designed to prevent the patient from reaching the anginal threshold. If anginal pain is not relieved within 15 minutes, emergency care should be sought because of the likelihood of having suffered an acute myocardial infarction. The classic symptom of acute myocardial infarction is retrosternal pain much like angina; however, in AMI, the pain lasts for more than 15 to 30 minutes. It is crucial to seek medical attention early because of the possibility of reversing the ischemia and preventing further infarction.

Acute myocardial infarctions can cause conduction problems that result in arrhythmias and ventricular fibrillation and, possibly, left ventricular failure. It is important to resume physical activity with caution.

Box 44–1

Guidelines for Resuming

Physical Activity after AMI

Intensity
- RPE < 13 (6–20 on Borg Scale)
- Post-MI: HR < 120 beats/min or HR_{rest} + 20 beats/min (arbitrary target)
- Postsurgery: HR_{rest} + 30 beats/min (arbitrary target)
- To tolerance if asymptomatic

Duration
- Intermittent bouts last 3–5 minutes
- Rest periods
  - At patient's discretion
  - Lasting 1–2 minutes
  - Shorter than exercise bout
- Total duration up to 20 minutes

Frequency
- Early mobilization: 3–4 times per day (days 1–3)
- Later mobilization: 2 times per day (beginning on day 3)

Progression
- Initially increase duration to 10–16 minutes of continuous exercise, then increase intensity

(From American College of Sports Medicine. *Guidelines for Exercise Testing and Prescription.* Baltimore: Williams & Wilkins; 1995:182.)

SUGGESTED READINGS

American College of Sports Medicine. *Guideline for Exercise Testing and Prescription.* Baltimore: Williams & Wilkins; 1995.

Blessey RL, Irwin S. Atherosclerosis: overview of the basic mechanism of atherogenesis, pathophysiology, and natural history. In: Irwin S, Tecklin JS, eds. *Cardiopulmonary Physical Therapy,* 3rd ed. St. Louis: Mosby-Year Book; 1996.

Braunwald E. Unstable angina: a classification. *Circulation* 1989; 80: 410.

Cahalin LP. Heart failure. *Phys Ther* 1996;76:516–533.

Cronqvist A, Faager G, Larsen F, Schenck-Gustafsson K. Stepwise versus symptom-limited in-hospital mobilisation after acute myocardial infarction. *Physiotherapy Theory and Practice* 1996; 12:67–75.

Dalen JE, Ockene IS, Alpert JS. Coronary spasm, coronary thrombosis, and myocardial infarction: a hypothesis concerning the pathphysiology of acute myocardial infarction. *Am Heart J* 1982;104:1119.

Gottlieb S, Moss AJ, McDermott M, et al. Interrelation of left ventricular ejection fraction, pulmonary congestion and outcome in acute myocardial infarction. *Am J Cardiol* 1992;69:977.

Irwin S, Blessey RL. Patient evaluation. In: Irwin S, Teaklin JS, eds. *Cardiopulmonary Physical Therapy,* 3rd ed. St. Louis: Mosby-Year Book; 1996.

Jaffe AS. Complications of acute myocardial infarction. *Cardiol Clin* 1984;2:79.

Klein RC, Vera Z, Mason DT. Intraventricular conduction defects in acute myocardial infarction: incidence, prognosis, and therapy. *Am Heart J* 1984;108:1007.

Krumholz HM, Friesinger GC, Cook EF, et al. Relationship of age with eligibility for thrombolytic therapy and mortality among patients with suspected myocardial infarction. *J Am Geriatr Soc* 1994;42:127.

Paciaroni E, Raffaeli S, Sirolla C, et al. Is age a predictor of mortality in patients with acute myocardial infarction? *Cardiol Elderly* 1994;2:15.

Pasternak PC. Acute myocardial infarction. In: Braunwald E, ed. *Heart Disease: A Textbook of Cardiovascular Medicine,* 4th ed. Philadelphia: W.B. Saunders; 1992.

Rich MW, Bosner MS, Chung MK, et al. Is age an independent predictor of early and late mortality in patients with acute myocardial infarction? *Am J Med* 1992;92:7–13.

Rotman M, Wagner GS, Wagner GS, Wallace AG. Bradyarrhythmias in acute myocardial infarction. *Circulation* 1972;45:703.

Siegel D, Grady D, Browner WS, et al. Risk factor modification after myocardial infarction. *Ann Intern Med* 1988;109:213.

Temes WC. Cardiac rehabilitation. In: Hillegass E, Sadowsky HS, eds. *Essentials of Cardiopulmonary Physical Therapy.* Philadelphia: W.B. Saunders; 1994.

Chapter **45**

Cardiac Arrhythmias and Conduction Disturbances

Joanne Dalgleish, M.D.
Pamela Reynolds, M.S., P.T., G.C.S.

INTRODUCTION

Cardiac rhythm originates from and is controlled by specific areas within the heart itself. These areas are called intrinsic pacemakers and are responsible for the propagation of electrical impulses that generally travel from the right atrium to the apex of the heart and activate both atria and ventricles in the process. Although these impulses can pass from cardiac muscle cell to adjacent cardiac muscle cell, there is a preferred route that follows as specialized conducting tissue situated within the myocardium and minimizes conduction time.

The primary intrinsic pacemaker is the sinoatrial (SA) node, situated at the junction of the superior vena cava and the right atrium (Fig. 45–1). Electrical impulses travel from the SA node through the atria to the atrioventricular (AV) node, which sits on the right side of the interatrial septum. The rate of SA node discharge is controlled by the autonomic nervous system. Sympathetic stimulation in-

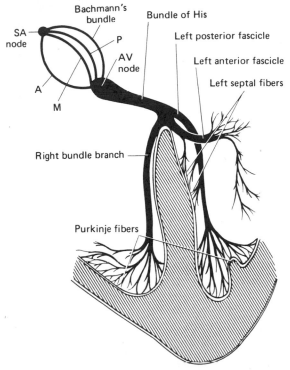

Figure 45–1 The conduction system. A, M, and p are the anterior, medial, and posterior interatrial tracts. (Reproduced with permission from Goldman MJ. *Principles of Clinical Electrocardiography,* 10th ed. Los Altos, Cal.: Lange Medical Books; 1979.)

creases the firing rate, whereas parasympathetic activity (vagal stimulation) lowers the rate.

The depolarization of the atria corresponds with the P wave on electrocardiogram (ECG) (Fig. 45–2). The impulse conduction is slowed as it traverses the AV node, allowing time for atrial contraction to be completed before ventricular contraction. This slowing, or delay, corresponds to the P-R interval on ECG. After passing through the AV node, the impulse passes into the bundle of His, then passes down the interventricular septum and divides into the right and left bundle branches that respectively supply impulses to the right and left ventricles. The ventricular depolarization corresponds to the QRS complex on the ECG. The ST segment and the T wave on ECG are produced by ventricular repolarization. Specifically, the ST segment is the absolute refractory period in which no depolarization of the ventricles can occur. T-wave repolarization is also known as the relative refractory period. During this time the ventricles can be stimulated to contract, but the heart is still electrically unstable and depolarization in this period can progress to ventricular tachycardia.

Each wave, segment, and interval has certain

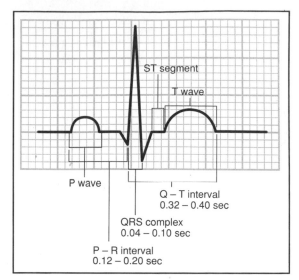

Figure 45–2 Graphic of ECG, all wave segments identified. Normal PR interval measures between .12 and .20 second. The normal duration for the QRS interval is between .04 and .10 second. Normal R-R intervals are regular and equally distanced; if irregular, the distance between the shortest and longest is <.12 second. Normal values for the Q–T interval depend on the heart rate. A normal ST segment is <1 mm elevated or depressed. (Reproduced with permission from Hillegass E. *Electrocardiography.* In: Hillegass E, Sadowsky HS. *Essentials of Cardiopulmonary Physical Therapy.* Philadelphia: W.B. Saunders; 1994.)

normal characteristics, which are identified in Figure 45–2. Variances are signs of a number of heart impairments. For instance, changes in the ST segment and T wave classically demonstrate some type of myocardial ischemia. ST segment depression greater than 0.1 mm is generally indicative of ischemia, which often results in symptoms of angina. T-wave inversion is usually a sign of ischemia or an evolving myocardial infarction or both. Other abnormalities are discussed in the following text.

Many areas of the heart can depolarize spontaneously and rhythmically. The rate of ventricular contraction is controlled by the area with the highest frequency of discharge. The SA node normally has the highest rate and therefore the ventricles follow the rate set by the SA node. This normal state of affairs is called normal sinus rhythm. Disturbances to cardiac rhythm and conduction can be classified in several ways—by heart rate; by the site of origin, delay, or block; by regularity or irregularity; by the mechanism of the arrhythmia; and by the ratio of atrial-to-ventricular depolarizations (P waves to QRS complexes).

RHYTHM DISTURBANCES

Abnormal cardiac rhythms can arise in the atrial muscle, in the junctional region between the atria

and ventricles, or in the ventricular muscle. These arrhythmias may be slow and sustained (bradycardias or bradyarrhythmias); or they can occur as early single beats (extrasystoles, or ectopic beats), or they can be sustained and fast (tachycardias or tachyarrhythmias). Rhythm disturbances may decrease cardiac output. If the ventricular rate is too fast, the volume of blood pumped with each contraction can be reduced. When the heart beats too slowly, there are not enough contractions to supply the body's demands adequately. In the normal resting adult, heart rates between 40 and 160 beats per minute are usually well tolerated, as physiological adaptations are able to maintain an adequate cardiac output and blood pressure. Problems can arise, however, in those with significant vascular disease if the heart rate drops below 50 beats per minute or goes above 120 beats per minute. These alterations in rate can cause tissue ischemia, with the heart being especially susceptible.

The advantage of having different parts of the heart able to initiate a depolarization sequence is that if the SA node fails, or conduction is blocked, another area will fire a depolarization and keep the heart beating. These secondary sites have lower depolarization frequencies than the SA node to avoid competition between pacing sites. As the heart is controlled by whichever site is discharging most frequently, the SA node, with a rate of about 70 beats per minute, is the primary site of impulse initiation. If the SA node fails, control will be assumed by a focus either in the atrial muscle or around the AV node (the junctional region). Both of these have spontaneous depolarization frequencies of 40 to 60 beats per minute. If these fail or if conduction through the bundle of His is blocked, a ventricular focus will take over, with a rate of about 30 to 40 beats per minute. Therefore, the major mechanisms that cause bradyarrhythmias are either depression of SA node activity or blocks within the conducting system. In both situations, a supplementary pacemaker takes over to control the heart rate. If these supplementary pacemakers are located above the bifurcation of the bundle of His, the rate will be sufficient to maintain cardiac output. Any bradyarrhythmia that causes hypoperfusion (inadequate bloodflow to the heart muscle) degenerates into a profound bradycardia, or asystole, which requires immediate treatment.

Junctional impulses arise from the AV node or above the bifurcation of the bundle of His. The impulse then spreads retrograde through the atria and antegrade toward the ventricles. Depending on the site of origin, the conduction velocity of the impulse, and the refractory periods of the atria and ventricles, activation of the atria may occur before, during, or after depolarization of the ventricle. AV

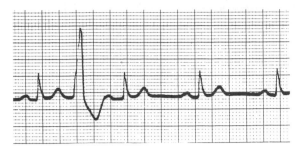

Figure 45–3 PVC. (With permission from Summerall CP III. *Lessons in EKG Interpretation,* 2nd ed. New York: Churchill Livingstone; 1991.)

dissociation can occur if the junctional pacemaker has a faster discharge rate than the SA node and the junctional impulse is blocked from retrograde conduction toward the atria.

Any part of the heart can depolarize earlier than it should, and if it initiates a heartbeat, it is called an extrasystole, or ectopic beat. Atrial ectopic beats cause abnormally shaped P waves on an ECG, whereas junctional ectopic beats may have no P wave or a P wave that arises immediately before or after the QRS complex, depending on the site within the junctional region of the ectopic focus. The QRS complexes for atrial and junctional ectopics are the same configuration as in normal SA rhythm. Ectopic beats arising in the ventricles do not travel down the normal bundle branches. Therefore, they evoke abnormally shaped QRS complexes that are frequently referred to as wide and bizarre QRS complexes. They are easily recognized on an ECG and are usually described as premature ventricular contractions (PVCs) (see Fig. 45–3).

"Tachycardia" refers to a clinical state in which the heart rate is over 100 beats per minute. Tachyarrhythmias are believed to result from three different mechanisms: ectopic foci, reentry, of triggered arrhythmias. Whether an ectopic focus is within the atria, the junctional (AV nodal) region, or the ventricles, it can fire rapidly and repeatedly, causing a sustained tachycardia. Reentry occurs when an impulse passes repeatedly through a defined route of conducting tissue at accelerated rates so as to induce tachycardia, with either a regular or disorganized rhythm. Triggered arrhythmias arc caused by changes in the potential myocardial cells have to initiate another depolarization during or immediately after repolarization and well before the next normal impulse. Urgent treatment is needed if hypoperfusion of the cardiac muscle results or rhythms develop that have the potential to become life-threatening.

The common types of rhythm disturbances are categorized according to the anatomical site of the disturbance—supraventricular (atrial), junctional, or ventricular. Each is then divided into the type of arrhythmia—slow, fast, or ectopic. Conduction blocks as a cause of bradycardia are discussed in the succeeding text.

Supraventricular (Atrial) Arrhythmias

Normal SA Rhythm

The impulse of the normal SA rhythm originates in the SA node and travels through the normal conduction system for depolarization. The heart rate is between 60 and 100. There is a P wave before each QRS complex, in other words the ratio is 1:1. When the intervals are normal, the P-R is 0.12 to 0.20 seconds, the QRS is 0.04 to 0.11 seconds, and the R-R interval is regular. The QRS complexes are identical to each other (see Fig. 45–4).

SA Arrhythmia

The rate of the SA node discharge can be altered by the vagal nerves and by changes in respiration.

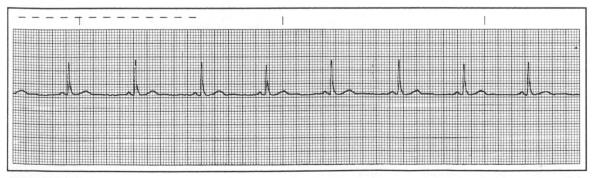

Figure 45–4 Normal sinus rhythm with a rate of approximately 62 beats per minute. (Reproduced with permission from Hillegass E. *Electrocardiography.* In: Hillegass E, Sadowsky HS. *Essentials of Cardiopulmonary Physical Therapy.* Philadelphia: W.B. Saunders; 1994.)

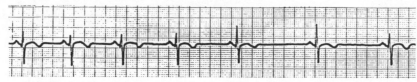

Figure 45–5 Sinus arrhythmia consisting of normal P-QRS-T configuration with increasing and decreasing intervals between complexes. (With permission from Thys D, Kaplan J. *The ECG in Anesthesia and Critical Care.* New York: Churchill Livingstone 1987.)

In SA arrhythmia, the ECG is normal except for the variability in the R-R interval (see Fig. 45–5). Variation is common, especially changes in rate with respiration which are very common in young people and tend to decline with aging. No treatment is required.

SA Bradycardia

SA bradycardia is a regular SA rhythm but with an SA node rate below 60 beats per minute. The ECG has normal P waves and PR intervals, and the AV conduction is 1:1, but the atrial rate is less than 60. It represents a suppression of the SA node discharge rate, usually in response to normal physiology in athletes, during sleep, and with stimulation of the vagus nerve. It may be drug-related, especially with narcotics, β-blockers, and calcium-channel-blockers. Pathologies that can produce a bradycardia include acute inferior myocardial infarction, increased intracranial pressure, hypersensitivity of the carotid sinus, and hypothyroidism. If evidence of hypoperfusion is present, treatment is needed. Drug treatment can be useful in the short term, but in those with symptomatic recurrent or persistent SA bradycardia, internal cardiac pacing is indicated (see Fig. 45–6).

SA Tachycardia

SA tachycardia is an acceleration of the SA node discharge rate. The ECG has normal P waves and PR intervals and a 1:1 conduction ratio between the atria and ventricles. The atrial rate increases to between 100 and 160 beats per minute (bpm). The tachycardia may be due to a normal physiological response as occurs in infants and children, with exertion or exercise, and emotions, especially anxiety. It may be drug-related as occurs with atropine, epinephrine, alcohol, nicotine, and caffeine. Also, it may reflect a pathological process such as fever, hypoxia, anemia, hypovolemia, or pulmonary embolism. In many of these conditions, the increased rate is an effort by the heart to increase cardiac output in an attempt to meet increased circulatory demands. Treatment of the underlying condition, especially in those with preexisting cardiac disease, is indicated, as increased cardiac output may further exacerbate heart problems (see Fig. 45–7).

Supraventricular Tachycardia, or Paroxysmal Atrial Tachycardia

Supraventricular tachycardia (SVT) is a regular, rapid rhythm that arises from any site above the bifurcation of the bundle of His. It is most likely

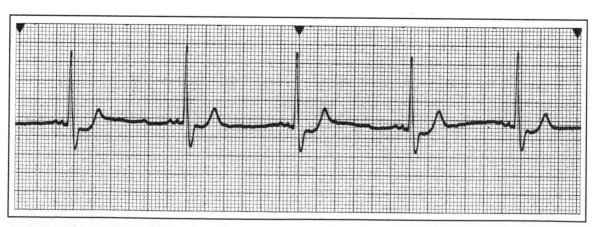

Figure 45–6 Electrocardiogram tracing illustrating sinus bradycardia with a rate of approximately 50 beats per minute. (With permission from Wiederhold R. *Electrocardiography: The Monitoring Lead.* Philadelphia: W.B. Saunders; 1989: 189.)

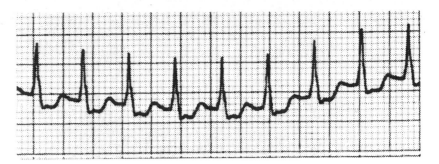

Figure 45–7 Atrial tachycardia. (With permission from Cohen M, Michel TH. *Cardiopulmonary Symptoms in Physical Therapy Practice.* New York: Churchill Livingstone; 1988:146.)

caused by reentry or an ectopic pacemaker (see Fig. 45–8). By far the most common type is reentry, with rates between 160 and 200 bpm. It may be tolerated for several days in the normal heart, but depression of cardiac output is inevitable. The ectopic form arises in the atria and has rates of 100 to 250 bpm. It is associated with acute myocardial infarction, chronic lung disease, pneumonia, alcohol intoxication, and dioxin toxicity. Reentrant SVT can occur in the normal heart or in association with rheumatic heart disease, pericarditis, myocardial infarction, mitral valve prolapse, and some of the preexcitation syndromes. Sensations of palpitations and lightheadedness are common with SVT. In those with coronary heart disease angina pain and dyspnea may occur as a result of the rapid heart rate, and in those with poor left ventricular function, heart failure and pulmonary edema are common occurrences. Treatment includes discontinuation of any causative drugs, use of a variety of antiarrhythmic medications to control the rate, and the use of vagal maneuvers (such as carotid sinus massage, valsalva, and immersion in cold water) to slow the atrial rate. Synchronized cardioversion should be done in any unstable patient with hypotension, pulmonary edema, or severe chest pain. These techniques should be performed only by those who have been properly trained.

Multifocal Atrial Tachycardia

Multifocal atrial tachycardia (MFAT) is an irregular atrial rhythm caused by at least two different sites of atrial ectopic foci (see Fig. 45–9). The ECG shows at least three or more differently shaped P waves; variable P-P, P-R, and R-R intervals, and an atrial rate between 100 and 180 bpm. MFAT is often confused with atrial flutter and atrial fibrillation. It is found in the elderly with chronic lung disease and may also be a complication of congestive heart failure, sepsis, and sometimes dioxin toxicity. Treatment is directed toward improving the underlying disease process.

Atrial Flutter

The exact mechanism involved in the development of atrial flutter is unknown, but the problem seems to involve a small area of the atrium only (see Fig. 45–10). The ECG characteristics include a regular atrial rate of 250 to 350 bpm, sawtoothshaped flutter waves in place of P waves that are especially noticeable in the inferior leads, and an AV block, usually with a 2:1 ratio, meaning the ventricular response is 125 to 175 bpm. Occasionally, the ratio is greater and the rhythm can be irregular. Atrial flutter can sometimes resemble ventricular tachycardia if conduction from the atria to the ventricles is aberrant, as this causes the QRS complex to widen. Carotid sinus massage is a useful technique to slow the ventricular response, increase the AV block, and unmask the flutter waves. Atrial flutter rarely occurs in the absence of preexisting heart disease. Incidence is highest in those with ischemic heart disease

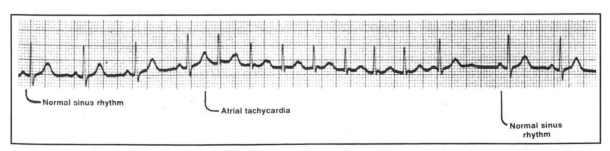

Normal sinus rhythm

Atrial tachycardia

Normal sinus rhythm

Figure 45–8 Paroxysmal atrial tachycardia (PAT); also known as supraventricular tachycardia (SUT). (Reproduced with permission from Phillips RE, Feeney MK. *The Cardiac Rhythms*, 3rd ed. Philadelphia: W.B. Saunders; 1990:154.)

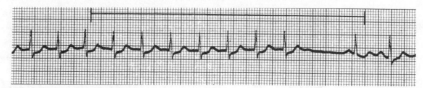

Figure 45–9 Multifocal atrial tachycardia. P waves vary in shape. Their timing is rapid and irregular. QRS complexes show narrow supraventricular configuration. (Reproduced with permission from Summerall CP III. *Lessons in EKG Interpretation*, 2nd ed. New York: Churchill Livingstone; 1991.)

or acute myocardial infarction, but it can also be a complication of congestive cardiomyopathies, myocarditis, pulmonary embolus, blunt chest trauma, and dioxin toxicity. Atrial flutter can occur as a transient arrhythmia between SA rhythm and atrial fibrillation. Treatment consists of cardioversion or medical therapy, depending on the clinical status of the patient.

Atrial Fibrillation

Atrial fibrillation occurs when there are multiple areas of the atrial myocardium continuously discharging and contracting. Depolarization and contraction are so disorganized and irregular that the atria quiver rather than contracting uniformly (see Fig. 45–11). The atrial rate is usually above 400 whereas the ventricular rate is slower because it is limited by the AV node refractory time. The ECG shows fibrillatory atrial activity (instead of P waves) and an irregular ventricular response. Disorders of atrial rhythm and drugs can slow the AV node conduction, whereas additional areas of conductive tissue called bypass tracts can increase the rate to over 200. Widening of the QRS complexes is seen whenever ventricular depolarization occurs via non-bundle-branch pathways.

There are primarily two problems in atrial fibril-lation. The atria do not depolarize; consequently, there is no contraction of the atria. Contraction of the atria can add as much as 30% to the ventricular volume, so without it, cardiac output can decrease up to 30%. Cardiac output is usually not affected in an individual who has a ventricular response of under 100 bpm. However, if the heart rate is more than 100 at rest or the person exercises, he or she may quickly demonstrate signs of decompensation. Second, there is a danger of blood coagulating in the fibrillating atria. Mural thrombi may form and subsequently lead to an embolus.

Atrial fibrillation can occur either as a paroxysmal burst or as a sustained rhythm. Rheumatic heart disease, hypertension, ischemic heart disease, and thyrotoxicosis are conditions in which atrial fibrillation commonly occurs. Less common causes include chronic lung disease, acute alcohol intoxication, and pericarditis. Treatment depends on the overall condition of the patient. In one with hemodynamic compromise, cardioversion is the best choice. Drugs can be used in the more stable patient. Response is best in the patient who is treated shortly after onset. Also, it is important to remember that in a person with a slow ventricular response secondary to drug treatment, atrial fibrillation can proceed to more serious problems like bradyarrhythmia or asystole.

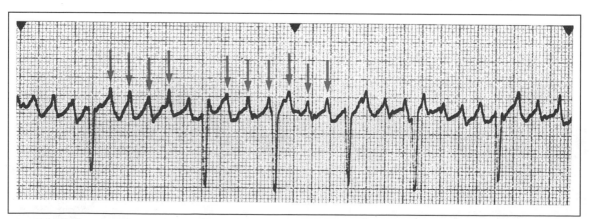

Figure 45–10 Electrocardiogram tracing of atrial flutter waves (arrows) with a variable block. (Reproduced with permission from Wiederhold R. *Electrocardiography: The Monitoring Lead*. Philadelphia: W.B. Saunders; 1989:218.)

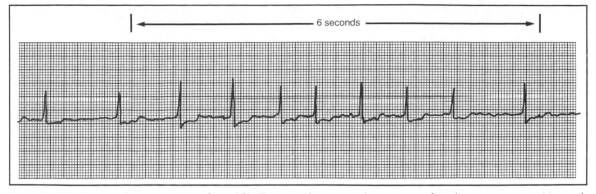

Figure 45–11 Electrocardiogram tracing of atrial fibrillation, with a ventricular response of 80 beats per minute. Notice the lack of P waves and the irregular rhythm. (Reproduced with permission from Hillegass E. *Electrocardiography.* In: Hillegass E, Sadowsky HS. *Essentials of Cardiopulmonary Physical Therapy.* Philadelphia: W.B. Saunders; 1994:377.)

Tachycardia-Bradycardia (Sick Sinus) Syndrome

Sick sinus syndrome occurs when there are problems with both impulse generation and conduction at or above the AV node region. Clinically, a variety of arrhythmias may be seen. Fortunately, most are transient. The main tachyarrhythmias include atrial fibrillation, junctional tachycardia, SVT, and atrial flutter. Intermittent SA bradycardia, prolonged SA arrest, and SA node block with AV node conduction abnormalities are the most common bradyarrhythmias. Symptoms reflect the presence of a fast or slow heart rate. A symptomatic bradyarrhythmia usually requires a permanent pacemaker. As many of the drugs used to treat tachyarrhythmias can worsen the AV block or SA arrest, insertion of a pacemaker is essential before drug therapy is begun.

Premature Atrial Contractions

Premature atrial contractions (PACs) originate from ectopic pacemakers located anywhere in the atrium other than the SA node. The ECG shows ectopic P waves that appear sooner than the next expected SA beat (see Fig. 45–12). The ectopic P wave has a shape or direction or both that is different from that of a normal P wave. The ectopic P wave will not be conducted if it reaches the AV node during the absolute refractory period, and it will be conducted with delay (a longer PR interval) during the relative refractory period. PACs that are conducted through the AV node, the bundle of His, and the bundle branches have typical QRS complexes. However, some may be aberrantly conducted through the infranodal system, which can distort the QRS shape. PACs may appear in all age groups and are often seen in the absence of heart disease. It is generally believed that stress, fatigue, alcohol, tobacco, and caffeine may precipitate PACs, although nothing has been proven yet. Frequent PACs are seen in chronic lung disease, ischemic heart disease, and digitalis toxicity. There is concern that PACs may trigger sustained atrial tachycardia, flutter, or fibrillation. Treatment involves cessation of precipitating causes and management of underlying disorders. If the PACs produce symptoms or sustained tachyarrhythmias, then the implementation of drugs aimed at suppressing the PACs is in order.

Junctional Rhythm

Under normal circumstances, the SA node discharges at a faster rate than the AV node, so the pacemaker at the AV junction is overridden. If the SA node discharge is slow or fails to reach the AV node then junctional escape beats may occur, usually at a rate of 40 to 60 bpm. Generally, these escape beats do not conduct back into the atria, so a QRS complex without a P wave is seen on the ECG (see Fig. 45–13). Whenever there is a long enough pause before an impulse reaches the AV node, the junctional pacemaker can elicit a junctional beat. This could happen in SA bradycardia,

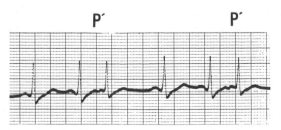

Figure 45–12 Premature atrial contractions. (With permission from Summerall, CP III. *Lessons in EKG Interpretation,* 2nd edition. New York: Churchill Livingstone; 1991:139.)

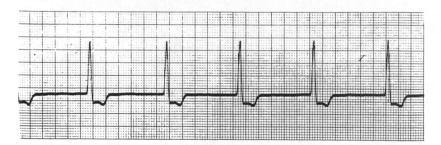

Figure 45–13 Junctional rate with sinus node arrest. (With permission from Cohen M, Michel TH. *Cardiopulmonary Symptoms in Physical Therapy Practice.* New York: Churchill Livingstone; 1988:151.)

in AV block, or during the prolonged pause after a premature beat. Sustained junctional escape rhythms may be seen with congestive heart failure, dioxin toxicity, and myocarditis.

Junctional Tachycardia

An enhanced junctional impulse may override the SA node and produce either an accelerated junctional rhythm with a rate of 60 to 100 bpm or a junctional tachycardia rate of more than 100 bpm. Accelerated junctional rhythm or junctional tachycardia can occur with inferior myocardial infarction or dioxin toxicity. If the enhanced rhythm is sustained and produces symptoms of hypoperfusion or ischemia, then therapy for the underlying cause is required. Also, acute therapy to increase the SA rate may be needed. At higher rates it is difficult to differentiate SVT from junctional tachycardia because if the P wave is present, it is lost in the QRS complex and not visible.

Junctional Premature Contractions

Junctional premature contractions (JPCs) arise from an ectopic pacemaker within the region of the AV node or the bundle of His prior to its bifurcation. ECG changes include premature ectopic QRS complexes and ectopic P waves with shapes and directions different from the norm and often inverted (see Fig. 45–14). The ectopic P wave may occur before or after the QRS complex, depending on how close to the bifurcation the ectopic P wave arises. The PR interval of the ectopic beat is shorter than the normal interval. QRS complexes are of normal shape unless there is aberrant conduction, too. The SA node is not usually affected so that the next beat is normal. JPCs may be single, multiple (such as bigeminy or trigeminy), or multifocal. They are uncommon in a normal heart and can occur with congestive heart failure, dioxin toxicity, ischemic heart disease, and acute myocardial infarction (especially of the inferior wall). Generally, treatment is reserved for those with frequent JPCs, symptomatic JPCs, or JPCs that initiate more serious arrhythmias.

Ventricular Arrhythmias
Premature Ventricular Contractions

Premature ventricular contractions (PVCs) are impulses that arise from a single or from multiple

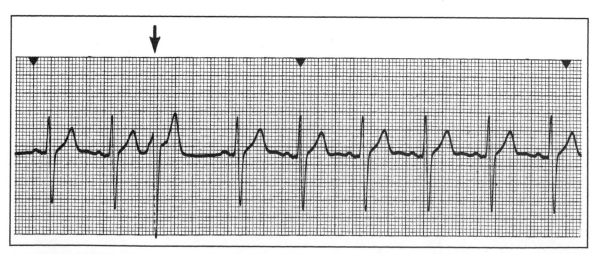

Figure 45–14 Electrocardiogram tracing of a premature junctional (or nodal) complex. The arrow points to the isolated premature beat, which has a QRS complex of normal width. The beat comes early, however, and the P wave is absent. (From Wiederhold R. *Electrocardiography: The Monitoring Lead.* Philadelphia: W.B. Saunders; 1989:61.)

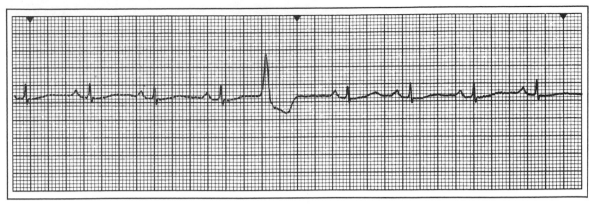

Figure 45–15 Electrocardiogram tracing of an isolated premature ventricular complex. (From Wiederhold R. *Electrocardiography: The Monitoring Lead.* Philadelphia: W.B. Saunders; 1989:82.)

areas within the ventricles. The ECG shows a premature, widened, and often bizarre QRS complex with no preceding P wave. The ST segment and the T wave of the PVC are opposite in direction from the major QRS deflection (see Figs. 45–3 and 45–15). Most PVCs do not affect the SA node discharge, so they trigger the next impulse after the refractory period. If conducted to the atria, a PVC causes a retrograde (inverted) P wave, and many times, a PVC has a fixed coupling interval (within 0.04 seconds) from the preceding SA beat. PVCs are common even in those without heart disease. However, they are frequent in people with ischemic heart disease and are universally found in those with acute myocardial infarction. This highlights the underlying electrical instability of the heart and the added risk of developing ventricular tachycardia. Other common causes of PVCs include congestive heart failure, hypoxia, dioxin toxicity, and hy-

pokalemia. Treatment of PVCs is important in patients with acute myocardial ischemia or infarction in whom maintenance of cardiac output is critical. The treatment of chronic ectopy (extra beats) depends on balancing the underlying heart disease, the origin of the ectopy, and the presence of symptoms against the risks of side effects of antiarrhythmic drugs.

Ventricular Tachycardia

Ventricular tachycardia (VT) is the occurrence of three or more consecutive PVCs at a rate greater than 100 bpm. The ECG findings are wide QRS complexes due to aberrant conduction, heart rates of more than 100 bpm (usually 150 to 200), regular rhythm, and a constant QRS axis. VT can occur in a nonsustained manner, usually as short bursts of a few seconds (see Fig. 45–16), that spontaneously

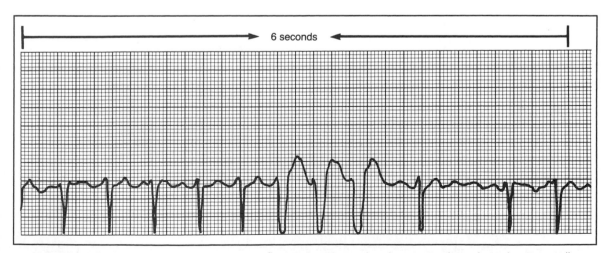

6 seconds

Figure 45–16 Electrocardiogram tracing of a triplet, otherwise known as a three-beat ventricular tachycardia. (From Hillegass E. Electrocardiography. In: Hillegass E, Sadowsky HS. *Essentials of Cardiopulmonary Physical Therapy.* Philadelphia: W.B. Saunders; 1994:387.)

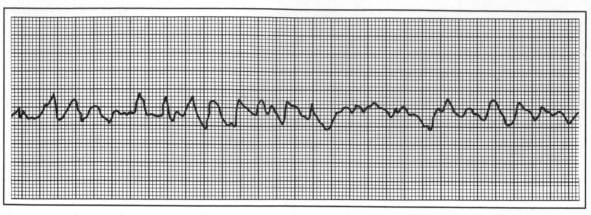

Figure 45–17 Electrocardiogram tracing showing ventricular fibrillation (coarse). (In Hillegass E, Sadowsky HS. *Essentials of Cardiopulmonary Physical Therapy.* Philadelphia: W.B. Saunders; 1994:389.)

terminate or in a sustained fashion with longer episodes and symptoms of hemodynamic instability. The latter form requires immediate treatment. A danger with sustained VT is that it can deteriorate into ventricular fibrillation. VT is rare in people without underlying heart disease. Ischemic heart disease and acute myocardial infarction are the most common causes of VT. Unstable patients are treated with cardioversion, whereas more stable patients receive intravenous antiarrhythmic drugs.

Ventricular Fibrillation

Ventricular fibrillation (VF) is the totally disorganized depolarization and contraction of the ventricular myocardium so that no effective ventricular output occurs. The ECG shows a fine to coarse zigzag pattern with no detectable P waves or QRS complexes (see Fig. 45–17). No blood pressure or pulse is detectable in VF. In an awake and responsive person, the ECG pattern of VF is usually due to loose lead artifact or electrical interference. VF is the most common complication of severe ischemic heart disease, with or without acute myocardial infarction. It can occur suddenly, without preceding hemodynamic deterioration or after a period of left ventricular failure or circulatory shock. Other causative factors include dioxin toxicity, blunt chest injury, hypothermia, severe electrolyte abnormali-

ties, and myocardial irritation from intracardiac catheter or pacemaker wires. Treatment is immediate defibrillation; several attempts may be necessary. Antiarrhythmic medications are used as adjuncts to cardioversion.

Accelerated Idioventricular Rhythm

Accelerated idioventricular rhythm (AIVR) is an ectopic rhythm that arises in the ventricle. Its rates vary from 40 to 100 bpm, which means that it is not a tachycardia. Findings on ECG include widened but regular QRS complexes (see Fig. 45–18). AIVR often begins with a fusion beat, and most runs are of short duration (3 to 30 seconds). This condition is found most commonly in a person with an acute myocardial infarction. It is also seen following successful thrombolytic therapy and in that case constitutes a reperfusion arrhythmia. AIVR itself causes no symptoms, but the loss of atrial contraction followed by a fall in cardiac output may lead to hemodynamic changes. AIVR has a variable association with ventricular tachycardia but apparently not with ventricular fibrillation. Treatment is not generally necessary, as most cases are self-limited. However, if sustained AIVR causes symptoms secondary to fall in cardiac output, then atrial pacing may be required.

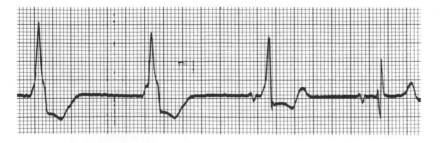

Figure 45–18 Idioventricular rhythm with fusion beat. (With permission from Summerall, CP III. *Lessons in EKG Interpretation,* 2nd edition. New York: Churchill Livingstone; 1991:81.)

CONDUCTION DISTURBANCES

Sinoatirial Disturbances

SA Node Block

The SA node discharge traverses the atria and paces the heart in normal sinus rhythm. SA node block can occur when the impulses are delayed or when their propagation is blocked. The block can fall into one of three categories; can be a first-, second-, or third-degree block. First-degree block is due to a delay in impulse conduction out of the SA node to the atria. With second-degree block, some impulses get through but others do not. Third-degree block occurs when the SA node discharge is completely blocked, meaning that no P waves originate from the SA node. SA node block can result from myocardial disease, especially acute inferior myocardial infarction. Drug toxicity and myocarditis can also cause this type of block. Treatment is dependent on the underlying cause, the associated arrhythmias, and whether hypoperfusion is present. Specific drugs can increase SA node discharge and aid conduction. Recurrent or persistent bradycardia, especially if symptomatic, may require an artificial cardiac pacemaker.

SA Arrest

SA arrest is failure of impulse generation within the SA node. If sustained, SA arrest can result in atrial standstill. Brief periods of SA arrest are a normal variation in healthy individuals and are caused by increased vagal tone. If the SA arrest is prolonged, junctional beats from the AV node can continue pacing the heart. Treatment is dependent on the underlying causes, which are the same as those that cause SA node block, the associated arrhythmias, and the presence of hypoperfusion. If symptomatic, specific drugs can increase the SA node discharge rate. Cardiac pacemaker insertion may be needed for persisting or recurrent bradycardia.

Atrioventricular Block

Atrioventricular (AV) block can be of the first-, second-, or third-degree type. The second-degree type is subdivided into Mobitz I (or Wenckebach) and Mobitz II.

First-degree AV Block

First-degree AV block is characterized by a delay in AV conduction. Although each impulse is conducted to the ventricles, the rate is slower than

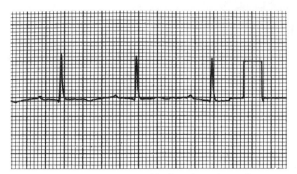

Figure 45–19 First-degree AV block with prolonged PR interval. (From Thys D, Kaplan J. *The ECG in Anesthesia and Critical Care.* New York: Churchill Livingstone;1987.)

normal, which leads to a prolongation of the P-R interval of more than 0.20 seconds (see Fig. 45–19). It is occasionally found in normal hearts but is more commonly seen with acute myocardial infarction, drug toxicity, and myocarditis. Many gerontologists consider first-degree heart block a normal variation in aging. Nerve conduction velocity is known to slow with the aging process, so first-degree heart block is viewed as a functional result of this decreased velocity. No treatment is required unless more serious conduction disturbances are also present.

Second-degree AV Block

The Mobitz type I, or Wenckebach phenomenon describes the progressive lengthening of the P-R interval, a dropped beat, and repetition of the cycle (see Fig. 45–20). There is progressive prolongation of AV conduction and of the P-R interval until an atrial impulse is completely blocked by a refractory AV node. After the dropped beat, which is seen as a P wave not followed by a QRS complex, the AV conduction returns to normal, and the cycle repeats itself with either the same (fixed) or a different (variable) conduction ratio. This block is usually transient and can be associated with an acute inferior myocardial infarction, dioxin toxicity, myocarditis, or cardiac surgery. Specific treatment is not required unless the ventricular rate is slow enough to reduce cardiac output and produce signs of hypoperfusion. Drugs can be used to increase the rate, but if they are unsuccessful, then transvenous ventricular demand pacing is needed.

In the Mobitz type II form of second-degree block, one or more beats may not be conducted at a single time; the PR interval, however, remains constant before and after the nonconducted atrial beats. This type of block occurs commonly with bundle-branch (or fascicular) problems, and the QRS complexes are consequently widened (see Fig.

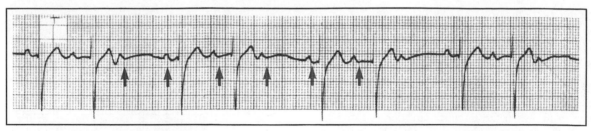

Figure 45–20 Electrocardiogram tracing showing type I second-degree heart block (Wenckeback's). The arrows identify the P waves. Notice the progressive lengthening of the P–R interval until finally a P wave exists without a QRS complex. (From Phillips RE, Feeney MK. *The Cardiac Rhythms,* 3rd ed. Philadelphia: W.B. Saunders; 1990:255.)

45–21). Type II block means that there is structural damage to the conducting system, which is usually permanent and may proceed suddenly to complete heart block, especially in the setting of acute myocardial infarction. Emergency treatment is required if the ventricular rate is slow enough to produce symptoms of hypoperfusion. If, in the acute setting, drug treatment is unsuccessful, then transcutaneous cardiac pacing is indicated. Most cases, especially those that occur in conjunction with acute myocardial infarction, require insertion of permanent transvenous cardiac pacemakers.

Third-degree (Complete) AV Block

In third-degree AV block there is no atrioventricular conduction. The ventricles are paced by an escape pacemaker at a slower rate than the atrial rate, which continues to originate from the SA node. If the block occurs at the level of the AV node, a junctional pacemaker (with a rate of 40 to 60) takes over. The resultant QRS complexes are narrow, as the rhythm originates before the bifurcation of the bundle of His. When the block occurs below the AV node, a ventricular rhythm at a rate less than 40 drives the ventricles. This is inadequate to maintain cardiac output. The QRS complexes are wide. Blocks, especially of the SA and AV nodes, often develop in the setting of acute myocardial infarction and although most are transient, they may persist for several days. Blocks that originate below the bifurcation of the bundle of His indicate structural damage to the distal conducting system and occur in cases of extensive acute anterior myocardial infarction. A third-degree block due to nodal disease is treated like a second-degree block, with drugs or a ventricular demand pacemaker. An infranodal third-degree block urgently needs a permanent ventricular pacemaker. External pacing or drugs may be used in the short term to accelerate the ventricular escape rhythm until insertion of a transvenous pacemaker can be completed.

Bundle-branch Blocks

Unifascicular

Bundle-branch, or fascicular, blocks can include one, two, or all three fascicles. A unifascicular block occurs when one of the major conduction

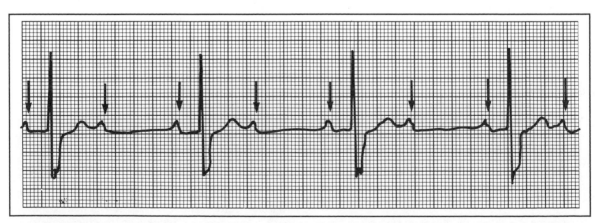

Figure 45–21 Electrocardiogram tracing of type II second-degree heart block (Mobitz II) with a heart rate of 37 beats per minute. Note the two P waves for every QRS complex. (In Hillegass E, Sadowsky HS. *Essentials of Cardiopulmonary Physical Therapy.* Philadelphia: W.B. Saunders; 1994:383.)

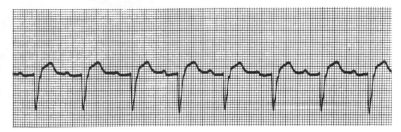

Figure 45–22 Bundle branch block demonstrating a wide QRS complex with a normal sinus rhythm. (From Cohen M, Michel TH. *Cardiopulmonary Symptoms in Physical Therapy Practice.* New York: Churchill Livingstone; 1988:157.)

pathways below the AV node and bundle of His has an obstruction that prevents passage of the depolarization impulse (see Fig. 45–22). As illustrated in Figure 45–1, the bundle of His bifurcates into a right bundle branch (RBB) and a left bundle branch (LBB). The left main bundle almost immediately divides into a left anterior superior fascicle (LASF) and a left posterior inferior fascicle (LPIF). Conduction block in the fascicles can be caused by a wide variety of conditions, such as ischemia, cardiomyopathies, valvular heart problems (especially aortic), myocarditis, cardiac surgery, and degenerative processes that affect the conduction tissue.

Bifascicular and Trifascicular Block

When conduction is blocked in two fascicles it is called a bifascicula block. Conduction blocks involving all three fascicles may be permanent or transient. Bifascicular and trifascicular conduction blocks indicate advanced heart disease. In spite of this, indications for permanent pacemaker insertion are persistent, especially for recurrent bradyarrhythmias with symptoms or signs of cardiac ischemia (angina). The risk of developing complete heart block during a myocardial infarction is much greater when bifascicular or trifascicular conduction blocks are present. They may have been present for some time or may have developed with the infarction. As the risk of complete heart block is high under these circumstances, the prophylactic placement of a ventricular pacemaker is indicated.

REHABILITATION CONSIDERATIONS FOR THE PERSON WITH CARDIAC ARRHYTHMIA OR CONDUCTION DISTURBANCE

The underlying reason for an irregular heart rate cannot be determined by palpation of a pulse. As discussed in prior text, some irregularities in rate can be relatively benign whereas others could lead to potentially lethal arrhythmias. It is imperative that the cause of the underlying arrhythmia be identified and understood so an appropriate treatment plan can be developed, either through a prudent chart review or by contacting the physician. It is

irresponsible to treat all people with cardiovascular disease with the same precautions and progressions.

Atrial arrhythmias without conduction disturbances are generally less serious than ventricular arrhythmias, which can decrease cardiac output, and the ranking is a reflection of the impairment they cause in the ventricles. Irwin and Blessey rank atrial arrhythmias from least serious to most serious as follows: (1) premature atrial contraction and premature junctional beats; (2) atrial fillbrilation; (3) supraventricular tachycardia; and (4) atrial flutter, which is considered a block. They rank ventricular dysrhythmias from least serious to most serious as follows: (1) unifocal PVCs; (2) multifocal PVCs; (3) coupled PVCs (R-on-T PVCs); (4) ventricular tachycardia; and (5) ventricular fibrillation. The relative and absolute contraindications for exercise training are shown in Cahalin's list in Table 45–1.

Table 45–1 Significant Arrhythmias and Contraindications for Exercise Training

Arrhythmia	Contraindications
Atrial	
PAC	None
JPC	None
Fibrillation	Relative
Paroxysmal tachycardia	Absolute
Flutter	Absolute
Ventricle	
Unifocal PVC	None
Multifocal PVCs	Relative
Coupled PVCs (R-on-T)	Relative
Tachycardia	Absolute
Fibrillation	Absolute
Other	
Bundle-branch block	None
AV node block	Relative

(Adapted from Cahalin LP. Exercise tolerance and training for healthy patients with cardiovascular disease. In: Hasson S, ed. *Clinical Exercise Physiology.* St. Louis: Mosby-Year Book; 1994:140.)

CONCLUSION

The most common disturbances in cardiac rhythms and conductions have been described and numerous examples have been shown. Some of these aberrations are more pathological than others. Differentiation between the less serious and the potentially lethal cannot be determined by taking a pulse; thorough cardiac evaluation is requisite to determine the type of arrhythmia or conduction disturbance. Before starting an exercise program with a patient with recognized cardiac pathology, the precise condition should be known. It is crucial that a physical therapist be aware of significant arrhythmias and contraindications to exercise training.

SUGGESTED READINGS

Brugada P, Brugada J, Mont L, et al. A new approach to the differential diagnosis of regular tachycardia with a wide QRS complex. *Circulation* 1991; 83:1649.

Cahalin LP. Exercise tolerance and training for healthy persons and cardiovascular disease. In: Hasson SM, ed. *Clinical Exercise Physiology* St. Louis: Mosby–Year Book; 1994:121–156.

Hillegas E. Electrocardiography. In: Hillegas E, Sadow H, eds. *Essentials of Cardiopulmonary Physical Therapy.* Philadelphia: W.B. Saunders; 1994; 335–401.

Irwin S, Blessey RL. Patient evaluation. In: Irwin S, Tecklin JS, eds. *Cardiopulmonary Physical Therapy,* 3rd ed. St. Louis: Mosby–Year Book; 1996:106–141.

Josephson ME. *Clinical Cardiac Electrophysiology,* 2nd ed. Philadelphia: Lea Febiger; 1993.

Mammen BA. Basic electrocardiography. In: Irwin S, Tecklin JS, eds. *Cardiopulmonary Physical Therapy,* 3rd ed. St. Louis: Mosby–Year Book; 1996:48–75.

Marriott HJL, Myerburg RJ. Recognition of cardiac arrhythmias and conduction disturbances. In: Hurst JW, ed. *The Heart, Arteries and Veins,* 7th ed. New York: McGraw-Hill; 1990:489.

Ochs GM, Ochs MA. *Recognition and Interpretation of ECG Rhythm,* 3rd ed. Stamford, Conn.: Appleton Lange; 1997.

Pritchett ELC. Management of atrial fibrillation. *N Engl J Med* 1991; 326:1264.

Roden DM. Treatment of cardiovascular disease: arryhthmias. In: Josephson ME, ed. *Clinical Cardiac Electrophysiology,* 2nd ed. Philadelphia: Lea Febiger; 1993.

Smith WM. Mechanisms of cardiac arrhythmias and conduction disturbances. In: Hurst JW, ed. *The Heart, Arteries and Veins,* 7th ed. New York: McGraw-Hill; 1990:473.

Waller BF. Anatomy, histology and pathology of the cardiac conduction system: III. *Clin Cardiol* 1993; 16:347.

Zipes DD. Specific arrhythmias: diagnosis and treatment. In: Braunwald E, ed. *Heart Disease: A Textbook of Cardiovascular Medicine,* 4th ed. Philadelphia: W.B. Saunders; 1992:667.

Chapter 46

Congestive Heart Failure and Valvular Heart Disease

Joanne Dalgleish, M.D.
Chris Wells, M.S., P.T., A.T., C.

INTRODUCTION

Heart failure is a pathophysiological state in which the heart is unable to pump blood at the rate required to meet the demands of body tissues or else the heart can do so only from an abnormally elevated filling pressure. The underlying problem in both situations is an abnormality in cardiac function. When evaluating people with heart failure, it is important to identify the underlying cause of the heart disease as well as any precipitating causes that may have contributed to the failure. A cardiac abnormality may exist for many years and produce minimal disability or none at all. That doesn't mean that the heart isn't overburdened, it means that physiological changes have compensated for the problem. Several of the valvular lesions, both congenital and acquired, fall into this group. In most cases, though, an acute problem places an additional load, or demand, on an already chronically overburdened heart, and heart failure occurs because there is no further cardiac reserve to deal with the additional requirements. The end result is further deterioration in cardiac function. Identifying the precipitating causes of heart failure is very important, as prompt treatment of those causes could be lifesaving. In the absence of underlying heart disease, it is rare for acute precipitants to lead to heart failure.

CONGESTIVE HEART FAILURE

Heart failure is a clinical syndrome that occurs when cardiac pump function is inadequate, at normal filling pressures, to meet the circulatory demands of the body. Often heart failure causes retention of fluid (congestion or edema) in many parts of the body—the lungs and legs are particularly affected—so the term "congestive heart failure" (CHF) is commonly used to describe this occurence. Heart failure can be categorized according to the rapidity of onset (acute versus chronic); the predominant side of ventricular impairment (right, left, or both); and the overall cardiac output (high, normal, or low).

CHF can result from many different diseases, and the clinical manifestations of failure are exacerbated by coexistent diseases and precipitating factors, so treatment focuses on the primary disease process and the other contributing factors.

Causes of Ventricular Failure

Right ventricular failure is most commonly caused by left ventricular failure. Isolated right-sided heart failure may occur as a result of pulmonary artery hypertension, mitral or tricuspid valve disease, restrictive or infiltrative cardiomyopathies, viral or idiopathic myocarditis, and some forms of congenital heart disease. Right-sided heart failure differs from left-sided failure in two respects: (1) in right-sided failure, the cardiac output and systemic blood pressure are decreased, and (2) the fluid accumulation occurs primarily in dependent areas of the body, not in the lungs.

The common causes of left ventricular failure are processes that result in lower cardiac output. They include hypertension, coronary artery disease, aortic or mitral valve disease, and dilated (congestive) cardiomyopathies. Less frequently, heart failure occurs because of an elevated cardiac output, when the left ventricle is unable to meet the very high circulatory demands. Conditions requiring an increased cardiac output include hyperthyroidism, septic shock, arteriovenous fistula, and Paget's disease. Acute left-sided heart failure usually produces pulmonary edema. Pulmonary edema can, however, be caused by noncardiac malfunctions, too.

Physiological compensatory mechanisms tend to preserve cardiac output, and most people remain asymptomatic, with only mild to moderate ventricular pump dysfunction as long as circulatory demands remain modest and stable. Other factors, however, may develop that demand increased cardiac output and therefore precipitate the clinical symptoms and signs of cardiac failure. The most common precipitating factors of heart failure are cardiac tachyarrythmias such as atrial fibrillation; acute myocardial ischemia or infarction; a discontinuation of preventive medications such as diuretics; an increased sodium intake; the administration of drugs that impair myocardial function, such as calcium-channel-antagonists; and physical overexertion. Please refer to Chapter 42 for guidelines on starting and stopping exercise training of patients with heart disease.

For a variety of reasons, arrhythmias are among the most frequent precipitating causes of heart failure in people with underlying but compensated heart disease. Tachyarrhythmias reduce the time available for ventricular filling, so the cardiac output is inadequate. The dissociation of atrial and ventricular contractions results in loss of the atrial booster pump mechanism. This loss prevents the normal topping up of the ventricle by the atria, so that the ventricle is underfilled and atrial pressure becomes elevated because of the additional blood remaining behind. Any arrhythmia with abnormal intraventricular conduction may further impair myocardial performance because of the loss of normal ventricle contraction synchronicity. Marked bradycardia, as seen in complete AV block, requires a greatly elevated stroke volume to maintain supply to the body, otherwise a marked reduction in cardiac output occurs.

In people with chronic but controlled ischemic heart disease, either angina or a new infarct can further impair ventricular function and precipitate heart failure, as can the cessation of medications for the treatment of heart failure.

Other Factors

When anemia is present, the oxygen demands of the metabolizing tissues can be delivered only by increasing the cardiac output. This increase can be sustained by a normal heart, but an impaired, overloaded heart that has compensated for an underlying heart problem may be unable to sufficiently augment the cardiac output to meet the requirements of the body's periphery. Anemia can precipitate ischemic heart disease because the cardiac output cannot increase enough to meet the demands of the myocardium. The combination of anemia and heart disease can lead to inadequate oxygen delivery and precipitate heart failure due to inadequate cardiac output. This is a particularly important factor after surgery in which blood loss is possible, especially in persons with hip fractures. At times these individuals may not be found until hours after the fracture injury and this delay also contributes to blood loss. Additionally, attempting to ambulate with a partial weight-bearing gait and a painful limb increases oxygen demand during rehabilitative mobility-training and exercise. Close monitoring of pulse rate and breathing is essential.

A rapid elevation in arterial blood pressure, as may be seen with undiagnosed or poorly controlled hypertension or after cessation of antihypertensive medication, can also precipitate heart failure due to cardiac decompensation. In this situation, the pressure beyond the heart is too high for the heart to pump against.

People with low cardiac output and physical inactivity are at increased risk of developing thrombi in the veins of the pelvis and lower limbs. These can embolize to the lungs, further increasing the pulmonary artery pressure which, in turn, can lead to or increase the degree of heart failure.

People with pulmonary vascular congestion are

more susceptible to pulmonary infections. The fever, tachycardia, hypoxemia, and increased metabolic demands of an infection may further overburden the diseased heart, taking it beyond the capabilities of its compensatory mechanisms so that the infection precipitates an episode of acute heart failure.

Excesses, whether physical, dietary, environmental, or emotional, can overburden a diseased heart, too (see Chapter 11, which considers thermoregulation). An increased sodium intake and excessive environmental heat or humidity can affect the cardiac output by changing the fluid volume of the body. Physical overexertion and emotional crises can increase the heart rate through activation of the sympathetic nervous system, but the cardiac output cannot increase because of the underlying disease, so output is inadequate to meet demands. The end result is cardiac decompensation and the precipitation of heart failure.

In addition to the above exacerbating causes of heart failure, other precipitants include thyrotoxicosis, which places demands on the heart similar to those made by anemia or infection; rheumatic fever and other forms of myocarditis from either inflammatory or immunological processes, that can have a direct effect on the myocardium and therefore on heart function; and finally, infective endocarditis, which incorporates valvular damage, fever, anemia, and myocarditis which individually or together can precipitate heart failure.

Clinical Features of Congestive Heart Failure

General signs of congestive heart failure include, tachypnea due to raised pulmonary pressures; central cyanosis due to pulmonary edema, peripheral cyanosis due to low cardiac output; hypotension also due to low cardiac output, and sinus tachycardia due to sympathetic stimulation, which is one of the compensatory mechanisms used to counteract the low output.

Edema, the classic sign of right-sided heart failure, generally occurs in the dependent parts of the body such as the feet, ankles, and pretibial area. Sacral edema is prominent in bedridden people. The genitalia, trunk, and upper limbs may be affected as well if massive edema occurs. If predominantly right heart failure is present, the patient is able to lie flat without dyspnea. Ascites is not common but can occur with right heart failure as a result of tricuspid valve disease or constrictive pericarditis.

Pleural effusions can occur with both right-sided and left-sided CHF; the effusion tends to be greater in amount when it is right-sided.

The first sign of left-sided failure is usually exertional dyspnea. As CHF progresses, dyspnea when lying flat develops. Interstitial edema causes a dry cough, whereas alveolar edema produces a cough with pinkish, frothy sputum.

Nonspecific but common complaints by those with heart failure, such as fatigue and muscle weakness, are thought to be due to reduced muscle perfusion. Others, such as anorexia, nausea, difficulty with memory and concentration, and headache may also reflect poor perfusion of involved regions.

In CHF, moist rales and the addition of third and fourth heart sounds are present on auscultation. Changes in chest x-rays vary depending on the severity of the heart failure, but an enlarged heart is an almost universal trait. After an episode of pulmonary edema it may be several days before chest x-rays show clear lungs, as they commonly lag well behind clinical improvement.

CHF increases exponentially with advancing age after the fifth decade. Treatment of chronic CHF includes reducing circulatory demands, correcting precipitating factors, decreasing vascular congestion, improving cardiac contractility, and controlling underlying myocardial diseases.

VALVULAR DISEASE

The heart has four valves, which function to keep blood flowing through the chambers of the heart in a unidirectional manner. Under normal conditions the valves permit the myocardial contraction to circulate blood efficiently. The atrioventricular valves are the tricuspid and mitral valves. These valves separate the atria and ventricles, respectively. The pulmonic and aortic valves, also known as the semilunar valves, assist in proper blood flow from the ventricles into the pulmonary trunk and aorta.

The valves function primarily according to pressure changes within the chambers. All valves are closed as the atria fill. Once the pressure within the atria exceeds the intraventricular pressure, the atrioventricular valves will open. As pressure in the atria falls below intraventricular pressure, the valves close. The same principle holds true for the aortic and pulmonic valves.

The atrioventricular valves have several components that can be damaged which results in various clinical signs and symptoms. The annulus is composed of fibrous rings that provide a secure attachment for the leaflets, or cusps. The space at the edge of the annulus where the leaflets insert is referred to as the commissure. The leaflets are made of a strong fibrous material and function as doors that allow unidirectional blood flow in the presence of a pressure gradient. The margins of the leaflets are thin and are stabilized by the chorda tendineae

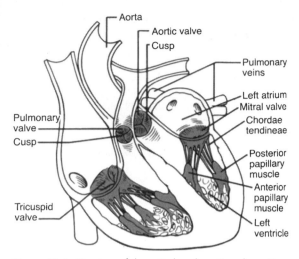

Figure 46–1. Structure of the mitral and aortic valves. (From Myers R: Saunders Manual of Physical Therapy Practice. Philadelphia: W.B. Saunders, 1995:196.)

cordis, which are strong fibrous cords that originate from the papillary muscle and insert into the leaflet margins. When myocardial contraction occurs, the papillary muscle contracts as well and makes the chorda tendineae cordis taut. It is this relationship that prevents the leaflets from inverting and causing a backwards flow of blood through the heart (see Fig. 46–1).

The semilunar valves are similar in function but are structurally different from the atrioventricular valves. There are three cusps per valve; they have a concave-convex shape, with the convexity facing the ventricles. After the ventricles begin to relax, there is a tendency for the blood to flow backwards toward the ventricles. The concavities of the cusps fill with blood, and the pressure from this blood secures the approximation of the cusps. The pulmonic valve is a more delicate structure than the aortic valve which must be rugged to function under the high pressure that exists.

The state of valvular dysfunction can be categorized as a stenosis or a regurgitation. The term "stenosis" refers to a narrowing of the valvular opening, which interferes with forward blood flow. The consequence of stenosis is an increasing myocardial oxygen demand and an increased workload that results in myocardial hypertrophy and dilation of the chambers. The end results of valvular stenosis are myocardial ischemia and congestive heart failure. Regurgitation, which is also referred to as a valvular insufficiency, is defined as backflow of blood across the valve. This causes an increase in blood volume in the chamber in front of the dysfunctional valve. The end results of regurgitation are also ischemia and heart failure. The two dys-

functions are not mutually exclusive of one another; a valve can be categorized as stenotic and insufficient.

Causes of Valvular Disease

Valvular dysfunciton has many causes. Rheumatic heart disease (RHD), one of the leading causes of valvular disease, is a complication of group A streptococcal infection that causes acute carditis. Typically, the patient does not present to the physician unless febrile and experiencing persistent dyspnea, fatigue, peripheral edema, or chest pain. Approximately 50% of cases are not diagnosed until the onset of progressive signs and symptoms of cardiac dysfunction. RHD results in fusion of the commissure, cuspids, and chorda tendineae cordis or in combined lesions involving multiple valve structures. RHD is the primary cause of mitral and aortic regurgitation and stenotic lesions. Valvular dysfunction can also be the result of myxomatous degeneration of the valve. This consists of primitive cells that spread into the central layer of the leaflets, within the annulus of chorda tendineae cordis, causing a thinning of the structure. Fibrotic changes are also occurring and they interfere with the compliance of the valve. Valvular dysfunction can also be attributed to congenital defects, trauma, or myocardial infarctions that damage the papillary muscle function. Finally, cardiovascular abnormalities such as dilation of the ascending aorta or right ventricular dilation can result in aortic and tricuspid regurgitation, respectively. A rise in pulmonary vascular resistance, as in pulmonary hypertension caused by congenital heart defect or connective tissue disorders, can result in pulmonary regurgitation.

Clinical Features

The signs and symptoms of valvular dysfunction vary according to which valve is malfunctioning and the severity of the malfunction. The ultimate key is the degree to which the malfunction affects cardiac output. With mitral regurgitation, the patient may present with complaints of excessive fatigue, dyspnea, or signs of right-heart failure. A dilated left atrium may result because of the increased amount of blood the atrium has to accept from the left ventricle at each contraction. The patient with mitral stenosis commonly presents with dyspnea on exertion, left atrium dilation, right-heart failure, hemoptysis, chest pain, and elevation of left atrial pressure. Aortic regurgitation is associated with left ventricular hypertrophy and dilatation, paroxymal nocturnal dyspnea, nocturnal angina, orthopnea, and palpitations. The patient may have an elevated systolic blood pressure, but a low diastolic pressure. The common signs and symptoms of aortic stenosis include left ventricular hypertrophy and failure, syncope, dyspnea, and pulmonary edema.

The end result of mitral or aortic valve dysfunction is the inability of the left ventricle to directly maintain cardiac output. A patient with this malfunction presents with low blood pressure, excessive fatigue, dyspnea, poor activity tolerance and, eventually, the experience of symptoms even when at rest. The degree of activity the patient can participate in is dependent upon the severity of the valve disease. Exercise is contraindicated in a patient with severe aortic or mitral valve disease, particularly aortic stenosis, who is symptomatic at rest. It is important that a cardiologist assist in establishing hemodynamic parameters as guidelines to direct the rehabilitation process.

Dysfunction of the pulmonic and tricuspid valves impairs filling of the left ventricle. Pulmonary and tricuspid regurgitation is the result primarily of right ventricular dilatation and dysfunction related to pulmonary hypertension. Infectious endocarditis can also result in regurgitation. A patient with tricuspid regurgitation presents with signs of right-heart failure—anorexia, jugular vein distension, cyanosis with dyspnea, and hepatic congestion. A patient with pulmonary regurgitation usually tolerates the dysfunction well unless it is associated with pulmonary hypertension. If pulmonary hypertension is present, the patient presents with the signs and symptoms of right-heart failure. Tricuspid stenosis is also the result of RHD and is associated with other valvular dysfunction. Congenital defects are the primary cause of pulmonary stenosis.

CONCLUSION

When recognized, the precipitating causes of heart failure can usually be treated more effectively than the underlying causes. The prognosis for people with heart failure in whom a precipitating cause can be identified is more favorable than the prognosis for those in whom progression of the underlying disease has advanced to the point of producing heart failure.

The management of a dysfunctional valve depends upon its cause and the degree of the patient's symptoms at the time of medical evaluation. Medical management includes treatment of hypertension, congestive heart failure, and dysrhythmia. When the valvular disease is severe and the patient is functionally limited, surgical intervention should be considered. A general description of the surgical intervention is presented in Chapter 48, "Invasive Cardiac Procedures."

SUGGESTED READINGS

Braunwald E. Heart failure. In: Isselbacher KJ, Braunwald E, Wilson JD, et al., eds. *Harrison's Principles of Internal Medicine,* 13th ed. New York: McGraw-Hill; 1994:998.

Bonow RO, Udelson JE. Left ventricular diastolic dysfunction as a cause of congestive heart failure: mechanisms and management. *Ann Intern Mech* 1992; 117:502.

Carabello BA. Valvular heart disease. *N Engl J Med* 1997; 337:32–41.

Grossman W. Clinical aspects of heart failure. In: Braunwald E, ed. *Heart Disease,* 4th ed. Philadelphia: W.B. Saunders; 1992:444.

Hicks GL. Cardiac surgery. *J Am Cell Surg* 1998; 186:129–133.

Kannel WB. Epidemiologic aspects of heart failure. In: Weber KT, ed. *Heart Failure: Current Concepts and Management, Cardiol Clinics Series* 7:1. Philadelphia: W.B. Saunders; 1989.

Rich MW. Congestive heart failure in the elderly. *Cardiol Elderly* 1993; 1:372.

Schultz S. Living with congestive heart failure. *Focus on Geriatric Care and Rehabilitation.* 1998; 12(2):1–12.

Chapter 47

Cardiac Pacemakers and Defibrillators

Chris Wells, M.S., P.T., A.T., C.
Joanne Dalgleish, M.D.

INTRODUCTION

The natural process of aging and the increased incidence of cardiac disease in the elderly result in the dysfunction or failure of the conduction system of the heart. With impairment of the intrinsic pacemaking structure, dysrhythmia becomes apparent. The type of dysrhythmia and its frequency determine the clinical significance of the dysfunction. Often, a disturbance in the conduction system results in the decreased ability of the heart to eject blood. The end result is a decrease in cardiac output, and the patient presents with clinical signs and symptoms of lightheadedness, visual disturbances, altered mentation, syncope, and balance dysfunction possibly contributing to falls.

Disruptions in the conduction system may be temporary or permanent. General causes for temporary dysfunction of the cardiac conduction system include increase in vagal stimulation during a cardiac catheterization, complications during or after open-heart surgery, and acute anterior or inferior wall myocardial infarction (AMI). Permanent conduction disturbances are caused by second- and third-degree heart blocks, sick sinus syndrome, recurrent tachycardia or bradycardia dysrhythmia, and frequent ventricular ectopy that compromises the patient's hemodynamics.

PACEMAKERS

One medical intervention used for conduction disturbances is a cardiac pacemaker, a device that delivers an artificial action potential to cause the myocardium to depolarize, which results in myocardial contraction and ejection of blood from the heart's chambers. The pacemaker has two components: (1) a pulse generator that contains the pacemaker's electronic program and the energy system that generates the electrical stimuli and (2) the lead, or wire, that delivers the impulse to the myocardium. The lead or leads can be described as endocardial or epicardial. Endocardial leads are inserted, along a transvenous route, inside the right atrium, the right ventricle, or both. Epicardial leads are attached directly to the surface of the right atrium or the right or left ventricle.

Temporary and Permanent Pacemakers

In the case of acute dysfunction of the conduction system a temporary pacer may be used to stabilize the patient until a permanent pacer can be inserted or until the rhythmics disturbance resolves. In an emergency, a temporary pacer with endocardial leads is typically inserted transvenously through the subclavian, internal jugular, or cephalic vein. Epicardial leads are commonly put in place at the end of open-heart surgery to be used for transthoracic pacing if it becomes necessary. In those cases the pulse generators are external to the body.

Once it is determined that a patient's conduction disturbance is irreversible and interferes with heart function, a permanent pacemaker is implanted. The pulse generator is inserted subcutaneously, usually in the region of the left pectodeltoid recess, and the leads may be either epicardial or endocardial.

The program in the pulse generator establishes the pace by sensing the intrinsic activity of the conduction system and the response of the pacemaker. Pacemakers work in three modes: (1) A fixed-rate, or asynchronous, mode paces the heart at a present rate, regardless of intrinsic electrical activity or physiological need. (2) In a demand, or inhibited, mode, the pacemaker senses intrinsic activity and inhibits the generator from releasing its electrical stimuli. (3) A triggered, or synchronous, mode paces when the conduction system fails to pace, but this mode also paces in unison with the conduction system when it senses intrinsic activity. This mode of dual pacing means that sensing and pacing occur in both the atria and the ventricles. This mode is desirable because it preserves the natural sequence of electrical conduction. The selected mode of pacing depends on the underlying pathology.

Pacemaker Universal Reference System

As the sophistication of pacemakers increased, a universal reference system was developed to describe the function of the device. The first two positions of this code refer to the location where the generator paces the heart and the location where an impulse is sensed, respectively. The code options are as follows: A = atrium, V = ventricle, D = dual, S = atrium or ventricle, and O = none. The third letter describes the response to pacing in which the options include O = none, I = inhibit, T = trigger, and D = dual. A pacemaker that is referred to as a VVI means that the generator paces and senses the ventricles and inhibits the firing of the generator when an intrinsic beat is recognized. A DDD pacer paces and senses atrial and ventricular activity, and the generator's response is to pace both the atrium and the ventricle, as indicated. Occasionally, there are forth and fifth letters in the code; they refer to the pacemaker's programmability and antitachyarrhythmia function, respectively.

Treatment Concerns

When working as a therapist with a patient who has a temporary pacemaker, it is important to monitor the patient's hemodynamic responses to the demand of the activity. The therapist should appreciate the underlying dysrhythmia that precipitated the use of the pacemaker. The connection of the external pacer should be protected during therapy using the same precautions that are used to ensure the integrity of intravenous lines during treatment or positioning. The transthoracic epicardial leads placed in the epicardium at the time of open-heart surgery are usually removed prior to discharge or when it is felt that external pacing is no longer necessary. The patient should be monitored for the next 72 hours for signs and symptoms of cardiac tamponade, which include tachycardia, decrease in systemic arterial blood pressure, dyspnea, orthopnea, and jugular venous distention.

The protocol for rehabilitation after the placement of a permanent pacemaker varies from facility to facility. Typically, the involved upper extremity is immobilized for the first 24 hours to decrease the pain, protect against bleeding, and decrease the risk of lead displacement. After the period of immobilization, range-of-motion, strengthening, and functional training can resume within the patient's tolerance. If a hematoma forms, rehabilitation may be delayed because of pain and the necessity of a longer period of immobilization. The patient may present with neurological symptoms because the hematoma is compressing on the brachial plexus, but this is an infrequent occurrence and symptoms usually subside as edema resolves. The therapist should confer with the cardiologist to verify the facility's protocol.

Before working with a patient who has a permanent pacemaker, the therapist should know which mode of pacing has been programmed into the device. The mode affects a patient's cardiovascular tolerance to exercise. Exercise tolerance is dependent on the underlying disease, the type of pacemaker, and the degree to which the patient is dependent on the pacer to maintain cardiac output. A patient who has a fixed-rate pacemaker is unable to elevate his or her heart rate to accommodate higher demand, so the therapist must recognize that limitation and adjust the treatment plan accordingly. A pacemaker set on dual mode, DDD, allows the patient's heart rate to vary according to demand. Such a patient would not be expected to have an exercise limitation because of the existing conduction abnormality. Exercise tolerance is also dependent on the patient's level of fitness.

There are special concerns the physical therapist must consider when working with a patient who has a pacemaker. Modalities like TENS, shortwave, and microwave diathermy, neuromuscular stimulators, and ultrasound should not be used in the region of the pacemaker. Superficial heat and cold should be safe to use once the surgical incision has healed, but the tissue directly over the generator should be insulated for tissue protection. In the case of temporary pacers, the site of the lead placement and the leads should be kept dry and clean. If there are any questions regarding the use of modalities or of a specific rehabilitation technique, the cardiologist should be consulted.

Pacemaker Complications

With the current use of lithium batteries, which have an 8- to 12-year life expectancy, the most common complications of pacemaker use include displacement or fracture of the leads and the device's failure to sense or pace. The myocardium can be punctured during electrode insertion, or an electrode may work its way through the myocardial wall into the pericardium which may lead to chest pain, pericardial effusion, or stimulation of the diaphragm. The myocardium can become irritated by the lead and that can cause further dysrhythmias. Local infection or hematoma formation may occur at the lead or generator site. As previously mentioned, cardiac tamponade can occur with the removal of a transthoracic temporary lead.

Failure to sense is the most common problem. Under-sensing refers to the generator's failure to recognize the intrinsic activity of the heart, whereas in oversensing, the generator interprets electrical activity that is not associated with atrial or ventricular depolarization as true intrinsic activity. The causes of inappropriate sensing include battery failure, lead malposition, improper sensitivity setting of the pacemaker, or changes in voltage of the intrinsic electrical activity, such as a high-voltage T wave.

Inadequate stimulus response refers to a situation in which the output of the generator is not sufficiently strong to cause a myocardial depolarization. This dysfunction can be caused by lead fracture or disconnection, battery depletion, or oversensing. It is more common in older pacemakers or when only one electrode is used, as in unipolar pacers.

Failure to pace is also known as loss of capture. This means the generator's electrical output, or spike, has not been followed by myocardial depolarization. Lead displacement in recently placed pacers, lead fractures, and disconnections can cause loss of capture. If the electrode site has become scarred, it requires a high output to be effective, and that can also cause loss of capture.

In working with a patient who has a pacemaker, it is important that the therapist monitor the patient's vital signs. Pacer malfunctions may result in an irregular heart rate determined by auscultation or palpation. The patient may also present with complaints of lightheadedness, syncope, lower blood pressure, and decreased tolerance to activity. With changes in the patient's compliance with exercise, the therapist should contact the physician so that pacemaker dysfunction can be ruled out or addressed.

DEFIBRILLATORS

In the case of a patient experiencing syncope due to sustained dysrhythmia or cardiac arrest, an automatic implantable cardiac defibrillator (AICD) may be the intervention of choice. The patient must be mature enough to remain complaint with medical follow-up and have at least a 6-month life expectancy. The use of an AICD has offered a 95%

survival rate of 5 years to patients with histories of life-threatening dysrhythmia such as ventricular tachycardia or ventricular fibrillation.

An AICD is a generator that is surgically implanted, usually into the submuscular or subcutaneous left upper quadrant of the abdomen. The generator can also be inserted by means of a left thoracotomy, medial sternotomy, or subcostal incision. Epicardial leads are used to monitor the function of the conduction system and deliver an electrical shock if necessary.

Most AICDs function in the following manner. The AICD monitors the heart's rate and rhythm for abnormalities. It is programmed to detect a preset rate. If that rate is exceeded, the device is activated. There is a delay in the response of the defibrillator in order to provide a chance for the abnormal rhythm to convert back to a normal rhythm. If the dysrhythmia continues beyond the delay, the generator charges. The generator then takes a second look at the rhythm and delivers an electrical shock if the abnormality is still present. The goal is to depolarize the myocardium and, it is hoped, return the patient's heart to a more stable rhythm. Some AICDs also have a feature known as antitachyarrhythmia pacing (ATP). When a tachyarrhythmia is detected, the AICD will overpace in order to break the dysrhythmia.

The therapist must be aware that she or he is working with a patient who has an AICD. In the acute phase, the incision must be protected during mobility like any abdominal incision. Good body mechanics and splinting should be taught. The therapist should know the rate at which the generator becomes activated as well as the length of time of the delay. If the patient's rate rises above the preset rate, the patient should sit down and be instructed to cough or perform a Valsalva maneuver. These maneuvers cause vagal stimulation and may cause the rate to break. The therapist should monitor the patient's vital signs and notify the cardiologist if the defibrillator delivers a shock. Complications involved in the use of an AICD are similar to the complications discussed for pacemakers.

CONCLUSION

Disturbance or dysfunction of normal heart conduction can result in decreased cardiac output, which leads to symptoms of lightheadedness, altered vision or mentation, syncope, and balance/fall dysfunction. Temporary and permanent conduction problems may be treated by inserting a pacemaker or, in cases of life-threatening dysrhythmia, an automatic implantable cardiac defibrillator. In such circumstances, the therapist must be aware of certain treatment concerns and must know the set mode of pacing prior to exercising a patient. Vital signs should be monitored during exercise to determine the patient's tolerance. TENS and diathermy should not be used in the region of a pacemaker. Superficial heat or cold may be used after the surgical incision has healed but should not be placed directly over the device.

SUGGESTED READINGS

Brannon FJ et al. *Cardiopulmonary Rehabilitation: Basic Theory and Application.* Philadelphia: F.A. Davis; 1993.

Cheitlin MD, Sokolow M, McIlroy MB. *Clinical Cardiology.* Norwalk, Conn.: Appleton & Lange; 1993.

Clochesy JM et al. *Critical Care Nursing.* Philadelphia: W.B. Saunders; 1993.

Farguson TB. Pacemakers. *Curr Prob Surg* 1997; 34:1–108.

Gillis AM. The current status of implantable cardioverter defibrillators. *Ann Rev Med* 1996; 47:85–93.

Hillegass EA, HS Sadowsky. *Essentials of Cardiopulmonary Physical Therapy.* Philadelphia: W.B. Saunders; 1994.

Morley-Davies A, Cobbe SM. Cardiac pacing. *Lancet* 1997; 349:41–46.

Wolfe DA, Kosinski D, Grubb BP. Update on implantable cardioverter defibrillators. *Postgrad Med* 1998; 103:115–130.

Chapter **48**

Invasive Cardiac Procedures
Chris Wells, M.S., P.T., A.T., C.
Joanne Dalgleish, M.D.

INTRODUCTION

Invasive procedures such as catheterization, angioplasty, and bypass surgery for the treatment of cardiac pathologies have become commonplace over the past 30 years. Elderly persons undergoing these procedures generally have a greater number of comorbidities and more extensive cardiac pathology than younger persons receiving the same diagnostic workup or treatment. Nevertheless, the technical success rate for angioplasty is approximately 90%. For coronary bypass surgery, survival rate at 5 years is nearly 75% for persons 75 years and older. A breakdown of survival rates by age group is shown in Table 48–1. Medical management and both acute and long-term rehabilitation contribute to a large degree to the success or failure of these procedures.

CATHETERIZATION

Cardiac catheterization has become a standard procedure in the diagnosis and assessment of the sever-

Table 48–1 Stratification by Age of Survival Rates after Coronary Bypass Surgery for 7,529 Patients

Age Group (y)	N	% Survival at 5 Years	% Survival at 10 Years	% Survival at 15 Years
≤45	402	92 ± 2	83 ± 3	56 ± 9
46–54	1470	94 ± 1	94 ± 1	69 ± 3
55–64	2520	91 ± 1	75 ± 1	57 ± 3
65–74	2112	84 ± 1	64 ± 2	40 ± 5
≥75	522	73 ± 3	41 ± 5	

From Cheitlin MD. Coronary bypass surgery in the elderly. *Clin Geriatr Med* 1996; 12:195.

ity of cardiac disease, and it is used to establish guidelines for the optimal management of heart disease. Catheterization is the best method to determine the extent of bloodflow in the presence of moderate valvular disease and the need for surgical intervention. The procedure can be used to evaluate the function of the myocardium, the pressures within the chambers of the heart, and the extent of coronary atherosclerosis.

A right-heart catheterization (RHC) is performed to measure hemodynamic stability and heart function. A catheter is introduced into the femoral, brachial, or internal jugular vein and extended through the right atrium and ventricle into the pulmonary artery. The physician can obtain pressures in the right side of the heart and pressure in the lungs. This provides information regarding blood volume, pulmonary vascular resistance, and preload, which is the volume of blood entering the ventricle. Cardiac output, oxygen saturation, and the function of tricuspid and pulmonic valves can be measured using an RHC. A temporary pacemaker lead can be inserted, if necessary, to control the electrical activity of the heart.

A left-heart catheterization (LHC) is performed by inserting a catheter into the femoral or brachial artery and advancing it up through the aorta and into the left side of the heart. Information regarding preload and mitral and aortic valve function can be obtained during an LHC. The most well-known reason for performing an LHC is to assess coronary atherosclerosis. From the data collected, a physician can determine the need for intervention and the best invasive method of managing the disease.

ANGIOPLASTY

Percutaneous transluminal coronary angioplasty (PTCA) is performed to enlarge a stenotic lumen of a coronary artery. A guide wire and catheter are inserted using the same procedure used in an LHC. The guide wire is advanced through the atherosclerotic lesion. Heparin is usually administered into the arterial system to decrease the risk of thrombus formation. Nitroglycerin may be administered into the coronary artery to prevent vasospasm. A dilation catheter balloon is inserted over the guide wire. The balloon is then inflated, with the goal of redistributing the atheromatous plaque. The intimal plaque is fractured and there is a disruption of the medial and adventitial layers of the vessel. The result is an enlargement of both the lumen and the overall diameter of the vessel. An angiography is repeated to assess the effectiveness of the PTCA.

The most common indication for performing a PTCA is the presence of a proximal, discrete, noncalcified lesion, this procedure has a success rate of over 90%. With advancements in the designs of guide wires and balloon catheters, clinical applications have broadened vastly to include multiple lesions in almost any part of the coronary vasculature, calcific lesions, and even totally occluded vessels. Other indications for PTCA include angina, recurrent ischemia due to atherosclerotic plaque, myocardial infarction, and ventricular dysrhythmia.

Although PTCA is a minimally invasive procedure, it is associated with several complications. Venous thrombosis and embolization may occur, causing a cerebrovascular (CVA) or occlusion accident of another coronary vessel and creating further ischemia or infarction. Perforation of the heart or coronary artery or dissection of the vessel could lead to tamponade and the need for an emergency surgical intervention. A catheter can cause life-threatening dysrhythmia. Bleeding, infection, and the development of a pseudoaneurysm may occur at the entrance site of the catheter, which is usually the femoral artery. The patient could experience an allergic reaction or renal failure due to the dye that is injected to perform the angiography. PTCA carries a 0.4 to 1.0% mortality rate.

Following the procedure, the patient is confined to bedrest for 6 to 12 hours with compression at the insertion site of the catheter. A PTCA can be performed as an outpatient procedure in an asymptomatic patient or in a 2- to 3-day admission to the hospital if the case is more complex. The clinician should monitor the insertion site for signs and symptoms of bleeding or infection. There is a 30% chance of restenosis within the first year after the PTCA; therefore, the patient should be educated regarding the recognition of ischemic signs and symptoms. It is believed that restenosis within 6 months after PTCA is due to platelet agitation, localized cell proliferation, and hyperplasia at the site of dilation. Restenosis after 6 months is theorized to be further progression of atherosclerotic disease.

ATHERECTOMY

Interventional cardiology is a relatively new field in which further advancement in technology has expanded the possible treatments for coronary disease beyond PTCA and conventional surgery. One such technique is atherectomy, which seeks to extract the plaque material. A catheter with directional (side-cutting), extraction (end-cutting), and rotational (abrasive) devices can be introduced at the site of the atherosclerotic plaque within the coronary artery. Atherectomy is used when traditional angioplasty is unsuccessful, and it is commonly used in conjunction with the PTCA procedure. Beyond the complications mentioned for PTCA, atherectomy can also cause a snow-plowing effect on embolized particles that can cause occlusion in distal arterial branches.

STENTS

In the case of acute or threatening closure after a PTCA or to seal a dissecting artery, a coronary stent may be put in place. A stent is a device that is positioned at the dilation site of the angioplasty and that either self-expands or is expanded by a balloon catheter. The purpose is to maintain the patency of the lumen. Within 8 weeks the stent will become covered with endothelial cells and may be incorporated into the vessel wall. Until this happens there is a high risk of thrombosis formation within the stent. The patient is typically placed on anticoagulation therapy.

LASERS

Finally, the atherosclerotic lesion can be managed by an ablative laser procedure. Direct ablation by a laser is indicated in the presence of a lesion in a saphenous vein graft, in aorto-ostial stenosis, in a fibrotic or calcified lesion, or in a lesion that affects a diffused area. To ablate the plaque, a wavelength that can be absorbed by the plaque is selected. The laser causes vaporization of tissue, ejection of debris, and a direct breakdown of the molecules of the plaque. The most common complication is perforation of the vessel.

BYPASS SURGERY (CABG)

The purpose of performing coronary arterial bypass graft surgery (CABG) is to restore perfusion to viable myocardium. The surgical approach is typically a median sternotomy. A vessel is harvested from another part of the body and is anastomosed between the aortic root and a point distal to the lesion or stenosis.

This procedure is indicated for various myocardial ischemic cases, particularly moderate vascular occlusion of the left main coronary artery and angina, with or without acute myocardial infarction. A patient experiencing angina who is unresponsive to medical therapy is also a candidate for a CABG. The procedure can also be performed in the presence of a failed PTCA or acute left ventricular (LV) dysfunction.

The vessels that are used to bypass the obstruction are called conduits. The most common is the saphenous vein because its diameter is relatively close to the diameter of the coronary arteries. When a vein graft is used, it is sutured to the aorta in the reverse direction so that the valves within the vein do not obstruct the bloodflow. The patency rate of the saphenous graft at 10 years is 81%. Another common conduit is the internal mammular artery (IMA), usually the left one, which is used to bypass anterior arteries like the left anterior descending artery. Other vessels have been explored in recent years because of the increase in the number of patients undergoing a second or third CABG. The basilic and cephalic veins and the radial artery are also being used, but they are associated with a high stenosis rate because of their small lumens. The splenic and right gastroepiploic arteries are other choices but are used infrequently because of the difficulty of the harvest procedures.

Certain risks are involved when a patient is undergoing a CABG. The surgery may be complicated by myocardial infarction, dysrhythmia, incisional and sternal infections, failure to wean from mechanical ventilation, bleeding, stroke, or acute renal failure. The procedure also carries a 1 to 3% mortality rate which can be higher in patients with postoperative complications or in patients with coexisting disease like diabetes or declining LV dysfunction.

Immediate Post-CABG Rehabilitation

The precautions taken and the care of the patient after surgery vary from facility to facility. Commonly, the incisions are covered with only a dry dressing in the immediate postoperative phase and in the presence of a draining wound. In terms of range of motion (ROM), activity is performed within the patient's tolerance unless the patient has a long history of diabetes associated with poor healing or is cognitively unable to report pain upon movement. In these cases, ROM may be restricted to activity below shoulder height. Acute care rehabilitation includes restoring functional mobility, increasing ambulation tolerance, and preparing for discharge. Strengthening and functional mobility exercises are also performed, within the patient's tolerance and using proper body mechanics to protect the sternum and incision. Care must be taken to educate the patient to avoid activities that position the arm in flexion, abduction, and external rotation until the surgeon is sure that the sternum is healing. Instructions in the use of the incentive spirometer and splinting techniques should be addressed to reduce the risk of atelectasis or pneumonia. Mobilization of the patient in an uncomplicated case usually occurs within the first 24 to 48 hours, and the goal for discharge from the hospital is within 5 days.

The focus of rehabilitation in the subacute phase is to restore the patient's ability to perform the activities of daily living and low-level aerobic exercise. Upper extremity ROM is progressed to within normal limits. Walking and cycling are the most common mode of exercise. The aerobic program usually begins with timed intervals based upon the patient's tolerance, with the goal of achieving 15 to 20 minutes of exercise daily. Referral to outpatient cardiac rehabilitation can occur as early as 2 to 3 weeks postoperatively. The goal of this phase of rehabilitation is to raise the patient's tolerance to the point where 40 minutes of aerobic exercise can be completed. Once the surgeon has confirmed that the sternum is healed, the patient can begin weightlifting at light to moderate levels. Questions about returning to work and recreational activities are entertained at this time. Typically, the patient should not drive for 6 to 8 weeks after a median sternotomy.

MINIMALLY INVASIVE DIRECT CORONARY ARTERY BYPASS

More advanced procedures have been developed with the goal of decreasing the surgical trauma caused by a median sternotomy, improving recovery, and reducing the length of the hospital stay. One such procedure is called a minimally invasive direct coronary artery bypass (MIDCAB). The surgical approach is through a small anterior thoracotomy incision in the left fourth or fifth intercostal space. Typically, the left IMA is the conduit of choice to bypass the left anterior descending artery. The inferior epigastric artery or the saphaneous vein can also be used as a conduit.

There are two major advantages to this surgical procedure. The patient does not have to be placed on cardiopulmonary bypass (CPB) during surgery and a median sternotomy is avoided. This procedure is also referred to as a keyhole procedure. It is usually selected over the traditional CABG in cases of isolated left anterior descending (LAD) artery disease with or without additional vessel stenosis that could be managed with PTCA. Patients who are at high risk for developing complications from cardiopulmonary bypass are candidates for a MIDCAB. Associated morbidities that are related to complications from CPB include renal failure, diffuse cerebrovascular or peripheral vascular disease, respiratory insufficiency, and age above 75.

TRANSMYOCARDIAL REVASCULARIZATION

A patient who suffers disabling angina but is not a candidate for the bypass procedure because of diffuse distal coronary disease may be a candidate for transmyocardial revascularization (TMR). The TMR procedure involves the use of a laser. An anterolateral left thoracotomy incision is made in the fifth or sixth intercostal space. When the LV is fully distended with blood and the LV depolarization has begun, a laser is fired through the myocardium. The laser makes a 1 mm channel through the wall of the LV. The laser beam is absorbed by the blood in the chamber. Several channels are made in through the myocardium. Direct pressure is applied to the epicardial surface to stop the bleeding into the pericardial sac. A suture may have to be placed at the entrance of the laser to control bleeding. TMR can be used alone or in conjunction with a CABG or MIDCAB.

The exact mechanism that enables TMR to improve myocardial perfusion is still unknown. One theory states that the perfusion is improved because blood is allowed to pass directly into the myocardium from within the chamber. The use of the laser may also stimulate the formation of collateral circulation, which further improves perfusion.

The rehabilitation process is similar to that recommended for the patient who has undergone a medial sternotomy, but with a few differences. With the incision in the intercostal space, no sternal precautions need be taken. Upper extremity ROM, strengthening, and functional mobility can progress within incisional tolerance. The rehabilitation progress may be slower for the patient who has undergone a TMR secondary to the extent of coronary arterial disease which has impaired overall myocardial perfusion.

VALVULAR PROCEDURES

In the case of moderate and severe valvular disease, the valve's diameter can be dilated, repaired, or replaced. Balloon valvuloplasty, a procedure done via catheterization for a noncalcified stenotic valve, places the balloon catheter across the valve. The balloon is inflated to dilate the lumen and thus decrease the pressure across the valve. The procedure may be complicated by hypotension, myocardial wall perforation, tamponade, dysrhythmia, an embolic event, rupture of the chorda tendineae cordis or papillary muscle, myocardial infarction, and valvular regurgitation. A valvotomy is a palliative procedure performed in the case of a younger patient with an uncomplicated, noncalcified stenotic lesion. This open procedure allows the surgeon to see the valve and to resect an atrial thrombus, a common finding. The surgeon can correct for fusion of the leaflets or chorda tendineae cordis and split the papillary muscles to improve the function of the valve. An annuloplasty involves the repair of the annulus, particularly necessary in cases of regurgitation. The annulus can be reduced in size to correct the insufficiency or a stent can be put in place to stabilize the valve function. Finally, a commissurotomy involves the surgical splitting of the commissure to correct a stenotic valve.

In the case of a complicated calcified lesion, a symptomatic patient with moderate to severe disease, or failure to repair a defect, the diseased valve can be replaced by either a mechanical or a biological valve. The mechanical valve, composed of metal or synthetic materials, is a ball or disk mechanism that responds to pressure changes. The most common valve is a St. Jude medical valve. It is highly durable and is the valve of choice for the younger patient. The disadvantage of the mechanical valve is that it makes an audible sound and requires that anticoagulation drugs be taken because of the risk of thromboembolic complications. Biological valves can be obtained from animal or human tissue. A heterograft is composed of porcine or bovine tissue. Human valves are harvested from cadavers, but the availability is low. The advantage of a biological valve is that it preserves the normal function of the valve and is fairly nonthrombogenic, but it is of limited durability and has a tendency to have a smaller orifice, which creates a stenotic state. The selection of the type of valve used depends on the age of the patient and the risk of anticoagulation. The rehabilitation of the patient who has undergone valvular repair or replacement is similar to that of patients who have undergone myocardial revascularization. See the above discussion under "Immediate Post-CABG Rehabilitation."

CONCLUSION

In the evaluation and treatment of cardiac pathology, various invasive techniques exist. Some of them are only minimally invasive, whereas others require extensive surgical techniques. Care-providers must be aware of the specific invasive techniques used and their associated precautions. Immediate postoperative wound care is a concern for all of the aforementioned techniques. In most cases, rehabilitation should commence within 24 to 48 hours after surgery. The goal of care is to return the patient to as normal a lifestyle as possible within weeks to months and within the limits of individual cardiac and coexisting pathologies.

SUGGESTED READINGS

Baum DS, Grossman W. *Cardiac Catheterization Angiography and Intervention.* Baltimore: Williams & Wilkins; 1996.

Braunwald E. *Heart Disease.* Philadelphia: W.B. Saunders; 1997.

Ellis SG, Holmes DR. *Strategic Approaches in Coronary Intervention.* Baltimore: Williams & Wilkins; 1996.

Calafiore AM et al. Left anterior descending coronary artery grafting via left anterior small thoracotomy without cardiopulmonary bypass. *Ann Thorac Surg* 1996; 61:1658–1663.

Calafiore AM et al. Composite arterial conduits for a wider myocardial revascularization. *Ann Thorac Surg* 1994; 58:185–190.

Cheitlin MD, Sokolow M, McIlroy MB. *Clinical Cardiology.* Norwalk, Conn.: Appleton & Lange; 1993.

Clochesy JM et al. *Critical Care Nursing.* Philadelphia: W.B. Saunders, 1993.

Cooley DA et al. Transmyocardial laser revascularization: clinical experience with twelve-month follow-up. *J Thorac Cardiovasc Surg* 1996; 111:791–799.

Horvath KA et al. Transmyocardial laser revascularization: operative techniques and clinical results at two years. *J Thorac Cardiovasc Surg* 1996; 111:1047–1053.

Chapter **49**

Pulmonary Diseases

Chris Wells, M.S., P.T., A.T., C.
Joanne Dalgleish, M.D.

INTRODUCTION

Lung disease can be classified based on presentation, into obstructive restrictive, also known as pulmonary fibrosis, or vascular disease categories. Chronic obstructive diseases of the pulmonary system include emphysema and chronic bronchitis, which have onset in the first to the sixth decade of life. Asthma and cystic fibrosis, which typically present early, from birth to early adolescence, are also obstructive pulmonary diseases. These diseases are all referred to as chronic obstructive lung disease (COLD) or chronic obstructive pulmonary disease (COPD). The term "pulmonary fibrosis" refers to hundreds of diseases that cause a scarring of lung tissue, such as interstitial pulmonary fibrosis, sarcoidosis, and coal workers' pneuomoceniosis. Pulmonary vascular diseases result in pulmonary hypertension. Pulmonary hypertension in the elderly is typically caused by mitral valve stenosis, long-standing obstructive or restrictive pulmonary disease, or pulmonary embolism. This chapter focuses on emphysema and chronic bronchitis as well as on the general characteristics of pulmonary fibrosis and pulmonary hypertension.

CHRONIC OBSTRUCTIVE PULMONARY DISEASE

Emphysema and Chronic Bronchitis

Emphysema is defined as irreversible anatomical enlargement of the airspaces that are distal to the terminal bronchioles and destructive of the alveolar walls (Fig. 49–1). There are four types of emphysema. Centrilobular emphysema is most commonly associated with smoking. The destruction of the lung architecture occurs at the proximal segments of the respiratory bronchioles. It more commonly affects the upper lobes. The central destruction of the acinus (the thin-walled air sac, or gas-exchange unit) involves the loss of many capillaries and leads to a mismatch between ventilation and perfusion. Panacinar emphysema is found in the elderly and in patients who are deficient in alpha 1 antitrypsin enzyme. This form of COPD affects all of the respiratory bronchioles in a uniform pattern. Localized or paraseptal emphysema presents with focal destruction of the alveolar ducts and sacs. Paracicatrical emphysema is characterized by irregular enlargement of the acinus, with fibrosis usually adjacent to a previous pulmonary lesion.

Emphysema is so prevalent that it is rare to find adult lungs completely free of this disease process. A definite increase in incidence occurs in the fifth decade and continues to increase through the seventh decade but very few changes occur after that. Approximately two thirds of males and one fourth of females will have well-defined emphysema, fortunately, most without recognized dysfunction. In most cases the emphysema is of limited extent; therefore, the majority of those with emphysema do not experience any symptoms or disability, unless under circumstances of moderate to high levels of exertion. The level of disability or impairment is dependent on the extent of destruction of the lung tissue, not the type of emphysema.

Chronic bronchitis is a condition that causes excessive mucus production within the bronchial tree in amounts sufficient to cause a productive cough for at least 3 months per year for 2 or more consecutive years (Fig. 49–2). The disease is characterized by hyperplasia of the mucus-secreting glands. The ratio between the thickness of the mucus-producing glands and the thickness of the bronchial wall is known as the Reid index. It is not diagnostic, but in the presence of chronic bronchitis, the Reid index is higher than 60%; the normal Reid index is lower than 25%. The ratio of goblet cells to ciliated cells is normally 1:20 whereas in chronic bronchitis the ratio is 1:1.

Although only a small number of males have clinically debilitating bronchitis, about 20% of adult males have symptoms that fit the definition of chronic bronchitis. Currently, males are affected more than females but with increasing cigarette smoking by women, the prevalence of chronic bronchitis is on the rise.

Contributing Factors

There are several contributing factors that have been linked to chronic bronchitis and emphysema. Cigarette smoking is the most commonly identified correlate with emphysema. Prolonged smoking impairs ciliary movement, inhibits alveolar macrophage function, and leads to hypertrophy and hyperplasia of the mucus-secreting glands. It is suggested that smoking produces an imbalance between protease and antiprotease activity. Smoking causes an inflammatory process. Neutrophils and macrophage necrosis liberate proteolytic enzyme. In industrialized countries where air pollution is prevalent, there is an increased incidence of emphysema and chronic bronchitis. Chronic bronchitis is more prev-

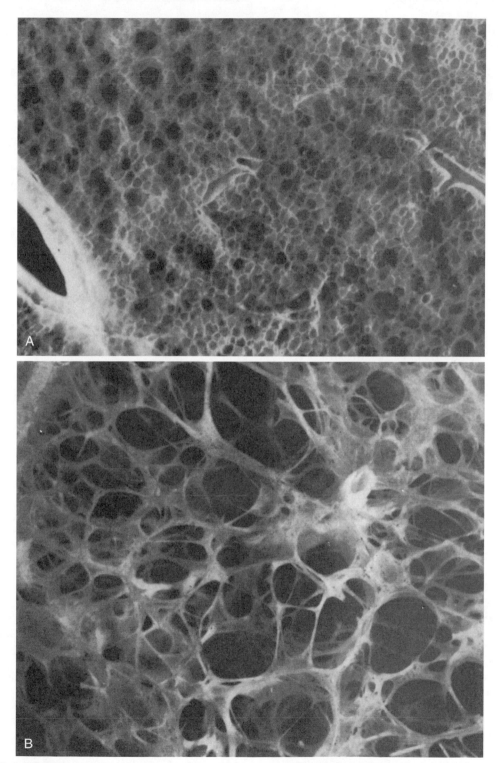

Figure 49–1 Comparison of the appearance of normal lung tissue (A) with the pathological changes observed in lung tissue damaged by emphysema (B). (From Heard B. *Pathology of Chronic Bronchitis and Emphysema*. London: Churchill Livingstone; 1969.)

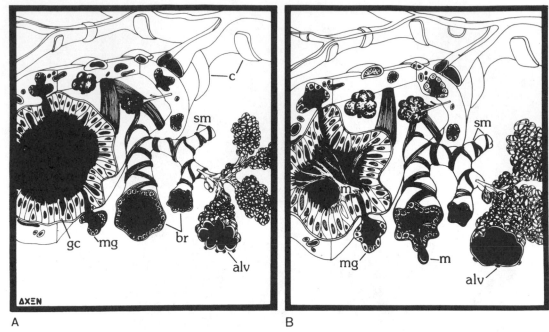

Figure 49–2 Comparison of normal airway (A) and chronic bronchitic airway (B); gc, goblet cell; c, cartilage; br, bronchi; mg, mucus gland; m, mucus; sm, smooth muscle; alv, alveoli. (From Des Jardins T. *Clinical Manifestations of Respiratory Disease.* Chicago: Year Book Medical Publishers; 1984. Redrawn by Kenneth Axen.)

alent in those with occupational exposure to organic or inorganic dusts and to noxious gases. Epidemiological studies suggest that the frequency of acute respiratory illness is a major factor associated with both the cause and progression of chronic airway obstruction. Finally, there are familial or genetic factors that have been linked with predisposition to emphysema and chronic bronchitis.

Clinical Manifestation

Chronic bronchitis and emphysema can exist without evidence of clinically significant obstruction. However, by the time the patient presents with dyspnea, obstruction is always demonstrable. Emphysema and chronic bronchitis result in limitation of airflow. Lumen size is decreased by smooth-muscle contraction and bronchial edema results from inflammation. With chronic inflammation, the smooth muscle may become hypertrophied. In chronic bronchitis the airway lumen may be partially occluded by excessive tenacious secretions and enlargment of the mucus-secreting glands. With emphysema there is destruction of the lung parenchyma, which may diminish the tethering forces exerted in the airway lumens. Moderate-sized airways that are not surrounded by cartilage become floppy and cause early closure of the airways, thus obstructing air flow. Narrowing of the airways is usually associated with an increase in airway resis-

tance and a decrease in maximal expiratory flow rates.

Gas exchange can be affected by the progression of an obstructive disease. Good bloodflow through the pulmonary capillary beds in areas that are poorly ventilated results in a widening of the alveolar-arterial gradient and shunting. In severe ventilation-perfusion mismatch, the result is arterial hypoxemia. Mismatch in which ventilation occurs in areas of poor perfusion results in an increase in dead space and impairment in the excretion of carbon dioxide.

With alterations in the relationship between ventilation and perfusion and disruption of the bronchioles, the end result is change in the control of breathing. The work of breathing increases as airway resistance increases. Deformation of the chest wall alters the length-to-tension relationship of muscles that contribute to respiration, and that increases the work of breathing. Control of breathing is also altered as blood gases are chronically changed, particularly as a result of the retention of carbon dioxide.

Dyspnea and impairment of the capacity for physical work indicate moderate to severe airway obstruction. Considerable variation exists among patients and, in general, those with predominant emphysema have greater levels of dyspnea and restriction of physical acitivity with lesser degrees of obstruction than do people in whom chronic bronchitis predominates. The great majority of patients have functionally mixed disease. They have exertional dyspnea when the forced expiratory volume in 1 second (FEV_1) falls below 50% of the predicted value for age, height, and weight. Dyspnea at rest occurs when FEV_1 equals 25% of the predicted value. By the time the FEV_1 is at 25%, both carbon dioxide retention and cor pulmonale may be present. Cor pulmonale is the enlargement of the right ventricle by dilation or hypertrophy or both. In those with severe obstruction and CO_2 retention, only about 20 to 30% will survive beyond 5 years.

Clinical Differences between Emphysema and Chronic Bronchitis

Although the majority of patients with COPD have a mixed disease with features of both emphysema and chronic bronchitis, certain clinical signs and symptoms are associated more with chronic bronchitis than with emphysema. Patients with emphysema as the predominant disease have a long history of dyspnea with exertion and a minimal cough, productive of small amounts of mucoid sputum. There is tachypnea with either a relatively long expiratory phase through pursed lips or a grunting sound at the beginning of expiration. These patients often position themselves leaning forward with their arms extended as though to brace themselves, which maximizes the use of accessory respiratory muscles. These patients maintain an elevated minute ventilation, which results in arterial oxygen concentration that is adequate to saturate hemoglobin. The results of pulmonary function tests document an increase in total lung capacity and residual volume as vital capacity is lowered. This overall retention of gas increases the diameter of the chest. The maximal expiratory flow rates, forced expiratory volume, and FEV_1 are diminished as a consequence of airway narrowing and increased resistance to flow. The lung's elastic recoil properties are severely impaired, which affects the ventilation-to-perfusion ratio, and the lungs' capacity to transfer carbon dioxide is proportionally lowered. Upon assessment, hyperresonance is found with percussion and there is a decrease in breath sounds, with faint, high-pitched rhonchi at the end of expiration. Radiographic assessment shows the diaphragm in a lower or flattened position. There is a decrease in bronchovascular markings in the peripheral lung fields, which is indicative of acinus destruction. There is also an increase in translucency in the lung fields which is consistent with hyperinflation.

Patients with chronic bronchitis usually have a long history of cough with copious sputum production. At the onset, the cough is present only during the winter months. Over the years, the cough becomes perennial and mucopurulent infections occur with increasing frequency, duration, and severity. By the time exertional dyspnea is experienced, a severe degree of obstruction is usually present. The patient with a predominance of chronic bronchitis is often overweight and cyanotic. Usually there is no apparent shortness of breath at rest. The respiratory rate is normal or sometimes only slightly increased. Percussion of the chest wall usually results in normal resonance and on auscultation, coarse rhonchi and wheezes are heard. Pulmonary function tests record a slightly diminished vital capacity, a marginally elevated residual volume, and usually normal total lung capacity. Maximal expiratory flow rates are lower in proportion to airway resistance. The chest x-ray illustrates an increase in bronchovascular markings in the lower lung fields due mainly to the presence of retained secretion.

Therapeutic Intervention

Medical treatment for patients with COPD consists of behavioral modifications that focus on weight management and smoking cessation. Brochodilators are often used to manage reactive airway symptoms, and corticosteroids are used to decrease airway inflammation. Antibiotics are used for the treatment of infections, and patients are encouraged to get flu vaccine shots each year. Oxygen therapy is used to correct hypoxemia, and chest physical therapy can be used to manage secretions.

Patients with COPD can benefit from rehabilitation, with the ultimate goal of improving quality of life. The therapy program should contain an educational component that addresses such issues as nutrition, weight management, and the specifics of the patient's disease process along with its medical management. It is important to educate the patient about the importance of aerobic exercise and light weightlifting, particularly for the upper body and antigravity muscles. The exercise program aids in the management of osteoporosis, which is a result of chronic corticosteroid use. The goal is to increase the efficiency of the peripheral musculature and thus increase work capacity. The patient's level of oxygen saturation should be monitored, and it may be necessary to adjust the level of supplemental oxygen during exercise. It is important not to exercise a patient who is being oxygenated ineffectively unless specific guidelines have been given by the physician. The level of perceived dyspnea typically goes down as the patient's exercise tolerance improves. The patient and family should be instructed in chest physical therapy or use of devices to aid in secretion management if the patient has a history of secretion retention and recurrent infections. The patient should be instructed in pursed-lip breathing and other breathing exercises to stengthen the respiratory muscles and improve the efficiency of the breathing pattern. As the pulmonary obstuction progresses, rehabilitation should begin to include job-simplification and energy-conservation. The exercise program should be periodically updated based on the progression of the disease and on the patient's tolerance.

PULMONARY FIBROSIS

Interstitial pulmonary fibrosis (IPF) has an insidious onset and makes slow progress during the fourth to seventh decades of life; dyspnea is the most common presenting symptom. IPF is a chronic inflammatory disorder of the lung parenchyma that progresses at a variable rate and results in widespread fibrosis.

Contributing Factors

The etiology of IPF is unknown and the pathophysiology is still under investigation, but several factors may contribute to the initiation and the progression of the fibrosis. Cigarette smoking has been linked to the worsening of the disease. Viral infections and collagen vascular diseases like lupus and scleroderma have been associated with the development of IPF. There also appears to be a genetic predisposition toward pulmonary fibrosis.

It is theorized that the immune system plays a vital role in the pathogenesis of pulmonary fibrosis. It is suggested that antigen-antibody compounds are deposited in the pulmonary capillary beds. This activates the complement system that in turn attracts macrophages to the site. A general pulmonary inflammatory process is activated. The complement system enhances the inflammatory response. Macrophages release various factors that stimulate fibroblast activity. Fibrotic material is deposited within the capillaries and the alveolar septum. As this process becomes chronic, plasma cells differentiate into lymphocytes. These mature cells produce new antibodies that bind to form new antigen-antibody compounds. The end product is the deposition of dense fibrotic tissue that replaces the alveolar walls.

Certain occupational exposures can be linked to the development of pulmonary fibrosis. Patients who have worked in poorly ventilated mines or quarries are at risk. Inhalation of dust particles of silica, copper, tin, and sandblasting materials results in the development of hard collagen nodules throughout the parenchyma. Coal workers' pneumonoconiosis, or black lung, affects the upper lobes primarily and is directly related to the degree of exposure. Asbestosis is another exposure-related disease that results in progressive fibrosis. The inhaled particles stimulate the inflammatory process. The pathogenesis of occupational-exposure diseases is thought to be similar to that of IPF.

Clinical Manifestation

Dyspnea is the most common presenting complaint. The patient usually reports a progressive dyspnea and a nonproductive cough. Physical capacity declines as the disease progresses as does anorexia. The patient is tachypneic and has a shallow breathing pattern. Upon examination, inspiratory or Velcro rales can be heard at the bases of the lungs and there is minimal expansion of the rib cage. Accessory muscle use will become necessary as the disease progresses. Most patients develop clubbing of the nail beds. The pulmonary function tests illustrate a decrease in lung volumes and diffusion capacity. Diffusion capacity decreases because of the increase in thickness of the alveolar septum due to fibrosis and the decrease in the pulmonary capillary bed. This results in hypoxia. A ventilation-perfusion mismatch occurs as ventilation declines. The chest x-ray shows a reticular infiltrate that is usually apparent in the lower lobes, and honeycombing develops in the later stages of the disease.

Therapeutic Intervention

Medical management focuses on controling the inflammatory process. Corticosteroids are the mainstay of treatment, but they have produced mimimal success. The patient should be removed from any environmental hazards, cigarette smoke, or occupational exposures that may contribute to respiratory distress or further disease progression. Supplemental oxygen therapy may assist in correcting hypoxemia.

Patients with pulmonary fibrosis can also benefit from rehabilitation. Once again, the ultimate goal is to improve the quality of life. The therapy program should address educational issues similar to those addressed with the patient with COPD. Aerobic exercise and strengthening are important components of the rehabilitation program, but patients with pulmonary fibrosis typically progress at much slower rates than do patients with COPD. The effectiveness of oxygen therapy should be monitored and adjusted as necessary during exercise. The level of perceived dyspnea typically goes down as the patient's exercise tolerance improves. The patient and family should be instructed in exercises and soft-tissue techniques that maintain or improve the mobility of the chest wall (see Chapter 25). The patient should be instructed in breathing exercises to strengthen the respiratory muscles and improve the efficiency of the breathing pattern. Pursed-lip breathing has a physiological benefit in patients with fibrosis. These patients do benefit from learning the inspiratory-pause breathing pattern. Typically, pulmonary fibrosis progresses more aggressively than does COPD; therefore, it is important to address job simplification and energy conservation early in the rehabilitation. The exercise program should be periodically updated based on the progression of the disease and the patient's tolerance.

PULMONARY HYPERTENSION

As pulmonary disease progresses to the point where the pulmonary capillary bed becomes affected, pulmonary pressure begins to rise. With the obstructive and restrictive diseases, pulmonary vascular resistance can become elevated as the architecture of the lung becomes destroyed. A significant amount of the lung parenchyma must be involved in order to cause pulmonary hypertension because the reserve capacity of the lungs is so vast. Precapillary arteries and aterioles become less distensible or are vasoconstricted. Early in the progression of pulmonary hypertension, the cardiac system begins to compensate by increasing cardiac output. If the pulmonary pressure is not relieved, the pulmonary vascular system becomes less distensible, and blood is shunted to the larger vessels, which causes a ventilation-perfusion mismatch. The right ventricle hypertrophies under the elevated pressures it has to overcome to eject its blood content into the pulmonary system. Eventually, the right ventricle dilates and fails.

Clinical Manifestation

Dyspnea becomes progressive, along with fatigability. Patients may begin to complain of presyncopal symptoms or may experience syncope. Chest pain, muscle fatigue, hypoxemia, and hemoptysis are other common systems related to pulmonary hypertension. As the patient develops cor pulmonale, the signs and symptoms of right-heart failure become present. Jugular vein distension, peripheral edema, and hepatic congestion become evident. Upon examination, the right ventricle may be palpable in the lower left sternal or subxiphoid area and abnormal heart sounds are present, including S4, S3 gallop, systolic ejection click, and tricuspid murmur.

Therapeutic Intervention

Treatment of pulmonary hypertension involves treating the primary cause of the hypertension. Drugs to decrease the strain on the right heart, such as digitalis and diuretics, and supplemental oxygen therapy to treat the hypoxemia may be effective. Anticoagulation medications may be used to decrease the risk of thromboembolic events because of the polycythemia that may develop as a compensatory mechanism to offset the hypoxemia.

Rehabilitation for patients with pulmonary hypertension typically focuses on functional mobility. Job simplification and energy conservation are important to review with these patients. They may tolerate an interval walking program. It is important to moniitor these patients closely for signs of chest discomfort, lightheadedness, or excessive fatigue. The therapist should also educate the patient about the adverse signs and symptoms that indicate distress and progression of the disease. The intensity of the walking program should not produce any distress. It is also vital that the therapist work directly with the physician to establish safe parameters for functional mobility activities (see Box 42–3 and Table 42–7 for guidelines).

C O N C L U S I O N

Emphysema is so prevalent after the fifth decade of life that it may be considered a primary aging factor, one that affects all persons with the passage of time. Clinically, emphysema and chronic bronchitits may exist without significant obstruction, and the conditions are usually concomittant. However, they may be differentiated by productivity of cough, history of presentation, pulmonary function tests, and radiographic findings. Patients with COPD do benefit from rehabilitation that involves education, appropriate strengthening and aerobic exercises, and proper breathing exercises and techniques. Similar rehabilitation approaches are beneficial for patients with pulmonary fibrosis or pulmonary hypertension.

SUGGESTED READINGS

Campbell EJ, Senioir RM. Emphysema. In: Fishman AP, ed. *Update: Pulmonary Diseases and Disorders.* New York: McGraw-Hilll; 1992:37.

Chermak NS. *Chronic Obstructive Pulmonary Disease.* Philadelphia: W.B. Saunders; 1991.

Clochesy JM et al. *Critical Care Nursing.* Philadelphia: W.B. Saunders; 1993.

Dantzker DR. *Cardiopulmonary Critical Care,* 2nd ed. Philadelphia: W.B. Saunders; 1991.

Frownfelter D, Dean E. *Principles and Practice of Cardio-pulmonary Physical Therapy,* 3rd ed. St. Louis: Mosby; 1996.

Fishman AP. *Pulmonary Diseases and Disorders,* 2nd ed. *Companion Handbook.* New York: McGraw-Hill; 1994.

Gurney JW. Pathophysiology of obstructive airways disease. *Radiol Clin North Am* 1998; 36:15–27.

Hillegass EA, Sadowsky HS. *Essentials of Cardiopulmonary Physical Therapy.* Philadelphia: W.B. Saunders; 1994.

Irwin S, Tecklin JS. *Cardiopulmonary Physical Therapy,* 3rd ed. St Louis: Mosby; 1995.

Kim WD, Eidelman DH, Lzquierdo JL, et al. Centrilobular and panacinar emphysema in smokers. *Am Rev Respir Dis* 1991; 144:1385.

Manaker S, Tino G. Natural history and prognosis of advanced disease. *Clin Chest Med* 1997; 18:435–455.

Stulbarg MS, Frank JA. Obstructive pulmonary disease: a clinic's perspective. *Radiol Clin North Am* 1998; 36:1–13.

BLOOD VESSEL CHANGES AND CIRCULATORY SKIN DISORDERS

Chapter 50

Diabetes

Carol Probst, M.S., P.T.
David E. Kelley, M.D.

INTRODUCTION

Diabetes mellitus is a prevalent disease, especially among the elderly. Age-related changes involving decreased insulin sensitivity in the peripheral tissues and reduced insulin control of hepatic glucose output, coupled with physical inactivity and increased obesity, contribute to higher incidences of abnormal glucose tolerances in the older population. Approximately 6.8% of the total U.S. population and 18.7% of people over age 65 have diabetes mellitus. It is estimated that half of these individuals are unaware of their disease state. Diabetes mellitus is a serious disease, and it causes a wide range of complications that account for nearly $1 of every $7 spent on health care.

DIAGNOSIS OF DIABETES MELLITUS

The diagnosis of diabetes mellitus has been revised and is based on the finding of elevated levels of plasma glucose. One or more of the following are the criteria for diagnosis: (1) a fasting plasma glucose (FPG) > 126 mg/dL; (2) a random plasma glucose > 200 mg/dL with classic diabetes symptoms; or (3) an oral glucose tolerance test (OGTT) that detects plasma glucose > 200 mg/dL 2 hours following ingestion of 75 grams of glucose.

Impaired glucose metabolism is considered to exist when fasting plasma glucose is > 110 but < 126, or > 140 but < 200 in a 2-hour sample OGTT.

The classic symptoms of diabetes mellitus are excess thirst and urination (polydipsia and polyuria). These are usually present if FPG > 200 mg/dL, but may be present at lower FPG levels. Unexplained weight loss (especially if accompanied by increased or normal food intake), poorly healing cuts, fatigue, vaginal yeast infections, and blurred vision are other common presenting symptoms.

TYPES OF DIABETES MELLITUS

There are several types of diabetes mellitus: (1) Type I (formerly known as insulin-dependent diabetes mellitus, or IDDM; (2) Type II (formerly known as noninsulin-dependent diabetes mellitus, or NIDDM; (3) gestational diabetes mellitus; and (4) secondary diabetes mellitus. By far, the most common type of diabetes in the older population is Type II. As secondary diabetes accounts for a very small number of cases, for the purposes of this Chapter, discussion will focus on Type I and Type II diabetes (see Table 50–1).

Type I

Type I diabetes is caused by autoimmune destruction of the insulin-producing beta cells of the pancreatic islets, so these patients have an absolute need for insulin therapy. Age of onset of Type I is most common during childhood or in young adults, but the onset of Type I can occur at any age. In the absence of insulin replacement, patients with Type I diabetes develop severe hyperglycemia, and metabolic acidosis results from the excess production of ketones—a by-product of fat breakdown in the absence of insulin. Diabetic ketoacidosis (DKA) is a medical emergency.

Type II

Of people with diabetes, 90% have Type II diabetes. This is nearly always a disease of adults, and its incidence increases with each decade of aging. A family history of Type II diabetes is common. Obesity is a major risk factor. Type II diabetes is regarded as a metabolic disorder tied to modern lifestyles involving stress, excess calorie intake (particularly fat), and inadequate physical activity. From a metabolic perspective, these patients generally have the twin defects of sluggish secretion of insulin following meals (and with long duration, poor overall insulin production) and peripheral insulin resistance of reduced cellular uptake and utilization of insulin.

Table 50–1 Type I and Type II Diabetes

	Type I Diabetes	Type II Diabetes
% of Diabetics	**2–5%**	**90–95%**
Onset of disease	Abrupt	Insidious
Age of onset	< 35 years	> 35 years
Symptoms at onset	Often in ketoacidosis	May be asymptomatic
Requiring insulin	Yes	In 25% of cases
Risk for ketoacidosis	Yes	Rare
Body type	Thin or normal	80% are overweight
Suspected cause	Autoimmune reaction with islet cell destruction	Insulin resistance/poor insulin secretion
Genetic predisposition	Yes	Yes

THERAPEUTIC INTERVENTION

Newly Diagnosed Diabetes

Patients newly diagnosed with diabetes mellitus have a special need for comprehensive education. The onset of diabetes can be precipitated by physical and emotional stress and other illnesses, and usually the diabetic state persists. Also, certain medications, most notably oral or parenteral steroid therapy, can trigger the onset of diabetes mellitus or upset metabolic control in a previously diagnosed patient.

Medical Treatment

Diet and exercise are the cornerstones of the treatment of diabetes mellitus. A comprehensive review of nutrition and diabetes appears in the *Handbook of Diabetes Medical Nutrition Therapy* (see "Suggested Readings" at the end of this chapter). Generally, it is not necessary to increase food intake prior to exercise of short duration or low intensity. Exercise of moderate intensity (1 hour of tennis, for example) may be preceded by 10 to 15 grams of carbohydrate, although this is often unnecessary with Type II diabetes.

Insulin Therapy for Type I Diabetes

Therapy for these individuals always includes insulin. Insulin is given by subcutaneous (SQ) injection or by use of an insulin pump, which also delivers insulin SQ. It is typical for patients with Type I diabetes to take at least two injections of insulin daily and not uncommon to administer insulin prior to each meal and at bedtime. Because blood glucose can fluctuate widely in a patient with Type I diabetes, it is recommended that blood glucose be monitored several times a day and that insulin levels be adjusted accordingly. Insulin preparations include regular, NPH (neutral protamine Hagedorn), or lente, and ultralente insulin; these differ in onset and duration of action. Patients with Type I diabetes typically use a combination of these preparations.

Treatment of Type II Diabetes

Treatment options for these patients are diverse. Patients with Type II diabetes can achieve control with diet and exercise therapy, especially if weight loss is achieved in an overweight patient. However, most Type II patients also require some pharmacological treatment. This can be oral medication or insulin. Oral medications include the sulfonylurea medications (e.g., glyburide, glipizide, chlorpropamide), metformin, which can be used in combination with a sulfonylurea, troglitazone, and acarbose.

When oral medications can no longer control plasma glucose, patients with Type II diabetes are usually placed on insulin therapy. The dose of insulin needed to control glucose levels in obese patients with Type II diabetes can be extremely large (up to 100 to 200 units daily).

Hypoglycemia

The main adverse effect of insulin or oral therapy is hypoglycemia (low blood glucose). In a patient with diabetes, symptoms of hypoglycemia generally have a rapid onset and occur when blood glucose is less than 70 to 80 mg/dL. A severe reaction can occur below 60 mg/dL. A patient may complain of shakiness and sweating or other symptoms created by increased epinephrine release, such as tachycardia and anxiety. Deprivation of glucose to the central nervous system causes blurred vision, weakness, confusion, slurred speech, and potentially seizure and coma, with permanent neurological damage. Symptoms of hypoglycemia may be blunted in a patient with long-standing diabetes, especially the early warning symptoms of nervousness, tremor, and sweating. Patients with long-standing diabetes mellitus may have disorientation as their initial symptom.

Hypoglycemia in a diabetic patient occurs because of too much insulin (or oral medications) insufficient food intake (relative to insulin or medication dose), or increased physical activity (again, relative to insulin dose). Treatment of hypoglycemia must be prompt. Mild hypoglycemia can usually be quickly reversed by ingesting something containing sugar. Handy sources of sugar include four ounces of orange juice, half a nondiet cola, a few hard candies, two glucose tablets, or two sugar packets.

Within 30 minutes after the symptoms disappear, the individual should eat a light snack such as half a sandwich and a glass of milk. Severe hypoglycemic reactions can require intravenous glucose or an intramuscular glucagon injection—and these are necessary if the patient is obtunded and cannot safely be given oral glucose because of risk of aspiration. A therapist who has treated a patient for a severe hypoglycemic reaction should always notify the physician. Hypoglycemia caused by sulfonylureas can be prolonged and has a higher risk of mortality than that caused by insulin; patients can require short-term hospitalization (see Table 50–2).

Exercise and Diabetes

Individuals without diabetes can maintain stable blood glucose levels during exercise. However, physical activity can have a marked effect on blood glucose in a person with diabetes. Exercise in-

Table 50–2 Comparison of Diabetic Complications

Characteristic	Hyperglycemia with Diabetic Ketoacidosis (DKA)	Hyperglycemia Hyperosmolarity Nonketosis Coma	Hypoglycemia
Precipitating factors	Absence of insulin	Illness, infections, steroid use, burns	Excessive exogenous insulin, decreased oral intake, stress
Onset	Gradual	Gradual	Abrupt
Initial effect	Lethargy	Lethargy	Agitation, shakiness
Skin	Hot, dry	Warm	Clammy, diaphoretic
Serum glucose levels	> 300 mg/dL	> 300 mg/dL	< 70 mg/dL
Hydration	Increased thirst, polyuria, dehydration	Rapid volume depletion with increased thirst, initial polyuria progressing to decreased urine output	Unchanged
Cardiopulmonary symptoms	Rapid deep breathing		Tachycardia
Early CNS symptoms	Headache		Headache, blurred vision, slurred speech
Later CNS symptoms	Confusion, coma, death	Confusion, coma, death	Confusion, coma, rarely death
Metabolic acidosis	Elevated serum acetone, ketone bodies in urine, fruity breath	No	No
GI symptoms	Abdominal pain	Abdominal pain	Hunger
Intervention required	Insulin, fluid and sodium bicarbonate replacement	Insulin, fluid and electrolyte replacement	4 oz. juice, nondiet soda, 2 glucose tablets or 2–4 hard candies

creases glucose use by muscle and improves muscle sensitivity to insulin. A regular program of exercise may lower requirements for insulin or oral medication. These are desirable effects, but it should be recognized that exercise can increase risk of hypoglycemia. Thirty minutes of interval or continuous exercise can decrease blood glucose regardless of fitness level. Glucose control does not always improve with exercise, so the effect must be evaluated for each patient. The first step is to increase glucose monitoring during exercise, especially when starting a program. This is essential for patients on insulin or oral medications. Blood glucose can be monitored with a glucose meter and a paper blood glucose strip. An individual who cannot afford a meter can use the kind of strips that can be read visually. At the beginning of an exercise program, particularly with Type I diabetic patients, glucose levels should be checked prior to exercise, every 15 to 30 minutes during exercise, and after stopping exercise. A final blood glucose check should be performed approximately 4 to 5 hours later. Occasionally, glucose levels can continue to fall for up to 24 hours after exercising.

Hyperglycemia

In Type I diabetes, exercising during insulin insufficiency can promote a hyperglycemic response and place the individual at risk for metabolic acidosis. Additional insulin may have to be administered and exercise deferred if the glucose level is higher than 250 mg/dL or if ketones are present in the urine. With Type II, the upper value for deferring exercise is higher (300 mg/dL) because ketosis is far less common and is unlikely to be provoked by exercise. Occasionally, especially with elderly Type II individuals, a medical crises of severe hyperglycemia and cellular dehydration may develop, often in response to the physiological stress of infections, burns, or illness. These individuals may progress to a hyperglycemic, hyperosmolar, nonketotic coma. Because of the absence of ketosis, the diagnosis may be overlooked, and treatment delay can easily result in mortality in this population (see Table 50–2).

If exercise substantially lowers blood glucose, particularly if it drops into the range where hypoglycemia is a risk, then some of the following strategies should be considered. The most fundamental options are to either reduce insulin (or oral medication dose) on exercise days or to take a supplemental snack prior to exercise. One rule of thumb is to reduce an insulin dose by approximately 20%, but the glucose response to exercise will provide additional information for this decision. If weight loss is a goal, then it is desirable to avoid supplemental calorie intake. It is also important to consider the timing of exercise with respect to the timing of insulin or oral medication administration and meals. Exercise should be done at least 1 to 2 hours after meals, and vigorous exercise should be undertaken when insulin levels are near the lower range. This might be in the morning, prior to injection, or four or more hours after injection of regular insulin. Also, consideration should be given to the site of the insulin injection. Insulin injected over an exercising muscle is absorbed more quickly, and this translates into more potent glucose-lowering effects. Because of this, if exercising within 30 minutes of injection, a patient should be advised to use the abdomen, not the arm or thigh, for SQ injection of insulin (see Table 50–3).

It is common for a patient initially referred for physical therapy to have a relatively low fitness level. This factor, together with the many medical complications that have to be considered, mandate a careful assessment prior to exercise and a cautious and gradual introduction of exercise. The metabolic perturbations of diabetes may further limit exercise tolerance.

DIABETIC COMPLICATIONS

Diabetes is a systemic disorder, and the function of every organ system in the body can be affected by diabetes. This material emphasizes the complications that have particular relevance to rehabilitation (see Table 50–3).

Delayed Wound Healing

Delayed wound healing is a complication of diabetes that is related to poor metabolic control, arterial insufficiency, neuropathy, and other factors. Diabetic foot ulcers are a principal cause of the high rate of lower extremity amputation in diabetics, which is 10 to 13 times more likely than in nondiabetic individuals. Prevention of foot ulcers is the best therapy, and prevention starts with a careful foot and lower extremity exam along with an aggressive program of patient education.

Neuropathy

Neuropathy is common, with sensory loss more prevalent than motor loss (see Chapters 35 and 36). Sensory loss typically presents in a stocking/glove pattern. Patients unable to perceive the touch of a Semmes Weinstein 5.07 monofilament on the plan-

Table 50–3 Precautions to Take During Exercise if Diabetic

Physical Feature	Precaution
Hypoglycemia	• Exercise 45 to 60 min after eating. • May need to increase dietary intake prior to and during exercise, if necessary. • Keep sugar supplements handy. • Be aware of delayed onset (up to 24 hours).
Insulin levels	• Exercise 1 h after injections. • Monitor glucose levels carefully. • Avoid exercise during peak insulin activity. • Use caution when injecting insulin over an exercising muscle.
Cardiovascular functioning	• Be aware that vital signs may not be an accurate indicator of exercise tolerance. • Utilize perceived exertion scale, note dyspnea with exertion. • Do not exercise with resting claudication.
Proliferative retinopathy	• Keep systolic pressure $<$ 170 mmHg. • Avoid isometrics, Valsalva maneuvers, head-jarring.
Autonomic nervous system dysfunction	• Be alert to signs of cardiac denervation syndrome (heart rate unresponsive to activity level). • Orthostatic hypotension. • Inability to perceive presence of angina or MI. • Distal anhidrosis. • Poor heat compensation.
End-stage renal disease	• Stay hydrated. • Avoid systolic BP $>$ 170 mmHg.
Peripheral neuropathy	• Wear proper footwear. • Avoid repetitive stresses. • Monitor distal extremities closely.

tar surface of the foot are at high risk for ulceration. Decreased proprioceptive input may cause balance and motor deficits that typically affect the smaller intrinsic muscles of the feet, thus altering foot structure and pressure dynamics. Patients with insensitive feet (see Chapter 53) are at increased risk for callus or blister formation, and this can be the trigger event that leads to serious infection (see Chapter 54), ulcer formation (see Chapter 52), and loss of limb or life (see Chapter 51). Education of patients should include a recommendation against walking barefoot and suggestions that water temperatures be tested with the elbow and that daily foot inspections be made. Although walking is the form of exercise many older people prefer, and it has the considerable advantage of being a low-intensity, low-cost type of exercise, a diabetic patient with marked neuropathy or foot deformity may be exposed to increased risk for foot ulceration with a walking program. These individuals may benefit more from a nonweight-bearing type of exercise such as bicycling or swimming. Proper footwear, commonly prescription footwear with orthotics, may alleviate some of the risk. Loose cotton socks

are preferable to tight nylon ones. Medicare has authorized payments for podiatry visits and specialized footwear for diabetic individuals. When a below-knee amputation does occur, 60% of diabetic patients lose the remaining leg within 5 years. Smoking significantly compounds the problem.

Physical therapists who are treating orthopedic problems should document the concomitant diagnosis of diabetes, as this may help to justify extended treatments. The healing of a foot ulcer can take weeks to months and a multidisciplinary approach is necessary to optimize conditions.

Vascular Complications

Vascular complications are the leading cause of death among individuals with diabetes, as they are at increased risk for coronary artery disease, stroke, peripheral vascular disease (PVD), and hypertension. An examination of the feet of a diabetic should include palpation of pulses and consideration of referral for noninvasive vascular testing if abnormalities are found. Symptomatic PVD often presents as intermittent claudication resulting from a burning, cramping sensation, usually in the calf, that is caused by activity-induced ischemia. These symptoms can be difficult to distinguish from painful diabetic peripheral neuropathy. Some patients may have significant arterial disease yet remain asymptomatic because of low levels of activity, and the demands of rehabilitation may unmask these problems. Physical rehabilitation should emphasize a graded program of exercise to encourage collateral circulation to the limbs. This entails encouraging patients to exercise the involved muscles to the point of pain but to avoid persisting once ischemia begins. For calf claudication, heel lifts might be a good exercise. It usually takes about 3 months for symptomatic relief through collateral circulation to occur. If the PVD has progressed to the point of constant pain and resting claudication in the foot, all lower extremity exercises are contraindicated, as such individuals are at risk for limb loss and require surgical revascularization. Whenever peripheral vascular disease is present, individuals should consult with a physician before using any over-the-counter medications for the foot.

Autonomic Neuropathy

Autonomic neuropathy develops in the sympathetic and parasympathetic nervous systems of 20 to 40% of persons with long-term diabetes. Exercise programs for diabetic patients with autonomic neuropathy should proceed cautiously. Autonomic neuropathy can result in distal anhidrosis, with poor heat dissipation as a result of decreased sweating in the extremities. Patients with this symptom should avoid overheating when exercising. Genitourinary autonomic dysfunction leads to impotence and risk of urinary infections. Gastrointestinal disturbances include constipation and diarrhea.

Some individuals with autonomic involvement may present with significant cardiac autonomic neuropathy. These individuals may be at risk for "silent" myocardial infarction and do not perceive anginal pain. Cardiac arrhythmias are not uncommon. Cardiac denervation syndrome, a result of autonomic dysfunction, produces a heart rate that is typically around 80 to 90 beats per minute and is unresponsive to activity levels, β-blockers, and antiarrhythmics. If a sustained grip, holding the breath, or a Valsalva maneuver produces no changes in vital signs, cardiac denervation syndrome may be present. The inability of the system to augment cardiac output places such individuals at risk for postural hypotension. Orthostatic problems superimposed upon cerebral arteriosclerotic changes may precipitate transient ischemia attacks. Whenever

cardiac autonomic changes are present, monitoring vital signs to assess exercise tolerance may not always produce accurate information. Individuals in this state should have thorough cardiac workups prior to initiating increased activity levels. If cardiac neuropathy is present, emphasis should be placed on perceived exertion rates, dyspnea, and other observed symptoms of distress, and not simply on pulse and blood pressure. Exercise warm-ups and cool-downs should be emphasized. Patients prone to orthostatic changes may benefit from minimizing changes in position during rehabilitation, wearing compressive stockings, and being sure to have adequate fluid intake.

Retinopathy

Retinopathy is a frequent complication of diabetes, and although most cases are of the nonproliferative variety (with only mild background changes in vision), some patients progress to proliferative retinopathy, which is a leading cause of blindness in adults. There are no convincing data that prove exercise accelerates retinopathy, but if retinopathy is present, caution suggests that systolic blood pressure be kept below 170 mmHg during exercise and that activities that might increase systolic pressure, such as isometrics, Valsalva maneuvers, and heavy lifting, be avoided. It would seem prudent, too, that head-jarring exercises and activities that lower the head also be eliminated.

Nephropathy

Nephropathy can culminate in renal failure and is a serious complication of diabetes. The first sign of diabetic nephropathy is proteinuria. Although exercise increases urinary protein excretion, there is no convincing evidence that links exercise with the progression of nephropathy. However, sustained hypertension is an aggravating factor and blood pressure should be monitored during activity. For patients on dialysis therapy, fluid replacement is a crucial issue that must influence the scheduling of exercise and rehabilitation. Also, dialysis patients are given heparin during infusions, and any wound care that is performed within 24 hours of dialysis should minimize aggressive débridement. Exercise programs should incorporate anticoagulant precautions such as guarding against skin trauma caused by weights, hand placement, or jarring, especially at IV sites, and there should be renewed vigilance against falling.

CONCLUSION

Diabetes mellitus is a common and chronic disease that includes multisystem involvement. Many patients with diabetes mellitus need medical and rehabilitative care because of complications resulting from the diabetes or for other illness. It is important that the health-care provider be aware of the significant influence diabetes has on rehabilitation.

SUGGESTED READINGS

Betts EF, Betts JJ, Betts CJ. Pharmacologic management of hyperglycemia in diabetes mellitus: implications for physical therapy. *Phys Ther* 1995; 75:415–425.

Bottini P, Tantucci C, Scionti L, et al. Cardiovascular response to exercise in diabetic patients: influence of autonomic neuropathy of different severity. *Diabetologia* 1995; 38:244–250.

Campaigne BN, Lampman RM. *Exercise in the Clinical Management of Diabetes.* Champaign, Ill.: Human Kinetics; 1994.

Diabetes 1998 Vital Statistics. Alexandria, VA: American Diabetes Association; 1998.

Handbook of Diabetes Medical Nutrition Therapy. Powers MA, ed. Gaithersburg, Md.: Aspen Publishers; 1996.

Horton ES. Role and management of exercise in diabetes mellitus. *Diabetes Care* 1988; 11:201–209.

Kumar S, Fernando DJS, Veves AA, et al. Semmes-Weinstein monofilaments: a simple, effective and inexpensive screening device for identifying diabetic patients at risk of foot ulceration. *Diab Res and Clin Pract* 1991; 13:63–68.

Zinman B, Ruderman N, Campaigne B, Devlin J, Schneider S. Diabetes mellitus and exercise. *Diabetes Care* 1998; 21[suppl 1]:540–544.

WEBSITES

http://www.Diabetes.org/professional.htm
http://www.Niddk.NIH.gov

Chapter 51

Amputations
Joan E. Edelstein, M.A., P.T., F.I.S.P.O.

INTRODUCTION

Amputation refers to removal of part of a body segment. Geriatric patients are much more likely to have lower, than upper, limb amputations. Peripheral vascular disease, with or without diabetes, is the leading cause of amputation in the United States. A few elders have lost a limb as a result of congenital anomalies, cancer, or trauma, and in most instances the loss has occurred years earlier.

These people have accommodated their lifestyles to cope with the interference with walking and other daily activities imposed by amputation. Insidious skin and musculoskeletal changes associated with aging are troublesome to adults with amputations, regardless of cause, because of the added stress on remaining tissues that limb anomaly and a prosthesis impose. (See Chapter 71 for details about evaluating the patient and prescribing prostheses).

The National Center for Health Statistics reported an annual vascular amputation census of 109,000. The rate of vascular amputation in the United States has remained relatively constant for the past decade. Nonvascular amputations account for less than 10% of the total number of amputations.

CLASSIFICATION OF AMPUTATIONS

Amputations are classified according to anatomical location. Partial foot amputations are very common among patients with peripheral vascular disease. The levels include phalangeal, ray, and transmetatarsal amputations. Removal of one or more phalanges compromises transition during late stance. If an entire toe, including the proximal phalanx, is absent, then the longitudinal arch of the foot will be flattened because the insertion of the plantar aponeurosis has been disrupted. A ray pertains to a metatarsal and its phalanges. Ray amputation interferes with late stance and the longitudinal arch; the foot will be narrowed. Transmetatarsal amputation has major effects on late stance, foot support, and balance; the patient tends to lean backwards on the heel. In all instances of partial foot amputation, the individual should be fitted with a shoe that has a rocker sole to aid late stance and, if needed, an arch support. The shoe insert for the individual with ray amputation must have a longitudinal segment to prevent the narrowed foot from sliding in the shoe.

Syme's amputation involves removal of the entire foot, except for the calcaneal fat pad and the malleoli. The fat pad is sutured to the distal tibia and fibula. The patient should be fitted with a Syme's prosthesis which replaces the shape and basic function of the foot. Syme's and partial foot amputations are end-bearing; the patient can stand on the distal end of the amputated limb, which provides good support and sensory feedback.

Transtibial (below-knee) amputation is the most common site for major (that is, proximal to the ankle) lower-limb amputation. The functional outcome for sitting and walking is encouraging because the patient retains the anatomical knee. Transfemoral (above-knee) amputation carries a poorer prognosis for prosthetic use. Older individuals with transfemoral amputation who have a prosthesis generally rely on a wheelchair for travel in the community. Ankle, knee, and hip disarticulations are uncommon, particularly among older adults.

The older patient with bilateral amputations due to vascular disease generally sustained one amputation prior to the second one. The presence of diabetes accelerates loss of the contralateral limb, so any patient with an amputation due to diabetes must be taught proper care of the residual and contralateral limbs (see the discussion of education and prevention in Chapter 50, "Diabetes").

RELATED CONDITIONS

Older adults who sustain amputation often have other evidence of vascular disease, especially cardiovascular disease, which may compromise their ability to tolerate vigorous exercise programs. Severe cardiovascular disease, in which the patient is dyspneic at rest, contraindicates prosthetic fitting. Cerebrovascular disease is a frequent concomitant. Hemiparesis, usually ipsilateral, is not uncommon. Paresis does not preclude prosthetic use, particularly if the amputation antedated the stroke. When peripheral vascular disease in one limb is severe enough to lead to amputation, circulation in the opposite limb is also compromised. Individuals may complain of intermittent claudication after a short walk. Prosthetic fitting reduces stress on the remaining limb. The remaining foot is vulnerable to pressure sores, which can lead to amputation. Vigilant foot inspection and hygiene, as well as suitable footwear, are essential.

Severe arthritis in the lower limbs or the hands makes prosthetic donning and use more difficult. When peripheral vascular disease is associated with diabetes, the patient may exhibit obesity, visual impairment, proprioceptive and tactile loss, and renal dysfunction, all of which complicate the wearing of a prosthesis.

TESTS AND RELATED DIAGNOSES

In addition to tests of the peripheral vascular system, including angiography and Doppler ultrasound, the patient with an amputation should be investigated for sensory diminution. Tactile sensation may be graded with Semmes-Weinstein monofilaments, and proprioception can be judged with balance testing. Heart rate and blood pressure should be monitored so that the rehabilitation program can be kept at a challenging level without overstressing the patient.

The amputation limb requires daily inspection to identify any incipient ulceration. A patient who has had recent amputation should have the surgical scar examined to ascertain whether healing is proceeding satisfactorily. Amputation limbs at or above the transtibial level are measured longitudinally and circumferentially. The longer the amputation limb, the less energy the individual consumes while walking with a prosthesis. The clinician should measure the girth of the limb. The proximal measurement of the transtibial limb is taken at the fibular head. For the transfemoral limb it is taken at a fixed distance below the greater trochanter. Additional distal measurements are taken at 4-cm intervals. Consistent circumferential measurements indicate that edema has subsided and the patient is ready for the fitting of a prosthesis.

Joint excursion and muscle strength in all limbs and the trunk are assessed periodically. Hip and knee flexion contractures compromise a prosthetic alignment and the patient's ability to stand and walk with a prosthesis. Weakness interferes with the ability to maintain sitting balance, to transfer from bed to wheelchair or to standing, and to manage a prosthesis. The clinician should ask the patient about the presence and intensity of phantom sensation and pain (awareness of the missing body part), which may be chronic. If the absent foot or leg is painful, then intervention must be sought to ameliorate the pain; otherwise, the patient may not be able to master self-care or tolerate a prosthesis.

The initial evaluation should also include inquiry regarding the individual's functional level prior to surgery, including the extent of use of assistive devices such as a cane. Assessment of the patient's cognitive status is important because dementia may contraindicate prosthetic fitting. The individual who is not able to don underpants independently is a very poor candidate for prosthetic rehabilitation, for the person lacks understanding of a very familiar task or is unable to maneuver the torso and legs appropriately. The individual with bilateral amputation who could not use a unilateral prosthesis is not suited to bilateral prostheses. Other factors that influence rehabilitation include pertinent features of the home, such as the number of steps at the entrance and within the home, the presurgical ability of the patient to drive an automobile, and the vocational and avocational interests of the patient. For example, the person who enjoyed golfing prior to surgery should be provided with a prosthetic foot that accommodates to the sloping terrain of a golf course.

CLINICAL RELEVANCE: MOBILITY AND REHABILITATION

Rehabilitation of the patient with amputation involves specific measures designed to improve the health of the amputation limb and interventions that increase the individual's independence with and without a prosthesis. Early care is ordinarily conducted without a prosthesis. The goals of treating the amputation limb are to reduce postoperative pain, foster healing, stabilize limb volume, and prevent complications such as contractures and skin disorders. The patient should be guided toward increasing self-care, including dressing, grooming, personal hygiene, maneuvering in bed, and various transfers, such as from bed to wheelchair, from wheelchair to toilet, and to standing. Some older individuals with unilateral amputation are able to negotiate short distances with a walker or a pair of crutches and the remaining leg. These activities should not be performed unless the patient is wearing a clean sock and a well-fitting shoe on the intact foot.

Most people with unilateral amputation or bilateral transtibial amputation receive prostheses (see Chapter 71, "Prosthetics"). Rehabilitation aims to enable the individual to don and use the prosthesis safely either as the sole mode of locomotion or as an alternative to wheelchair mobility, particularly indoors. A preparatory prosthesis for balance during transfers or for cosmetic value may be considered. The clinic team, consisting of physician, physical therapist, and prosthetist, should select the prosthetic design and components that will provide the patient with the best opportunity to accomplish meaningful activities and that are within the individual's functional capacity. Prior to training a person in the use of a prosthesis, the physical therapist should evaluate the fit and function of all its components.

THERAPEUTIC INTERVENTIONS

Early Care

Reducing postoperative edema has the triple benefit of diminishing pain, fostering healing, and stabilizing limb volume. Elastic bandaging of the amputation limb is intended to promote resorption of interstitial fluid. Most patients can learn to bandage a partial foot, Syme's, or transtibial amputation limb, but it is exceedingly difficult for a person of any age to apply an effective bandage to the transfemoral amputation limb. Regardless of amputation level, the elastic bandage loosens as the patient moves in bed or transfers into and out of the wheelchair. Consequently, the bandage must be reapplied several times a day. Elastic shrinker socks are easier to apply and can be used at the transtibial and transfemoral levels, although suspension on the thigh is difficult to maintain. As limb volume re-

duces, successively smaller socks are needed. They are used until limb girth stabilizes.

Elastic bandages and shrinker socks are the least effective ways of controlling edema. A rigid plaster dressing applied at the time of surgery is a much more effective way to control edema, particularly for transtibial amputation. Unless signs of infection are evident, the dressing is left in place until the time of suture removal. An aluminum or plastic pylon and a prosthetic foot can be attached to the rigid dressing to create an immediate postoperative prosthesis, although this modification is rarely used with older patients. However, age alone should not be the criterion for this procedure. Plaster dressings are more difficult to apply, require suspension from a waist belt, and usually prevent inspection of the operative wound. Sometimes the distal portion of the dressing over the scar is cut so that the plaster can be removed and replaced easily. Alternatively, a removable rigid dressing can be used, and it, too, allows for wound inspection. Removal of the plaster requires a cast cutter.

The Unna semirigid dressing is zinc oxide, calamine, gelatin, and glycerine in a gauze bandage. It combines the best features of an elastic bandage and a plaster dressing. The Unna dressing is easy to apply and remove, adheres to the skin and thus requires no waist belt, and promotes healing; it is well suited to amputations at every level, including transfemoral. The dressing remains on the limb until the sutures are removed. The semirigid dressing by itself cannot support a pylon and foot. After removal of the rigid or semirigid dressing, most patients wear a shrinker sock to resolve residual edema.

Additional Therapeutic Care

In addition to the use of the semirigid or rigid dressing, other interventions that focus on the amputation limb are those that reduce phantom pain, including ultrasound, transcutaneous electrical nerve stimulation (TENS), bilateral resistive exercise, and percussive massage. An educational program and peer support may help the patient accept the phenomenon of phantom sensation. Contractures can be prevented by encouraging the patient to alternate positions rather than remain seated. A bivalved plaster or a canvas knee splint and a wheelchair knee support retard development of a knee flexion contracture. Resistive exercises should emphasize hip and knee extension. After it has healed, the scar can be massaged to prevent adherence.

Independence is fostered by interventions that enable the patient to resume self-care and mobility.

Most times, the patient is fitted with a wheelchair. It is important that the chair be neither too large nor too small. The seat should have a firm foundation and a proper cushion to distribute pressure. A lumbar support to overcome the slingback effect of a flexible backrest is helpful. The brakes must be operative.

Leg amputation shifts one's center of gravity posteriorly. Consequently, either a special model with posteriorly offset wheels should be obtained or an adapter should be bolted to the rear wheels of a standard wheelchair. The wheelchair will then have an increased base of support, preventing upset of the wheelchair and its occupant when ascending steep ramps. The person with unilateral amputation should have a wheelchair with swing-out footrests so that the remaining foot and the prosthesis can be supported. The individual with bilateral amputations who is not a candidate for prostheses will have a less difficult time transferring if the wheelchair does not have footrests, but removable armrests may be facilitative.

The physical therapist should demonstrate the safest way of transferring into and out of the wheelchair and the most efficient ways of maneuvering it. The home may require modification to accommodate the wheelchair, such as rearrangement of furniture to create a pathway for the wheelchair and removal of throw rugs and saddle boards at doorways to ease the rolling of the wheelchair. If the wheelchair cannot fit through the bathroom door, then a commode and alternative bathing facilities will be needed.

Aerobic conditioning exercises are beneficial. Special attention should be paid to improving the flexibility, coordination, and strength of the hands, shoulders, and trunk. All patients should be provided with a suitable shoe and should be taught how to inspect and clean the foot. Peer support helps many patients and their families cope with the emotional and practical problems associated with amputation.

Rehabilitation

The basic rehabilitation program emphasizes the correct donning of the prosthesis, transfer into and out of chairs, standing balance, and walking. Instruction in care of the amputation limb and the prosthesis is imperative. Some older adults are able to climb stairs and ramps, drive a car, and engage in a wide range of recreational activities once they become used to the prosthesis.

Applying a partial foot prosthesis generally involves slipping the prosthesis into the shoe, donning the appropriate sock, making sure that it is not wrinkled, and finally inserting the foot into the shoe. The sequence for donning the usual transtibial prosthesis is to put the sock and shoe on the prosthetic foot, drape the trouser around the prosthesis, don the amputation limb sock, insert the amputation limb into the socket, and secure any straps or other fastenings. Some people prefer to don the amputation limb sock and the socket liner and then enter the socket. The entire sequence can be performed while sitting.

Donning the transfemoral prosthesis is begun while sitting. The patient applies the amputation limb sock, removes the suction valve from the prosthetic socket, then places the thigh in the socket. At that point the patient stands and pulls the distal end of the sock through the valve hole in order to smooth superficial tissues into the socket. The patient tucks the sock end into the socket, installs the valve, and fastens the belt around the torso. If the prosthesis has total suction suspension, the easiest method is to lubricate the thigh, insert it into the socket while sitting or standing, and install the valve.

Teaching the patient to move safely from various chairs to the standing position and back again is the most critical aspect of prosthetic rehabilitation for the older adult. Regardless of amputation level, a patient has the easiest time moving from an armchair with a firm seat, such as the wheelchair. Both feet should be on the floor, with the sound foot placed slightly posterior. Initially, the patient may use the armrests to assist in rising.

Balancing with a prosthesis may begin at the parallel bars or at the side of a sturdy table. The latter approach prevents the individual from forming the habit of pulling, rather than pushing, on the supporting structure. The therapist should guide the patient in shifting from side to side, forwards and backwards, and diagonally while maintaining upright posture. Eventually, the patient should be able to shift weight without holding onto a support. Advanced balancing exercises include stepping on a low stool with the sound foot, thus prolonging weight-bearing on the prosthesis.

Gait training may involve the use of a cane, forearm crutch, or a walker, depending on the patient's ability to master balance exercises. Proper adjustment of the assistive device and instruction in its use are essential to promote safe walking. The goals of gait training are safety, symmetrical step length, and equal time spent on each leg. The therapist should be certain that the prosthesis fits well and that the adjustment of the prosthetic foot and knee unit remains appropriate for the patient. Gait training should include practice in walking on various surfaces, such as smooth flooring, carpets, and grass.

People who are able to walk safely on level surfaces should have an opportunity to climb stairs and ramps. The easiest task is ascending stairs that have a handrail on the contralateral side. Most individuals with transtibial or more distal amputations ascend and descend in a foot-over-foot manner, alternating feet on each step. In contrast, people with transfemoral prostheses ascend leading with the sound foot and descend leading with the prosthesis. A few exceptionally agile individuals learn to descend in a foot-over-foot pattern. Stair climbing by those who wear bilateral transfemoral prostheses is exceedingly rare. They may choose to ascend and to descend seated on the buttocks. Maximal assistance is often necessary. Two handrails may be facilitative, or an electric stair seat may be appropriate. Ramps pose a problem for those who wear prostheses, because most prosthetic feet have limited ranges of dorsiflexion and plantarflexion. Diagonal (sideways) climbing may be more practical for older adults.

Driving a car involves two concerns, namely transferring into and out of the car and operating the vehicle. The individual with a right amputation has an easier time entering the passenger side. With a left prosthesis, the patient should first sit sideways on the passenger's seat and then lift the prosthesis to the forward-facing position while pivoting on the buttocks. Operating an automobile that has automatic transmission is easier for the individual with left amputation. The adult with a right prosthesis may choose to cross the left leg so that the sensate left foot moves the accelerator and brake pedals. Others install an extension to the accelerator so that the left foot can reach it comfortably. Individuals with transtibial amputation often require no special adaptation or equipment for driving.

Many recreational pursuits are popular with older adults who have amputations. Some sports such as swimming require no prosthesis. Other activities such as golfing demand good balance and rotational control on uneven terrain and may be attainable by some.

CONCLUSION

Amputation of a body segment in an aging person is usually the result of peripheral vascular disease. The incidence of amputation due to vascular problems has remained essentially unchanged for the past 10 years. Rehabilitation of an older person who has had an amputation should be focused on independence. In a few instances, coexisting pathologies may preclude prosthetic fitting or aggressive efforts in rehabilitation, but with proper care and environmental modifications, some older patients with amputations are able to resume full independence, including driving a vehicle and participating in recreational activities and sports.

SUGGESTED READINGS

Bowker JH, Michael JW, eds. *Atlas of Limb Prosthetics*, 2nd ed. St. Louis: C.V. Mosby; 1992.

Burgess EM, Rappoport A. *Physical Fitness: A Guide for Individuals with Lower Limb Loss.* Washington, D.C.: Department of Veterans Affairs; 1992.

Edelstein JE. Prosthetic assessment and management. In: O'Sullivan SB, Schmitz TJ, eds. *Physical Rehabilitation Assessment and Treatment*, 3rd ed. Philadelphia: F.A. Davis; 1994:397–422.

Greive AC, Lankhorst GJ. Functional outcome of lower-limb amputees: a prospective descriptive study in a general hospital. *Prosthet Orthot Int* 1996; 20:79–87.

Isakov E, Burger H, Krajnik J, et al. Double-limb support and step-length asymmetry in below-knee amputees. *Scand J Rehabil Med* 1996; 29:75–79.

Karacoloff LA, Hammersley CS, Schneider FJ. *Lower Extremity Amputation: A Guide to Functional Outcomes in Physical Therapy Management*, 2nd ed. Gaithersburg, Md.: Aspen Publications; 1992.

Roth EJ, Park KL, Sullivan WJ. Cardiovascular disease in patients with dysvascular amputation. *Arch Phys Med Rehabil* 1998; 79:205–215.

Sanderson DJ, Martin PE. Lower extremity kinematic and kinetic adaptation in unilateral below-knee amputees during walking. *Gait Posture* 1997; 6:126–136.

Chapter **52**

Wound Management

Pamela G. Unger, P.T.

INTRODUCTION

The integument (the skin) is a vital organ. When a human being sustains an injury to the integument a break has occurred in the protective barrier between the organs and the outside environment. This principle is crucial to the survival of the elderly. It is fairly common knowledge that chronic dermal wounds occur most frequently in the elderly. The human body's ability to heal is altered by various health problems—diabetes mellitus, circulatory problems, hypertension, and chronic obstructive pulmonary disease (COPD). Normal age-related changes in the skin also affect the rate and quality of healing (see Chapter 54, "Skin Disorders"), and there may be additional risk factors, including inadequate nutrition, limited mobility, and muscle atrophy.

WOUNDS AND THE HEALING PROCESS

The normal healing process has three phases. The body's natural response to injury is to activate the inflammatory response. The inflammatory response extends from injury to 4 to 6 days after the injury. The process follows a normal sequence of events, including vasoconstriction, fibrin clots, vasodilation, and the presence of neutrophils and macrophages that remove bacteria and debris. The proliferative phase occurs approximately 7 days after injury. This phase includes the utilization of growth factors—endothelial cells, fibroblasts, new blood vessels, and collagen. The growth factors also generate keratinocytes that cause reepithelialization. In the remodeling phase, there is no longer an open wound. During this phase the connective tissue becomes better aligned and tensile strength increases. This process can take up to a year to complete.

Wounds are generally classified according to the predominant underlying cause. Common categories include arterial insufficiency, venous insufficiency, pressure ulcers, neurotrophic ulcers, traumatic wounds, and burns. There are several wound classification systems. Box 52–1 presents pressure ulcer classification stages I–IV, burn degrees, and partial- and full-thickness differentiation for all wounds not included in the other classifications. The Wagner system is another important assessment tool (Box 52–2).

EVALUATING THE PATIENT

The evaluation of a patient with a wound should be completed by a multidisciplinary team (physician, nurse, therapist, social worker). The physical therapist on the wound care team plays an important role and must have expertise in dealing with the integument. This expertise should include not only

---

Box 52–1

Wound Classification Systems

PRESSURE ULCERS

Stage I:	Nonblanchable erythema of intact skin, the heralding lesion of skin ulceration
Stage II:	Partial-thickness skin loss involving epidermis and/or dermis; ulcer is superficial and presents clinically as an abrasion, blister, or hollow crater
Stage III:	Full-thickness skin loss involving damage or necrosis of subcutaneous tissue that may extend down to, but not through, underlying fascia; ulcer presents clinically as a deep crater with or without undermining of the adjacent tissue
Stage IV:	Full-thickness skin loss with extensive destruction, tissue necrosis, or damage to muscle, bone, or supporting structures (for example, tendon or joint capsule)

BURNS

1st-degree:	Involves the superficial epidermal layer; skin is pink or red, dry and painful, and sheds within a week without residual scar
2nd-degree:	Involves the epidermis and the dermis; wound is immediately blistered and wet, local edema is present; if superficial, will heal within 2–3 weeks and will not scar if not infected or unduly traumatized; if deep, may require skin grafting to achieve optimal healing
3rd-degree:	Involves the entire thickness of the skin; wound varies in color from white to black and may present with dark networks of thrombosed capillaries that do not blanch with pressure; surface is usually dry, but may be wet; these wounds require skin grafting for closure if more than 1 in in diameter

Burns are also designated, at times, by partial- and full-thickness; 1st- and 2nd-degree burns are synonymous with partial-thickness. Full-thickness burns are those in which the entire epidermis has been destroyed. Parts of the dermis may also be destroyed, along with injury into the subcutaneous structures.

VENOUS, ARTERIAL, AND TRAUMATIC WOUNDS

Partial-thickness:	Penetration into the epidermis or into the beginning of the dermis
Full-thickness:	Penetration into the subcutaneous tissue, muscle, or bone

Box 52-2

Wagner Classification System
of Ulcer Stages

STAGE	DESCRIPTION
0	Intact skin
1	Superficial ulcer involving skin only
2	Deep ulcer involving muscle and, perhaps, bone and joint structures
3	Localized infection; may be abscess or osteomyelitis
4	Gangrene, limited to forefoot area
5	Gangrene of the majority of the foot

active range of motion of all joints, bed mobility, transfers, and gait status, but also the classification of wounds. This information can then be processed to establish a plan of care that optimizes wound homeostasis and healing.

When initiating the evaluation, the following elements should be included (see Figs. 52–1, 52–2, and 52–3):

- Obtain a thorough medical history; the patient's past medial history may predispose him or her to a nonhealing wound (e.g., diabetes mellitus or peripheral vascular disease).
- Encourage the patient's primary care physician to evaluate the patient's medical status extensively (e.g., blood sugars, albumin, hemoglobin, and medications).
- Assess the patient's physical mobility. Contractures may predispose a patient to pressure ulcers. Immobility limits a patient's ability to change positions in bed or a chair.
- Assess the integument. Is it well hydrated? Is there good turgor?
- Assess nutrition. What and how much is your patient eating?
- Assess the patient's support surface. What type of bed, chair, and shoes does the patient use regularly?
- Review the patient's personal care (hygiene).
- Assess peripheral pulses.
- Assess the wound:
  - specific location of the wound
  - size of the wound—length, width, depth
  - wound classification
  - wound odor
  - percentage of necrotic tissue
  - drainage—amount, odor, color, consistency
- presence of undermining or tunneling
- wound color
- periwound condition
- girth measurements (when applicable).

Distinguishing among Types of Ulcers

In order to appropriately intervene it is crucial to distinguish among the various categories of ulcers (Table 52–1).

Venous insufficiency is defined as a disturbance in the forward flow of blood in the lower extremities that may progress to increased hydrostatic pressure, venous hypertension and, ultimately, dermal ulceration. The etiology includes valvular incompetence of lower extremity veins, obstruction of the deep venous system, congenital absence or malformation of valves in the venous system, and regurgitation from the deep to the superficial venous system. To assess venous insufficiency clinically, see Table 52–1. The treatment of venous insufficiency involves four major areas: (1) control of underlying medical and nutritional disorders, (2) education of the patient, (3) control of edema, and (4) topical therapy.

Arterial insufficiency is defined as insufficient arterial perfusion to an extremity or a particular location. The cause may be arteriosclerosis. Pain is a significant symptom associated with arterial insufficiency. The pain may be described as intermittent claudication or as resting, positional, nocturnal, or decreased in response to analgesia. A few simple tests for perfusion can be used: (1) Check for peripheral pulses; are they absent or diminished? (2) Check for a decrease in skin temperature. (3) Check for delayed capillary refill time (more than 3 seconds). (4) Check color; is there pallor on elevation or dependent rubor? The treatment of arterial insufficiency involves seven major focuses: (1) control underlying medical and nutritional disorders; (2) educate the patient; (3) manage the pain; (4) have the patient stop smoking; (5) control edema; (6) encourage ambulation to tolerance; (7) use topical therapy.

Neuropathic ulcers (also referred to as neurotrophic ulcers) have a direct correlation with peripheral neuropathy. Peripheral neuropathy is defined as an altered function in the extremities that may involve diminished or absent sensation in response to touch, pain, or temperature, absence of sweating, foot deformities, and altered gait and weight-bearing. Causes include damage to sensory, motor, and autonomic nerves of the lower extremities. The physical examination of the patient should include (1) palpation of peripheral pulses, (2) notation of skin temperature, (3) notation of skin color,

Physical History

Name _____ Date _____

Brief history: _____

_____

_____

_____

Past medical history:

  Major illness

        Cardiovascular: Coronary disease _____ Angina _____

                           Congestive heart failure _____ Arrhythmia _____

                           Myocardial infarct _____ Hypertension _____

                           Hypercholesterol _____

                           Other _____

        Pulmonary: COPD _____ Pneumonia _____

                           TB _____ Asthma _____

                           Other _____

        Diabetes mellitus: Insulin-dependent _____

                           Noninsulin-dependent _____

        Vascular: Claudication _____ Rest Pain _____

                           Varicose veins _____ DVT _____

                           Other_____

        Musculoskeletal: Arthritis _____ Muscle weakness _____

                           Fractures _____

        GI: Peptic ulcer disease _____ Cirrhosis _____

                           Bleeding _____ Hepatitis _____

                           Pancreatitis _____ Other _____

        GU: Kidneys _____

                           Bladder _____

                           Other _____

        Hematology: Anemia _____ Bruisability _____

                           Sickle cell anemia _____

                         Bleeding tendency _____

        Neuro: TIA _____ Stroke _____ RIND _____

                         Other _____

        Malignancies: _____

                      _____

                      _____

        Operations: _____

                      _____

                      _____

                      _____

        Injuries: _____

                      _____

                      _____

                      _____

        Hospitalizations: _____

                      _____

                      _____

                      _____

                      _____

                      _____

Figure 52-1 *See legend on opposite page*

Medications: _____

Allergies: _____

Social history: _____
  Occupation _____
  Smoke _____
  Alcohol _____
  Drugs _____
Family history: _____

Family physician: _____
Other physicians: _____

Reviewed by: _____ RN

_____ PT

_____ MD

Figure 52–1 Sample form for taking a patient history.

(4) assessment of capillary refill (less than 3 seconds), and (5) assessment of motor, sensory, and autonomic neuropathy. The treatment of the neuropathic ulcers involves six major areas: (1) control of underlying medical and nutritional disorders, (2) patient education, (3) cessation of smoking, (4) good control of diabetes, (5) no weight-bearing on the affected area, (6) topical therapy.

Pressure ulcers are a serious problem that can affect patients regardless of their usual living environments. Pressure ulcers lead to pain, longer hospital stays, and slower recovery. They are defined as lesions caused by unrelieved pressure that results in damage to underlying tissue and usually develop over bony prominences. The staging system for pressure ulcers classifies the degree of tissue damage. It is important to note that pressure ulcers do not necessarily progress from stage I to stage IV, and they do not heal from stage IV to stage I. The treatment of pressure ulcers involves six major areas: (1) control of underlying medical and nutri-

tional disorders, (2) management of tissue loads, (3) ulcer care, (4) topical therapy, (5) management of bacterial colonization and infection, and (6) education. Individuals with limited mobility should always be assessed for additional factors that increase the risk for developing pressure ulcers. These factors include immobility, incontinence, nutritional factors, and altered levels of consciousness. The multidisciplinary team should adopt a validated risk assessment tool such as the Braden Scale or the Norton Scale (Tables 52–2 and 52–3). The results recorded on the scales should be documented and used periodically to reassess the patient's risk.

THERAPEUTIC INTERVENTION

A wide variety of adjunctive procedures are used by physical therapists to treat patients with chronic dermal wounds (see Tables 52–4 and 52–5). When physical therapy intervention is utilized, the two

Physical Assessment

General

Alert _____ Oriented _____ Ht. _____ Wt. _____

Vital signs

Temp _____ Pulse _____ Resp _____ BP _____

_____ RN

HEENT

Normal _____ Abnormal _____

Neck

JVD _____ Nodes _____ Bruits _____ Thyroid _____

Heart

Regular _____ Irregular _____

Lungs

Clear _____ Rhonchi _____ Rales _____ Wheezes _____

Abdomen

Tenderness _____ Masses _____ Hernias _____ Organs _____

Extremities

Edema _____ Cyanosis _____ Clubbing _____

Other _____

Pulses (0–4+)

Radial Femoral Popliteal Dorsalis Pedis Post Tibial

RT

LT

Description of wound: _____

_____

_____

_____

Impression: _____

_____

_____

_____

Plan: _____

_____

_____

_____

_____ MD

Figure 52–2 Sample physical assessment form.

primary goals are (1) to directly amplify the body's natural healing process and (2) to eliminate factors that block the activity of the body's natural healing processes.

Hydrotherapy is the oldest known modality of physical therapy. Its use is crucial to the cleansing of wounds. Over the years, hydrotherapy has taken various forms, such as whirlpools, water piks, and pulsatile lavage. The combination of water, heat, and agitation is successful in cleansing, softening necrotic tissue, assisting with the debridement process, and removing residues left after the application of topical agents (see Table 52–4).

Compression therapy is the primary modality used to control edema. Edema is major factor in the lack of healing of lower extremity ulcers complicated by venous insufficiency. Compression devices assist in decreasing interstitial fluid. The pressure shift encourages the movement of fluid and proteins from the interstitial spaces into the veins and lymphatics. Compression therapy can be provided by a variety of devices, among them intermittent/sequential compression pumps, custom-made elastic stockings, Unna's boots, elastic bandages, and ready-made elastic stockings. The goal of compression is to provide sufficient compression to stimulate fluid resorption. The compression found in elastic garments ranges from 8 mmHg to 60 mmHg. Pressure greater than 40 mmHg may occlude blood flow, so caution is necessary if arterial insufficiency is suspected. In general practice, the compressive stocking is donned prior to getting out of bed and removed prior to bedtime. One common occurrence in the geriatric population is the inability to pull on

Text continued on page 264

Name _____

Date _____

Pulses: (R) Post. Tib. _____ Dorsalis Pedis. _____ Popliteal _____

   (L) Post. Tib. _____ Dorsalis Pedis. _____ Popliteal _____

Location: _____

Type of wound: _____

_____

_____

                Stage:

Partial/full thickness: _____

_____

Size/depth: _____

_____

Exposed tendon: _____

Exposed bone: _____

Color: _____

_____

_____

Percent of necrosis: _____

_____

_____

Drainage: _____

_____

_____

Odor: _____

_____

Undermining: _____

_____

_____

Periwound condition: _____

_____

_____

_____

Assessment: _____

_____

_____

_____

Plan: _____

_____

_____

_____

_____

Figure 52-3 Sample wound evaluation form.

Table 52-1 Clinical Typing of Ulcers

	Pressure	Venous	Arterial	Neuropathic
Location	Bony prominences	Medial aspect lower leg/ankle Superior to med. malleolus	Between toes, tips of toes Around lateral malleolus Over phalangeal heads	Plantar aspect of foot Metatarsal heads Heels Altered pressure points Site of repetitive trauma
Wound appearance	Redness present Tunneling/undermining present Necrotic tissue may be present Maceration present Induration present Pain present Odor present	Irregular wound margins Ruddy base (color) Shallow depth Moderate to heavy exudate Granulation present	Pale or necrotic base Granulation absent or minimal Minimal exudate Gangrene/necrosis Infection	Even, well-defined wound margins Variable depth Variable exudate Variable extent of necrotic tissue Granulation present
Surrounding skin	Erythema Possible induration	Erythema Possible induration Cellulitis Hemosiderin stains	Erythema Possible induration Cellulitis	Erythema Possible induration Cellulitis Callus frequently present
Pain	Frequent pain	Minimal unless infected or desiccated	Frequently painful	Usually painless
Prevention	Education Identify at-risk patients Improve tissue tolerance Protect against pressure	Patient education No smoking Adequate nutrition Skin care Optimize venous return Take medications Constant compression	Patient education No smoking Take medications Diabetes control Avoid leg crossing, cold, moisture Professional foot care Well-fitting footwear Pressure reduction	Patient education No smoking Take medications Control diabetes Avoid cold, moisture Daily footcare Appropriate footwear Avoid extreme temperatures Avoid external heat

Table 52-2 Braden Scale for Predicting Pressure-Sore Risk

Patient's Name	Evaluator's Name		Date of Assessment			
Sensory Perception Ability to respond meaningfully to pressure-related discomfort	**1. Completely limited:** Unresponsive (does not moan, flinch, or grasp) to painful stimuli due to diminished level of consciousness or sedation *or* limited ability to feel pain over most of body surface	**2. Very limited:** Responds only to painful stimuli; Cannot communicate discomfort except by moaning or restlessness *or* has a sensory impairment that limits the ability to feel pain or discomfort over ½ of body	**3. Slightly limited:** Responds to verbal commands but cannot always communicate discomfort or need to be turned *or* has some sensory impairment that limits ability to feel pain or discomfort in 1 or 2 extremities	**4. No impairment:** Responds to verbal commands; has no sensory deficit that would limit ability to feel or void pain or discomfort		
Moisture Degree to which skin is exposed to moisture	**1. Constantly moist:** Skin is kept moist almost constantly by perspiration, urine, etc. Dampness is detected every time patient is moved or turned	**2. Moist:** Skin is often but not always moist; Linen must be changed at least once a shift	**3. Occasionally moist:** Skin is occasionally moist, requiring an extra linen change approximately once a day	**4. Rarely moist:** Skin is usually dry; linen requires changing only at routine inervals		
Activity Degree of physical activity	**1. Bedfast:** Confined to bed	**2. Chairfast:** Ability to walk severely limited or nonexistent; cannot bear own weight and/or must be assisted into chair or wheelchair	**3. Walks occasionally:** Walks occasionally during day but for very short distances, with or without assistance; spends majority of each shift in bed or chair	**4. Walks frequently:** Walks outside the room at least twice a day and inside room at least once every 2 hours during waking hours		
Mobility Ability to change and control body position	**1. Completely immobile:** Does not make even slight changes in body or extremity position without assistance	**2. Very limited:** Makes occasional slight changes in body or extremity position but unable to make frequent or significant changes independently	**3. Slightly limited:** Makes frequent though slight changes in body or extremity position independently	**4. No limitations:** Makes major and frequent changes in position without assistance		

Table continued on following page

Table 52–2 Braden Scale for Predicting Pressure-Sore Risk *Continued*

Patient's Name		Evaluator's Name	Date of Assessment		
Nutrition Usual food intake pattern	**1. Very poor:** Never eats a complete meal; rarely eats more than ⅓ of any food offered; eats 2 servings or less of protein (meat or dairy products) per day; takes fluids poorly; does not take a liquid dietary supplement or is NPO[a] and/or maintained on clear liquids or IV[b] for more than 5 days	**2. Probably inadequate:** Rarely eats a complete meal and generally eats only about ½ of any food offered; protein intake includes only 3 servings of meat or dairy products per day; occasionally takes a dietary supplement, or receives less than optimum amount of liquid diet or tube feeding	**3. Adequate** Eats over ½ of most meals; eats a total of 4 servings of protein (meat, dairy products) each day; occasionally refuses a meal, but will usually take a supplement if offered or is on a tube feeding or TPN[c] regimen, which probably meets most of nutritional needs	**4. Excellent:** Eats most of every meal; never refuses a meal; usually eats a total of 4 or more servings of meat and dairy products; occasionally eats between meals; does not require supplementation	
Friction and Shear	**1. Problem:** Requires moderate to maximum assistance in moving; complete lifting without sliding against sheets is impossible; frequently slides down in bed or chair, requiring frequent repositioning with maximum assistance; spasticity, contractures, or agitation leads to almost constant friction	**2. Potential problem:** Moves feebly or requires minimum assistance; during a move skin probably slides to some extent against sheets, chair, restraints, or other devices; maintains relatively good position in chair or bed most of the time but occasionally slides down	**3. No apparent problem:** Moves in bed and in chair independently and has sufficient muscle strength to lift up completely during move; maintains good position in bed or chair at all times		
					Total score

[a] NPO, nothing by mouth
[b] IV, intravenously
[c] TPN, total parenteral nutrition
Braden BJ, Bergstrom N. A conceptual schema for the study of the etiology of pressure sores. *Rehabil Nurs* 1987;12:8–12.

Table 52-3 Norton Scale

Physical Condition		Mental Condition		Activity		Mobility		Incontinent		Total Score
Good	4	Alert	4	Ambulant	4	Full	4	Not	4	
Fair	3	Apathetic	3	Walk/help	3	Slightly Limited	3	Occasional	3	
Poor	2	Confused	2	Chairbound	2	Very Limited	2	Usually/urine	2	
Very Bad	1	Stupor	1	Bed	1	Immobile	1	Doubly	1	

Name	Date										

Source: Doreen Norton, Rhoda McLaren, and A.N. Exton-Smith. An investigation of geriatric nursing problems in the hospital. London, National Corporation for the Care of Old People (now the Centre for Policy on Ageing); 1962. Reprinted with permission.

Table 52–4 Treatment Suggestions

Electrical stimulation (high-voltage pulse current)	Initially ($-$) polarity, 50–80 pps, 100–150 volts
	After 5 visits (or when wound is clean), ($+$) polarity, 80–100 pps, 100 volts
	Electrode placement: dispersive pad proximal, foil electrode saline-soaked or conductive hydrogel pad directly into the wound
Hydrotherapy	
Whirlpool	10–20 min per treatment session (daily)
	Temperature 92–99°F
Pulsatile lavage	10–30 minutes in entirety, periodic placement of tube throughout the wound
	Room-temperature saline solution
Ultrasound: 3 MHz pulsed	
Partial-thickness wounds	0.5–1.5 W/cm^2 for 1 min/cm^2 area of wound
	Pulsed, 20–40% duty cycle
	Use hydrogel medium or conductive gel
	Use over the wound or around the wound periphery
1 MHz	
Full-thickness wounds	0.5–1.5 W/cm^2 for 1 min/cm^2 area of wound
	Pulsed, 20–40% duty cycle
	Use hydrogel medium or conductive gel
	Use over the wound or around the wound periphery
Compression	
Sequential/Intermittent	Ideally, patient is supine with lower extremity elevated
	Use mmHg pressure at least 20 mmHg below the diastolic reading of the blood pressure taken in the treatment position
	Treat for a minimum of 1h
	Treat in morning if possible
	Follow with static compression wrap
Static	Wrap bandage from MTP joints to two fingers below the fibula head
	Be certain to apply equal pressure
	Overlap bandage at least ⅔ with each wrap
	Cover with protective stocking or additional elastic wrap
Pulsed electromagnetic fields	
Thermal	5-min warm-up—5/10 cycle
	20-min treatment—10/12 cycle
	5-min cool down—5/10 cycle
	Treat once per day
Nonthermal	
Acute wound	30 min cycle, cycle 6
Chronic wound	45 min, cycle, cycle 4
	Treat once per day

the custom-made compression stockings. Therefore, compression pumps are a great help in fluid resorption.

Ultrasound (nonthermal) has been found to be effective in enhancing wound healing, particularly when venous insufficiency is a major factor. The 3 MHz unit is proposed to be the most effective frequency because with it, the most energy is absorbed by the superficial tissues. Ultrasound has been found to enhance the body's ability to move through the inflammatory to the proliferative phase. It has also been associated with less dense, more resilient scar tissue. Ultrasound must be adminis-

tered through a medium such as a hydrogel or a hydrogel sheet. The treatment can be administered either along the periphery or directly over the wound bed (see Table 52–4 for parameters).

Electrical stimulation has been advocated over the years for the enhancement of wound healing, regardless of the underlying cause. More than 20 studies address the effectiveness of electrical stimulation in enhancing wound healing. Unfortunately, the ideal parameters have yet to be defined. The majority of the protocols indicate the use of a pulsed, monophasic waveform. Electrical stimulation has been reported to be very successful in the

Table 52–5 Treatment Interventions

Treatment	Clinical Applications	Physiological Response
Hydrotherapy/Pulsatile lavage Dx: Neurotrophic 　　Venous 　　Arterial 　　Pressure ulcers 　　Diabetic 　　Burns 　　Acute trauma	Cleanse Debride Soak off dressings	Superficial heat/cold Micromassage Increased moisture
Ultrasound Dx: Neurotrophic 　　Venous 　　Arterial 　　Diabetic	Debride Promote clean wound bed	Increase microcirculation Edema absorption Superficial/deep heat
Compression Dx: Venous 　　Arterial 　　Diabetic 　　Burns	Reduce edema	Decrease venous hypertension Increase venous return
Electrical stimulation Dx: Pressure ulcers 　　Arterial 　　Diabetic 　　Neurotrophic 　　Venous 　　Acute Trauma 　　Burns	Debride Decrease infection Increase circulation Decrease pain Promote closure	Increase circulation Bactericidal effects Increase fibroblasts activity Decrease edema
Pulsed electromagnetic fields Dx: Diabetic 　　Arterial 　　Acute Trauma 　　Venous 　　Pressure Ulcers	Reduce pain Reduce edema	Edema reduction Increase transport of 　cutaneous oxygen

treatment of pressure ulcers. The current must be transmitted through a medium, such as a foil, carbon, self-adhesive, or conductive gel electrode. The electrode is placed directly into the wound, with a dispersive pad proximal. It is also recommended that the dispersive pad be of a larger size (see Table 52–4).

Pulsed electromagnetic fields are a relatively new entity in wound care. Solid-state equipment generates a radio-wave frequency into the tissues, creating an electrical charge in the tissues. The specifications include a 27.12 MHz frequency. To date, conclusive scientific evidence has not been established, although several clinical trials have been completed in the United States (see Table 52–4 for parameters).

Total contact casting is used primarily for the treatment of patients with neuropathic plantar ulcers that are classed as grades I and II. The goal of this treatment is to remove weight-bearing forces from inflamed tissues and immobilize them so healing can occur. Following the application of a total contact cast, a patient must be instructed in partial weight-bearing with an appropriate assistive device. Generally, these patients have altered sensation, which makes an exact fit crucial. The total contact cast is generally reapplied every 1 to 2 weeks, but loosening of the cast, large amounts of drainage, or damage to the cast require premature removal. In some cases a bivalve cast is appropriate. The patient must understand that the bivalve cast is not to be removed until bedtime.

CONCLUSION

Effective intervention for wound care requires a thorough evaluation and an individualized treatment plan established by a multidisciplinary team. The team must coordinate a plan that focuses on removing the factors that are contributing to the nonhealing status and on choosing an intervention that will foster healing. This plan may require constant revisions before healing is achieved. When healing has been attained, the patient, family, and caregivers must be educated in continued care and prevention.

SELECTED READINGS

Brown G. Diathermy: a renewed interest in a proven therapy. *Phys Ther Today* 1993; 78–80.

Gogia P. *Clinical Wound Management.* Thorofare, N.J.: Slack; 1995.

Guccione A. *Geriatric Physial Therapy.* St. Louis: Mosby-Year Book; 1993.

Kloth L, McCulloch J, Feedar J. *Wound Healing: Alternatives in Management.* Philadelphia: F.A. Davis; 1990.

Krasner D. *Chronic Wound Care.* King of Prussia, Pa.: Health Management Publications; 1990.

Mayrovitz H, Larsen P. Effects of pulsed electromagnetic fields on skin microvascular blood perfusion. *Wounds* 1992; 4:197–202.

Mulder G, Fairchild P, Jetter K. *Clinician's Pocket Guide to Chronic Wound Repair.* Highlands Ranch, Co.: Wound Healing Publications; 1995–1996.

Pressure Ulcers in Adults: Prediction and Prevention. U.S. Department of Health and Human Services, Agency for Health Care Policy and Research. Pub. No. 92-0050; May 1992.

Pressure Ulcer Treatment. U.S. Department of Health and Human Services, Agency for Health Care Policy and Research. Pub. No. 95-0653; December 1994.

Salzberg C, Cooper-Vastola SA, et al. The effects of non-thermal pulsed electromagnetic energy (diapulse) on wound healing of pressure ulcers in spinal cord-injured patients: a randomized, double-blind study. *Wounds* 1995; 7:11–16.

Tung S, Khaski A. The application of diapulse in the treatment of decubitus ulcers: case reports. *Contemp Surg* 1995; 47:27–31.

Venous Insufficiency, Arterial Insufficiency, Peripheral Neuropathy, Clinical Fact Sheet. Costa Mesa, Ca.: Wound Osteotomy Continence Nurses' Society.

Chapter 53

The Insensitive Foot

Jennifer M. Bottomley, Ph.D., M.S., P.T.

INTRODUCTION

Insensitivity of the foot is the usual end result of numerous pathological conditions that affect the elderly. Chronic diseases such as diabetes mellitus, Hansen's disease, peripheral vascular disease, Raynaud's disease, deep-vein thrombosis, spinal cord injury (e.g., spinal stenosis, tumors), peripheral nerve injuries, hormonal imbalances, and vitamin B complex deficiencies produce breakdown of the microvascular structures with diminution of sympathetic nerve endings and somatic sensory receptors leading to neuropathic conditions of the foot. These pathologies lead to a decrease in circulatory and peripheral nerve integrity, which results in edema, discoloration, diminished skin status, increased pain, absence of sensation and, ultimately, a decrease in functional mobility.

Typical warning signs such as changes in gait patterns and pain associated with foot pathologies are absent in the insensitive foot. Repetitive stress coupled with the loss of protective sensation are primary causes of foot ulcerations. The lack of a warning system for pain and abnormal stress on the plantar surface of the foot predispose the neuropathic foot to injury and ulceration. However, if the mechanisms of injury and the risk factors are recognized (Box 53–1), foot ulcerations are preventable and treatable injuries.

Neuropathic changes in the insensitive foot are a heterogeneous mixture of disorders that includes progressive distal polyneuropathy, ischemic mononeuropathy, amyotrophy, and neuroarthropathy. A combination of sensory, autonomic, and motor neuropathies of the foot results in symmetrical or asymmetrical loss of perception of pain and temperature. Sympathetic denervation can lead to a progressive mixed-fiber neuropathy with a loss in light touch and vibratory sensation and motor loss in the intrinsic muscles of the foot. Characteristic foot deformities such as hyperextension of the metatarsophalangeal joints, clawing of the toes, and distal migration of the fibroadipose cushions under the heel and metatarsal heads result in abnormal weight-bearing patterns and increased plantar pressures. Tissue damage to the insensitive foot may result from continuous pressure that causes ischemia or from concentrated high pressure, heat or cold, repetitive mechanical stress, or infection of the tissues.

Amyotrophic changes result from a lack of nourishment to the musculature. There is a progressive weakening and wasting of muscles accompanied initially by an aching or stabbing pain and resulting in the total loss of muscle function due to atrophy, paresthesia, paralysis, and loss of sensory input.

Neuropathic arthropathy results from joint erosions, unrecognized fractures, demineralization, and devitalization of the bones and articulations of the foot. Typically, these changes result from routine weight-bearing activities in the absence of normal protective proprioceptive and nociceptive functions of the peripheral sensory system. In the limb with intact sensation, pain inhibits functional activities and further trauma to the joints so that the hypertrophic or reparative phases of callus formation can commence. In the insensate limb, however, the injured part is repeatedly traumatized, leading to increased hyperemia and resorption of damaged bone.

Box 53–1

Risk Factors in the Neuropathic Foot

RISK FACTOR	POSSIBLE INJURY
Loss of protective sensation	Absence of pain-warning input
High plantar pressures	Ulcers occurring at peak pressure sites
Autonomic neuropathy	Dehydrated, inelastic skin
Previous ulceration or amputation	Concentration of stress over scar or lesion
Foot deformities	Increased local pressures
Neuropathic fractures	Increased plantar pressures and foot instability
Abnormal foot function	Abnormal load application
High activity level	Increased cumulative stress
Vascular disease	Devitalized tissue susceptible to injury, poor healing
Inadequate footwear or footcare	Decreased protection, instability, poor hygiene
Visual loss	Inappropriate assessment of environment, inability to inspect feet
Poor insulin regulation	Complications of diabetes

Text continued on page 272

Box 53–2

Risk Classification

0—No loss of protective sensation

1—Loss of protective sensation with no deformity or history of ulcer

2—Loss of protective sensation and deformity with no history of ulcer

3—Loss of protective sensation with history of ulceration

Loss of sensation in the joints and bones of the foot predisposes the neuropathic foot to bony destruction. Midtarsal fractures or dislocations and hypertrophic bone formation may lead to a Charcot's deformity, which is the collapse of the foot into severe rocker-bottom foot deformity. Charcot's fracture is evidenced by swelling and increased temperature in the area of bone involvement. Clinically, neuropathic fractures should be suspected in all patients with signs of inflammation in the absence of an open wound. Differential diagnosis, in addition to osteomyelitis, would include cellulitis, pyarthosis, and reflex sympathetic dystrophy.

EVALUATION OF THE NEUROPATHIC FOOT

Regular and comprehensive screening of the neuropathic foot is essential for early identification of risk factors that may predispose an elderly individual to injury (Fig. 53–1). The foot screening is a brief examination to identify the history of any previous ulceration, motor weakness, sensory dysfunction, or deformities that would predispose the foot to local areas of high stress. Circulatory status, color, temperature, general condition, and the presence of edema or skin lesions should be assessed. Based on the foot screening, the relative risk of foot complications can be determined for each individual.

The level of sensory loss that places an individual at risk for foot injury is referred to as loss of protective sensation. The use of nylon monofilaments calibrated to bend at 10 grams of force (Semmes-Weinstein monofilaments) is a precise method of determining loss of sensation. The inability to feel a monofilament of 5.07 grams has been determined to be the level at which loss of protective sensation occurs. A risk classification scheme identifies the individuals most likely to develop plantar ulceration and, therefore, most likely to benefit from protective footwear and education (Box 53–2).

FOOT SCREENING EVALUATION

Date _____

Name _____

Address _____

Phone (   ) _____

Sex _____ DOB _____

Language or Communication problems: No   Yes   (describe) _____

Primary Doctor/Podiatrist _____

Address _____

Phone (   ) _____

SUBJECTIVE DATA

Medical History: _____

_____

1. Do you have:
   - Arthritis _____
   - Circulatory Problems _____
   - Heart Disease _____
   - Diabetes Mellitus _____
   - Kidney Problems _____
   - High Blood Pressure _____
   - Foot Problems _____
   - Eye Problems _____
   - Thyroid Problems _____
   - Hearing Problems _____
   - Vertigo _____
   - Dizziness _____
   - Fx hip _____

2. Did you have an injury in the:

		Left Leg		Right Leg	
		Sprain	Fx	Sprain	Fx
No					
Yes	hip				
	knee				
	ankle				
	foot				
	back				

3. Are you experiencing any leg pain?

		Left Leg	Right Leg
No			
Yes	Hip		
	Knee		

Figure 53–1 Foot-screening evaluation guide.

FOOT SCREENING EVALUATION

4. Are you experiencing any foot pain?

		Left Leg	Right Leg
No			
Yes	Aching		
	Burning		
	Stabbing		
	Nail Pain		
	Shoe Pain		
	Met Heads		
	Toes		

Pain increased:

	Left Leg	Right Leg
when Standing		
when Walking		
when Wearing Shoes		
in the Morning		
in the Afternoon		
at other times (describe)		

OBJECTIVE DATA

1. Ambulates without assistance?   No   Yes

2. Ambulates with assistive devices?   No   Yes

cane	
walker	
crutches	
other	

3. Falls? No Yes   describe _____

4. Distance Ambulated?   Home   1 Block   2 Blocks   5 Blocks   1 Mile   Unlimited

5. Regular Exercise?   No   Yes

6. Examination of Feet (Removing shoes and stockings)

	Left Foot		Right Foot	
	Unacceptable	Acceptable	Unacceptable	Acceptable
Cleanliness of foot?				
Socks/stockings a good fit?				
Proper fitting shoes? ____	Short		Short	
	Long		Long	
	Narrow		Narrow	
	Worn down		Worn down	
Shoe Wear: Heel ____				
Sole ____				
Lateral Counter ____				

Figure 53–1 *Continued*

Illustration continued on following page

FOOT SCREENING EVALUATION

7. Problems

• Bunions

	Left Foot	Right Foot
HAV		
Taylor		

		Left Foot					Right Foot				
		I	II	III	IV	V	I	II	III	IV	V
• Calluses	Spin										
	Pinch										
	IPK										
	Sub										
	Shear										
• Corns	Met Heads										
	Heloma Molle										
	Heloma Duram										
• Involuted Nails											
• Ingrown Toenails											
• Nail Trophic Changes											

• Circulatory Problems

Left Foot		Right Foot	
DPP: 0	PTP: 0	DPP: 0	PTP: 0
1+	1+	1+	1+
2+	2+	2+	2+
3+	3+	3+	3+

		I	II	III	IV	V	I	II	III	IV	V
• Toe Clubbing											
• Toe Deformities	Hammer										
	Claw										
	Mallet										
	Overlap										
	Hallux										
		I	II	III	IV	V	I	II	III	IV	V

	Left Leg	Right Leg
• Foot/Ankle Deformities		
• Dermatitis (PI) Fungus Infection		
• Dry, Scaly Skin		
• Edema Foot		
Ankle		
Extremity		

• Infection (Describe) _____

• Other _____

Figure 53–1 *Continued*

FOOT SCREENING EVALUATION

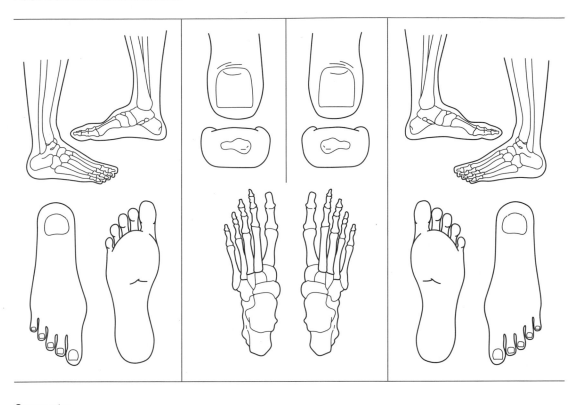

Comments:

_____

_____

_____

ASSESSMENT

_____

_____

_____

Recommend: • None
                    • Refer to Orthotics Clinic   Date: _____ Time: _____
                    • Refer for Shoes
                    • Refer to Pediatrist
                    • Refer to Podiatrist
                    • Educated in _____
                    • Orthotics Fabricated   Date: _____ Time: _____

                           _____

                           _____

         2-month follow-up: Date: _____ Time: _____
         6-month follow-up: Date: _____ Time: _____

Figure 53–1 _Continued_

Evaluating Sensation and Neurological Involvement

Protective sensation, as defined by Nawcozenski and Birke, is 5.07 grams of pressure using the Semmes-Weinstein monofilaments. Specific evaluation of the entire plantar surface of the foot determines areas of sensory loss that are vulnerable to breakdown.

Vibratory and temperature sense are diminished very early in the process of peripheral vascular disease, and that loss compromises proprioception, kinesthesia, and awareness of temperature gradients.

The neurological examination requires a reflex hammer, a tuning fork (128 cps), and Semmes-Weinstein monofilaments. Testing for vibratory, proprioceptive, temperature, and protective sensation should be done with the patient's eyes closed. Distinguish the boundaries of any hyper- or hypoesthesias and determine whether these patterns are symmetrical or asymmetrical. The absence or presence of sweating should be noted. Reflexes to be tested include the patellar reflex and the ankle jerk. As the ankle jerk is increasingly difficult to elicit with increasing age, it may appear to be absent. To aid this reflex, gently pronate and dorsiflex the foot to put tension on the Achilles tendon and gently tap the tendon. Test for the Babinski reflex to determine whether there is a superficial plantar response. To determine if there is clonus, forcibly dorsiflex the foot at the ankle. To test for loss of balance, have the individual stand with eyes closed and feet close together and compare this to the same stance with the eyes open (Romberg's sign).

Muscle strength should be tested in all lower extremity muscles using a graded manual muscle test. Again, symmetry should be noted. Gait evaluation is a helpful adjunct to muscular evaluation to determine unsteady gait patterns, foot-drops, or the presence of a "steppage" gait. Range of motion and joint mobility should be evaluated and any deformities (e.g., Charcot joints, hammer, claw, or mallet toes, hallux abductus valgus) should be noted, as these abnormalities are usually indicative of intrinsic foot muscle weakness. Trophic nail changes should also be evaluated.

The Semmes-Weinstein monofilaments have been found to be a reproducible and accurate way to test sensation, and it is reliable in predicting which individuals are at risk for ulceration due to loss of protective sensation. The Carville group of the G. W. Long Hansen's Disease Center in Carville, La. measured protective sensation using the Semmes-Weinstein monofilaments and found that individuals who could not feel the 5.07 monofilament were at greater risk for skin breakdown than were those who could feel this level of stimulation. They demonstrated that 5.07 was the threshold of protective sensation. Standardization of sensory testing is crucial in evaluation so that adequate protective measures can be taken to prevent feet at risk from developing ulcers.

Evaluation of Circulatory Status

Vascular evaluation should include the palpation and grading of the femoral, popliteal, dorsalis pedis, and posterior tibial pulses and the observation of other clinical signs and symptoms indicating vascular compromise in the lower extremities. These include intermittent claudication, foot temperature (i.e., cold feet), nocturnal pain, rest pain, nocturnal and rest pain relieved by dependency, blanching on elevation, delayed venous filling time after elevation, dependent rubor, atrophic skin, absence of hair growth, and presence of gangrene. Any lesions or areas of hyperkeratosis or discoloration should be observed.

Palpating for the pedal pulses can yield a qualitative measure of the dorsalis pedis or posterior tibial circulation, but the examiner must realize that there can be a substantial decrease in flow to the extremity even though arterial ankle pulses are good.

To differentiate an organic disorder such as blockage of the lumen of the vessel from a vasospastic condition, temporary dilation of the vessel in question is a useful vascular test. This is accomplished by using an arterial tourniquet for 3 minutes and then releasing it. The perfusion distal to the tourniquet should increase if the condition is due to vasospasm.

Observation of blanching and filling times is accomplished by using the Buerger-Allen vascular assessment (see Figs. 53–2, 53–3, and 53–4). A stopwatch is used to determine the time it takes the veins in the dorsum of the foot to fill with blood after they have been drained by elevating the leg. Basically, this is a means of appraising the general circulation in the foot. The arterial blood being pumped into the dependent leg diffuses into the arterioles, the capillaries, and the venules and then into the veins of the foot. The time of venous filling is subject to several variables: the arterial blood pressure, the caliber of the arteries, the volume of blood reaching the capillary bed of the foot with each thrust of the heart, and the rate of venous return. A filling time of up to 20 seconds indicates reasonably good collateral circulation. A venous filling time longer than 20 seconds is indicative of a compromised peripheral vascular system and of venous insufficiency.

The rubor of the skin should be noted. Depen-

BUERGER-ALLEN INITIAL EVALUATION[1]

PATIENT_____ AGE_____ SEX_____ RM#_____
DIAGNOSIS_____ PHYSICIAN_____
DATE INITIAL EVAL_____ THERAPIST_____
Signature

	RIGHT LE	LEFT LE
APPEARANCE:		
SKIN INTEGRITY:		
SKIN TEMP:		

EDEMA PRESENT: 0☐ +1☐ +2☐ +3☐   0☐ +1☐ +2☐ +3☐

CIRCUMFERENTIAL:

	RIGHT	LEFT
☐MET HEADS		
☐ARCH		
☐ANKLE		
☐SUPRA MALLEOLAR		
☐MID CALF		
☐SUB PATELLAR		

PULSES:

		RIGHT	LEFT
	DORSAL PEDALIS	0☐ +1☐ +2☐ +3☐	0☐ +1☐ +2☐ +3☐
	POST TIBIALIS	0☐ +1☐ +2☐ +3☐	0☐ +1☐ +2☐ +3☐
	POPLITEAL	0☐ +1☐ +2☐ +3☐	0☐ +1☐ +2☐ +3☐
	FEMORAL	0☐ +1☐ +2☐ +3☐	0☐ +1☐ +2☐ +3☐

SENSORY TESTING:

VIBRATORY SENSE: ☐PRESENT   ☐PRESENT
☐DIMINISHED   ☐DIMINISHED
☐ABSENT   ☐ABSENT

PROTECTIVE SENSATION:

1 = 01 gr (4.17 for Normal)
2 = 10 gr (5.07 Protective Sense)
3 = 75 gr (6.10 Loss Protective Sense)
4 = No Protective Sensation

DORSUM:	1☐ 2☐ 3☐ 4☐	1☐ 2☐ 3☐ 4☐
PLANTAR DIGIT 1:	1☐ 2☐ 3☐ 4☐	1☐ 2☐ 3☐ 4☐
PLANTAR DIGIT 3:	1☐ 2☐ 3☐ 4☐	1☐ 2☐ 3☐ 4☐
PLANTAR DIGIT 5:	1☐ 2☐ 3☐ 4☐	1☐ 2☐ 3☐ 4☐
MET HEAD 1:	1☐ 2☐ 3☐ 4☐	1☐ 2☐ 3☐ 4☐
MET HEAD 3:	1☐ 2☐ 3☐ 4☐	1☐ 2☐ 3☐ 4☐
MET HEAD 5:	1☐ 2☐ 3☐ 4☐	1☐ 2☐ 3☐ 4☐
PROXIMAL HEAD 5:	1☐ 2☐ 3☐ 4☐	1☐ 2☐ 3☐ 4☐
ARCH:	1☐ 2☐ 3☐ 4☐	1☐ 2☐ 3☐ 4☐
HEEL:	1☐ 2☐ 3☐ 4☐	1☐ 2☐ 3☐ 4☐

STRENGTH:

RIGHT		LEFT
	Anterior Tibialis	
	Extensor Hallucis Longus	
	Flexor Hallucis Longus	
	Posterior Tibialis	
	Peroneus Longus	
	Gastroc / Soleus	
	Intrinsics (S / W / A)	

DEFORMITIES:

	RIGHT	LEFT
Hammer/Claw:		
Boney Prominence:		
Drop Foot:		
Charcot Foot:		
Hallux Limitus		
Rear/ForeFt Varus:		
Plantar flexed 1st:		
Equinus:		
Amputation:		

FOOTWEAR: ☐STANDARD   ☐SPECIAL   DESCRIBE_____
☐ADEQUATE   ☐INADEQUATE   DESCRIBE_____

BLANCHING/FILLING TIMES: _____ ELEVATED _____ HORIZONTAL _____ DEPENDENT

TREATMENT RECOMMENDATIONS:[2]
☐BUERGER-ALLEN EXERCISES   CYCLES_____   TIMES/DAY_____   MODIFIED   Yes / No
☐PATIENT EDUCATION   ☐SKIN CARE   ☐FOOTWEAR   ☐ORTHOTICS

[1] BUERGER-ALLEN EVALUATION FORM CREATED BY: JENNIFER M. BOTTOMLEY, Ph.D, MS, PT © 1996
[2] REFER TO BUERGER-ALLEN TREATMENT FLOWSHEET FOR INITIAL BLANCHING/FILLING TIMES etc.

Figure 53–2 Buerger-Allen Initial Evaluation form.

BUERGER-ALLEN FOLLOW-UP EVALUATION[3]

PATIENT_____ AGE_____ SEX_____ RM#_____ MD_____

DIAGNOSIS_____ INITIAL EVAL_____ F/U EVAL_____

TOTAL # TREATMENTS_____ THERAPIST_____

Signature

	RIGHT LE	LEFT LE
APPEARANCE:	_____	_____
SKIN INTEGRITY:	_____	_____
SKIN TEMP:	_____	_____
EDEMA PRESENT:	0☐ +1☐ +2☐ +3☐	0☐ +1☐ +2☐ +3☐

CIRCUMFERENTIAL:

	RIGHT	LEFT
☐MET HEADS	_____	_____
☐ARCH	_____	_____
☐ANKLE	_____	_____
☐SUPRA MALLEOLAR	_____	_____
☐MID CALF	_____	_____
☐SUB PATELLAR	_____	_____

PULSES:

		RIGHT	LEFT
DORSAL PEDALIS		0☐ +1☐ +2☐ +3☐	0☐ +1☐ +2☐ +3☐
POST TIBIALIS		0☐ +1☐ +2☐ +3☐	0☐ +1☐ +2☐ +3☐
POPLITEAL		0☐ +1☐ +2☐ +3☐	0☐ +1☐ +2☐ +3☐
FEMORAL		0☐ +1☐ +2☐ +3☐	0☐ +1☐ +2☐ +3☐

SENSORY TESTING:

VIBRATORY SENSE:
☐PRESENT ☐DIMINISHED ☐ABSENT (RIGHT)
☐PRESENT ☐DIMINISHED ☐ABSENT (LEFT)

1 = 01 gr (4.17 for Normal)
2 = 10 gr (5.07 Protective Sense)
3 = 75 gr (6.10 Loss Protective Sense)
4 = No Protective Sensation

PROTECTIVE SENSATION:

	RIGHT	LEFT
DORSUM:	1☐ 2☐ 3☐ 4☐	1☐ 2☐ 3☐ 4☐
PLANTAR DIGIT 1:	1☐ 2☐ 3☐ 4☐	1☐ 2☐ 3☐ 4☐
PLANTAR DIGIT 3:	1☐ 2☐ 3☐ 4☐	1☐ 2☐ 3☐ 4☐
PLANTAR DIGIT 5:	1☐ 2☐ 3☐ 4☐	1☐ 2☐ 3☐ 4☐
MET HEAD 1:	1☐ 2☐ 3☐ 4☐	1☐ 2☐ 3☐ 4☐
MET HEAD 3:	1☐ 2☐ 3☐ 4☐	1☐ 2☐ 3☐ 4☐
MET HEAD 5:	1☐ 2☐ 3☐ 4☐	1☐ 2☐ 3☐ 4☐
PROXIMAL HEAD 5:	1☐ 2☐ 3☐ 4☐	1☐ 2☐ 3☐ 4☐
ARCH:	1☐ 2☐ 3☐ 4☐	1☐ 2☐ 3☐ 4☐
HEEL:	1☐ 2☐ 3☐ 4☐	1☐ 2☐ 3☐ 4☐

STRENGTH:

RIGHT		LEFT
_____	Anterior Tibialis	_____
_____	Extensor Hallucis Longus	_____
_____	Flexor Hallucis Longus	_____
_____	Posterior Tibialis	_____
_____	Peroneus Longus	_____
_____	Gastroc / Soleus	_____
_____	Intrinsics (S / W / A)	_____

DEFORMITIES:

	RIGHT	LEFT
Hammer/Claw:	_____	_____
Boney Prominence:	_____	_____
Drop Foot:	_____	_____
Charcot Foot:	_____	_____
Hallux Limitus	_____	_____
Rear/ForeFt Varus:	_____	_____
Plantar flexed 1st:	_____	_____
Equinus:	_____	_____
Amputation:	_____	_____

FOOTWEAR: ☐STANDARD ☐SPECIAL DESCRIBE_____
☐ADEQUATE ☐INADEQUATE DESCRIBE_____

TREATMENT RECOMMENDATIONS:[4]
☐BUERGER-ALLEN EXERCISES CYCLES_____ TIMES/DAY_____ MODIFIED Yes / No
☐PATIENT EDUCATION ☐SKIN CARE ☐FOOTWEAR ☐ORTHOTICS

[3] BUERGER-ALLEN EVALUATION FORM CREATED BY: JENNIFER M. BOTTOMLEY, Ph.D, MS, PT © 1996
[4] REFER TO BUERGER-ALLEN TREATMENT FLOWSHEET FOR INITIAL BLANCHING/FILLING TIMES etc.

Figure 53–3 Buerger-Allen Follow-up Evaluation form.

dent rubor is the reddish-blue color of the toes and forefoot caused by reduced blood flow in the capillaries. When there is diminished arterial flow, peripheral resistance drops with arteriocapillary dilatation and maximum oxygen extraction by the tissues. With dependency, this is exaggerated. The actual degree of rubor can be noted when measuring venous filling time. Maximum rubor is usually evi-dent in 2 to 3 minutes; it manifests as a dusky red color when severe ischemia is present.

The evaluation of skin temperatures and circumferential measures is another means of assessing circulatory insufficiency and determining the presence of infection.

Skin temperature measurements are useful if the circulatory problem is asymmetrical, although test

BUERGER-ALLEN TREATMENT FLOW SHEET[5]

PATIENT________________ AGE_____ SEX _____ RM#_____ THERAPIST INITIALS_____

DIAGNOSIS______________ ☐ DIABETES ☐ PVD ☐ AMPUTEE__________ ☐ CARDIAC ☐ HTN

WOUND: ☐ PRESENT ☐ NOT PRESENT DESCRIBE________________

BUERGER-ALLEN PROTOCOL: CYCLES__________ TIMES/DAY__________ MODIFIED__________

PARAMETER	INITIAL EVAL	FOLLOW-UP	FOLLOW-UP	FOLLOW-UP	NOTES
DATE / THERAPIST INITIALS					
RESTING HEART RATE (Supine)					
BLOOD PRESSURE (Supine)					
RESPIRATORY RATE (Supine)					
PLANTAR SKIN TEMPERATURE	L / R	L / R	L / R	L / R	
DORSAL PEDALIS PULSE LEFT	☐0 ☐+1 ☐+2 ☐+3	☐0 ☐+1 ☐+2 ☐+3	☐0 ☐+1 ☐+2 ☐+3	☐0 ☐+1 ☐+2 ☐+3	
DORSAL PEDALIS PULSE RIGHT	☐0 ☐+1 ☐+2 ☐+3	☐0 ☐+1 ☐+2 ☐+3	☐0 ☐+1 ☐+2 ☐+3	☐0 ☐+1 ☐+2 ☐+3	
POST. TIBIALIS PULSE LEFT	☐0 ☐+1 ☐+2 ☐+3	☐0 ☐+1 ☐+2 ☐+3	☐0 ☐+1 ☐+2 ☐+3	☐0 ☐+1 ☐+2 ☐+3	
POST. TIBIALIS PULSE RIGHT	☐0 ☐+1 ☐+2 ☐+3	☐0 ☐+1 ☐+2 ☐+3	☐0 ☐+1 ☐+2 ☐+3	☐0 ☐+1 ☐+2 ☐+3	
EDEMA (Supine)	☐0 ☐+1 ☐+2 ☐+3	☐0 ☐+1 ☐+2 ☐+3	☐0 ☐+1 ☐+2 ☐+3	☐0 ☐+1 ☐+2 ☐+3	
CIRCUMFERENTIAL MEASURES					
MET HEADS	L / R	L / R	L / R	L / R	
ARCH	L / R	L / R	L / R	L / R	
ANKLE (figure 8)	L / R	L / R	L / R	L / R	
SUPRA MALLEOLAR	L / R	L / R	L / R	L / R	
MID CALF	L / R	L / R	L / R	L / R	
SUB PATELLAR	L / R	L / R	L / R	L / R	
BLANCHING TIME ELEVATED					
FILLING TIME HORIZONTAL					
FILLING TIME DEPENDENT					-

[5] © 1996 JENNIFER M. BOTTOMLEY, Ph.D, MS, PT

Figure 53–4 Buerger-Allen Treatment Flow Sheet.

results may be variable because of ambient temperature. In an individual with peripheral vascular disease, the extremities are often cool to the touch, and in the presence of infection, there may be hot spots. The use of a skin temperature monitoring device to obtain precise temperature measures is helpful, but the therapist can also evaluate skin temperature by touch, grading it cold, cool, warm, or hot.

Circumferential measurements of the lower leg and foot also aid in the assessment of an individual with peripheral vascular involvement. Edema is often present when the peripheral vascular system is involved because of the inability of the involved vessels to efficiently remove waste materials from the interstitial tissues. This edema will increase in the dependent position owing to gravity. Measurement of circumference can be accomplished by using Jobst measurement tapes (which are free from your local vendor) to measure around the metatarsal heads, the midfoot, in a figure eight around the ankle, and incrementally every 3 inches up the lower leg from the malleolar level to the subpatellar level. Another means of determining the degree of edema is volume displacement; using a bucket of water with a ruler taped to the inside, measure the amount of water that is displaced upward when the lower extremity is submerged. This method will provide an objective and reproducible means of assessing edema in the lower extremity.

Evaluating Wound Status

In the presence of foot lesions it is helpful to grade the lesion for objective monitoring. Wagner's classification grades vascular dysfunction from 0 to 5, as follows (also see Box 52–2):

Grade 0 Foot: The skin is without ulceration. No open lesions are present, but potentially ulcerating deformities, such as bunions, hammer toes, and Charcot's deformity, may be present. Healed partial-foot amputations may also be included in this group.

Grade 1 Foot: A full-thickness superficial skin loss is present. The lesion does not extend to bone. No abscess is present.

Grade 2 Foot: An open ulceration is noted; it is deeper than that of grade 1. It may penetrate to tendon or joint capsule.

Grade 3 Foot: The lesion penetrates to bone, and osteomyelitis is present. Joint infection or plantar fascial plane abscess may also be noted.

Grade 4 Foot: Gangrene is noted in the forefoot.

Grade 5 Foot: Gangrene involving the entire foot is noted. This is not salvageable by local procedures.

In the presence of an ulceration, objective documentation of wound size is best accomplished by tracing the wound on sterilized x-ray film or by photographing it on line-graphed film. This is helpful in monitoring improvement or decline in wound status.

THERAPEUTIC INTERVENTION

Preventive Management

A management plan for the neuropathic foot patient is based on the risk classification scheme. Patients in risk categories 1 through 3 are given education in foot inspection, skin care, and selection of footwear. Footwear recommendations are dependent on level of risk and on the specific needs of each individual. For example, category 1 patients benefit from a shoe with a leather (or other compliant material) upper and a toe-box that accommodates the shape of the foot. A cushioned insole may be added. Category 2 and 3 patients may need customized insoles and shoe modifications appropriate for their deformities. Once a patient is assigned a level of risk through the screening process, a program of routine follow-up is recommended: once a year for risk 0, biannually for risk 1, every 3 months for risk 2, and monthly for those in the risk 3 category.

Treatment of Plantar Ulcers

The treatment of choice for plantar ulcers is the total contact cast (see Coleman et al.). In this casting technique, foam padding encloses the toes; felt pads provide protection over the malleoli, tibial crest, posterior heel, and navicular tuberosity; and local padding provides relief at the ulcer site. The initial cast should be changed within the first week to prevent injury due to an improper fit, as edema resolves. The effectiveness of walking casts in healing diabetic and nondiabetic foot ulcers has been demonstrated in numerous studies. Walking casts promote plantar wound healing by (1) reducing plantar pressures, (2) reducing leg edema, and (3) protecting the area from traumatic reinjury.

Not every patient will accept, or is a candidate for, a walking cast. Infection and fragile skin are contraindications for casting. For these cases, alternatives to casting should be employed. A walking splint is a posterior cast secured to the leg by an elastic wrap. The shell is made of plaster reinforced by fiberglass taping, and relief for the posterior heel and plantar lesion is provided by adhesive-backed padding.

The ulcer-relief (cut-out) sandal is another device that can be used as an alternative to casting.

The footbed of molded plastazote is cut out or cut in relief to reduce pressure beneath the plantar lesion.

Prevention and Treatment

The challenge is to prevent reulceration. The patient must be provided with temporary protective footwear at the time of healing and protective footgear following the healing of the ulceration and then gradually allowed to resume activities, avoiding those that may have contributed to the ulcer formation. A sandal molded from thermoplastic materials is an acceptable device during this critical period. Individuals who resume activity too quickly after a period of casting or other immobilization by protective footwear are at risk of developing a neuropathic fracture. The best way to monitor progression is by comparing temperature differences between the involved and uninvolved foot. Temperatures increase due to stress-induced inflammation by as much as one degree. A skin-surface temperature monitor can be employed to evaluate differences in temperature between the inflamed area and the noninflamed areas of the foot. The patient must be aware that the first evidence of injury to the bones of the foot is swelling and warmth.

When the ulcer site is fully healed, footwear is progressed to modified shoes fitted with accommodative orthotics. With mild deformities, molded insoles are added to extra-depth shoes or sneakers. For healed forefoot ulcers, a rocker sole is applied to the sole of the shoe to assist with push-off. If the foot is significantly shortened or deformed, custom shoes may be required. Custom shoes are made by pedorthists or orthotists over plaster models of the patient's feet and extra depth is incorporated in the shoe to accommodate a soft, molded interface beneath the foot.

Charcot fractures often result in serious deformity of the foot. Acute Charcot fractures may require surgery or long periods of immobilization in a cast. Additional immobilization and temperature-monitoring are required. The length of time of casting and immobilization varies based on the individual rate of healing. Custom shoes are prescribed for the individual when there is no longer a difference in skin temperature between the fractured and the uninvolved foot.

Buerger-Allen Exercise Protocol

Buerger-Allen exercises are performed according to the protocol displayed in Figures 53–5 through 53–7. The individual lies supine with the legs elevated at an angle of 45 degrees until blanching

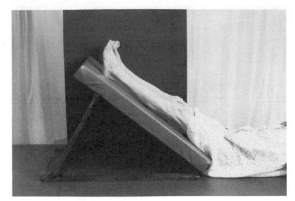

Figure 53–5 Buerger-Allen protocol: legs elevated.

occurs or for a maximum time of 3 minutes (Fig. 53–5). Active pumping and circling of the feet and isometric quadriceps and gluteal contractions are performed for the first minute or more in the elevated position. Once the blanching has occurred, the subject sits up and hangs the lower leg over the edge of the bed (Fig. 53–6). (Note: If the individual is subject to orthostatic hypotension, the leg should be held horizontally between being held in the elevated and the dependent positions.) While the leg

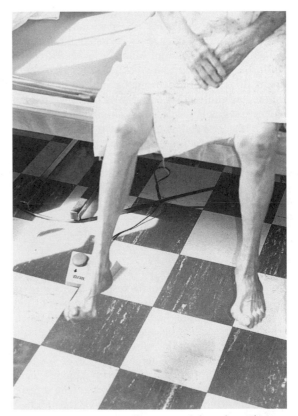

Figure 53–6 Buerger-Allen protocol: legs dependent.

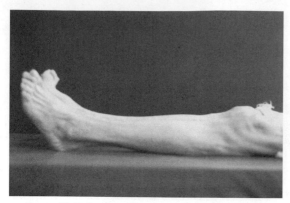

Figure 53-7 Buerger-Allen protocol: legs horizontal.

is in the dependent position, the individual is encouraged to actively plantarflex, dorsiflex, and circle the foot. This position is maintained for a minimum of 3 minutes, or until rubor has occurred. Finally, the individual lies supine with the lower extremities flat for 3 minutes (Fig. 53-7). Again, active contraction of the leg muscles is performed for at least 1 minute in this position. One note of caution: In the presence of severe physiological compromise of the cardiovascular system, the author recommends assuming the supine position between the elevation and dependent phases as well as between the dependent and elevation phases to prevent the consequences of orthostatic hypotension. The entire sequence is repeated three times in each exercise session. Buerger-Allen exercises should be performed twice each day for maximum benefit. If peripheral neuropathy is present and active muscle contraction is not possible, the clinician can passively plantarflex and dorsiflex the foot in each of the respective positions to increase blood flow, which is facilitated by the pumping action of the surrounding musculature. The author has successfully employed high-frequency electrical stimulation to elicit threshold muscle contractions in the lower extremities of elderly patients with peripheral neuropathy.

CONCLUSION

The insensitive foot, which results from various pathological conditions, is far too common and problematic for aging persons. The key to good care is proper evaluation, which leads to appropriate therapeutic intervention. Several evaluation tools are presented and the Buerger-Allen exercise routine is described. In conjunction with patient education, which is crucial for prevention, effective care can mitigate the deleterious effects of the insensitive foot.

SUGGESTED READINGS

Bailey TS, Yu HM, Rayfield EJ. Patterns of foot examination in a diabetes clinic. *Am J Med* 1985; 78:371–374.

Birke JA, Sims DS. The insensitive foot. In: Hunt GC, ed. *Physical Therapy of the Foot and Ankle*. New York: Churchill Livingstone; 1988:133–168.

Birke JA, Sims DS, Theriot SM. *Foot Screening Examination*. Instructional videotape. Carville, La.: G.W. Long Hansen's Disease Center; 1985.

Bottomley JB, Herman H. Making simple, inexpensive changes for the management of foot problems in the aged. *Top Geriatr Rehabil* 1992; 7:62–77.

Bottomley JM, Schwartz N. The diabetic foot. In: Donatelli RA, ed. *The Biomechanics of the Foot and Ankle*, 2nd ed. Philadelphia: F.A. Davis; 1996:189–222.

Brand PW. Management of the insensitive limb. *Phys Ther* 1979: 59:8.

Breuer U. Diabetic patient's compliance with bespoke footwear after healing of neuropathic foot ulcers. Diabète Métab 1994; 20:415–419.

Coleman WC, Brand PW, Birke JA. The total contact cast: a therapy for plantar ulceration on insensitive feet. *J Am Podiatr Med Assoc* 1984; 74:548–552.

Graham S, Theriot S, Birke JA. *Comparison of Sensory Testing Methods in the Neuropathic Foot*. Carville, La.: G.W. Long Hansen's Disease Center; [unpublished].

Gramuglia VJ, Palmarozzo PM, Rzonca EC. Biomechanical concepts in the treatment of ulcers in the diabetic foot. *Clin Pod Med Surg* 1988; 5:613–626.

Kaye RA. The extra-depth toe-box: a rational approach. *Foot Ankle Int* 1994; 15:146–150.

White J. Custom shoe therapy: current concepts, designs, and special considerations. *Clin Podiatr Med Surg* 1994; 11:259–270.

Chapter **54**

Skin Disorders
Randy Berger, M.D.
Barbara A. Gilchrest, M.D.

INTRODUCTION

As the skin ages, many structural and functional changes take place. These alterations include a flattening of the dermal-epidermal junction, and in the epidermis, a decreased number of Langerhans cells, which are responsible for immune recognition, a decreased number of melanocytes, which are responsible for protective pigmentation, and a variation in the size and shape of keratinocytes. The dermis is characterized by a decrease in thickness, cellularity, and vascularity and a degeneration of elastic fibers. In general, the hair follicles, sebaceous glands, and eccrine glands decrease in number, and there is a loss of hair bulb melanocytes, which accounts for the graying of hair. Functional changes in aging skin include altered permeability, diminished sebum production, decreased inflammatory and immunological responsiveness, and attenuated thermoregulation, with decreased sweating. There is impaired wound healing, reduced elasticity, decreased vitamin D production, and impaired sensory perception. In addition to these normal changes, known as intrinsic aging, additional changes take place in response to cumulative ultraviolet irradiation that are known as photoaging. These changes include atrophy of the epidermis, epidermal dysplasia and atypia, further decrease in Langerhans cells, increased and irregular distribution and activity of melanocytes, dermal elastosis (deposits of abnormal elastic fibers), and further decrease in inflammatory and immunological responsiveness.

GENERAL PRINCIPLES

In evaluating a patient with a skin disorder, it is important to ascertain what topical home remedies and other products, such as alcohol or detergents, are being applied, as these products often exacerbate the primary skin condition. A full medical history that includes particular attention to medications, is essential. The chronicity of the condition and whether others in the patient's environment have a similar condition may also provide clues to the diagnosis.

Management of skin conditions must be tailored to the patient's physical capabilities and circumstances. Limitations in movement of the geriatric rehabilitation patient can make application of topical treatments difficult, and common remedies used in younger patients, such as oil in bath water, may be quite dangerous for the elderly. To avoid errors, treatment regimens should be made as simple as possible. Moreover, the elderly are two to three times more likely to experience adverse reactions to antihistamines and corticosteroids, drugs frequently used to treat skin disorders. These drugs should be prescribed reluctantly and always with clear, written instructions.

Most dermatological agents are applied topically, and the choice of a base for the active ingredient is important. Ointments, greasy preparations containing little water, are most useful for treating conditions in which the skin is dry, scaly, or thickened. In general, a medication in an ointment base is better absorbed and therefore is more potent than the same medication in a cream or lotion vehicle. Creams, semisolid emulsions of water in oil, are more cosmetically appealing but can be drying, and are thus useful in treating exudative conditions. Most creams, however, contain stabilizers or preser-

vatives that can induce allergic sensitization. Lotions, usually suspensions of fine powder in an aqueous base, are useful in evaporative cooling and drying of the skin and are preferred on hair-bearing areas because of their ease of application. Powders are useful for absorbing moisture from weepy or intertriginous skin. Soaks and compresses, which are very drying as they evaporate, are soothing and thus appropriate for highly exudative and vesicular lesions.

Topical steroid medications are commonly used in the treatment of dermatological conditions. Numerous preparations are available; they are classified by their potency. A few representative medications are listed in Table 54–1. This chapter offers guidelines as to the appropriate potency of topical steroids indicated for the various conditions discussed; however, certain basic principles should be emphasized. Overuse of topical steroids can result in local side effects of skin atrophy, telangiectasia, hypopigmentation, and tachyphylaxis. The higher the potency of the drug and the longer the duration of use, the greater the risk. Only mild-potency topical steroids should be used on the face, genitalia, and intertriginous areas. Finally, application of topical steroids over a large area of the body's surface results in systemic absorption, which can lead to possible adrenal suppression and other sequelae.

TREATMENT OF INFECTIONS

Viral Infections

Herpes Simplex

Herpetic infection appears clinically as grouped vesicles on an erythematous base. Vesicles can become pustules and eventually crusts and erosions, with a characteristic punched-out appearance. Herpes simplex virus (HSV) infection can be accompanied by pruritus, burning, or pain. The diagnosis can be confirmed either by the presence of multinucleated giant cells on a Tzank smear or by viral culture. Herpes simplex eruptions can be either primary or secondary; secondary eruptions can be provoked by stress, infection, trauma, or ultraviolet radiation. They are most commonly seen in the perioral and anogenital regions, though they can be seen in any location. Herpetic whitlow refers to a herpes simplex infection of the finger, classically seen in health-care workers as a result of inoculation by a patient's lesions. In the immunocompetent host, HSV is a self-limited infection that does not necessarily require treatment, as is often the case with perioral herpes. If treatment is desired, as in the case of genital herpes, oral acyclovir 200 mg five times a day is effective (treat for 10 days for

Table 54–1 Examples of Topical Corticosteroid Preparations[a]

Potency	Compound	Formulation
Very high	Clobetasol proprionate	Cream or ointment 0.05%
	Halobetasol proprionate	Cream or ointment 0.05%[b]
High	Betamethasone diproprionate	Cream or ointment 0.05%
	Betamethasone valerate	Ointment 0.1%
	Fluocinonide	Cream or ointment 0.05%
	Halcinonide	Cream or ointment 0.1%
Medium	Betamethasone valerate	Cream 0.1%
	Fluocinolone acetonide	Cream or ointment 0.025%
	Hydrocortisone valerate	Cream or ointment 0.2%
	Triamcinolone acetonide	Cream, ointment, or lotion 0.1% or 0.025%
Low	Hydrocortisone	Cream, ointment, or lotion 2.5% or 1.0%

[a]Many equally effective compounds and formulations are not listed.

[b]Ointments are more potent than creams containing the same corticosteroid in the same concentration because of their enhanced penetration.

Modified, with permission, from Gilchrest BA. Skin changes and disorders. In: Abrams WB, Beers MH, Berkow R, Fletcher AJ, eds. *The Merck Manual of Geriatrics,* 2nd ed. Whitehouse Station, N.J.: Merck Research Laboratories; 1995:1255.

primary infection, 5 days for recurrent infection). When indicated, acyclovir can be used for chronic suppression of HSV with 400 mg twice a day. A severe herpes simplex infection in an immunocompromised host should be treated with intravenous acyclovir 5 mg/kg every 8 hours until resolution.

Herpes Zoster

Otherwise known as shingles, herpes zoster is an acute eruption caused by a reactivation of latent varicella virus in the dorsal root ganglia. Although it may occur at any age, elderly patients are at greater risk. Other, often additive, factors that predispose to zoster include immunosuppressive drugs, corticosteroids, malignancies, local irradiation, trauma, and surgery. A common sequela of herpes zoster infection is postherpetic neuralgia, for which the incidence, duration, and severity increase with age. Other complications include encephalitis, ophthalmic disease when the first branch of the trigeminal nerve is involved, facial paralysis and taste loss when the second branch of the trigeminal nerve is involved (Ramsay-Hunt syndrome), motor neuropathies, Guillain-Barré syndrome, and urinary or fecal retention when sacral nerves are involved.

Clinical presentation of herpes zoster infection is sometimes preceded by prodromal symptoms of pain, pruritus, or paresthesia along the affected dermatome. Fever, chills, malaise, and gastrointestinal symptoms can also occur. Usually, red papules appear along a dermatome within 3 days. These rapidly progress to grouped vesicles on an erythema-

tous base that may become hemorrhagic vesicles or pustules. After about 5 days, the vesicle formation ceases and crusts form. Gradual healing occurs over the next 2 to 4 weeks, sometimes resolving with pigmentary disturbances or scarring. In patients with underlying malignancy or immunodeficiency, disseminated herpes zoster infection can occur. This is a potentially life-threatening infection that requires hospitalization and intravenous acyclovir (10–12 mg/kg every 8 hours).

Not all cases of herpes zoster require treatment. If treatment is to be instituted, it should be started within 72 hours of the onset of symptoms. Two antiviral drugs are currently available: acyclovir 800 mg five times a day for 7 to 10 days (note that a much higher dose is needed than for herpes simplex) and famcyclovir 500 mg three times a day for 7 days. Other antivirals are currently undergoing testing. Antiviral therapy has been shown to hasten the resolution of the acute disease; however, its role in decreasing the incidence of postherpetic neuralgia is controversial. In addition, the use of systemic steroids has been in and out of favor in recent years. Certainly, antiviral therapy has a more favorable side-effect profile, and if systemic steroids are prescribed, they must be used with care in the elderly. Topical soaks with an astringent solution such as Burow's solution (aluminum acetate) can help dry up vesicles and soothe the affected area. Analgesics are commonly required. It should be kept in mind that vesicle fluid is contagious to those who have never had varicella and to immunocompromised individuals. Thus, care-givers should wear gloves to avoid direct contact with the lesions. Pregnant women should likewise avoid contact. Once the lesions have crusted over, they are no longer infectious.

Fungal Infections

Superficial fungal infections may be caused by yeast or dermatophytes. Deep fungal infections of the skin are rare and occur mainly in severely immunocompromised patients. They will not be discussed here.

Tinea

Tinea, the name given to superficial dermatophyte infection of the skin, is further classified by anatomical location—that is, tinea pedis (foot), tinea cruris (groin), tinea manuum (hand), tinea corporis (body), tinea unguium or onychomycosis (nails). Tinea cruris characteristically spares the genitalia, as opposed to candidiasis, in which the scrotum and penis in men and the vulva in women usually are involved. Tinea capitis, or fungal infection of the scalp, is rare in older adults. Heat and moisture predispose to fungal infection. Tinea clinically manifests as scaly patches or plaques with annular or serpiginous, often slightly raised, borders. Varying degrees of erythema may be present. Tinea pedis and tinea manuum may present as diffuse scaling of the plantar or palmar surfaces. Often, one hand and two feet are affected. Tinea pedis may also present with toe-web maceration. Nails, too, are commonly involved, showing thickening and yellow discoloration of the nail plate, onycholysis (separation of the nail plate from the nail bed), and hyperkeratotic debris under the nail plate. Greenish discoloration indicates pseudomonal superinfection of the nail. When fungal infections are mistakenly treated with topical steroids, they initially appear to improve and show diminished scaling and inflammation. Nevertheless, fungal organisms flourish and infected areas enlarge (tinea incognito). Discontinuation of steroids results in a flare of the affected area. The infection can invade the hair follicle, resulting in a deeper infection known as Majocchi's granuloma.

Diagnosis of a fungal infection is made by culture or by direct microscopic visualization of fungal hyphae in scales after treatment with potassium hydroxide (KOH). Most cutaneous dermatophyte infections can be treated with a 4-week course of topical antifungal medication (Box 54–1). Affected areas should be kept as dry as possible, particularly the groin and toe-web spaces. The exceptions to topical treatment are tinea unguium, tinea capitis, and often tinea manuum and Majocchi's granuloma,

---

Box 54–1

Examples of Antifungal Preparations[a]

Compound	Formulation
Clotrimazole	Cream or lotion 1.0%
Ketoconazole	Cream 2.0%
Nystatin	Cream or powder[b]
Terbinafine hydrochloride	Cream 1.0%[c]

[a]Many equally effective compounds and formulations are not listed.
[b]Effective against candida but not against dermatophytes.
[c]Fungicidal against dermatophytes (others are fungistatic), thus allowing shorter duration of treatment; activity against candida is variable.

---

which require oral antifungal agents. Until recently, the only agent approved for the treatment of cutaneous dermatophyte infection was griseofulvin, which is quite effective for infections of the scalp and skin. Ultramicrosized griseofulvin 3.3 mg/kg/day given once or twice a day for 4 to 6 weeks is usually curative. Nails, however, are best treated with itraconazole. Because the drug is retained in the nail plate for extended periods, controlled trials support a pulsed regimen of 200 mg twice a day for 1 week of each month, but current FDA guidelines recommend 200 mg/day for 3 months. Other agents undergoing FDA review for use in onychomycosis include fluconazole and terbinafine. In patients with both tinea pedis and onychomycosis, recurrence of tinea pedis is common if the nails are not also treated, often necessitating indefinite topical treatment.

Candidiasis

Candida albicans thrives in warm, moist areas, such as the groin, the axilla, and the inframammary regions. Diabetic and immunosupressed patients, as well as those receiving systemic antibiotic therapy that reduces competing surface bacteria, are at increased risk. The organism may be carried asymptomatically in the bowel, mouth, and vagina. Cutaneous candidal infection is characterized by beefy red, often moist plaques with satellite pustules and papules. As mentioned above, unlike tinea cruris, candidiasis involves the skin of the genitalia. Oral candidiasis, or thrush, presents as creamy white plaques on the tongue, palate, or buccal mucosa that can be easily scraped off. Perleche, or angular cheilitis, is a candidal infection of the corners of the mouth characterized by erythema, fissuring, and a white exudate. Predisposing factors are dental malocclusion, poorly fitting dentures, and deep folds at the corners of the mouth with consequent retention of saliva and food particles in the affected area. Candida paronychia is an infection of the skin proximal and lateral to the nails, characterized by erythema, tenderness, and swelling, with separation of the nail plate from the adjacent nail folds. This condition is chronic and should be distinguished from acute paronychia, which is usually bacterial in origin. Frequent immersion of hands in water is a predisposing factor.

Confirmation of cutaneous candidal infection is by culture or KOH preparation. Topical antifungal medication is usually curative, and attempts should be made to keep affected areas clean and dry.

Bacterial Infections

Impetigo

Impetigo is a superficial bacterial infection of the skin most commonly caused by either *Staphylococcus aureus* or group A streptococcus. Vesicles or pustules in the early stages break down to form golden-colored crusts that often adhere to the underlying skin. The infection can occur on previously normal, intact skin, or it can present as a superinfection of a primary skin disorder (e.g., eczema, neurodermatitis, herpes zoster) in which breaks in the cutaneous barrier allow bacteria to penetrate.

In managing impetigo, a skin swab should be sent for culture and sensitivity. Single or localized lesions can be treated topically with mupirocin ointment applied three times a day, but more extensive impetigo requires systemic antibiotics, such as dicloxacillin 250 to 500 mg four times a day for 7 to 10 days. Wet lesions can be soaked in an astringent such as Burow's solution that also has antimicrobial properties.

Folliculitis

Infection of the hair follicle is manifested by follicularly based, erythematous papules and pustules. Lesions can be either superficial or deep. Areas of predilection are the scalp and extremities, although the eruption can occur anywhere. Sweating and occlusion, such as under a splint, predispose to folliculitis, although as long as therapy has been initiated, exercise and splints are not contraindicated in patients with this condition. The most common causative organism is *Staphylococcus aureus.* However, gram-negative organisms (as in hot-tub

folliculitis caused by *Pseudomonas*), candida, and *Pityrosporum* yeast can also be pathogenic. Due to the variety of potentially causative organisms, it is advisable to send pustule contents for culture and sensitivity. Treatment is a 1- to 2-week course of antibiotics. Given that most cases are caused by *S. aureus,* it is reasonable to start antistaphylococcal treatment, such as dicloxacillin 250 to 500 mg four times a day, pending culture results. Mild cases can be treated with topical antistaphylococcal antibiotics, such as erythromycin, clindamycin, or mupirocin. Antibacterial soaps, such as Hibiclens, pHisoHex, and Lever 2000, help maintain a lower bacterial count on predisposed hosts. Treatment of candidal infection has been discussed previously. *Pityrosporum* folliculitis occurs mainly on the trunk and is often associated with diabetes mellitus, antibiotic therapy, or immunosupression. Treatment is with a 2-week course of selenium sulfide 2.5% lotion applied daily for 10 minutes and then washed off. Topical antifungal creams are also effective (see Box 54–1).

Erysipelas

Erysipelas is a superficial infection of the skin caused by group A or group C hemolytic streptococci. The organism may enter the skin through minor cuts, wounds, or insect bites. Lesions of erysipelas are characterized by warm, edematous, erythematous plaques with well-defined, often rapidly advancing margins. Vesicles and bullae may be present and can even be hemorrhagic. Fever, malaise, and lymphadenopathy accompany cutaneous infection. The face is the most common location for erysipelas, but infection can occur anywhere. Treatment is with oral or intravenous antistreptococcal antibiotics such as penicillin or erythromycin (in penicillin-allergic patients). A typical outpatient regimen is 250 to 500 mg four times a day for 2 weeks. Clinical judgment and continuous evaluation of the clinical course determine the treatment setting and route of administration of antibiotics. Because infection continues to spread during the first 12 to 24 hours of oral therapy, patients with facial lesions often require hospitalization and intravenous antibiotics to prevent the complication of cavernous sinus thrombosis.

Cellulitis

Cellulitis is a deeper infection of the skin, most commonly caused by group A streptococci and occasionally by *S. aureus* or gram-negative organisms. It can occur as a complication of an open wound, a venous ulcer, or tinea pedis, or it can develop on intact skin, particularly on the legs. Clinically, it presents as erythema, tenderness, swelling, and warmth. Fever and lymphadenopathy may also occur. Treatment is with oral or intravenous antibiotics, depending upon the severity of infection and the background health of the patient. Streptococcal cellulitis is best treated with penicillin, as outlined above; however, if *S. aureus* is suspected or the causative agent is unclear, broader coverage, such as with dicloxacillin or cephalexin 250 to 500 mg four times a day, should be instituted and adjusted according to clinical response. Patients with diabetes mellitus or peripheral vascular disease will probably need close monitoring and intravenous therapy. Diabetic patients are more likely to have gram-negative, anaerobic, and mixed microbial infections. Treatment of any underlying predisposing condition should also be undertaken. If the cellulitis does not respond to antimicrobial therapy, gram-negative or resistant organisms or an alternative diagnosis should be considered.

Swelling, pain, and open lesions may necessitate modification or temporary suspension of physical rehabilitation, but cellulitis is not a frank contraindication to physical exercise. Clinical judgment must be used, and the effects of disuse must be weighed against the need for rest. Aggravating the condition is to be avoided.

TREATMENT OF INFESTATIONS

Scabies

Scabies is an intensely pruritic eruption caused by the *Sarcoptes scabiei* mite. The female mite burrows into the skin and deposits eggs, which hatch into larvae in a few days. Scabies is easily transmitted by skin-to-skin contact and can be readily spread between residents of the same household, nursing home, or institution. Pruritus is due to a hypersensitivity reaction, so infestation has usually been present for weeks before it manifests clinically. Pruritus is severe and often worse at night. The hallmark of scabies is the burrow, a linear ridge, often with a tiny vesicle at one end; however, these lesions may be obscured by scratching. Other cutaneous signs of scabies are papules, nodules, and vesicles. Lesions are characteristically found in the interdigital web spaces, the flexor aspects of the wrists, the axilla, the umbilicus, around the nipples, and on the genitalia. The skin is almost always excoriated, and lesions are susceptible to secondary impetiginization. In elderly and physically or mentally disabled patients, scabies may present less typically because of the inability to scratch, and often has been a long-standing infestation. The condition may mimic eczema or exfoliative dermatitis,

and widespread hyperkeratotic and crusted lesions may be present.

The diagnosis is confirmed by observation of the scabies mite, eggs, or excretions in a skin scraping placed in mineral oil and examined under a microscope. A typical patient has only 10 to 12 adult female mites at one time, so confirmation of scabies is not always possible, and diagnosis is often presumptive. Several antiscabitic creams and lotions are effective in treating scabies. The two most commonly used drugs today are 5% permethrin cream and 1% lindane lotion or cream. Lindane, particularly if overused, can have neurotoxic side effects, including headaches, dizziness, nausea, and, rarely, seizures. Permethrin is thought to be a safer treatment for infants and pregnant women. Successful treatment requires the treatment of all close personal contacts. In an inpatient or residential facility, all clinical staff, patients, selected visitors, and their household contacts should be treated. As mentioned earlier, infestation can be subclinical for weeks, so infested contacts may be asymptomatic. The medication should be applied to the entire body, from the neck down (in infants the head is also treated). Particular attention should be paid to applying the cream or lotion under the fingernails and to the external genitalia. The medication should be washed off 8 hours later, and at that time all clothing and linens should be washed in hot water, dry-cleaned, or placed in a hot dryer. This process should be repeated again in 1 week to kill any newly hatched larvae. Unlike lindane, permethrin has the advantage of killing scabies eggs, as well as the mites and larvae, so in theory, only one application is necessary; however, two applications are usually performed to ensure cure. It must be kept in mind that because pruritus is due to allergic sensitization and not to viable organisms, it may continue for 1 to 2 weeks after successful treatment. This can usually be controlled with mild to midpotency topical steroids (see Table 54–1) and oral antihistamines, if necessary. Itching that continues beyond a few weeks may indicate treatment failure, reinfestation, or an incorrect diagnosis.

Pediculosis

Three species of lice infest humans: *Pediculus humanus* var. *capitis* (head lice), *Pediculus humanus* var. *corporis* (body lice), and *Phthirius pubis* (pubic lice, also known as crab lice). Transmission is by close person-to-person contact or by sharing clothing, hats, or combs. Elderly persons who have poor personal hygiene or who live in an overcrowded environment are at risk for head and body lice. Pediculosis capitis presents with scalp pruritus which can progress to eczematous changes with impetiginization. Localized lymphadenopathy can occur. Examination reveals small, gray-white nits (ova) adherent to hair shafts. Adult lice can occasionally be found. *Pediculosis corporis* should be considered in a patient who presents with generalized pruritus. Again, secondary eczematous changes, excoriation, and impetiginization can occur. Lice and nits are usually not found on the body but rather in the seams of clothing. Pediculosis pubis is usually spread by sexual contact but may also be transmitted via clothing or towels. The bases of pubic hairs should be examined for lice and nits in a patient complaining of pubic pruritus.

Head lice are treated with 1% lindane shampoo, which is applied for 4 minutes, then washed off. Treatment should be repeated in 7 to 10 days. Close contacts should also be examined and treated. Combs and brushes should be soaked in lindane shampoo for 1 hour. The presence of nits after appropriate treatment does not signify treatment failure. They can be removed from the hair with a fine-tooth comb dipped in vinegar.

Body lice are treated by washing the affected clothing in hot water, dry-cleaning them, or placing them in a hot dryer and then ironing the seams. Alternatively, the clothing can be disinfected with an insecticidal powder such as DDT 10% or malathion 1%. If lice or nits are found on the skin, the patient can wash with lindane shampoo as above. Pubic lice are treated identically to head lice, with local application of lindane shampoo. In all forms of infestation, pruritus and dermatitis can be treated with emollients and topical steroids, and impetiginization may require antibiotics.

TREATMENT OF INFLAMMATORY SKIN CONDITIONS

Pruritus

Pruritus, or itching, is a common complaint. It can occur in the presence or absence of objective cutaneous findings; associated skin eruptions may be causative (primary) or secondary. Patients who complain of pruritus should be examined for inconspicuous primary skin lesions because some pruritic skin diseases, such as bullous pemphigoid and scabies, may show little if any cutaneous signs initially. Systemic disorders associated with generalized pruritus without primary skin lesions include liver and renal disease, polycythemia vera, iron deficiency anemia, lymphomas, leukemias, parasitosis (usually of the GI tract), and psychiatric disease. Some drugs (e.g., barbiturates, narcotics) can also cause itching without a skin eruption. Disorders rarely associated with itching include diabetes mellitus, hyperthyroidism, hypothytroidism (where pruritus is usually secondary to xerosis), and solid malignancies. Nevertheless, the most common cause of pruritus is xerosis (dry skin) and, regardless of cause, most patients complaining of pruritus benefit from treatment for xerosis (see the following section). Antihistamines can be helpful in some cases but should be used cautiously in the elderly.

If no skin disease is evident, patients should be examined for evidence of systemic disorders, such as lymphadenopathy, hepatosplenomegaly, jaundice, and anemia. Appropriate laboratory tests for screening include a complete blood count, erythrocyte sedimentation rate, electrolytes, including urea nitrogen and creatinine, urine glucose, thyroid function tests, and liver function tests. If indicated by history or physical examination, a chest x-ray may be obtained or stool tested for occult blood, ova, and parasites. When itching begins suddenly and is severe and unrelenting, an underlying disease should be strongly suspected, and laboratory evaluation should be thorough.

Xerosis

Xerosis is quite common in the elderly, and it is the most common cause of pruritus. Symptoms are often worse in the winter when central heating decreases the humidity indoors, and the skin is exposed to cold and wind outdoors. Patients should be advised to avoid very hot baths or showers as well as irritants such as harsh detergents and topically applied alcohol. Emollients should be applied liberally and frequently, especially immediately after bathing when the skin is still moist. Severely dry skin may become inflamed (see asteatotic eczema in the next section).

TREATMENT OF DERMATITIS

Often used interchangeably with the term *eczema*, dermatitis indicates a superficial inflammation of the skin due to exposure to an irritant, allergic sensitization, genetically determined factors, or a combination of these factors. Pruritus, erythema, and edema progress to vesiculation, oozing, crusting, and scaling. Eventually, the skin may become lichenified (thickened and with prominent skin markings) from repeated rubbing or scratching.

Allergic Contact Dermatitis

Allergic contact dermatitis is an immune-mediated, type IV, delayed type of hypersensitivity reaction.

The prototype is *Rhus* dermatitis, or poison ivy. Acute lesions tend to be vesicular, whereas chronic contact dermatitis appears scaly and lichenified. Clues to an allergic contact dermatitis are bizarre shape or location or linear arrangement of lesions. Common contact allergens include nickel, fragrance additives, preservatives in cosmetics or medications, rubber, lanolin, chromates (used in tanning leather), topical antibiotics (especially neomycin, which is used, for example, on chronic ulcers), and topical anesthetics such as benzocaine. Treatment consists of identifying and removing the causative agent and applying mid- to high-potency topical steroids (see Table 54–1). Soaks such as Burow's solution dry acute vesicular lesions, whereas emollients soothe dry, chronic lesions and resolving acute lesions. Pure petrolatum has no fragrances or preservatives and is advised when a fragrance or preservative allergy is suspected or when the allergen is unknown. If a contact dermatitis is suspected, and a causative agent is not apparent by history and physical examination, patch-testing, usually performed by a dermatologist, can aid in making the diagnosis. All cutaneous allergies should be documented on the patient's chart because systemic exposure (e.g., via oral medication) to chemically related compounds may result in severe systemic allergic reactions.

Irritant Contact Dermatitis

Unlike allergic contact dermatitis, irritant contact dermatitis is not immune-mediated. Given enough contact with an irritant, any patient will develop a dermatitis. Common irritants are soaps and detergents. Although the elderly have a less pronounced inflammatory response to most irritants than do younger patients, chronic irritant dermatitis is a common occurrence in the elderly. Clinical manifestations are identical to those of allergic contact dermatitis, and treatment is similar.

Atopic Dermatitis

Atopic dermatitis, commonly referred to as eczema, is a chronic, pruritic condition commonly associated with other atopic features, such as asthma, allergic rhinitis, and xerosis. Atopic dermatitis is often referred to as "the itch that rashes," highlighting pruritus as the hallmark of this condition. Atopic dermatitis rarely begins in adulthood and usually improves with age. However, it can be exacerbated by environmental factors such as the dry environment that occurs in the winter due to central heating as well as by woolen clothing, harsh detergents,

and prolonged bathing. Treatment centers around altering habits to avoid the aforementioned and aggressively using emollients and midpotency topical steroids (see Table 54–1).

Nummular Dermatitis

Nummular dermatitis consists of nummular (coin-shaped), pruritic, erythematous, scaly, and sometimes crusted plaques found most often on the extremities. Dermatophyte infection must be excluded by KOH preparation or culture. Treatment is similar to that of other forms of chronic dermatitis.

Lichen Simplex Chronicus

Also known as neurodermatitis, lichen simplex chronicus is a localized, pruritic eruption that results from chronic scratching and rubbing, eventuating in a scratch-itch-scratch cycle. Clinically, lesions appear erythematous or hyperpigmented, lichenified, and scaly. High-potency topical steroids are often required to break this cycle. Steroid-impregnated tape, such as flurandrenolide (Cordran), applied at bedtime or after bathing and left in place up to 24 hours also protects the lesions from being scratched. When symptoms improve, the potency can be reduced (see Table 54–1). Topical doxepin relieves pruritus and also helps to break the scratch-itch cycle, but systemic absorption and drowsiness sometimes limit its use. If applicable, lesions can be covered with dressings such as an Unna's boot to prevent the patient from scratching. More nodular lesions are termed prurigo nodularis.

Asteatotic Eczema

When skin becomes excessively dry and scaly, fissures and excoriations allow environmental irritants to penetrate and further worsen the condition, adding inflammation to dryness. This commonly occurs on the lower legs and is characterized by scaly, erythematous plaques with a "cracked porcelain" appearance caused by superficial fissures and scale-crust, referred to as eczema craquele. Treatment consists of aggressive use of emollients and, initially, additional use of a low- to midpotency topical steroid ointment (see Table 54–1).

Stasis Dermatitis

Stasis dermatitis, commonly seen in the aging population, occurs in the context of chronic venous hypertension. Scaling and erythema are seen on a background of edema, varicosities, and hemosiderin hyperpigmentation. At times, stasis dermatitis may be confused with cellulitis, but it is usually chronic and bilateral. When severe and chronic, the condition may induce sclerosis beginning at the ankles and progressing proximally (termed lipodermatosclerosis). Another complication of severe venous statis is ulceration. Successful treatment of stasis dermatitis is contingent upon treating the underlying venous hypertension with leg elevation and compression therapy, if not contraindicated by concomitant arterial disease. Low-potency topical steroids (see Table 54–1) and emollients relieve the dermatitic component and the frequently associated pruritus. Potential contact allergens, such as neomycin, should be avoided.

Seborrheic Dermatitis

Seborrheic dermatitis is a common scaly erythematous eruption of the central part of the face (particularly eyebrows, glabella, eyelids, and nasolabial folds), postauricular and beard areas, body flexures, and scalp, where it is known in lay terms as dandruff. The central chest and interscapular areas can also be affected. Seborrheic dermatitis affecting the eyelids causes blepharitis and sometimes associated conjunctivitis. Seborrheic dermatitis is especially prevalent among patients with neurological conditions, particularly Parkinson's disease, facial nerve injury, poliomyelitis, syringomyelia, and spinal cord injury. Neuroleptic drugs with Parkinsonian side effects can also bring about seborrheic dermatitis. More recently, severe seborrheic dermatitis has been found with increased frequency in HIV-infected individuals. Although still a controversial theory, an inflammatory response to an overgrowth of the normally resident lipophilic yeast *Pityrosporum ovale* is thought to be the cause. Treatment can focus on suppressing inflammation by means of a mild-potency topical steroid such as hydrocortisone or on killing the yeast with a topical antifungal such as ketoconazole. Topical ketoconazole also exerts some anti-inflammatory effects. Seborrheic dermatitis of the scalp responds to shampoos containing selenium sulfide, zinc pyrithione, salicylic acid, and tar. Ketoconazole shampoo and mild topical steroid solutions can also be helpful.

Intertrigo

Intertrigo is an inflammation of intertriginous skin as a result of irritation, friction, and maceration. It appears as moist, erythematous, and sometimes scaly areas in the flexures. Patients may complain of pruritus or soreness. Contributing factors include obesity, poor hygiene, hot weather, irritating or occlusive products applied locally, and clothing made of synthetic fabrics that do not breathe. Secondary candidal or dermatophyte infection is common and should be treated with an antifungal cream (see Table 54–1). Treatment should focus primarily on eliminating the contributing factors mentioned above. The affected areas should be kept as dry as possible. A low-potency topical steroid such as hydrocortisone is used initially to decrease inflammation and allow restoration of an intact skin barrier. Lotrisone, a commonly prescribed combination antifungal and topical steroid cream, should not be used for this condition, as the steroid it contains (betamethasone diproprionate) is too strong for use in intertriginous locations.

TREATMENT OF PSORIASIS

Psoriasis is a common, chronic papulosquamous condition that follows an unpredictable, waxing and waning course. The cause of psoriasis is not known, although a genetic predisposition to it has been noted. Clinically, it is characterized by well-demarcated, pink plaques with adherent, thick, "silvery" scales. Areas of predilection are the extensor surfaces of both upper and lower extremities, the scalp, the gluteal cleft, and the penis. Psoriatic plaques commonly occur at areas of trauma, such as scars or burns. This is referred to as the isomorphic response, or Koebner's phenomenon. Nails are often involved, with pitting of the nail plate, areas of yellowish discoloration known as oil spots, onycholysis (separation of the nail plate from the nail bed), and subungual debris. Psoriatic arthritis accompanies skin lesions in 5 to 8% of patients. Factors that exacerbate psoriasis include stress, streptococcal infection, cold climate, and certain medications, such as β-blockers, antimalarials, nonsteroidal anti-inflammatory drugs, lithium, and alcohol. Systemic steroids should be used with care and tapered slowly in a psoriatic patient, as a severe flare can occur with discontinuation. Psoriatic variants include inverse psoriasis of intertriginous areas, guttate psoriasis, pustular psoriasis, and erythrodermic psoriasis.

Treatment is suppressive, not curative. The most commonly used medications are the topical steroids. In general, mid- to high-potency steroids are needed (see Table 54–1). The vitamin D derivative calcipotriene (Dovonex) ointment is often effective and lacks the side effects of atrophy, tachyphylaxis, and (rarely) adrenal suppression due to systemic absorption that are associated with topical steroid use. A maximum of 100 grams can be used per week, and it is contraindicated in patients with hypercalcemia, vitamin D toxicity, or renal stones. Tar-containing bath additives, shampoos, and ointments are good adjunctive therapy, though they can be messy, and baths are often not feasible for the elderly or disabled. Treatment of a coexisting streptococcal infection often results in improvement of the psoriasis. Emollients should be used liberally. Other treatment modalities used by dermatologists include anthralin, phototherapy, oral retinoids, and methotrexate.

ULCERS

The topic of ulcers, or wounds, is discussed at length in Chapter 52. It is important to keep in mind that atypical or nonhealing ulcers should be referred for biopsy to exclude less common causes such as malignancy, vasculitis, and infection before assuming arterial or venous insufficiency alone is responsible.

TREATMENT OF DRUG ERUPTIONS

Drug eruptions can present in a wide variety of clinical manifestations. They typically appear 1 to 10 days after starting a drug and last up to 14 days after discontinuation of the drug. A rechallenge results in more rapid development of a rash. Rarely, drug eruptions can occur after weeks, months, or even years of using a medication. The drugs most commonly implicated are penicillins, sulfonamides, cephalosporins (10% crossreactivity with penicillins), anticonvulsants, blood products, quinidine, barbiturates, isoniazid, and furosemide. However, any medication, including over-the-counter preparations and sporadically used drugs, can cause eruptions.

The most common morphology is the morbilliform, or maculopapular, eruption which is a symmetrical pruritic eruption of coalescing erythematous macules and papules distributed on the trunk and extending peripherally onto the extremities. Other forms of drug eruptions are urticaria, photosensitivity, lichenoid drug eruption, vasculitis (discussed below), and fixed drug eruption (a single or a few localized, red-to-violacious, round plaques that resolve with hyperpigmentation and recur in the same location with rechallenge). Treatment of a drug eruption requires discontinuation of the culprit drug. Medium-potency topical steroids (see Table 54–1), antihistamines, and antipruritic lotions, such as calamine and Sarna lotion, give symptomatic relief.

Potentially life-threatening drug eruptions are exfoliative erythroderma, anticonvulsant hypersensitivity syndrome, erythema multiforme major (Stevens-Johnson syndrome), and toxic epidermal necrolysis. These are dermatological emergencies requiring hospitalization and supportive care. Exfoliative erythroderma is characterized by generalized erythema and scaling. Inability to maintain fluids or to regulate electrolytes and temperature and high-output cardiac failure are complications. Anticonvulsant hypersensitivity syndrome is a multiorgan reaction that occurs with phenobarbital, carbamazepine, and phenytoin, all of which crossreact with each other. In addition to cutaneous findings, which can be of any type, fever, lymphadenopathy, hematological abnormalities, and hepatitis are seen. Other organs can also be affected. In erythema multiforme major, the pathognomonic target lesions, which have red peripheries and cyanotic or bullous centers, are accompanied by erosion of the mucous membranes. This can sometimes be seen on a continuum with toxic epidermal necrolysis, which is characterized by a tender skin eruption that rapidly progresses to blistering and sloughing of skin. Applying lateral force to the skin causes the overlying epidermis to shear off (Nikolsky's sign). This condition, with its 50% mortality rate, is best treated in a burn unit.

TREATMENT OF URTICARIA

Urticaria, or hives, is characterized by pruritic, edematous, usually erythematous papules and plaques often surrounded by a red halo (flare). Angioedema or deeper subcutaneous swellings may accompany urticaria. By definition, individual lesions last no longer than 24 hours; if lesions are longer-lasting, then urticarial vasculitis or other diagnoses should be considered. Urticaria has a variety of causes, the most common of which is an allergic reaction to foods (e.g., strawberries, nuts, shellfish) or drugs (e.g., penicillin, contrast dye). Physical factors, such as cold, pressure, or sunlight; emotional stress; or infections (e.g., dental abscess, streptococcal upper respiratory infection, parasitic infection) can also induce urticaria. Certain medications, such as aspirin and narcotics, can cause direct, nonimmunological degranulation of mast cells, which result in urticaria. Bullous pemphigoid (see below) can initially mimic urticaria. Urticaria usually resolves spontaneously within days to a few weeks; if lesions continue to appear for more than 6 weeks and if no allergen can be identified, a workup for systemic disease is warranted. Whenever possible, the causative agent should be identified and eliminated. Antihistamines are the mainstay of treatment. Examples of commonly prescribed antihistamines are the nonsedating H_1 blocker loratadine, 10 mg each day, and the sedating antihistamines diphenhydramine 25 mg and hydroxyzine 10 to 25 mg every 4 to 6 hours until lesions cease appearing. In cases of anaphylaxis or laryngeal edema, emergency resuscitation measures should be undertaken, including the administration of epinephrine, support of blood pressure, and maintenance of a patent airway.

DIFFERENTIAL DIAGNOSIS AND TREATMENT OF BLISTERS

Bullous eruptions in an elderly patient can range from those due to benign physical factors to life-threatening, immune-mediated bullous disorders. A flattening of the dermal-epidermal junction with aging results in increased skin fragility and susceptibility to blistering. Edematous skin is even more likely to develop blisters. The following is a partial list of diagnoses to consider:

Pressure Blisters. Lesions can occur over pressure points such as the heels and maleoli in a patient with a diminished level of consciousness or with sensory deficits. Macular erythema often precedes blistering. Treatment is to relieve the causative pressure, usually by frequent repositioning, protective cushioning, or both.

Burns. Chemical, thermal, and ultraviolet-light injury can cause blisters in affected areas. Usually, history points to this cause. Treatment is supportive, employing cool soaks for thermal and ultraviolet burns as well as antibiotic ointments such as silver sulfadiazene and protective dressings. Nonsteroidal anti-inflammatory drugs, such as aspirin or indomethacin, can also be beneficial early in the treatment of sunburns.

Contact Dermatitis. As discussed above, an acute contact dermatitis can result in such serious inflammation and edema as to result in frank vesiculation. Clues to contact dermatitis are linear arrangements of vesicles, odd-shaped lesions, and sharply demarcated lesions. Treatment is outlined above.

Herpetic Infection. As discussed above, herpes is characterized by grouped vesicles on an erythematous base that evolve into pustules, erosions, and crusts. Acyclovir (200 mg five times a day for herpes simplex or 800 mg five times a day for herpes zoster) is the gold standard of treatment.

Bullous Impetigo. This superficial staphylococcal infection presents as flaccid bullae that easily rupture, leaving yellowish crusts. Treatment is with antistaphylococcal antibiotics such as dicloxacillin 250 to 500 mg four times a day.

Bullous Pemphigoid. This is a chronic, immunologically mediated bullous disorder characterized by tense bullae on normal or erythematous skin. Pruritus is common, and mucous membrane involvement occurs in approximately 20 to 50% of cases. As mentioned above, bullous pemphigoid can have a prebullous phase that presents as urticaria or as pruritus without distinct skin lesions. Men and women are equally affected, and most patients are over 60 years old at the onset of disease. Diagnosis is made by skin biopsy for routine pathology and for immunofluorescence. Immunofluorescence reveals IgG and complement (C3) deposits at the dermal-epidermal junction of perilesional skin. Traditionally, bullous pemphigoid has been treated with systemic corticosteroids and immunosuppressive therapy. Recently, tetracycline and nicotinamide have been shown to be effective in some patients. Consultation with a dermatologist is strongly advised.

Pemphigus Vulgaris. Much less common than bullous pemphigoid, pemphigus vulgaris is another chronic, immunologically mediated bullous disease that presents with flaccid rather than tense bullae. Often only ruptured bullae (erosions and crusts) are present. Mucous membranes are almost always affected and may sometimes be the only manifestations of the disease. Again, the diagnosis is made by skin biopsy and immunofluorescence, which shows IgG and C3 deposited on the surface of keratinocytes. Before the advent of corticosteroids, pemphigus vulgaris was universally fatal. Today, it is treated aggressively with corticosteroids and other immunosuppressives, leading to long-lasting remissions.

TREATMENT OF PURPURA

When blood extravasates into cutaneous tissue, purpura results. One can classify purpura as disorders of hemostasis, increased fragility of blood vessels and their supporting connective tissue, and vasculitis, or inflammation of the blood vessels.

Disorders of Hemostasis. Purpura can be a manifestation of bleeding disorders, such as idiopathic thrombocytopenic purpura, thrombotic thrombocytopenic purpura, disseminated intravascular coagulation, liver disease, thrombocythemia, or bone marrow dysfunction secondary to leukemia or drugs. Anticoagulants, such as heparin, coumadin, aspirin, or nonsteroidal anti-inflammatory drugs, can also be associated with purpura, usually in response to some injury to the skin. Often in such patients, other dermatitides such as drug eruptions can become purpuric. Treatment is directed at the underlying problem.

Fragility of Blood Vessels. The most common cause of this purpura is actinic (Bateman's) purpura. The combination of aging and chronic sun damage leads to degeneration of the collagen that surrounds and supports small vessels. Minor trauma, often not even noted by the patient, results in slowly resolving purpuric macules. Chronic corticosteroid administration can produce similar changes.

Vasculitis. Palpable purpuric papules should point to the possibility of vasculitis, although lesions of vasculitis need not always be palpable. Causes of vasculitis include drug allergy, blood-borne infection (e.g., streptococcus, meningococcemia, viral hepatitis, endocarditis), serum sickness, collagen vascular diseases, and cryoglobulinemia. Wegener's granulomatosis and polyarteritis nodosa are examples of vasculitis involving larger, medium-sized vessels. When vasculitis is present in the skin, it is important to rule out systemic involvement with a urinalysis, renal and liver function tests, and a stool guaiac. Whenever possible, treatment is directed to the underlying condition. Treatment is generally supportive, though some forms of vasculitis, particularly those with systemic involvement, may require treatment with corticosteroids or other anti-inflammatory or immunosuppressive drugs.

Pigmented Purpuras. In this disorder, there are several idiopathic purpuric eruptions, unrelated to any systemic disease, that affect primarily the lower legs. Lesions may be predominantly red-purple (of recent onset) or brown to golden-brown (chronic hemosiderin deposits). No treatment is necessary and, indeed, none is very effective.

CUTANEOUS TUMORS

A variety of benign, premalignant, and malignant tumors can arise in the skin. They are covered in detail in Chapter 40.

CONCLUSION

Age-related changes occur in the skin's structure and function. Viral, fungal, and bacterial infections as well as infestations and inflammatory conditions are possible, and the use of some common treatment interventions can be affected by the advanced age of the patient, so precautions must be taken. Proper care of the skin of an aging person is confounded by coexisting pathology; thus, special considerations may be necessary.

SUGGESTED READINGS

Beutner KR, Friedman DJ, Andersen PL, et al. Valaciclovir compared with acyclovir for improved therapy for herpes zoster in immunocompetent adults. *Antimicrob Agents Chemother* 1995; 39:1546–1553.

Fitzpatrick TB, Eisen AZ, Wolff K, et al. *Dermatology in General Medicine,* 5th ed. New York: McGraw-Hill; 1998.

Gilchrest BA. Skin changes and disorders. In: Abrams WB, Beers MH, Berkow R, Fletcher JA, eds. *The Merck Manual of Geriatrics,* 2nd ed. Whitehouse Station, NJ: Merck Research Laboratories; 1995:1255.

Goldstein SM, Wintroub BU. A Physician's Guide—Adverse Cutaneous Reactions to Medication. New York: CoMedia; 1994.

Wood MJ, Kay R, Dworkin RH, Soong SJ, Whitley RJ. Oral acyclovir therapy accelerates pain resolution in patients with herpes zoster: a meta-analysis of placebo-controlled trials. *Clin Infect Dis* 1996; 22:341–347.

AGING AND THE PATHOLOGICAL SENSORIUM

Chapter 55

Functional Vision Changes in the Aging Eye

Bruce Rosenthal, O.D.

INTRODUCTION

Many normal vision changes take place in the aging eye on physiological, functional, and pathological levels.

One of the first effects of aging is a gradual and irreversible decrease in the ability to accommodate, or focus on, nearby objects. This reduction in accommodative ability that occurs as part of the normal aging process[1] is known as presbyopia, which literally translated means "the eyesight of the aged."[2] Borish[3, 4] has described presbyopia as a decrease in accommodative amplitude as compared to the normal accommodative amplitude predicted for a given age.

The first symptoms of presbyopia usually include the blurring of print, headaches, and the inability to sustain reading. The onset of the first symptoms may appear earlier in life in persons of short stature because the print has to be held closer, where the accommodative demand is higher. Age is the primary risk factor of presbyopia, but accommodation can also be affected by medications, nutrition, systemic conditions such as diabetes or myasthenia gravis, stroke, and farsightedness (hyperopia).

The onset of presbyopia, which is generally accepted as occurring between the age of 40 and 50, results in the need for a reading correction or reading aid for those already wearing corrections for myopia, hyperopia, or astigmatism. The prescription for close work and all close-up tasks increases as the accommodative amplitude decreases.

Correction for reading can be incorporated into a pair of glasses, contact lenses, bifocals (which are a combination of distance and reading prescriptions), or trifocals (which cover the distance, intermediate, and near ranges).

Individuals who have had cataract extraction lose the ability to accommodate, as the natural lens is replaced with an intraocular implant (IOL). As a result, postoperative treatment of individuals who have undergone cataract surgery with IOLs includes an examination for a prescription for reading glasses.

THE FUNCTIONAL CHANGES IN VISION

Visual Acuity

Static Visual Acuity   Static visual acuity, as determined by stationary test types or test objects such as a visual acuity chart, appears to decline with age, according to Weymouth using data from Hirsch.[4–6] In general, static visual acuity declines very little with age other than when it can be accounted for by miosis or the increased density of the lens.[7]

Dynamic Visual Acuity   Dynamic visual acuity is tested when the target is moving. Burg and Reading reported that with aging, there is a decline in dynamic visual acuity as target velocity increases.[8, 9]

Visual Field

A decrease in visual field size with age, in the absence of pathology, may be attributed to an increase in the density of the lens due to reduced retinal illuminance. It has been stated that there is a reduction of 1 to 3 degrees per decade; others have found a reduction of 0.5 dB to 1.0 dB per decade in static testing of the visual field.

Contrast Sensitivity Function

The degree of blackness to whiteness of a target is known as contrast.[10] Contrast testing gives some indication of how a person sees under nonideal conditions and may give a more realistic indication of how a person sees. The findings of a test of the contrast sensitivity function can be plotted as a contrast sensitivity curve. This curve plots the contrast sensitivity function (the inverse of contrast threshold) against the spatial frequency (size) of the target. Contrast sensitivity function changes have been attributed to neuron loss within the visual pathway, not to lenticular changes.[11]

Color Vision

It has been established that ability to see color declines with age because of the changes in absorption of light by the ocular media such as the lens as well as because of a reduction in pupil size.[12]

Acquired color vision loss in older people is different from congenital (present at birth) defects in which altered characteristics of cone photopigments lead to color confusion. One way of classifying acquired color vision defects is Köllner's law, which describes the location of the color vision loss. The law states that lesions in the outer retinal layers give rise to blue-yellow defects, whereas lesions in the inner retinal layers and optic nerve give rise to red-green defects.

Individuals with cataracts that have only a nuclear yellowing commonly have blue-yellow confusion as do individuals with age-related macular degeneration and glaucoma. Other individuals, those with optic neuritis (inflammation of the optic nerve), may report a red-green defect.

Persons who are taking medications or combinations of drugs may also experience a change in perception of color. Drugs that can affect color perception are sedatives, antibiotics, and antipsychotics.

Color vision tests are often clinically relevant, in conjunction with other clinical findings, as part of diagnostic profiles. Color vision is also important for certain tasks such as seeing a traffic light when driving or crossing the street.

Recovery from Glare

The elderly are more sensitive to glare and often take longer to recover when exposed to a source of glare.[13] It is important for a person to be aware of this change when moving from an area of low light to one of high light such as when going outside on a very bright day, as this response to glare may increase the risk for falls. Among the clinical applications of glare testing is its use as a significant preoperative test in persons with cataracts or corneal opacities. It is also used to monitor the progression of a cataract and is an indicator of visual function.

Glare testing has also been useful in the postoperative evaluation of persons who have undergone cataract extraction, corneal transplants, and some of the laser procedures for correction of myopia.

Changes in Adaptation to Darkness

With age, a decline can occur in the ability to function well in poorly illuminated surroundings. This may be attributed to media (cornea, lens, vitreous) and neural changes. The clinical significance of problems with adaptation to darkness is that some people may have difficulty entering a movie theatre or a dimly lit restaurant because the eye does not adapt quickly enough to the lower level of light.

PHYSIOLOGICAL CHANGES IN THE EYE

Various structural changes can occur in the aging eyelid that may cause pain and decreased vision. Among the changes are entropion, which is an inward turning of the lower eyelid due to atrophy and loss of tone and elasticity. There is a sensation of

discomfort in entropion that is caused by the lashes rubbing against the cornea.

Ectropion is an outward turning of the lower lid margin due to a loss of muscle tone in the supporting tissue. One of the consequences of ectropion is that tears may run down the cheek because they are not properly drained into the nasal lacrimal duct. However, a more serious effect of ectropion is the possibility of exposure keratitis (inflammation of the cornea).

Blepharoptosis is a drooping of the upper eyelid that generally results in a narrowing of the space between the eyelids (palpebral fissure) when the eye is open. The clinical significance of this is that it may result in less light entering the eye, as the upper lid may be obscuring the pupil. Treatment includes a "ptosis crutch" or surgery to support the upper lid.

Additional age-related physiological changes include the thinning and yellowing of the conjunctiva.[14] The eye tends to dry as tear production decreases and tear film loses stability with increasing age.[15] The cornea does not appear to be affected greatly by the normal aging process, although there is increased light scatter and an overall flattening.[15]

The pupil generally decreases in size by about 2.5 mm as a person ages from 20 to 80.[17] The clinical significance of this smaller pupil is that illumination may be inadequate under certain conditions. For example, mobility may be difficult at night or when reading restaurant menus because inadequate light is reaching the retina as a result of the smaller pupil.

The density and the weight of the lens increases with age. The lens also yellows and fluorescence is greater with age. The number of retinal pigment epithelial (RPE) cells in the posterior pole decreases with age.[18] Lipofuscin accumulates in the RPE cells with age and displaces the melanin.[18] Also, it is estimated that a 70-year-old person has lost 25% of the axons in the optic nerve.[15, 19] The clinical relevance of changes in the optic nerve is that there is a decrease in the contrast sensitivity function which may result in the need for greater illumination when reading and difficulty seeing in an area that is poorly lit.

MAJOR PATHOLOGICAL EYE CHANGES ASSOCIATED WITH AGING

Cataracts

A cataract is a clouding of the lens of the eye, which may lead to a host of common signs and symptoms,[20] including problems with glare and blurry distance vision. Streaks or rays of light may seem to come from light sources such as headlights and stop lights, especially at night. The individual instinctively shades his or her eyes from the sun and feels more comfortable wearing a visor. Reflections of light from the metal on a car or from road pavement and bright or hazy skies may cause excessive glare that results in the loss of color perception and difficulty in reading. Fluorescent ceiling lights and bright reading lamps may also cause glare. Print may appear faded and lacking in contrast and may be difficult to read in dim light. When outdoors, a person may find that sunglasses appear to reduce vision. Highway signs, particularly on bright days, are difficult to read. There is night blindness. Also, there may be an improvement in vision known as second sight, which is generally due to refractive changes in the eye. Cataracts can affect mobility by decreasing proprioception of the edges of stairs and curbs. Depth perception may also be impaired.

Risk Factors, Evaluation, and Intervention

Risk factors for cataracts include diabetes, drugs, especially long use of steroids, ultraviolet radiation, smoking, alcohol abuse, malnutrition, injury to the eye, and hypercholesterolemia or elevated triglycerides.

When evaluating cataracts it is important to obtain a functional case history, including visual acuity and glare brightness acuity testing. The pupils should be dilated, and tonometry for intraocular pressure should be performed. Additional investigation should include contrast sensitivity, potential acuity meter (PAM), laser interferometry, and preoperative tests.

Therapeutic intervention includes cataract removal, and correction of aphakia (lack of a lens) through the use of an intraocular lens of some type, cataract glasses, or contact lenses. After cataract surgery, the best corrected visual acuity drops one line on the eye chart for each 3.4 years.[21]

The prevalence of cataracts increases with age as can be seen in Tables 55–1, 55–2, and 55–3. It should be noted that in the Framingham study, a cataract was defined as a lens change that cannot be ascribed to specific causes and is accompanied by a visual acuity of 20/30 or worse.

Age-Related Macular Degeneration

Macular degeneration results from any degenerative, inflammatory, toxic, vascular, or dystrophic condition that affects primarily the foveomacular area. There may be atrophy, hemorrhage, fibrovas-

cular scarring, or degenerative or localized cystic changes in the macula or the perimacular area.[22, 24]

Symptoms of macular degeneration include diminished central vision, blurred reading vision even with current reading glasses, and loss of detail such as facial features. Straight lines may appear distorted, for example, telephone poles may look crooked. Colors may seem faded, and colors or objects may appear different through each eye. These visual problems can create problems with depth perception, and objects may disappear from the field of vision, which may lead to difficulty in mobility.

Risk Factors, Evaluation, Intervention

The risk factors for macular degeneration include smoking, hypertension, and excessive exposure to ultraviolet light, and there may be a possible hereditary link. Soft drusen are found; these are yellowish or white dots located in the retina that are colloid deposits or hyaline bodies. Elevated levels of cholesterol over time and poor diet, specifically a lack

---

Table 55–1 Prevalence of Cataract[a] According to the Framingham Study

Age	Percentage
52–64	5%
65–74	18%
75–84	91%

[a]Cataract, as defined by the study, is a lens change that cannot be ascribed to specific causes and is accompanied by a visual acuity of 20/30 or worse.

Data from Kahn HA, Leibowitz HM, Ganley JP, Kini MM, Colton T, Nickerson RS, Dawber TR. The Framingham Eye Study. I. Outline and major prevalence finding. *Am J Epidemiol* 1977; 106(1):17–32.

Table 55–2 Lens Opacities According to the National Eye Institute[23]

Age	Percentage
65–74	74%
75–84	91%

Table 55–3 Estimated Incidence of Cortical and Nuclear Cataracts: Waterman Eye Study[a]

Age	Cortical Cataract	Nuclear Cataract
30–39	1%	<1%
40–49	3%	2%
50–59	8%	12%
60–69	17%	32%
70–79	32%	51%
80 +	32%	55%

[a]Data from Taylor HR, West SK, Rosenthal FS, Munoz B, Newland HS, Abbey H, Emmett EA. Effect of ultraviolet radiation on cataract formation. *N Engl J Med* 1988; 319(22):1429–1433.

of vitamins and minerals in the retina, are additional risk factors.

There are three types of macular degeneration: atrophic (dry), wet, and pigment epithelial detachment. The diagnosis of macular degeneration should be confirmed by using tests of visual function in-

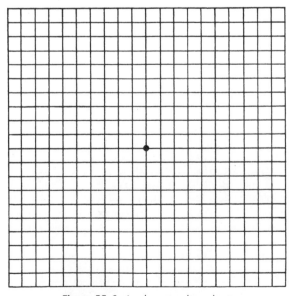

AMSLER RECORDING CHART
A replica of Chart No. 1, printed in black on white for convenience of recording

Figure 55–1 Amsler recording chart.

cluding acuity and contrast sensitivity, color vision, and the Amsler grid (see Fig. 55–1).

Treatment of macular degeneration includes laser photocoagulation and the use of low-vision devices, which are listed Box 55–1. Photos of these devices are shown in Figure 55–2. In addition, several treatments are under investigation, including radiation, thalidomide, and RPE transplants.

The prevalence of macular degeneration, like that of cataracts, increases with age. As can be seen in Table 55–4, one third of persons 75 years old or older have signs of this condition.

Glaucoma

Glaucoma is a condition in which defective aqueous outflow due to increased resistence in the drainage canals results in high intraocular pressure.[24] The signs and symptoms of glaucoma depend upon the progression of the condition; they may include seeing rainbow-colored halos around lights and poor contrast sensitivity. There may be sensitivity to glare and excessive tearing, with pain or redness in the eyes. The pupils may be dilated and mobility may be jeopardized because of blind spots in the visual field, poor peripheral vision, and poor night vision, which can cause a person to bump into objects.

Evaluation and Intervention

In the evaluation of glaucoma it is important to obtain the patient's medical history and to measure intraocular pressure with tonometry. Ophthalmoscopy of the optic nerve is important. A flashlight, slit-lamp, visual fields assessment, gonioscopy and tomography are additional evaluation tools.

Therapeutic intervention may include drug therapy with cholinergic and anticholinesterase agents and with β-adrenergic agents. Additionally, carbonic anhydrase inhibitors, hyperosmotic agents,

Box 55–1

Types of Low-Vision Devices

High plus or microscopic lenses
Hand magnifiers
Stand magnifiers
Hand-held and spectacle-mounted telescopes
Absorptive lenses
Closed-circuit television and electronic devices
Nonoptical devices
Field-expanding devices

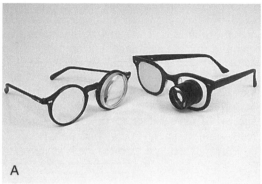

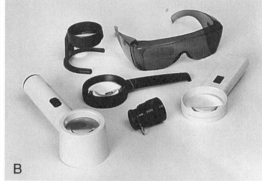

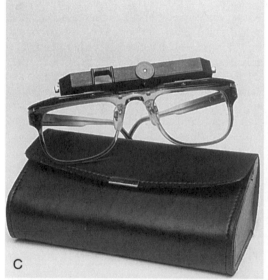

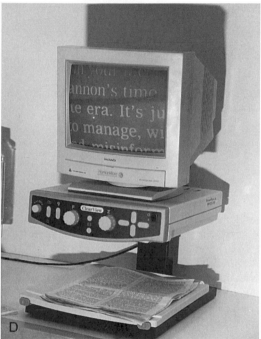

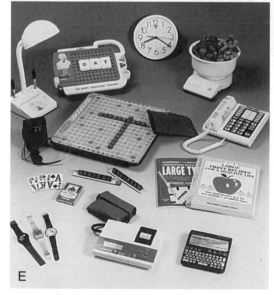

Figure 55–2 Types of low vision devices: (A) *left,* doublet microscopic reading lens for the left eye, *right,* very high-powered microscopic lens in the left eye; (B) *clockwise from the center,* hand magnifier, stand magnifier, absorptive lenses, another hand magnifier, handheld telescopic system, another stand magnifier; (C) Keplerian (prism) spectacle-mounted telescope; (D) closed-circuit television—note the reverse polarity on the screen, i.e., white letters on a black background; (E) Nonoptical low-vision devices. (Courtesy of The Lighthouse, Inc.)

Table 55–4 Prevalence and Signs of Macular Degeneration

Age	Number	Percentage
40 and older[a]	1.2 million	1.4%
65 and older[b]		5% have some signs of visual impairment as a result of macular degeneration
75 and older[c]		33% have signs of the condition

[a]*The Lighthouse National Survey on Vision Loss: The experiences, attitudes, and knowledge of middle-aged and older Americans.* New York: The Lighthouse; 1994.
[b]Chang YP, Bassi LJ, Javitt JC. Federal budgetary costs of blindness. *Milbank Q* 1992; 70:319–340.
[c]National Society to Prevent Blindness (*Prevent Blindness America* 1980). *Vision Problems in the US.*

and prostaglandins are used in the nonsurgical treatment of glaucoma. Laser surgery is invaluable in treating of glaucoma. Low-vision devices as shown in Figure 55–2, are helpful. Rehabilitation services should include orientation to furniture and living situations. Mobility and ability to perform the activities of daily living should be evaluated.

The prevalence of glaucoma is somewhat varied, as can be seen in Table 55–5.

Diabetic Retinopathy (Type II Adult-Onset)

Diabetic retinopathy is hemorrhagic, proliferative, exudative, or occlusive retinopathy secondary to diabetics mellitus. The signs and symptoms include seeing a fluctuating image, blurring, distortion, and decreased vision. There may be a change in refractive correction. Diplopia, loss of color vision, and the presence of floaters also occur.

Approximately 12.7 million Americans over the age of 40 have diabetes;[29] diabetic retinopathy affects approximately 5% of that population. About 8,000 new cases are reported each year.[25]

Risk Factors, Evaluation, Intervention

Risk factors for diabetic retinopathy include high blood sugar levels, hypertension, obesity, smoking, and duration of diabetes, as visual changes generally appear approximately 15 years after the onset of diabetes. Diabetic retinopathy should be assessed with the full battery of vision function tests, including visual acuity, contrast sensitivity, Amsler grid and visual fields, ophthalmoscopy, slit-lamp evaluation, and fluorescein angiography. Treatment includes laser surgery, possible vitrectomy, use of low-vision devices, and rehabilitation, which should include orientation to the living area and to means of mobility. A patient may have to be given training in ways of performing the activities of daily living.

Visual Impairment and Blindness

Functional visual impairment is a significant limitation of visual capability resulting from disease, trauma, or congenital condition, that cannot be fully ameliorated by standard refractive correction, medication, or surgery. The prevalence of self-reported

Table 55–5 Prevalence of Glaucoma

Age	Number	Percentage
All ages	3–4 million	4–5%
40 and over (African-Americans)[a]	500,600; 4 to 6 times higher among blacks than whites[27b]	6%
40 and over[a]	1,477,904	2%
All ages worldwide	50,000,000[a]	

[a]*Prevent Blindness America.*

Table 55–6 Prevalence of Self Reported Visual Impairment[a]

Age	Percentage	Number (million)
45–64	15%	7.2
65–74	17%	3.1
75 and older	26%	3.5

[a]*The Lighthouse National Survey on Vision Loss: The experiences, attitudes, and knowledge of middle-aged and older Americans.* New York: The Lighthouse; 1994.

visual impairment, as shown in Table 55–6, increases with age; it affects one in four persons aged 75 years years and older. Visual impairment is manifested by one or more of the following[30]:

1. Insufficient visual resolution (worse than 20/60 in the better eye with best correction of ametropia);

2. Inadequate field of vision (worse than 20 degrees along the widest meridian in the eye with the more intact central field; or homonymous hemianopsia);

3. Reduced peak contrast sensitivity (< 1.7 log CS binocularly);

4. Insufficient visual resolution or peak contrast sensitivity (see 1 and 3) at high or low luminances within a range typically encountered in everyday life.

LEGAL BLINDNESS is defined as visual acuity of 20/200 or less or a visual field of 20 degrees or less in the widest meridian. According to the 1990 census, there are 912,000 individuals over the age of 40 who are legally blind. The problem increases with age, as the number of legally blind people over the age of 65 was estimated to be 713,000, according to a 1992 study.[32] The leading causes of legal blindness are shown in Table 55–7.

CONCLUSION

Many age-related changes (presbyopia) occur in the eye and result in reduced vision. Pathological changes such as cataracts, macular degeneration, glaucoma, and diabetic retinopathy compound the effects of presbyopia and lead to further visual impairment, which is self-reported by over 25% of persons 75 years old and older. This reduced vision is a significant factor in rehabilitation, as it minimizes mobility, increases the risk for falls and injury, and degrades the quality of life. Many of the visual problems are treatable with medications, low-vision devices, and surgery.

Table 55–7 Leading Causes of Legal Blindness

Number	Pathology	Percentage
1	Glaucoma	12.5%
2	Macular degeneration	11.7%
3	Senile cataract	8.3%
4	Optic nerve atrophy	7.0%
5	Diabetic retinopathy	6.6%
6	Retinitis pigmentosa	4.7%
7	Myopia	4.0%
	All others, including albinism, corneal dystrophy, macular holes and cysts, vascular occlusions, toxoplasmosis, uveitis, and visual field defect	45.2%

REFERENCES

1. Cline D, Hofstetter, Griffin JR, *Dictionary of Visual Science,* 3rd ed. Radnor, Pa.: Chilton; 1980.
2. Weale RA. Presbyopia and its occurrence in different parts of the world. In: Stark L, Obrecht G, eds. Presbyopia, Recent Research and Reviews from the Third International Symposium. New York: Fairchild Publications; 1985: 2.
3. Borish IM. *Clinical Refraction,* 3rd ed. Chicago: Professional Press; 1970.
4. Borish IM. Accommodation, Presbyopia and Anomalies in Clinical Refraction, 1st ed. Chicago: Profession Press; 1954: 367.
5. Morgan MW. Changes in Visual Function in the Aging Eye. In: Rosenbloom AA, Morgan MW. *Vision and Aging.* New York: Professional Press Books; 1986; 121.
6. Weymouth F. Effect of age on visual acuity. In: Hirsch MJ, Wick RE, eds. Vision of the Aging Patient. Philadelphia: Chilton; 1960: 37–62.
7. Pitts DG. Visual acuity as a function of age. *J Am Optom Assoc* 1982; 53: 117–124.
8. Burg A. Visual acuity measured by dynamic and static tests: a comprehensive evaluation. *J Appl Psychol* 1966; 50: 460–466.
9. Reading VM. Visual resolution as measured by dynamic and static tests. *Pflugers Arch* 1972; 338:17–26.
10. Arden GG. The importance of measuring contrast sensitivity in cases of visual disturbance. *Br J Ophthalmol* 1978; 62:198–209.
11. Owsley C, Gardner T, Sekuler R, Lieberman H. Role of the crystalline lens in the spatial vision loss of the elderly. *Invest Ophthalmol Vis Sci* 1985; 26:1165–1170.
12. Aston SJ, Maino JH. *Clinical Geriatric Eyecare.* Boston: Butterworth-Heinemann; 1993:58–59.
13. Paulson LE, Sjostrand J. Contrast sensitivity in the presence of a glare light. *Invest Ophthalmol Vis Sci* 1980; 19:401–406.
14. Michaels DD. Ocular disease in the elderly. In: Rosenbloom AA, Morgan MW, eds. *Vision and Aging.* Boston: Butterworth-Heinemann; 1993.

15. Horn MJ, Maino JH. Normal vision problems of the elderly. In: Aston SJ, Maino JH. *Clinical Geriatric Eyecare* Boston: Butterworth-Heinemann; 1993.
16. Marmor MF. Visual changes with age. In: Caird FI, Williamson J, eds. *The Eye and Its Disorders in the Elderly.* Bristol, Scotland: Wright; 1986:28–36.
17. Morgan MW. Changes in visual function in the aging eye. In: Rosenbloom AA, Morgan MW, eds. *Vision and Aging.* New York: Fairchild Publications; 1986:121–134.
18. Dorney CK, Wu G, Ebenstein D, et al. Cell loss in the aging retina. *Invest Ophthalmol Vis Sci* 1989; 30:1691–1699.
19. Balazsi AG, Bootman J, Drance SM, et al. The effect of age on the nerve fiber population of the human optic nerve. *Am J Ophthalmol* 1984; 97:760–766.
20. Faye EE, Rosenthal BP, Sussman-Skalka CJ. Cataract and the aging eye. New York: Lighthouse National Center for Vision and Aging; 1995.
21. Murrill CA, Stanfield DL, VanBrocklin MD, et al. Care of the adult patient with cataract. St. Louis: American Optometric Association; 1995.
22. Jay JL, Mammo RB, Allan D. Effect of age on visual acuity after cataract extraction. *Br J Ophthalmol* 1987; 71:112–115.
23. Cataract Management Guideline Panel *Cataracts in Adults: Management of Functional Impairment.* Rockville, Md: U.S. Dept. of Health and Human Services, Agency for Health Care Policy and Research. AHCPR Pub. No. 93-0542.
24. Faye EE. Clinical Low Vision, 2nd ed. Boston: Little, Brown; 1984: 281.
25. Prevent Blindness America. *Vision Problems in the U.S.* Glaucoma. 1994.
26. National Eye Institute. Vision Research: A National Plan 1994–1998: A report of the National Advisory Eye Council. (NIH Publication No. 95-3186) 1993.
27. Tielsch JA, Sommer K, Witt K, et al. Blindness and visual impairment in an American urban population: the Baltimore Eye survey. *Arch Ophthalmol* 1990; 108:286–290.
28. The Glaucoma Foundation Information located in fact sheets located at: www.glaucoma.foundation.org/info. 1996.
29. American Diabetes Association *Diabetes Facts and Figures.* Cedar Rapids, Iowa: 1995.
30. Arditi A, Rosenthal B. Hacia una definición objectiva del término "deficiencia visual." Entre do mundo, O.N.C.E. Centro Bibliografico y Cultura, Madrid, 1996.
31. The Lighthouse National Survey on Vision Loss: The experience, attitudes, and knowledge of middle-aged and older Americans. New York: The Lighthouse; 1994.
32. Chiang YP, Bassi LJ, Javitt JC. Federal budgetary costs of blindness. *Milbank Q* 1992; 70:319–340.
33. National Society to Prevent Blindness (Prevent Blindness America 1980). *Vision Problems in the U.S.* Schaumberg, Ill.: Author.

Chapter **56**

Functional Hearing Changes in the Aging Ear

Kristen D. Alexander, M.A., CCC/A
Paula Curliss, M.A., CCC/A

INTRODUCTION

Two professions are primarily involved in the diagnosis and management of ear and hearing disorders. The first is otolaryngology, the medical and surgical management of ear, nose, and throat disorders. Physicians in this field may be referred to as otologists, otolaryngologists, otorhinolaryngologists, or ear, nose, and throat specialists (ENTs). The second profession is audiology. An audiologist specializes in the differential diagnosis of ear, hearing, and balance disorders. During an audiological assessment, an attempt is made to determine the physiology and severity of and the prognosis for a hearing loss or to determine the need for medical referral. When an individual experiences dizziness, disequilibrium, lightheadedness, or gait disturbances, a balance evaluation is performed in order to differentiate between inner ear/vestibular and central pathologies. The selection and dispensing of hearing aids is also within the scope of the audiologist's practice. Both professions frequently work together to provide comprehensive management.

According to the National Center for Health Statistics Survey of 1995, hearing loss is one of the most prevalent chronic health conditions in the United States. The same survey indicated that the incidence of hearing loss for those 65 to 74 years of age is 22.9%, and among those 75 years of age and older, it is 31.9%.

Unfortunately, most laypeople and some healthcare providers are unaware of the communication difficulties that plague the geriatric population experiencing hearing loss. Hearing loss is an invisible handicap. The behaviors that accompany hearing loss can be misinterpreted or misdiagnosed as dementia, cognitive impairment, forgetfulness, or confusion. A hearing evaluation assists in differentiating between hearing loss and other such diagnoses. The progression of hearing loss is often gradual, occurring over a period of years. Therefore, it is not always obvious to those around an individual that hearing sensitivity is becoming compromised.

CAUSES OF HEARING LOSS IN ADVANCED AGE

The term "presbycusis" was initially coined to identify hearing loss due to aging. This loss occurs gradually and affects the high-pitch range of hearing in both ears. However, it has become common knowledge that the hearing loss of many older adults is the cumulative result of many factors, the most widespread of which is exposure to excessive noise. This includes exposure not only to military and industrial noises, but also to common, everyday noises from motor vehicles, household appliances, power equipment, and other sounds that permeate an industrialized society.

There are various otologic pathologies that can result in temporary or permanent hearing loss. These may include bacterial or viral infections of the hearing or balance mechanisms. A medical examination is necessary to diagnosis and treat these disorders.

Damage to the balance or hearing mechanisms on a permanent or temporary basis by certain medications is referred to as ototoxicity. These medications include but are not limited to a variety of intravenous antibiotics, some chemotherapy agents, loop-inhibiting diuretics, antimalarial agents, salicylates, and analgesics (see Box 56–1). The pharmacological mechanisms of ototoxicity are not entirely understood and may vary with the classification of medication. The combination of impaired renal function and the use of ototoxic medications potentiates the risk for hearing loss. Noise exposure also has a synergistic effect with the use of ototoxic medications, and therefore individuals receiving such medications must be advised to use ear protection. Audiological baseline testing and regular monitoring can assist in the early detection and possible reversal of ototoxicity. The American Speech-Language-Hearing Association, in 1994, advised its audiologists to implement an ototoxicity monitoring program.

Some additional factors that contribute to loss of hearing in members of the older population are cardiovascular disease, cerebrovascular accidents, transient ischemic attacks, and atherosclerosis. These conditions can also cause a decrease in an individual's ability to understand speech and can impair the processing of spoken language, regardless of a person's actual hearing ability. This is attributed to damage of the auditory structures in the central nervous system.

OTHER AUDITORY CONDITIONS

A common complaint of the aged that may exist alone or in conjunction with hearing loss is that of tinnitus, a ringing or other noise in the ears. Tinnitus may be the symptom of a treatable disease and therefore can resolve upon the identification and management of the specific condition. However, the

---

Box 56–1

Medications That Are Potentially Ototoxic

AMINOGLYCOSIDES

Amikacin	Vancomycin
Streptomycin	Netilmicin
Tobramycin	Gentamicin
Kanamycin	Neomycin

DIURETICS

Furosemide (Lasix)	Bumetanide
Ethacrynic Acid	

SALICYLATES

Aspirin

CHEMOTHERAPEUTIC AGENTS

Cisplatin

OTHER AGENTS

Quinine	Quinidine

The incidence of ototoxicity varies significantly among these medications and with each patient. This list does not necessarily include all possible ototoxic agents. Consult with a physician or pharmacist regarding the ototoxic effects of these and other medications.

---

source of tinnitus frequently cannot be identified, and its exact mechanism remains unknown. In some cases, its severity is enough to significantly interfere with daily functioning. Various treatments are available and many strategies are recommended for the management of tinnitus, including but not limited to medications, dietary changes, nutritional supplements, stress reduction and relaxation therapy, cognitive therapy, biofeedback, hearing aids, tinnitus maskers, and tinnitus retraining therapy. An individual complaining of tinnitus should first receive an audiological and otological evaluation.

Some of the aged experience greater difficulty understanding spoken language than would be expected based on their hearing sensitivity alone. They may not be able to process speech accurately in the presence of background noise, where there are multiple speakers, while listening to rapid speech, or in poor acoustical environments. A practical solution to this problem is to optimize the listening environment; this will be discussed in the next section.

MANAGEMENT AND REHABILITATION

Upon the identification of permanent hearing loss, the rehabilitation process can begin. This is imperative because an individual's ability to communicate effectively is critical to his or her social and emotional well-being. A decreased ability to communicate may cause an individual to become depressed and may contribute to thoughts of morbidity and worthlessness. Adequate hearing is obviously necessary for daily activities such as watching television and communicating with friends and family in person and on the telephone. Moreover, senior citizens have become a more vital and integral part of their communities than ever before, and sufficient hearing is crucial for their continued involvement.

Modifying the listening environment is not only the most important intervention strategy, it is also the most accessible and advantageous strategy. One method of optimizing communication is to reduce background noise and improve environmental acoustics. This can be done simply by removing or turning off the noise source or reducing its volume by physically increasing one's distance from it. Sound-absorbing materials such as carpeting, cloth window treatments, upholstery, and acoustic tiles can be utilized to improve the acoustical environment. Another means of improving communication is by training the hard-of-hearing to capitalize on visual cues, such as lip movements, facial expressions, and body movements. These individuals must also learn to be more assertive about creating the best possible listening environment for themselves. Counseling the hard-of-hearing about the changes in their environment that may optimize their listening abilities is a necessary component of rehabilitation. An individual should not hesitate to ask a person to speak louder or to stand face to face, to inform the speaker of interfering noise, to move his or her seat or position if necessary, or to ask that changes in lighting be made if visual cues are compromised.

Many devices are available to assist the hard-of-hearing. The most common is the hearing aid, which amplifies sound according to an individual's particular hearing loss. Because hearing aids are selected and customized for an individual's ear and hearing loss, they should not be shared or given to others experiencing hearing difficulties. It is not wise for an individual to use a hearing aid that was not specifically prescribed for him or her. It can be dangerous and further damage hearing, or it can provide little or no benefit.

The use of a hearing aid alone may not be sufficient for some. Assistive listening devices are available to improve specific listening situations. Among them are telephone amplifiers, teletypewriters and relay systems, television amplifiers and decoders, alerting systems for doorbells, smoke detectors, incoming telephone signals, and alarm clocks, and other devices for monitoring auditory signals such as a crying infant. Also available are systems designed to improve listening situations in public and group settings, including FM, infrared, induction loop, and hardwired systems. If there are any questions about the suitability or appropriateness of a hearing aid or assistive listening device for an individual, the advice of an audiologist, hearing aid dispenser, or assistive listening device specialist should be sought.

CONCLUSION

The consumer, the public, and the members of the health-care profession must be educated about hearing loss. As this knowledge increases, so will the diagnostic and rehabilitation services available to the geriatric population. Further information is available from the American Speech-Language-Hearing Association, 10801 Rockville Pike, Rockville, MD 20852–3279; (301) 897–5700, and from the American Tinnitus Association, P.O. Box 5, Portland, OR 97207; (503) 248–9985.

SUGGESTED READINGS

Adams PF, Marano MA. *Current Estimates from National Health Interview Survey, 1994*. National Center for Health Statistics; Vital Health Statistics. 10 (193), 1995; 83–84.
Guidelines for the audiologic management of individuals receiving cochleotoxic drug therapy. *American Speech-Language-Hearing Association* 1994; 36[suppl]:11–19.
Haybach PJ. Tuning into ototoxicity. *Nursing* 1993; 34–40.

Chapter 57

Considerations in Elder Patient Communication

Carolyn Marshall, M.P.H., Ph.D.

INTRODUCTION

For health-care professionals to deliver the best possible treatment to their older patients, some special considerations must be discussed. In order to understand the patient's expectations concerning proposed treatment or procedures, and his or her ability to follow through with prescribed self-care both during and after treatment, a mutually understandable, accurate, and satisfying communication between practitioner and patient should be established.

The health-care provider and staff have to identify what communication skills are necessary to reach each older individual. They must know the patient's physical assessment in order to learn whether there are hearing or visual deficits. Knowledge of a patient's educational level and reading ability is also necessary in order to determine how to most effectively present information concerning treatment and self-care. There are creative alternatives to pamphlets and other written patient education materials that can be used. Cultural differences should be considered as well.

If there is a question concerning the patient's status, simple evaluation tools can be used. If a barrier does exist, how is it determined whether there is a short-term confusional state or long-term dysfunction? Executive dysfunction and its implications for treatment is another important aspect to consider. Specific communication techniques can be used with patients who exhibit executive dysfunction.

CULTURAL CONSIDERATIONS

Health-care professionals must consider how those receiving care should be informed in order to reduce their future risk. To understand and to reach a patient, it is necessary to look at each individual's physical and genetic histories (Hispanic, African-American, Asian, Anglo, and so forth) as well as cultural beliefs, myths, and customs concerning diet and health. The patient's attitude toward the specific health-care setting can strongly affect interactions with care-givers.

For example, how is someone who has held health-care professionals in great respect or awe to be convinced that it is proper to ask questions and even to ask for another opinion at times? No matter what the culture, the accepted health professional/patient relationship usually can be described as one of dependence. In the Mexican-American culture, the one with which the author is most familiar, *respeto* (respect) is valued highly. Health professionals are greatly respected and usually are not questioned even if the patient does not understand the explanation of the illness or the treatment prescribed.

Health professionals who do not understand the Mexican-American culture often mistake the polite smile and nod of the head for understanding when a patient is asked if he or she understands what has been explained. In fact, it may mean that the patient does not want to admit lack of understanding either for fear of insulting the provider of the information by implying that a poor explanation has been given, or for fear of being considered ignorant. When a patient does not follow a prescribed treatment regimen, he or she is described as being "not compliant." Compliance is understood to mean the act of conforming or yielding, a tendency to yield readily to others, especially in a weak or subservient way.

"Adherence," a term much preferred by this author and one used by others concerned with health-care and effective adult patient education, is defined as "a mutually agreed-upon course of action." A person is more likely to make behavioral changes if situations are explained in a manner that can be understood both intellectually and emotionally. The possible or probable outcomes are put forward by the health-care provider and the expectations of both provider and patient can be discussed. Then, the *mutually agreed-upon* course of action is clear, and the patient assumes a measure of control and responsibility for the outcomes.

Similarly, how should an issue as culturally sensitive and culturally based as diet be addressed when a patient is to follow a specific diet? In addressing the role of diet and the importance of nutrition in health-care, Payne[1] says that nutrition considerations are not yet an integral part of most provider/patient office experiences. This is so in spite of the fact that no custom is more universally shared then the ritual of eating a meal together. The ritual symbolizes family traditions, close relationships, friendship, and sentiment, and definite dietary and cultural habits, passed on from generation to generation, have emerged from the custom. Attitudes about food and dietary practices within cultural groups can often be related to attitudes and beliefs that influence diet and consequently have an impact on health. Therefore, although a clinician may not be able to be fully armed with knowledge of the intricacies of diet among a particular cultural group, there should be at least some awareness of cultural dietary practices when managing a patient whose culture is different from the clinician's own.

To answer some of the preceding questions, a practitioner must go beyond the traditional methods of patient education used in most settings and look at each person as an individual.

Literacy

The unabridged edition of *The Random House Dictionary of the English Language* (1973) defines "literate" as (1) able to read and write; (2) having an education; (3) having or showing knowledge of literature, writing, and so forth. The same reference defines "illiterate" as (1) unable to read and write; (2) lacking education; (3) showing lack of *culture*, especially in language and literature.

The preceding definitions create the necessity of defining the words "culture" and "knowledge" as they are used in the context of this chapter. "Culture" can be defined as (1) a particular form or stage of civilization, as that of a certain nation or period; (2) the sum total of ways of living built up by a group of human beings and transmitted from one generation to another. "Knowledge," on the other hand, is defined as (1) acquaintance with facts, truths, or principles, as from study or investigation; (2) the body of truths or facts accumulated by humankind in the course of time; (3) the sum of what is known.

Although the ability to read is probably assumed when literacy is mentioned, the preceding definitions of culture and knowledge do not depend on that ability. When considering the concept of literacy, it is important to realize that of the tens of thousands of languages spoken during human history only 106 have ever been committed to writing to the degree of producing literature, and most have never been written down at all. Of the 3000 spoken languages that exist today, only 78 have a literature.[2]

Although the generally held concept is that lack of reading ability means that the individual cannot produce abstract thought, this notion is emphatically wrong. The inability to read is often the result of the circumstances in which the individual has lived and is not an indicator of lack of intelligence. For example, Mexican-American elders have worked in a predominately literate (reading) world where another language is the norm. Most did not have the opportunity to go to school on a regular basis but have supported and reared children who probably live in a cultural world different from theirs. Most people would be hard-pressed to function in

today's world without the ability to read and write. Yet despite the fact that their health status is generally lower than that of the Anglo population, Mexican-American elders see themselves as competent and functional members of their culture and the world in which they live.[3]

The way in which educators and health-care providers approach older individuals must honor their culture. For any culturally sensitive population, instructional materials should validate the life experiences and coping skills that have been developed to survive without the ability to read. In order to produce materials relevant to a particular culture, the developers must always pay close attention to detail and learner analysis, be aware of limited abilities, and be sensitive to cultural norms.[4]

World View

World view, as described by Kearney,[4] is the way human societies look at reality and make sense of their world. A world view consists of basic assumptions that may or may not be accurate, but are more or less coherent. Geertz[5] identified world view as "their picture of the way things in sheer actuality are; their concept of nature, of self, of society." For example, according to Kearney, every society has a time orientation. For the dominant Anglo culture in the United States, it is a future orientation; but for most Mexican-American elders, and in many other cultures, the orientation is that of the timeless present. The changes practitioners often recommend are seen as applying to something that might occur in the future. The concepts of chronic disease, risk factors, and the prevention of complications are based in a future orientation.

An article by Hamadeh[6] reveals an excellent example of a practitioner of Western medicine who recommended going beyond what some consider to be customary practice in order to understand his patient and the patient's situation. He used what he described as the Ecological Framework approach as a means of generating hypotheses about the patient's responses. Hamadeh described several levels of analysis: (1) the individual level, on which psychological problems, stress, and depression all may be contributing factors to poor response; (2) the family level, on which the factors affecting the patient's illness include family myths and beliefs about disease and the family's experience with the medical profession; and (3) the cultural level, on which factors affecting illness behavior may be misunderstood by the health-care provider unless he or she is aware of the larger context of the patient's background. This background includes knowledge about the economic, social, and religious factors affecting the patient's life.

Hamadeh's article concludes with a list of pertinent questions to be asked when a health-provider is new to a community and wishes to understand the patients:[6]

1. What is good health, in the community's understanding?
2. When is a member considered ill?
3. What are common explanations of cause of illness in the community?
4. What usual modes of treatment and *alternative* health-care systems are available?
5. How much is the patient responsible for illness, cure, or prevention?
6. Who is the medical decision-maker in the family?
7. What are the attitudes about death and dying?

To understand and treat elders who have lived a life of tradition within their culture, health-care professionals of all disciplines should learn about the traditions of their patients and relate to them with understanding and acceptance. The way in which educators and health-care providers approach individuals must honor their culture. Is it ethical to keep on insisting on behavior change when people demonstrate that they understand their care-givers' intentions but don't wish to change? The attitude of the provider can exert a great impact on the acceptance of a course of action depending on whether rigid compliance is expected, or whether a course of action toward change is recommended and mutually agreed upon (adherence). The attitude of the provider can greatly affect the likelihood that a change in behavior or lifestyle will occur.

PHYSICAL AND COGNITIVE CONSIDERATIONS

Hearing Impairment

When considering the cultural setting in which providers observe patients, it is important to remember the physical and cognitive barriers that can stand in the way of good communication. Hearing impairment or loss may have a major impact on rehabilitation (this problem is described in detail in Chapter 56). The negative effects of a hearing loss on elderly persons may lead to disengagement and paranoia if impairments are severe and continue for any length of time. Additionally, loss of hearing may create a sense of loneliness and isolation and possible emotional distress as a result of anxiety or depression.

Certain behavioral compensations by a patient may lead a care-provider to suspect a hearing loss. These compensations are listed in Box 57–1.

Vision Impairment

An additional sensory impairment that leads to communication barriers is the loss of vision (presbyopia and various visual pathologies are described in chapter 55). Simple compensations can be used to assist persons with visual loss such as increasing print size and boldness in all printed material, including medical and personal history forms. Glare should be minimized and bold primary colors should be used for all written materials, especially for directions.

It is not uncommon to find older individuals who have a combination of hearing and visual loss which leads to typical behaviors such as squinting, frowning, or grimacing during conversation. Often individuals with this type of impairment rely more on touch for reassurance. At times they appear to be distrusting or withdrawn. Additionally, they may seem worried about being awkward and may exhibit reluctance to communicate. This may lead to fearful behavior even in normal activities. Methods that help in communicating with patients who have im-

---

Box 57–1

Behavioral Compensations Indicative of Hearing Impairment

1. Leaning closer to the speaker
2. Cupping an ear
3. Speaking in a loud voice
4. Positioning the head so the "good" ear is near the speaker
5. Asking for phrases to be repeated
6. Answering questions inappropriately
7. Looking blank
8. Being inattentive
9. Isolating self or refusing to engage in conversation
10. Having a shorter attention span
11. Not reacting
12. Showing emotional upset

pairments in seeing or hearing or both are shown in Box 57–2.

Short-term Cognitive Dysfunction

In addition to the sensory impairments and cultural problems that lead to communication barriers between health-care providers and elderly patients, there are a host of short-term confusional states that can impede effective communication during rehabilitation. These include distortion of time and space cues so that the patient becomes confused as a result of being in an unfamiliar room and having no familiar objects in view. The hospital schedule is often totally asynchronous with the individual's normal schedule.

Hospital conditions may lead to depersonalization, as the individual loses a sense of self. A patient may simply become "the woman in room 410, bed 1." The loss of continuity with life history may also lead to some short-term confusional states. This occurs because the individual's cohorts have all died or been institutionalized, so there is no one to whom he or she can say "Do you remember . . . ?" Also, the individual may be living alone and the loss of human companionship can result in withdrawal and disengagement from social activities. Furthermore, hyperthermia and hypothermia,

---

Box 57–2

Aids to Communication for Those with Hearing and/or Visual Impairments

1. Cut down on background noise such as music or other distractions to assist a patient with hearing deficits or a hearing aid.

2. Get the person's attention before beginning to speak.

3. Do not stand with glare behind you.

4. Face the patient.

5. If you are wearing a mask, take it down before speaking to the patient; he or she has to be able to see your lips.

6. Speak slowly and distinctly; avoid long, complex sentences.

7. Ask questions to confirm that the patient understands.

8. Communicate one idea or instruction at a time.

---

electrolyte imbalance, and certain medications may lead to acute short-term states of confusion.

Long-term Cognitive Dysfunction

In the presence of cognitive dysfunction, communication takes on a whole new meaning. There are various common reasons for long-term cognitive dysfunction in aging patients, including stroke, dementia, head injuries resulting from falls or other accidents, and developmental disabilities.

When working with a patient with cognitive dysfunction or aphasia, verbal and nonverbal behavior that makes the individual feel guilty for not speaking should be avoided. It is important to accept the individual at his or her level of function and build on that. It is crucial to point out progress so that the patient grasps the idea that gains are being made. The health-care provider should try not to answer questions for the aphasic patient but should require the patient to answer them. If the individual cannot find the proper words and becomes frustrated, empathy and understanding should be expressed, but it is unwise to pretend to understand an individual when what he or she is trying to say has not been comprehended. The provider should get the person's attention before speaking, and should speak according to the individual's ability, avoiding long sentences, rapid speech, or difficult and uncommon words. It is helpful to communicate one idea at a time in clear, short sentences, using everyday words and to avoid speaking in a loud voice unless the individual has suffered a hearing loss. Facing the aphasic individual when speaking, and using gestures are useful practices too, and it is wise to avoid asking too many questions at one time or repeating a question immediately.

Sometimes there exists the possibility of using the written language; it may be a better and more understandable method of communicating for a particular individual. A communication board may be of value.

It is crucial that care-givers not discuss an individual in his presence as if he or she were not there. The person should have every opportunity to hear speech and should be encouraged to participate in normal home and community social activities at whatever level is best for his or her abilities.

An individual should be allowed to occupy himself or herself with enjoyable activities, even if an activity seems meaningless and futile to the care-provider. The patient should always be informed of what has happened and what will be happening next. An attempt should be made to include the individual's input into major decisions while avoiding unnecessary details.

It is important to recognize that everyone is an important member of the team, including the patient. Family and friends should be educated as to the nature of the aphasic individual's problems and the ways in which they can be helpful. A tendency among family and friends to prescribe therapy for the aphasic patient should be guarded against. The care-giver's own needs and feelings must not be allowed to become confused with those of the patient, nor should the care-giver—or the family—expect the patient to appreciate all of their efforts.

It is of utmost importance to avoid letting other persons' lives revolve around the needs of the individual patient. For family members, particularly, the best counsel is that they should take care of their own physical and emotional health. Taking care of themselves means that they will be in the best possible position to help their loved one, the patient.[7]

Executive Cognitive Function

Dr. Donald R. Royall proposes that dementia might be better understood as a syndrome of executive dyscontrol: "The executive control functions are the cognitive processes that orchestrate relatively simple ideas, movements, or actions into complex goal-oriented behaviors (such as cooking a meal) [see Box 57–3]. They help maintain goal-directed behavior in the face of both internal and external distractions. Without them, behaviors important for independent living can be expected to break down into their component parts. Direction and purpose are lost, undermining the independence of demented patients. This situation can lead to problem behaviors in a variety of settings."[8]

Many problem behaviors can be construed as examples of disordered executive cognitive function (ECF).

Treatment outcomes and function are indirectly affected by ECF impairment. Patients are often given responsibilities that are goal-directed and require executive control. Diabetic patients are often required to self-administer insulin based on the outcome of glucose monitoring. Psychologists call this a "go/no-go" paradigm; it is especially sensitive to ECF impairment in humans. Synthesis is required to bring all the pieces together and administer the correct dosage.

In patients with ECF impairment, the ability to synthesize is simply not there. Even those patients who have successfully completed the Mini Mental Status Exam (MMSE) (see Box 31–1) may not be properly diagnosed with ECF dysfunction and may appear simply to fail to follow their insulin regimen or their dietary restrictions. "Poor adherence to prescribed diet or medication is a well-known cause of poor outcomes in chronic medical conditions such as diabetes or congestive heart failure."[9]

When patients are expected to keep appointments made weeks in advance, to remember to refill prescriptions, or to file for insurance, they are calling on ECF behaviors. Executive impairment that goes unrecognized interferes with treatment, expected outcomes, access to care, and follow-up.

There is no single comprehensive test of executive function. Dr. Royall and his colleagues have developed the EXIT25 and the CLOX instruments in an attempt to operationalize ECF testing at the bedside.[10] With training, lay personnel can administer EXIT25. EXIT25 and CLOX have demonstrated ECF impairment in a variety of conditions, including association with problem behaviors.

When there is a diagnosis of ECF dysfunction, or if the patient is unable to go from step one to step two in a procedure in which he has received proper instruction, the family or formal care-giver must be taught the procedure. Instructing a care-giver allows the patient to maintain a feeling of control and self-worth.

Including the care-giver in treatment planning has many positive features: "Studies indicate that care-giver descriptors are stronger predictors of functional status and level of care than the severity of the patient's dementia or problem behavior. Early in dementia, a patient's executive control allows for his or her participation in decision-making. Once executive control is lost, the care-giver's role in these decisions becomes more important. The main-

---

Box 57–3

Components of Executive Cognitive Function

1. Simple elements make up complex goal-setting behavior.

2. Planning involves selecting simple, appropriate behaviors and sequencing them into a coherent, complex whole.

3. The judgment of which behaviors are appropriate is made in the context of the current external situation and relevant internal drives, motives, or goals.

4. The execution of a complex series of behaviors requires continuous reappraisal of the situation and of the individual's own progress toward the goal.

tenance of adequate supervision, a safe environment, treatment adherence, and the avoidance of unwitting cues for inappropriate behavior are all under the care-giver's control. Ritualizing the patient's daily routine early in the course of the dementia may help the care-giver as the disease progresses."[11]

In the home or in any other treatment setting, the following suggestions can help those who care for patients with ECF:

- Work to establish a daily ritual.
- Use new routines to develop new habits and to break old habits.
- Build good new habits through repetition.
- Listen to what the patient's environment is "saying" to the patient.
- Use social and environmental cues to the patient's advantage.
- Remove or alter cues that seem to trigger problem behaviors.

CONCLUSION

All health-care disciplines can develop techniques to help patients learn to take personal responsibility in planning and implementing their own care by looking at adherence, not compliance. It is important to work with the whole family within its cultural framework and to determine who is the medical decision-maker. Health-care professionals must consider the expectations of outcome of the individuals being served rather than their own outcome expectations.

The personal touch is needed. It takes more time, but it is so important when working with those of other cultures, especially older individuals who may also have problems in seeing and hearing. Often overlooked is the fact that some older individuals do not read in any language. Technology is a necessary element in modern health-care, but it is up to all practitioners to treat those with whom they work with patience and respect. But to treat all elders, especially those of other cultures and ethnicities, as a homogeneous group makes no more sense than treating all children from birth to age 18 as a unit of like individuals. The best role is one of patient advocacy and support. Listening and observation should be common practice.

REFERENCES

1. Payne ZA. Diet and folk remedies: the influence of cultural patterns on medical management. *Urban Health* 1980; Dec:24–28.
2. Greenlaw MJ. *The Quest for Literacy* (Report No. CS–009–11). Washington, D.C.: U.S. Department of Education (ERIC Document Reproduction Service No. ED 290129); 1987.
3. Smith F. Overselling literacy. *Phi Delta Kappan* 1989; Jan:353–359.
4. Kearney M. *World view.* Novato, Cal.: Chandler & Sharp Publishers; 1984.
5. Geertz C. Ethos, world view, and the analysis of sacred symbols. In: Geertz C, ed. *The Interpretation of Cultures.* New York: Basic Books; 1973:126–141.
6. Hamadeh G. Religion, magic, and medicine. *J Fam Pract* 1987; 25:561–568.
7. Tigard, Ore.: C.C. Publications; 1983.
8. Royall DR. Precis of executive dyscontrol as a cause of problem behavior in dementia. *Exp Aging Res* 1994; 20:73–94.
9. Royall DR. Cognitive dysfunction and need for long-term care: implications for public policy. Washington, D.C.: American Association of Retired Persons; 1994.
10. Royall DR, Mahurin RK. Neuroanatomy, measurement, and clinical significance of the executive cognitive functions. *Rev Psychiatr* 1990; 15.
11. Rueben DB, Yoshikawa TT, Besdine RW, eds. *Geriatrics Review Syllabus: A Core Curriculum in Geriatric Medicine.* New York: American Geriatrics Society; 1996.

UNIT IV

SPECIFIC PROBLEMS

Chapter **58***

Dysphagia
Colleen Reynolds
Shelley Slott

INTRODUCTION

Eating is more than just a biological function—eating is an important part of the quality of life. When an individual loses the ability to eat safely, medical as well as social complications can arise.

Dysphagia, or the inability to swallow, can affect patients with a variety of disorders. Stroke, cancer, burns, and trauma are often associated with dysphagia; however, other disease processes may induce a dysphagia disorder too, including diabetes, cardiac dysfunction, neurodegenerative diseases, chronic obstructive pulmonary disease (COPD), and, on rare occasions, cervical hypertrophic osteoarthropathy, as the osteophytes encroach at the C-6 cricoid cartilage area. Also, medications such as carbidopa-levodopa and some antibiotics may cause dysphagia. A patient may be at risk for a swallowing problem simply because he or she is deconditioned, agitated, or lethargic. Many of these conditions are commonly found in aging persons.

THE THREE STAGES OF INGESTION

The process of ingestion involves three interrelated stages: oral, pharyngeal, and esophageal. The oral stage of ingestion refers to the coordinated functions of the jaws, lips, teeth, and tongue. Foods and liquids are accepted into the mouth, prepared or chewed as needed, and then efficiently transferred to the pharynx. During the pharyngeal stage of ingestion, foods and liquids are moved through the throat and into the esophagus. Airway protection is an important component of this stage of swallowing, and most immediately recognizable symptoms of dysphagia are indicative of a pharyngeal-stage dysphagia (e.g., coughing, choking, multiple swallows). The esophageal stage of ingestion refers to the process by which foods and liquids are transported from the throat to the stomach.

Dysfunction may occur in any one or in all stages of the ingestion system, and problems in one stage may affect all other stages. For example, a patient with oral symptomatology—loss of labial sensation and lingual weakness—may have pharyngeal dysphagia resulting from the inability to keep foods and liquids from leaking into the pharynx

*Copyright of this chapter is held by Crozer-Chester Medical Center, Upland, Pennsylvania

prematurely. A patient with compromised esophageal transport and emptying may feel the sensation of foods sticking in his throat or may become used to overmasticating foods.

A patient diagnosed with a swallowing disorder may face medical complications. In some instances these medical problems can even be life-threatening. A dysphagia disorder may put a patient at risk for aspiration, which is when foods, liquids, or secretions enter the airway. Aspiration pneumonia may ultimately result. Aspiration presence or risk can be identified and reduced or eliminated by a speech/language pathologist experienced in dysphagia management.

Swallowing problems can also result in decreased oral intake. Inadequate fluid intake and nutrition can lead to further medical complications. Alternative or supplemental feeding or hydration may then have to be put into place. It can be intravenous feeding or the use of a nasogastric tube that is inserted into the nose and passed through to the stomach. A longer-term means of providing nutrition is by means of percutaneous endoscopic gastrostomy (PEG) or jejunostomy (PEJ), a feeding tube placed in the stomach or jejunum. If a feeding tube cannot be placed endoscopically (through the mouth, into the esophagus, and out through the wall of the stomach), it may be placed surgically through an incision made into the stomach. This may be a temporary or a long-term solution, depending on the severity of the dysphagia disorder.

DYSPHAGIA SYMPTOMS

Symptoms of a swallowing disorder may be easily identifiable (overt) or may be subtle and harder to detect (covert). Asking a patient directly about any swallowing problems he or she may be experiencing can be very helpful to the clinician during the evaluation process. The following questions may isolate specific dysphagia symptoms, as well as any concerns a patient has with regard to his feeding or swallowing status.

- Do you have difficulty keeping food, liquid, or saliva in your mouth?
- Do you have difficulty chewing food that is coarse in texture (e.g., tough meat, vegetables)?
- Do you find food remaining in your mouth after you've swallowed?
- Do you frequently cough, choke, and turn red or blue in the face during meals?
- Do you frequently clear your throat during meals?
- Do you feel as if food or liquid sticks in your throat?

- Do you have difficulty starting your swallow?
- Do you frequently feel full or bloated immediately after a meal (even a small meal)?
- Do you have the sensation of food or liquid being stuck in your chest?
- Do you frequently feel as if food or liquid will come back up into your mouth?
- Do you have frequent belching, hiccupping, or vomiting during or after meals?

With direct observation, the speech/language pathologist may identify the following overt dysphagia symptoms: coughing, choking, vomiting, throat-clearing, complaint of food being stuck in the throat or chest area, multiple swallows, food residue anywhere in the mouth after the swallow, absent chewing, absent swallowing, drooling, watering eyes, runny nose.

With direct observation, the speech/language pathologist may identify the following covert dysphagia symptoms: mildly delayed cough or throat-clearing, wet voice quality following the swallow, mildly delayed swallow initiation, eructations, frequent indigestion or heartburn, early satiety, or decreased oral intake.

Behaviors observed during eating that may signal a potential risk for dysphagia include verbalization throughout a meal despite the presence of food in the mouth, inability to attend to food in the mouth to ensure adequate mastication, impulsivity, and reduced ability to regulate rate and amount of ingestion of foods and liquids.

DYSPHAGIA IDENTIFICATION AND THE ROLE OF THE SPEECH/LANGUAGE PATHOLOGIST

Family members, nurses, or aides may be the first to suspect that a patient has a dysphagia disorder, based on symptoms observed during feeding. Physicians may suspect dysphagia based on the patient's clinical presentation, and nutritionists may question the cause of any observed changes in a patient's oral intake.

At this time, the speech/language pathologist is usually consulted by the patient's attending physician. It is the role of the speech/language pathologist to diagnose and treat swallowing disorders. The speech/language pathologist also coordinates the interdisciplinary dysphagia team, which may include physicians, nurses, respiratory therapists, occupational therapists, physical therapists, and clinical nutritionists. Patient and family involvement are also crucial.

After a complete case history is obtained, a bedside swallowing assessment is completed by the speech/language pathologist. Any dysphagia symp-

toms are identified, and therapy techniques are implemented to remediate or compensate for the disorder. Box 58–1 highlights some remedial and compensatory procedures and their effects on the ingestion system.

Box 58–1
Compensatory Swallowing Techniques and Their Benefits

Head Posture

- Chin tuck
  Widens vallecular space
  Holds material in the widened valleculae until the swallow is triggered
  Epiglottis diverts material away from the airway
- Turn head to weaker side
  Directs material down the stronger side while weaker side is closed
- Tilt head to stronger side
  Directs the material down stronger side by gravity
- Tilt head backward
  Increases oral transport of bolus by gravity

Body Posture

- Upright at 90 degrees
  Reduces risk of aspiration
- Lying on one side
  Reduces risk of aspiration of pharyngeal pooled material

Manner of Oral Intake

- Decrease rate of intake
  Increases patient control of bolus
  Decreases risk of aspiration
- Multiple swallows per bolus
  Increases clearance of pharyngeal residue
  Decreases risk of aspiration
- Alternate solids with liquids
  Increases clearance of pharyngeal residue
  Decreases risk of aspiration
- Decrease bolus size
  Decreases risk of aspiration
- Liquids by spoon
  Decreases risk of aspiration
  Bypasses oral stage
- Liquids or puree by syringe
  Increases oral control of bolus

From Abeloff MD, Armitage JO, Lichter AS, Niederhuber JE, eds. *Clinical Oncology.* New York: Churchill Livingstone; 1995.

Because of their medical status or levels of alertness, some patients may not be candidates for a bedside swallowing assessment. In that case, the speech/language pathologist begins the process of dry swallow training, which prepares the patient and his ingestion system for a full evaluation when his status improves.

Upon completion of the bedside evaluation, the speech/language pathologist determines whether the patient is a candidate for oral feeding. The appropriate diet level is designated at this time. If the patient is not a candidate for oral feedings, NPO (nil per ora, or nothing by mouth) status is recommended, pending completion of further diagnostic testing of the swallow. NPO status is usually recommended if the presence of or risk for aspiration (the descent of foods or liquids below the level of the vocal cords) exists. A full evaluation under videofluoroscopy is usually the next step in the management of the dysphagic patient.

A videofluoroscopic swallowing function study is a radiological procedure performed by a radiologist and speech/language pathologist. This dynamic or moving x-ray of the swallow examines the oral, pharyngeal, and esophageal stages of ingestion. This study enables the speech/language pathologist to identify the cause of the symptoms that were observed during the bedside evaluation. Once the cause is known, appropriate therapeutic techniques can then be implemented.

DISCHARGE GOAL

The goal for discharge from dysphagia intervention is usually the patient's return to his or her previous feeding and diet level without the need for supplemental or alternative nutritional support. In cases in which this is not possible, the patient is returned to a diet level at which swallowing is safe and nutritional needs can be maintained. Sometimes supplemental nutritional support is necessary as either temporary or long-term assistance in meeting nutritional needs. The patient who is unable to return to any oral feedings is a candidate for a long-term nutritional support device such as a PEG or a PEJ.

APPROPRIATE CONSULTS

The Crozer Keystone Health System protocol for appropriate dysphagia service consultation includes the following individuals:

• Any patient with acute onset of feeding or swallowing disorders,

• Any patient with parenteral or enteral feeding systems,
• Any patient with a history of observed or reported oral, pharyngeal, or esophageal dysphagia symptoms,
• Any patient with early satiety, decreased PO feeds, dehydration, aspiration (confirmed or suspected), or deconditioning as the admitting diagnosis,
• Any patient with a history of endotracheal intubation, tracheostomy, or ventilator/vent wean, and
• Any patient with identified vocal cord anomalies, including paresis, paralysis, or laryngospasm.

Contraindications to treatment by the dysphagia team include the following conditions:

• Unstable medical or respiratory status or change in same,
• Inability to remain alert or awake during feeding,
• Sudden change in body temperature of unknown cause,
• Inability to maintain upright or side-lying at 90 degrees in bed or chair,
• Active GI bleed, and
• Active vent wean.

CONCLUSION

Together with the support of the patient's family, the dysphagia team's goal is to restore functional swallowing and feeding skills in order to return the patient as closely as possible to the level he or she demonstrated prior to hospitalization. Nutrition, health, and quality of life are impacted negatively if the ability to swallow has been disrupted and is left untreated. All members of the health-care team should be aware of the symptoms of dysphagia so that if it is suspected or observed, proper consultation can be sought.

SUGGESTED READINGS

Groher ME, ed. *Dysphasia: Diagnosis and Management*, 2nd ed. Boston, Mass.: Butterworth-Heinemann, 1992.

Jaradeh S. Neurophysiology of swallowing in the aged. *Dysphasia* 1994;9: 218–220.

Upper gastrointestinal tract disorders. In: Castell D, Just R. *The Merck Manual of Geriatrics*, 2nd ed. Whitehouse Station, N.J.: 1995; 642–649.

Wheeler D. Communication and swallowing problems in the frail older person. *Top Geriatr Rehabil* 1995; 11(2):11–23.

Chapter **59**

Incontinence of the Bowel and Bladder

Scott Paist, M.D.

INTRODUCTION

Incontinence of bowel or bladder has a major impact on home care and social activities and is one of the primary reasons for the institutionalization of people. Fecal incontinence varies by degree and appears to increase with age, with 16 to 60% of institutionalized older persons having some problems. Urinary incontinence ranges between 15 and 35% in noninstitutionalized persons 60 years old and older, with twice the incidence among women as among men. Up to 53% of homebound elderly are incontinent.

INCONTINENCE OF THE BOWEL

Normal Control

Incontinence of the bowel is usually defined as involuntary loss of stool severe enough to have hygienic or social consequences. This definition is, by its nature, a functional one, not a purely physiological one, because it is the function of the bowel that is important here. Thus, this subject must be considered from a functional and social point of view, as the loss of this control may lead to institutionalization.

The leakage of feces from the anus is normally prevented by the smooth muscle control of the internal anal sphincter and the voluntary striated muscle of the external anal sphincter. In response to rectal stimulation by filling, parasympathetic nerves initiate strong peristaltic waves that move the fecal content along. At the same time, other body actions such as the Valsalva maneuver and upward and outward contraction of the pelvic floor musculature help to move the feces downward and outward. The final response is voluntary relaxation of the external anal sphincter.

With increasing age, the role of the pelvic floor musculature in controlling bowel evacuation may become more important. Age-related loss of strength as well as possible changes in tissue elasticity and resting pressures are probably important, too. These changes occur because decreased distension of the bowel may inhibit anal sphincter tone and encourage rectal urgency.

Causes of Incontinence

The causes of stool incontinence in the elderly are shown in Box 59–1. The treatable causes are, unfortunately, few. Fecal incontinence results from leakage of liquid stool or from loss of stool secondary to loss of sensation or loss of muscle tone. Finally, stool loss may occur as a result of change in the overall level of consciousness.

Loss of sensation to the perineum causes the patient not to sense the need for emptying the rectum until natural forces have done so, resulting in involuntary loss. Such perineal anesthesia may commonly result from spinal cord injury, tumor, or stroke.

Loss of all muscle tone in the muscles of continence, described briefly above, changes the balance of forces such that the expulsive force of the colon exceeds any voluntary attempt by the patient to impede such force. These kinds of losses, like those of sensation, commonly are the result of tumor, stroke, spinal cord injury, or pudendal neuropathy.

Stool leakage around an obstruction is very often found in older people. For a small percentage of them, cancer or a benign polyp is the cause, but most will have been chronically impacted with

---

Box 59–1

Causes of Fecal

Incontinence in the Elderly

Fecal Impaction	Decreased Rectal Sensation
Funtional Impairment	• Diabetes mellitus
• Mental (dementia, confusion)	• Megarectum
• Physical (weakness, immobility)	• Fecal impaction
	Impaired Anal Sphincter and Puborectal Muscle Function
Decreased Reservoir Capacity	• Idiopathic (perineal descent)
• Aging	• Trauma, surgery
• Radiation	• Spinal cord or pudendal lesions
• Tumor	
• Ischemia	
• Surgical resection	

From Wald A. Constipation and fecal incontinence in the elderly. *Gastroenterol Clin North Am* 1990; 19:405–418. Used with permission.

Box 59–2

Costs of Urinary Incontinence

Direct Costs

- Diagnostic and evaluation costs
  Physician consultation and examination
  Laboratory
  Diagnostic procedures
- Treatment costs
  Surgery
  Drugs
- Routine care costs
  Nursing labor
  Supplies
  Laundry
- Rehabilitation costs
  Nursing labor
  Supplies
- lincontinence consequence costs
  Skin breakdowns
  Urinary tract infection
  Falls
  Additional nursing home admissions
  Longer hospital stays

Indirect Costs

- Time costs of unpaid care-givers for treating
  and caring for incontinent elderly persons
- Loss of productivity because of morbidity
- Loss of productivity because of mortality

From Hu T-W. The economic impact of urinary incontinence. *Clin Geriatr Med* 1986; 2:676.

ment—anatomical, physiological, mental, or a combination—and who is in some way impeded from establishing a usable stooling position may only appear to be incontinent. These patients may actually be able to manage easily with some re-arrangement in the environment.

Diagnosis and Therapeutic Intervention

If the situations described above are kept in mind, diagnosis and treatment are not difficult. First, a careful history must be obtained (from the patient, from the nursing staff or physician, or from the chart) and action to reverse the condition sought. The following rhetorical questions may be helpful:

- Is the patient delirious, demented, or suffering from a condition that produces watery stool?
- Is there a history of constipation with obstruction?
- Is there blood in the stool (suggesting a neoplasm or certain infections)?
- What has a recent rectal exam shown?
- Are patient mobility and level of understanding well-matched with obstructions to mobility (side rails, restraints, casts)?

Box 59–3

Reversible Incontinence

Delirium or other confusional state

Infection, urinary tract, symptomatic

Atrophic urethritis or vaginitis

Pharmaceuticals
- sedative/hypnotics, especially long-acting
- alcohol abuse
- loop diuretics (e.g., Bumex, Lasix, Edecrin)
- anticholinergic agents (e.g., antipsychotics, antidepressants, antihistamines, antiparkinsonian agents, antiarrhythmics, antispasmodics, opiates, antidiarrheal agents

Psychological disorders (especially depression)

Endocrine disorders (hyperglycemia or hypercalcemia)

Restriction mobility

Stool impaction

From Clinical Practice Guideline: Urinary Incontinence in Adults. U.S. Department of Health and Human Services, Public Health Service, Agency for Health Care Policy and Research.

stool, often as a result of chronic laxative abuse and poor bowel habits. In either case, liquid stool from higher in the colon will leak past the hard, immovable obstruction and drain from the anus despite the best efforts of the patient. Finally, a patient who has a condition that has led to especially loose stool (drugs, inappropriate diet, infection) may suffer involuntary loss of this watery fecal material. This is also seen in the bedridden patient who has poor muscle tone, especially when attempting to perform mobility and range-of-motion exercises. A change of gravitational force may cause additional physiological and social demands on these patients who are starting to transfer to bipedal and gait activities.

Finally, a patient may lose stool because he or she is either too demented or too delirious to realize what is happening. Such a patient may have forgotten how properly to manage stool (as in dementia) or may not be sufficiently oriented to manage it (as in delirium). A patient who has some impair-

In the nondemented patient without fecal impaction, proctological evaluation is important.

One of the reversible conditions, diarrhea, should be controlled no matter what its cause. The use of antibiotics such as cephalosporins and extended-spectrum penicillins or chemotherapy may lead to a common nosocomial diarrhea produced by the cytotoxin *Clostridium difficile*. This is a contagious condition and can impede rehabilitation efforts. The implicated drug should be stopped and treatment with clindamycin or Flagyl instituted. Unfortunately, relapse is common in up to 25% of cases.

INCONTINENCE OF URINE

Many of the same ideas already discussed are important when considering urinary incontinence, which is a much more common occurrence. Again, the definition is a functional one: involuntary loss of urine so severe as to have social or hygienic consequences. These considerations are listed in Table 59–1. Additionally, the monetary costs of urinary incontinence have been estimated to be over $15 billion annually (Agency for Healthcare Policy and Research Publication 96–0686). The enormity of this problem may be determined by the direct and indirect costs as shown in Box 59–2.

Types of Incontinence

It is useful to consider urinary incontinence according to how it presents to the patient. Although in many cases these presentations are mixed, three distinct types can be identified: urge incontinence, stress incontinence, and overflow incontinence.

Urge incontinence is described by patients as feeling the need to empty the bladder but having insufficient time to do so in a socially acceptable way. In urge incontinence, involuntary loss of urine may be large and postvoid residual volume small. Postvoid residual volume is measured by having the patient void as completely as possible and then immediately placing a straight catheter into the bladder and measuring the remaining urinary volume. The most common cause of this type of incon-

Table 59–1 Summary of Consequences of Urinary Incontinence

Individual	Family	Health-Care Professional

Psychological symptoms
  Insecurity
  Anger
  Apathy
  Dependence
  Guilt
  Indignity
  Feeling of abandonment
  Shame
  Embarrassment
  Depression
  Denial
Sense of self
  Loss of self-confidence/self-esteem
Sexual difficulties
Lack of attention to personal hygiene
Social interaction
  Reduction in social activities
  Socially disengaged
  Socially isolated
Physiological and functional decline
Potential for institutionalization
	Care-giver burden and emotional stress
	Impaired interpersonal relationships
	Economic worries
	Health deterioration of primary care-giver
	Potential for abuse or neglect
	Decision to institutionalize
	Delay of discharge from institutional care
		Negative feeling and behaviors toward patients with urinary incontinence
		Reaction formation
		  Overindulgence
		  Excessive permissiveness
		  Excessive caring
		Extra care responsibilities
		Staff frustration, depression, and guilt
		Reduction in staff morale
		Burn-out syndrome

From Ory M et al. Psychosocial factors in urinary incontinence. *Clin Geriatr Med* 1986; 2:661.

Box 59–4

Treatment Options Available to Physical Therapists

Bladder Training (retraining)

Indications
- Best used to manage incontinence because of urgency or frequency or urge incontinence caused by detrusor instability or bladder hypersensitivity
- Very good for people who practice "just in case" toileting
- Not suitable for patients with stress incontinence or overflow incontinence

Components
- Patient is educated about the anatomy and pathophysiology of the lower urinary tract
- A voiding schedule that incorporates progressively longer periods between voiding is adopted.
- Delaying is accomplished by trying to suppress the urge to urinate by:
  Sitting or standing still rather than rushing to the toilet
  Doing pelvic floor exercises
  Pressing on the perineum
  Performing breathing exercises
  Performing various mental distractions
  The initial interval may be as short as 1 hour

Habit Training (timed voiding)

Indications
- Can be useful for nursing home residents
- Unlike bladder training, there is no systematic effort to motivate the patient to delay voiding or resist the urge to void.

Components
- Determine the patient's natural voiding pattern over a 72-hour time span
- The care-giver takes the patient to the toilet at times that match the patient's normal intervals

Pelvic Floor Exercises (often called Kegel exercises)

Indications
- The goal is to strengthen the voluntary periurethral and pelvic floor muscles and thereby increase muscle support to the pelvic floor and improve urethral resistance

Components
- Using the pelvic floor muscles. The patient should be instructed to:
  Sit well back on a chair
  Lean forward with forearms on thighs
  Concentrate on the vaginal, urethral, and rectal areas
  Tighten the pelvic floor muscles
  Feel the tension in the pelvic floor muscles
  Hold the contraction. The goal is 10 seconds
  Relax and feel the muscles softening
  Tighten the muscles again. Beware of incorrect contractions (i.e. do not hold breath)
  Relax. Feel the difference between the contracted state and the relaxed state
  Contract the muscles briefly and let go
  Do three repetitions to start. Weak muscles tire easily

From Adams C, Frahm J. *Genitourinary system*. In: Myers RS, ed. *Saunders Manual of Physical Therapy Practice*. Philadelphia: W.B. Saunders; 1995:485–487.

tinence is an overactive bladder detrusor muscle (detrusor instability).

Stress incontinence occurs when the patient coughs, strains, laughs, sneezes, or otherwise initiates a Valsalva maneuver. Trunk flexion exercises and possibly the sit-to-stand movement may provoke stress incontinence. At such times, a few drops to a few ounces of urine escape from the bladder. Most common in females, postvoid residual volume is small.

Overflow incontinence occurs when the bladder is overly distended (either from outlet obstruction or from bladder atony), causing bladder pressure to exceed urethral pressure no matter what the patient may attempt. Another cause of overflow symptoms is the loss of the bladder sphincter secondary to surgery or injury. Loss of urine occurs in small amounts but may occur nearly continuously, and postvoid residual is high (potentially liters!).

Diagnosis and Therapeutic Intervention

Many cases of urinary incontinence may be largely irreversible, but it is important to obtain a good diagnostic evaluation. The history of the complaint should include active medical conditions, medications, fluid intact pattern, past history, present complaints, and environmental factors. In addition to a standard physical examination, a urinalysis and culture should be performed. Selected patients may benefit from a urological examination that includes urodynamic tests. The DIAPPERS mnemonic shown in Box 59–3 is important to consider. Some of the treatment options available to physical therapists are discussed in Box 59–4.

CONCLUSION

Constant efforts must be made to find and treat reversible causes of incontinence. It must *never* be assumed that incontinence is a result of aging. It isn't. Although many people with bowel and bladder incontinence are not completely treatable, most can be helped significantly if the health-care team takes the time to think about possible causes and to institute treatment plans based on careful diagnosis.

SUGGESTED READINGS

Adams C, Frahm J. Genitourinary system. In: Myers RS, ed. *Saunders Manual of Physical Therapy Practice*. Philadelphia: W. B. Saunders; 1995.
Busby-Whitehead J, Johnson T: Urinary incontinence. *Clin Geriatr Med* 1998; 14: 285.
The Merck Manual of Geriatrics, 2nd ed. White House Station, N.J.: Merck Research Laboratories; 1995:15, 53, 55.
Managing acute and chronic urinary incontinence. Agency for Health Care Policy and Research, Pub. 96–0686, 1996.

Chapter **60**

Iatrogenic Effects
LaDora V. Thompson, Ph.D., P.T.

INTRODUCTION

Mobility is critical for the well-being and quality of life of the elderly. A common threat to the elderly is bedrest or immobility. Many physical, psychological, pathological, and environmental factors can result in bedrest or immobility. Box 60–1 summarizes the usual causes of immobility in the elderly.

Box 60–1

Causes of Immobility in the Elderly

Musculoskeletal Disorders
• Arthritis
• Osteoporosis
• Fractures (especially femur)
• Podiatric problems (bunions, calluses)
• Pain

Neurological Disorders
• Stroke
• Parkinson's disease
• Alzheimer's disease

Cardiovascular Disease
• Congestive heart failure
• Coronary artery disease (frequent angina)
• Peripheral vascular disease (with frequent claudication)
• Pulmonary disease
• Chronic obstructive pulmonary disease

Environmental Causes
• Forced immobility
• Inadequate aids for mobility (canes, walkers, appropriately placed railings)
• Being wheelchair bound

Other
• Fear (fear of falling)
• Malnutrition
• Deconditioning
• Drug side effects

Bedrest can be beneficial during an illness, but it can have negative consequences that complicate the return to independence. Bedrest may contribute to iatrogenic complications (defined as physician-induced illnesses) if activity is not resumed as soon as possible. During a period of immobility there are pathophysiological alterations that occur in the major organ systems. Box 60–2 outlines the major changes that can occur in the cardiovascular, musculoskeletal, nervous, pulmonary, metabolic, skin, genitourinary, psychological, and gastrointestinal systems. The alterations occur to varying degrees depending on the organ system, the prior level of fitness of the individual, and the extent of immobility. Bedrest-induced alterations can begin within the first 24 hours and, if immobility continues can result in new illnesses.

There are challenges in understanding the consequences of bedrest in older persons because they have diminished physiological reserves secondary to age-related changes and disease processes. Every organ system is altered when a person is immobile, so it is critical that health-care professionals recognize the negative consequences of bedrest or immobility for the older individual. The return to independence by the elderly can be speeded up if they understand the deleterious consequences of immobility, the relative time frame in which those consequences can develop, and the potential value of therapeutic interventions.

THE CONSEQUENCES OF IMMOBILITY ON MAJOR ORGAN SYSTEMS AND FUNCTIONS

The Musculoskeletal System

Joint Range of Motion

Immobility results in loss of weight-bearing forces on joints. When joints are unloaded, there is a rapid change in the cellular biochemical and mechanical properties that results in alterations in periarticular and articular structures. The joint capsule becomes thickened and the synovium hyperemic. There is fibrofatty proliferation of connective tissue within the joint space. Collagen becomes denser and develops a more random arrangement, which results in the shortening of tendons. The ligaments of the joint atrophy, which results in a decline of tensile strength. Functionally, there is an increase in joint stiffness, a decrease in the flexibility of joints, and a decrease in joint range of motion (ROM). The alterations in the cellular biochemical and mechanical properties can occur in as few as 5 days of immobilization, with measurable losses in joint ROM occurring within a week. Long-term immobilization produces significant reductions in ROM; there can be as much as a 45% decrease after 5 weeks, and that can lead to the development of contractures.

All joints are susceptible to immobility but the hip, knee, and ankle are particularly sensitive to immobilization. Impairment of the ROM in the hip, knee, and ankle can lead to problems with sitting, functional positioning, walking, and balance stability.

Physical and occupational therapies are very beneficial in counteracting joint ROM deterioration secondary to immobilization because they enable continued movement of joints. Decreased ROM (especially in shoulder external rotation, hip extension, knee extension, and ankle dorsiflexion), limited

---

Box 60–2

Pathophysiological Alterations of Immobility

Musculoskeletal
- Decreased range of motion
- Decreased joint flexibility
- Development of contractures
- Loss of muscular strength (muscular atrophy)
- Loss of muscular endurance (deconditioning)
- Loss of bone mass
- Loss of bone strength

Cardiopulmonary
- Decreased ventilation
- Atelectasis
- Aspiration pneumonia
- Deterioration of the respiratory system
- Increased cardiac output
- Increased resting heart rate
- Increase of orthostatic hypotension

Skin
- Development of pressure sores
- Skin atrophy
- Skin tears

Genitourinary
- Urinary infection
- Urinary retention
- Bladder calculi

Psychological/Neurological
- Depression
- Perceptual ability
- Social isolation
- Learned helplessness
- Altered sleep patterns, anxiety, irritability, hostility

Metabolic
- Negative nitrogen balance
- Loss of calcium

joint flexibility, and the development of contractures can be counteracted by therapeutic heating. Therapeutic heating increases the compliance of collagen fibers and is followed by ROM exercises, strengthening exercises, and stretching. Normal loading of the joints (weight-bearing exercises) may be very important in attenuating the changes in articular cartilage. The objectives of the exercises are to improve mobility and flexibility and to relieve stiffness. The older individual is taught to perform these exercises independently as soon as possible. General body stretching for a period of 15 minutes increases flexibility. Appropriate positioning, splinting, and early ambulation are good therapeutic techniques that assist in maintaining functional ROM of joints. Appropriate resting and night splints can prevent a dropped-foot condition and pressure ulcers.

Muscular Strength and Endurance

Inactivity causes a significant decline in muscle strength and muscle endurance. The muscles most affected by immobility are the antigravity muscles that facilitate locomotion and assist in maintaining an upright position (quadriceps, glutei, erector spinae, and gastrocnemius-soleus muscles). Generally, 10 to 15% of muscle strength is lost each week, and it may be that as much as 5.5% is lost in each day of immobility. The greatest loss of strength occurs during the initial period of inactivity. Inactivity-induced loss of muscle strength is not linear; bedrest for 4 to 5 weeks has been known to decrease strength of lower limb extensor muscle groups 20 to 25%. In addition to a decrease in physiological and functional muscle strength, muscles atrophy and change resting lengths—shortening leads to loss of motion and lengthening leads to stretch weakness.

As muscle strength decreases there is a concomitant decline in endurance. The decrease in endurance has a profound influence on the ability to sustain any activity of daily living. Fatigue is a common complaint because of the decreased endurance and diminished exercise tolerance. Adaptations of the muscle system interfere with mobility, performance of the activities of daily living, posture, and gait. The amount of strength and endurance lost by the elderly during bedrest is variable.

Rehabilitative services are essential treatment strategies for disuse atrophy and muscle weakness. Therapeutic exercise is designed to increase muscle strength and endurance. Progressive resistive exercises (isometric and isotonic contractions) are particularly important because they are muscle-specific but have crossover effects on other muscle groups. An exercise program that requires development of maximal muscular contraction intermittently (30- to 60-second contractions) is beneficial in attenuating the decline in muscle strength. Ideally, the exercise program is initiated at 60% of a maximum lift (3 to 4 sets of 8 to 10 repetitions per muscle group) with a rest period between each set. The Valsalva maneuver should be avoided because it may elevate blood pressure and jeopardize the cardiovascular response.

Bone Mass and Strength

Immobility causes a loss of bone mass. With bedrest there is a decline in the gravitational forces superimposed on bones which leads to bone demineralization and a loss in trabeculae volume. Bones become thin, porous, and fragile because of a relative increase in osteoclastic activity and greater resorption of bone. Bone loss occurs as early as the third day of immobilization. Bone alterations induced by immobilization predispose the elderly patient to fractures of the hip, spine, and extremities. The elderly are especially vulnerable because bone loss resulting from inactivity or limited mobility is compounded by bone loss resulting from age-related osteoporosis. Complications such as urolithiasis and heterotrophic calcification can occur.

Rehabilitative treatment techniques for enhancing bone mass and strength consist chiefly of increasing muscle strength, mobility, and ambulation as soon as possible. Restoring weight-bearing forces is essential in maintaining bone mass and reversing bone loss. Ambulation exercise has been found to restore bone mineral at a rate of 1% per month. In addition to early standing and ambulation, isotonic and isometric contractions (muscle-strengthening programs) assist in the prevention of bone wasting.

Cardiovascular System

The cardiovascular system undergoes significant changes during bedrest. Many of the changes are immediate and they are probably the most serious. When a patient is in the supine position, approximately 11% of the total blood volume is redistributed from the circulatory system of the lower extremities to the thorax. An increase in volume enters the thoracic circulation and results in an increase in cardiac output. Thus, there is increased cardiac workload as the heart works harder to circulate the extra volume.

With bedrest, there is cardiovascular deconditioning—an increase in resting heart rate and a decrease in maximal oxygen uptake. It has been reported that by the end of 3 weeks of bedrest, resting heart rate increases by 20%, averaging one beat for every 2 days of bedrest. Bedrest diminishes physical work capacity by blunting the exercise-induced increase in stroke volume and cardiac output. Maximal oxygen uptake goes down, leading to diminished exercise tolerance (manifested by weakness, fatigue, and shortness of breath). Peak maximal oxygen uptake (Vo_2) decreases by an average of 7.5% with 10 to 20 days of bedrest, with a range of 0.3 to 26% in young subjects.

Orthostatic hypotension is a common cardiovascular complication of immobility. When moving from a supine to a vertical posture, a redistribution of blood occurs. Venous return is reduced, and central venous pressure, stroke volume, and systolic blood pressure decrease concomitantly. Baroreceptors in the autonomic nervous system typically elicit sympathetic stimulation to counter the effects; however, during bedrest, position changes do not elicit postural vascular responses, and orthostatic hypotension results. Orthostatic hypotension can occur in the elderly when they are immobilized for as little as 1 week. Signs and symptoms of orthostatic intolerance include tachycardia, nausea, diaphoresis, and syncope. Functionally, orthostatic hypotension can significantly enhance the risk of falls and stability during standing and ambulation. Orthostatic blood pressure changes become more exaggerated after prolonged immobilization, leading to orthostatic intolerance and diminished exercise tolerance.

Recovery from orthostasis is very slow after bedrest. Orthostatic hypotension may not only impair rehabilitative efforts but also predispose the elderly to serious cardiovascular events such as stroke and myocardial infarction.

The development of venous stasis predisposes the patient to the development of both pelvic and peripheral venous thrombosis. Pulmonary emboli can occur as a serious complication of venous stasis. The seated position encourages flexion of the hips, knees, and elbows. This position forces the feet to remain dependent and predisposes the patient to the development of venous stasis also.

The Valsalva maneuver, an increase in intrathoracic pressure produced by forceful exhalation against a closed glottis, is common in patients with inactivity. The Valsalva occurs because of straining when turning in bed, lifting oneself, pushing oneself up and so forth. With the increase in intrathoracic pressure, venous blood flow is inhibited, causing an increase in pulse rate and a transient increase in systemic blood pressure.

Rehabilitation and Exercise

Anticoagulants, elastic stockings, changes in position, including sitting, and early rehabilitative intervention can prevent or limit the extent of deconditioning and orthostatic hypotension. Intermittent sitting during the period of immobility attenuates the great decline in maximal oxygen uptake and the development of orthostatic hypotension. Therapeutic exercise consisting of aerobic conditioning is important for cardiopulmonary fitness. Exercise in an upright position or use of a reverse gradient garment prevents or reduces the decline in maximal oxygen uptake. Both isometric and isotonic exercises incorporating large muscle groups are essential. In the deconditioned patient therapeutic exercise should be started at a very low intensity. It may be initiated with active and weight-bearing or resistive exercises in the bed or in a chair. For example, adequate sitting tolerance can be established by increasing the frequency and duration of sitting. If orthostatic hypotension is a problem, the traditional treatments (elastic hose, elevation of the head of the bed at night, and progressive mobility training) are necessary. For the severely deconditioned patient, early mobilization requires monitoring the patient's symptoms and vital signs (see Box 42–3, "Guidelines for Termination of an Exercise Session"). A target heart rate is 20 beats above the resting heart rate if the latter is not excessively elevated. If the patient tolerates this for 1 to 2 days, and is medically stable, the target may be increased. Guidelines for ambulation frequency are not well established, but having a patient walk until mild fatigue is present and doing that three times a day is a reasonable level. In addition, it is vital to educate patients and their care-givers about the importance of exercise.

Respiratory System

The supine position leads to changes in lung volumes and in the mechanics of breathing. These changes are significant in the elderly, who already have diminished lung recoil. With immobilization, the vital capacity and tidal volume of the lungs decrease, secretions increase, and expectoration decreases. There is insufficient clearance of the airway, which results in the pooling of secretions and increased bacterial growth distal to the obstruction, predisposing the elderly patient to pneumonia and local atelectasis. Atelectasis and pneumonia are common complications of immobility in all patients, and pulmonary embolism and aspiration pneumonitis can also occur. Impaired ventilation-perfusion, the widening of the alveolar-arterial gradient, and the decrease in arterial oxygen lead to oxygen desaturation.

Prevention measures include mobility at the earliest possible time and respiratory muscle training, which is taught to the patient so he or she can incorporate it independently throughout the day.

The Integumentary System

Pressure Sores

Decubitus ulcers are serious consequences of immobilization. With prolonged compression, skin circulation and skin perfusion decrease over bony prominences, which causes infarction of the skin. The skin becomes more vulnerable to the forces of pressure, shear, friction, and moisture, and tissue injury results. The extent and duration of immobilization are crucial factors in the development of impaired tissue integrity. If tissue injury does occur, healing is slowed by the fact that the body's metabolism is impaired, particularly with respect to nitrogen imbalance. Large decubitus ulcers may lead to even more serious infections such as osteomyelitis.

The older individual is particularly susceptible to the development of pressure sores when immobile. With aging, the skin becomes a less resistant barrier. It is predisposed to injury because of age-related decreases in amount of subcutaneous adipose tissue, number of sweat and sebaceous glands, and elasticity of connective tissue (see Chapter 54, "Skin Disorders").

Appropriate beds and bed materials (air, fluid, alternating pressure, egg-crate mattresses) that distribute pressure are essential. Changes in position relieve pressure and thus decrease the risk of pressure sores, so a turning schedule should be instituted. Protective clothing and the incorporation of rehabilitation exercises as soon as possible aid in prevention. All care-providers must practice appropriate preventive measures, giving extra attention to patients who have recently had anesthesia or are taking medications that induce relaxation and deep sleep. The effects of these medications increase the risk of pressure sores as do repeated transfers, armrests, footpedals, and the sling effects from a soft pliable chair back or seat.

Urinary Function

In a recumbent patient, loss of gravitational emptying of the renal pelvis leads to stagnation in the calyces. Impaired renal drainages, changes in urinary calcium levels, and decreased pH predispose the elderly to calculus formations, aggregation of crystalloids, and urinary tract infections. The increased time of urinary stasis in both the kidney and bladder allows for bacterial growth.

Risks can be lessened by frequent turning, sitting up in a chair, and use of a bedside commode or the bathroom rather than a bed pan. Adequate fluid intake and early mobility can be beneficial, too, as can isotonic and isometric exercises performed daily during bedrest to attenuate and stabilize fluid shifts.

Gastrointestinal Function

During bedrest, the elderly may have limited fluid intake, a diminished appetite, and alterations in ingestion, digestion, and elimination. The ability to digest and use nutrients is interrupted because of a reduction in the cellular exchange of nutrients that occurs with slowed metabolic activity. Constipation and fecal impaction can occur because of less intestinal motility (peristalsis decreases), inadequate ingestion of fiber and fluid, and difficulty in defecating because of weakness. Swallowing may be difficult in a supine position. Eating habits are disrupted, which can cause clinical malnutrition and loss of weight. Early standing and ambulation are valuable in minimizing any decline in gastrointestinal function.

Neurological Function and Others

Compression neuropathies can occur with lengthy bedrest. Ulnar, radial, median, sciatic, and peroneal nerve compression injuries have been observed. Falling asleep while leaning against the wheelchair armrest can cause a radial nerve injury.

Sleep patterns are altered and this can cause tiredness, depression, and lack of motivation. Distortion of time perception, mood changes, poorer sense of well-being, and learned helplessness occur. Loneliness and longing for signs of recognition have been noted in healthy young persons during only 3 hours of immobility. Bedrest causes a decrease in coordination and a marked increase in body sway, resulting in altered balance and altered stability and thus an increased risk of falls. Balance decrements occur after 2 to 3 weeks of bedrest.

Variable high- and low-intensity, short-duration isotonic training during bedrest has been shown to assist with sleep patterns and mental concentration. Early mobility, especially standing and ambulation, improve balance.

Metabolic Imbalances

Loss of calcium and the development of a negative nitrogen balance occur during immobility. Hypercalcemia can result and cause further problems such as anorexia, nausea, vomiting, abdominal cramping, constipation, muscle weakness, and lethargy. Negative nitrogen balance secondary to muscle breakdown can occur within 5 days of immobilization. Metabolic balance is particularly important if tissue injury such as a burn or laceration has occurred because the success of repair of damaged tissue tissue is dependent on an optimal metabolic environment. Rehabilitative exercises for mobility and strength attenuate any metabolic imbalances.

THERAPEUTIC INTERVENTIONS

The longer an individual remains inactive, the more pronounced the negative consequences are and the longer it takes for the body to return to a healthy status. Major physiological changes that occur early in immobility involve the fluid-electrolyte and venous compliance systems, and these changes can be life-threatening. Immobility cannot be avoided, but many of its adverse effects can be prevented by means of therapeutic intervention (Box 60–3).

Patients' mobility should be assessed and reassessed on an ongoing basis. Optimal management of immobile elderly patients necessitates thorough assessments, specific diagnoses, and multimodal treatment by multidisciplinary geriatric consultation teams. Physical and occupational therapists assess and manage immobility and associated functional disabilities and should be consulted as early as

Box 60–3

Strategies for Minimizing Negative Consequences of Bedrest

Minimize duration of bedrest

Avoid strict bedrest unless absolutely necessary

Allow bathroom privileges or bedside commode

Let the patient stand 30 to 60 seconds whenever transferring (bed to chair)

Encourage the wearing of street clothes

Encourage taking meals at a table

Encourage walking to hospital appointments

Encourage passes out of the hospital on evenings and weekends

Involve physical therapy, occupational therapy, and restorative nursing

Encourage daily exercises as a basis of good care

Involve use of protective splinting

Box 60–4

Physical Therapy in the Management of Immobile Elderly Patients

- Assess the need for and teach the use of assistive devices for ambulation.
- Evaluate, maintain, and improve joint ROM.
- Evaluate and improve strength, endurance, motor skills, and coordination.
- Evaluate and improve mobility, gait, and stability.
- Evaluate and improve ability to perform ADLs.
- Assess mobility: bed mobility, transfers, ambulation.

Goals
- Relieve pain
- Restore, maintain, and improve the ability to function independently

Treatment/Interventions
- Exercise (active and passive) isometric or isotonic
- Heat (hot packs, paraffin, etc.)
- Cold
- Hydrotherapy
- Ultrasound
- Transcutaneous electrical nerve stimulation

possible in cases that involve immobile elderly patients. Even relatively small improvements in mobility can decrease the incidence and severity of complications and improve the well-being of older individuals. When full activity is not possible, limited activity such as movement in bed and intermittent sitting and standing reduce the frequency of some complications of bedrest. Proactive nursing care to prevent the sequelae of bedrest is crucial, as is ongoing nutritional assessment.

Specific rehabilitation objectives involve controlling disease activity, decreasing pain, correcting deformities, restoring or improving efficient function, and preventing future episodes (Box 60–4). Therapeutic techniques include analgesic modalities and therapeutic exercises to mobilize joints, strengthen muscles, and enhance endurance and fitness—ROM exercises, graded strengthening exercises, positioning, mobility skills, and transfers to ambulation are all important. The graded strengthening exercise sessions are designed to provide optimal stimulation while allowing sufficient recovery intervals so that excessive fatigue and injury are avoided. Specific goals must be individualized, and in some older individuals these goals will involve preventing the complications caused by immobility and adapting the environment to the individual.

CONCLUSION

The older individual, especially the frail, are particularly susceptible to the deleterious effects of immobility. The onset of these negative consequences can occur within the first 24 hours and may impact the major organ systems and normal physiological functions. Additionally, immobility accentuates age-related changes that impair physiological reserve. Management depends on the health-care provider's awareness of the effects of bedrest and the importance of rehabilitation. Mobility is a critical issue that pertains to all the functions and the very quality of life.

SUGGESTED READINGS

Dudley GA, Hather BM, Buchanan P. Skeletal muscle responses to unloading with special reference to man. *J. Fla Med Assoc* 1992;79:525–529.

Gorbien MJ, Bishop J, Beers MH, et al. Iatrogenic illness in hospitalized elderly people. *J Am Geriatr Soc* 1992;40:1031–1042.

Greenleaf JE. Intensive exercise training during bed rest attenuates deconditioning. *Med Sci Sports Exerc* 1997;29:207–215.

Harper CM, Lyles YM. Physiology and complications of bed rest. *J Am Geriatr Soc* 1988;36:1047–1054.

Mobily PR, Kelley LS. Iatrogenesis in the elderly. *J Gerontol Nurs* 1991;17:5–10.

Chapter 61

Estrogen Replacement Therapy

Chris Stabler, M.D.

INTRODUCTION

Estrogen therapy has been riding the roller coaster of public opinion since 1963 when Robert Wilson published *Feminine Forever*. Touted as the fountain of youth, estrogen used in uncontrolled amounts was thought to revitalize and rejuvenate menopausal women. The tidal wave of interest in estrogen replacement came to an abrupt halt 12 to 15 years later with the publication of an article that provided first clinical evidence that estrogen therapy may increase a woman's risk of endometrial cancer. Ten years later, estrogen regained some of its luster with the support of clinical data that demonstrated its efficacy and safety when used in a combined regimen with progesterone. Research demonstrating the protective effects of hormone therapy against the development of osteoporosis, heart disease and, po-

tentially, colon cancer and Alzheimer's disease has strengthened its support among clinicians and patients alike.

THE BENEFITS OF HORMONE REPLACEMENT THERAPY

Despite overwhelming evidence that hormone replacement therapy (HRT) can increase both life expectancy and quality of life for postmenopausal women, only a fraction of those with clear indications take advantage of this intervention. Misperceptions of the risk of hormone replacement therapy far outweigh the public's knowledge of its therapeutic benefits. The role of the clinician is to educate patients regarding the risks of taking hormone replacement therapy and of not taking hormone replacement therapy, and to provide a clear overview of its broad benefits.

Menopause can be looked at as an endocrinopathy in which a specific endocrine organ, the ovary, has failed. Although every woman experiences menopause, readily available replacement therapy can eliminate the degenerative effects associated with estrogen deficiency.

Side Effects of Menopause

It is the physiological side effects of menopause that cause women to visit their clinicians. Hot flashes, sleep disturbances, mood abnormalities, skin and hair changes, and urinary incontinence are direct results of estrogen deficiency.

Hot flashes occur in 75% of women going through menopause. In fully one third of these women, the hot flashes persist for more than 5 years. Hot flashes can occur as infrequently as once a week or up to 20 to 30 times a day. Obese women experience fewer hot flashes, which is thought to be a direct effect of endogenous estrogen produced in peripheral adipose tissue. In placebo-controlled studies, estrogen produced a marked reduction in hot flashes in both obese and nonobese individuals. In the concomitant crossover study, cessation of estrogen prompted a rapid return of hot flashes. Sleep disturbances, early morning awakening, and night sweats are equivalents of hot flashes and respond equally well to estrogen replacement therapy.

The skin is an end organ for estrogen activity. Research reports have demonstrated the response of skin collagen to oral estrogen replacement therapy in menopausal women. Untreated patients experienced significant drops in skin collagen and skin thickness, whereas estrogen-treated individuals maintained a higher skin collagen content. This correlates with the loss of elasticity of skin at menopause that is reversed with estrogen replacement therapy.

Menopausal women experience more urinary stress incontinence than premenopausal women. Causes of this phenomenon are multiple, but subjectively, patients improve on estrogen replacement therapy. Objectively, urethral pressure profiles also improve with hormone replacement. Vaginal epithelial thickness also improves, and there is less colonization of the vagina with anaerobic and gram-negative bacteria, therefore less local inflammation and incontinence.

Bone Density

Yet it is the intangible benefits that hormone replacement therapy offers to women that are most important. Repeated, conclusive studies have shown that estrogen replacement therapy decreases the lifetime probability that a woman will develop osteoporosis and may reduce the risk of vertebral fractures by up to 50% and the risk of hip fractures by more than 25%. In a classic study, patients were given either an estrogen and progestin combination or placebo. For the first 24 months, patients taking HRT gained a slight amount of bone and those on placebo lost bone. Patients were rerandomized at 24 months. The patients maintained on estrogen therapy continued to gain bone, whereas those who were discontinued began to lose bone in a fashion parallel to that of patients who had never been on estrogen therapy.

Considering that women may lose as much as 10% of their total bone mass in the first year of menopause, estrogen replacement therapy should begin as early as possible. In high-risk groups, women with family histories of osteoporosis, smokers, patients receiving corticosteroid therapy, patients receiving thyroid hormone replacement, patients with prolonged immobility, and women with fair skin and blue eyes should receive estrogen replacement therapy even before menses cease (Box 61–1). Estrogen should be maintained as long as the patient has no contraindications. Cessation of hormone replacement therapy reinstitutes bone loss. The incidence of fracture is related to bone density—the lower the bone density the higher the probability of fracture. Therefore, maintaining bone density with estrogen should decrease fractures in the hip, vertebral column, and long bones.

When the dose of conjugated equine estrogens was compared with the total change in bone density, it was found that bone density was maintained at a dose of the equivalent of 0.625 mg daily. Increased doses yielded no significant increase in bone den-

> **Box 61–1**
> ### Women at High Risk for Osteoporosis Who Are Candidates for Estrogen Replacement Therapy
>
> - Women with histories of osteoporosis
> - Smokers
> - Patients on corticosteroids
> - Patients on thyroid hormone replacement therapy
> - Patients with prolonged immobility
> - Women with fair skin and blue eyes
> - Women with thin builds

sity. Numerous other studies have confirmed that other forms of estrogen, including transdermal and micronized estradiol, also yielded significant increases in bone density in women receiving these preparations. Calcium intake of 1000 to 1500 mg/day (see Box 19–3) is also an essential part of the prevention of osteoporosis, but researchers have found that calcium alone yields insignificant changes in bone mass when compared to placebo. It is only when combined with estrogen that calcium ingestion produces significant increases in bone density. Combinations of estrogen and progesterone seem to increase bone density at a higher rate than estrogen alone, especially at lower-than-standard doses.

Bone density assessment may be helpful in determining who is at risk for osteoporosis, hence encouraging early initiation of hormone replacement therapy. It also may be a marker to convince women at risk to continue hormone replacement therapy.

Cognitive Function

Estrogen receptors are found in many areas of the human brain. Evidence indicates that estrogen may play a role in the cognitive functioning of women. Verbal memory is enhanced by estrogen use. Far more interesting are studies suggesting a reduced risk of Alzheimer's disease in estrogen users. A prospective study of 2529 women who died between 1981 and 1997 showed that postmenopausal women who took estrogen had a 30% reduction in the risk of Alzheimer's disease and other dementias. These data are preliminary but extremely encouraging. In addition, recent studies have suggested a reduction in risk of colon cancer in postmenopausal estrogen users. Research to clarify this finding continues.

Cardiovascular Disease

The rate of cardiovascular disease in women is often underestimated. Cardiovascular disease accounts for 36% of all deaths of women and is the leading age-adjusted cause of death of women. In contrast, 4% die of breast cancer, 2.5% of osteoporotic fractures, and 2% of cancers of the reproductive organs. The risk factors for cardiovascular disease in women are similar to those in men—smoking, hypertension, family history, and elevated lipids. However, only in women do we see a significant increase in risk of cardiovascular disease related solely to an endocrinological effect, menopause (Box 61–2).

Age and postmenopausal status are independent risk factors in women. The effects of menopause on the cardiovascular system include:

1. Vasoreactivity — a shift from normal vasodilation to vasoconstriction of arteries and arterioles.
2. Coagulation — increased fibrinogen levels, increased platelet aggregation, increased risk of clot formation.
3. Lipid profile — increased levels of low-density lipoprotein, cholesterol, and lipoprotein (a), as well as increased aortic cholesterol accumulation and deposition.

In multiple observational studies published between 1974 and 1987, estrogen therapy demonstrated a reduction in cardiovascular disease of between 30 and 90% in postmenopausal women. The average reduction in risk was 50%. Concomitantly, a total mortality reduction of 35 to 45% has been shown in estrogen users. The data regarding stroke

---

Box 61–2

Risk Factors for Cardiovascular Disease in Women

- Smoking
- Hypertension
- Family history
- Elevated lipids
- Menopause

---

prevention seem to be less clear; evidence from the Nurses' Health Study indicated no evidence of risk reduction.

The Postmenopausal Estrogen/Progestin Interventions (PEPI) Trial measured the effects of estrogen and estrogen plus progestin against placebo on risk factors for cardiovascular disease in healthy postmenopausal women. This encouraging study found that estrogen users experienced significantly increased levels of serum high-density lipoprotein and lowered levels of low-density lipoprotein cholesterol. Fibrinogen levels were also reduced in all treatment groups. Insulin levels and blood pressure were not affected in estrogen users.

One area of concern regarding the cardiovascular benefits of hormone replacement therapy is the belief that progestin may diminish the effects of estrogen receptors and potentially negate the beneficial cardiovascular effects of estrogen. Recent studies have shown that low-dose medroxyprogesterone acetate results in no change in beneficial cardiovascular effects of estrogen.

Another interesting benefit of estrogen may be its antioxidant action. Along with vitamins E, C, A, and beta-carotene, estrogen seems to reduce the peroxidation of lipoproteins, an important step in the incorporation of LDL into macrophages during the formation of foam cells that trigger arteriosclerotic plaque formation.

RISK ASSOCIATED WITH HORMONE REPLACEMENT THERAPY

Evidence to support the benefits of estrogen replacement therapy for postmenopausal women is overwhelming. With any benefit comes associated risk. The risks of estrogen replacement therapy, although overshadowed by its benefits, must be explained and understood fully.

Previous concern regarding an association between the estrogens in hormone replacement therapy and thrombosis have been reviewed and rebutted. According to the Boston Collaborative Drug Surveillance Program, estrogen replacement therapy at common doses is not associated with an increased risk of venous thrombosis, thrombophlebitis, or pulmonary embolism.

Risk for endometrial cancer has consistently been shown to increase with the use of unopposed estrogen; that risk is three to five times greater in users of unopposed estrogen. Conversely, the risk for endometrial cancer when using combined estrogen and progesterone is significantly less than it is for women receiving no hormones at all. This ground-breaking finding has been supported by study after study. The increased risk of endometrial cancer shown with unopposed estrogen was, in essence, neutralized by the addition of progesterone. This reassuring point should be emphasized to women considering estrogen replacement therapy. In fact, stage I endometrial cancer is not considered a contraindication to the use of estrogen replacement therapy.

Other estrogen-dependent tumors may be telling another story. The most significant risk of ERT is the theoretical association between estrogen use and breast cancer. It has generated a notable amount of controversy among epidemiologists, physicians, and patients. The largest epidemiological study conducted to date, the Nurses' Health Study, indicates there may be a relationship between duration of estrogen therapy in older women and the development of breast cancer. This study of over 100,000 women, many of whom are now in their 50s or 60s, shows that the risk of breast cancer may increase as duration of hormone replacement therapy increases. The calculated risk approaches 1.3. Not all studies have found this association to be true; a 1995 report showed no increased risk for any user of unopposed estrogen for up to 15 years. Another study by the American Cancer Society showed that women who took estrogen for up to 11 years had a 16% lower mortality rate from breast cancer than those who had never taken estrogen. Similarly, the Western Washington study failed to find any relationship between exogenous hormones and breast cancer.

CONCLUSION

Controversy continues. A meta-analysis of over 50 studies showed conflicting results. At this time, the truth is a moving target and clinicians must continue to stay current with the literature in order to provide patients with accurate information. It is clear that definitive data from randomized controlled studies are needed before this issue an be resolved completely. Analysis of the risks and benefits of HRT clearly shows that use of hormone replacement therapy in the postmenopausal years is beneficial. Counseling each patient on an individual basis and providing her with a clear picture of her personal risks and benefits will allow patients to become an integral part of the decision making. Alternative therapies, including exercise, diet modification, vitamin E, and aspirin for cardiovascular protection, and frequent screening for osteoporosis may be a viable option for patients.

SUGGESTED READINGS

Birge SJ. The role of estrogen in the treatment and prevention of dementia: proceedings of a symposium. *Am J Med* 1997; 103:1s–50s.

Boston Collaboration Drug Surveillance Program, Boston University Medical Center. Surgically confirmed gallbladder disease, venous thromboembolism, and breast tumors in relation to postmenopausal estrogen therapy. *N Engl J Med* 1974; 290:15–19.

Colditz G, Stumpfer M, Willett W, et al. Type of postmenopausal hormone use and risk of breast cancer: 12-year follow-up from the Nurses' Health Study. *Cancer Causes Control* 1992; 3:433–439.

Mack T, Pike M, Henderson B, et al. Estrogens and endometrial cancer in a retirement community. *N Engl J Med* 1976; 294:1262–1267.

Paganini-Hill A, Dworsky R. Krauss R. Hormone replacement therapy, hormone levels and lipoprotein cholesterol concentrations in elderly women. *Am J Obstet Gynecol* 1996; 174:897–902.

Stanford J, Weiss N, Voigt K, Polins J, Habel L, Rossing M. Combined estrogen and progestin hormone replacement therapy in relation to risk of breast cancer in middle-aged women. *JAMA* 1995; 274:137–142.

Chapter **62**

Dizziness
Susan L. Whitney, Ph.D., P.T., A.T.C.

INTRODUCTION

Dizziness is a frequently occurring disorder of older individuals, and it is one that can result in serious functional deficits. Older adults often visit their physicians with nonspecific complaints of dizziness; it is the most common complaint of adults over the age of 75 and the third most common complaint to physicians in outpatient settings, regardless of age. As dizziness is a subjective experience, it is difficult to determine whether the patient and the examiner agree on what the symptoms are.

PRESENTATION AND DIAGNOSIS

Dizziness is interpreted differently by various people and is often difficult to describe. Commonly, people complain of a sense of giddiness, floating, or lightheadedness or a sensation of being drunk. Table 62–1 includes other common descriptors associated with dizziness and used by patients to explain their complaints to their practitioners.

Some patients who experience dizziness have nystagmus which is a nonvoluntary rhythmic oscillation of the eyes in either the lateral or the superior/inferior direction. The nystagmus usually manifests with a fast and a slow component to the eye movements in opposite directions.

Table 62–1 Common Complaints of Persons Experiencing Dizziness

Chief Complaint	History	Physical Exam
Head alignment abnormalities		x
Difficulty controlling their center of mass within their base of support	x	x
Difficulty orienting their bodies to vertical	x	x
Problems with selecting the most appropriate sensory information to make decisions		x
Eye movement abnormalities	x	x
Abnormal motion perception	x	x
Physical deconditioning	x	x
Gait abnormalities	x	x
Swimming sensation in the head	x	x
Imbalance	x	x
Blurred vision	x	x
Tinnitus	x	Sometimes
Aural fullness	x	Sometimes
Hearing loss	x	x
Oscillopsia (an illusory movement of the visual world that occurs with high-frequency head movement)	x	x
Confusion, especially in rich sensory environments	x	
Lightheadedness	x	x
Anxiety	x	Sometimes
Headache	x	
Fatigue	x	x
Falling	x	Sometimes
Clumsiness	x	Sometimes
Neck pain	x	x

Besides nystagmus, some patients also describe having symptoms of vertigo, which is classically defined as an illusion of movement that usually has a rotatory component. People who experience vertigo often have a sensation of turning. Vertigo has been described as rotational, as translational, and as a sense of being tilted.

Most patients who experience dizziness or vertigo modify their activity levels even when they are not experiencing symptoms. Fear of falling is often associated with the symptoms of dizziness or imbalance in elderly people. They commonly become noticeably less active over time because of the fear of experiencing dizziness or gait imbalance, especially in unfamiliar environments. This fear leads to inactivity, which can start a downward decline in function in older people.

Ideally, no patient should be treated in physical or occupational therapy for dizziness without a thorough evaluation by a physician. There are numerous possible causes of dizziness, as noted in Box 62–1, rendering it impossible to determine the cause without testing. Laboratory and clinical tests that are performed in the attempt to diagnose the cause of the dizziness are included in Table 62–2. Although thorough testing is crucial to obtain an accurate diagnosis, the home health-care patient may not have the benefit of such an extensive workup. By being aware of the various causes of and tests for dizziness, the home health-care provider is more likely to make appropriate clinical decisions about referrals and care.

Dizziness History

A complete history of a patient's dizziness is essential so that the physician can make the medical diagnosis and the physical therapist can develop the best individualized exercise program. Some of the common questions that should be asked concern the characteristics of the dizziness, how long the patient has had the symptoms, how the first incident would be described, what makes the symptoms worse or better, any associated otological or neurological symptoms, and the frequency of the incidents or

Box 62-1

Common Causes of Dizziness

Peripheral vestibular disorders	Benign paroxysmal positional nystagmus and vertigo (BPPN or BPPV)
	Meniere's disease
	Endolymphatic hydrops
	Perilymph fistula
	Vestibular neuritis
	Bilateral vestibulopathy
Central disorders	Cervical vertigo
	Vestibular ocular dysfunction
	Traumatic head injury
	Labyrinthine concussion
	Posttraumatic anxiety symptoms
	Stroke/transient ischemic attacks
	Multiple sclerosis
Psychiatric disorders	Panic disorders
	Agoraphobia
	Hyperventilation syndrome
Others	Low blood pressure
	Medication
	Presyncope
	Arrhythmias
	Migraines
	Vertebral artery trauma
	Alternobaric vertigo
	Diabetes mellitus
	Thyroid dysfunction
	Renal disease
	HIV
	Syphilitic labyrinthitis
	Epstein-Barr virus
	Brain stem hemorrhage
	Friedreich's ataxia
	Hyperventilation disorders
	Recent diplopia

Table 62-2 Common Testing Provided to Older Persons Who Experience Chronic Dizziness

Test	Performed by Physician	Performed by Physical Therapist
Caloric testing	x	
Rotational testing: assesses the vestibulo-ocular reflex independent of vision and can assess the visual/vestibular interaction	x	
Oculomotor testing: smooth pursuit movements, saccades	x	x
Neurological examination	x	x
Optokinetic screening	x	
Electronystagmography: a test for vestibulo-ocular asymmetry and includes caloric testing, positional testing, and ocular motor function	x	
Audiogram	x	
Electrocochleography	x	
MRI or CT scan	x	
Brain stem auditory evoked potential	x	
Visual evoked potential	x	
Posturography	x	x
Standing and lying blood pressure measures	x	x
Hallpike maneuver	x	x
Fistula test	x	
Romberg/tandem Romberg test	x	x
Electrocardiogram	x	
Holter monitoring	x	
Cervical spine x-rays	x	
Testing for positional nystagmus with Frenzel glasses	x	x
Biochemical metabolic evaluation	x	
Glucose tolerance test	x	
Electroencephalogram	x	

attacks. A thorough history of past and present functional activities is also important. Specific activities of daily living (ADLs) may exacerbate the symptoms. This functional history is helpful in designing a treatment program based on symptoms. Others use the Dizziness Handicap Inventory (DHI) which provides a numerical score that ranges from 0 to 100 to specify how handicapped the patient perceives himself or herself to be because of the dizziness (Fig. 62–1). A "yes" answer scores 4; "sometimes" scores 2; and "no" is 0. The higher the total score, the greater the dizziness handicap. The DHI has also been used to document a patient's self-rating of improvement or lack of progress.

Many times, a patient with a chief complaint of dizziness receives an anti-dizziness medication, which can decrease the ability of the central nervous system (CNS) to compensate. Most anti-dizziness medications are depressants of the central nervous system and may limit the ability of the CNS to adapt to change caused by an insult to or dysfunction in the balance mechanism. If possible, it is best

to provide physical therapy when the patient is on a low dose of vestibular suppressants or none at all, but as some patients are unable to function without a vestibular suppressant, that may not be possible.

FUNCTIONAL DEFICITS

Dizziness can severely limit a patient's ability to perform ADLs. Each person's dizziness is unique, but complaints often heard include having difficulty with transitional movements and with moving quickly. Transitional movements include activities such as rolling, moving from a supine position to sitting, moving from sitting to standing, and walking while making certain head movements. Even standing while moving the head can increase symptoms in some patients. Walking while making head movements is often the most difficult of activities because the patient is unstable and may feel unsafe.

A patient may complain of having difficulty when movement is perceived with peripheral vision or when watching television or reading. A patient

Name: _____

MRN: _____   Date: _____/_____/_____

Referred by: _____   Age: _____

DIZZINESS HANDICAP INVENTORY (DHI)

Instructions: The purpose of this scale is to identify difficulties that you may be experiencing because of your dizziness. Please answer "yes," "no," or "sometimes" to each question. *Answer each question as it pertains to your dizziness problem only.*

Questions	Yes	Sometimes	No
P1. Does looking up increase your problem?			
P2. Because of your problem do you feel frustrated?			
P3. Because of your problem do you restrict your travel for business or recreation?			
P4. Does walking down the aisle of a supermarket increase your problem?			
P5. Because of your problem do you have difficulty getting into or out of bed?			
P6. Does your problem significantly restrict your participation in social activities such as going out to dinner, going to the movies, dancing, or going to parties?			
P7. Because of your problem do you have difficulty reading?			
P8. Does performing more ambitious activities like sports, dancing, or household chores such as sweeping or putting dishes away increase your problem?			
P9. Because of your problem are you afraid to leave your home without having someone to accompany you?			
P10. Because of your problem have you been embarrassed in front of others?			
P11. Do quick movements of your head increase your problem?			
P12. Because of your problem do you avoid heights?			
P13. Does turning over in bed increase your problem?			
P14. Because of your problem, is it difficult for you to do strenuous housework or yardwork?			
P15. Because of your problem are you afraid people may think that you are intoxicated?			
P16. Because of your problem is it difficult for you to go for a walk by yourself?			
P17. Does walking down a sidewalk increase your problem?			
P18. Because of your problem is it difficult for you to concentrate?			
P19. Because of your problem is it difficult for you to walk around your house in the dark?			
P20. Because of your problem are you afraid to stay home alone?			
P21. Because of your problem do you feel handicapped?			
P22. Has your problem placed stress on your relationship with friends or members of your family?			
P23. Because of your problem are you depressed?			
P24. Does your problem interfere with your job or household responsibilities?			
P25. Does bending over increase your problem?			

Figure 62–1 Dizziness handicap inventory (DHI). With permission from Jacobson GP, Newman CW. The development of the dizziness handicap inventory. *Arch Otolaryngol Head Neck Surg* 1990; 116:424.

may have dizziness when driving or when a passenger in a car. Clinically, it is noted that patients report less dizziness when they themselves are driving. For some older adults, losing the ability to drive can cause significant psychosocial dilemmas.

One characteristic symptom of patients with dizziness is having difficulty walking down the aisle of a grocery store or department store because of the constant input of extraneous visual information from both sides. This optic flow can be disorienting and can contribute to increased dizziness, nausea, and headaches; thus, people with severe dizziness often limit the amount of time they spend out of the home. Indeed, dizziness has been associated with agoraphobia and depression. It is a problem that can limit function even when the dizziness is not present, for the fear of becoming dizzy in a stressful situation is often enough for some people to limit their activities.

Not all patients with dizziness are easily treated. Patients with unilateral vestibular dysfunction often do the best with exercise programs. Patients with central vestibular dysfunction have more difficulty with exercise because of CNS involvement, and those with fluctuating symptoms have the most difficult time with exercises. Some of the fluctuating disorders, such as Meniere's disease and perilymph fistulas, may have to be surgically repaired in order for symptoms to disappear. Dizziness can be sequela to multiple sclerosis and stroke. In these patients, dizziness can lessen but may not completely resolve. Dizziness may be decreased or eliminated through surgery, yet some patients continue to experience tinnitus, which can be a disabling symptom, as it is often described as a dull roar or loud noise in the ear.

People with dizziness often have difficulty explaining their symptoms to family members because there are no externally obvious signs of the disorder, and family members can find it hard to comprehend the physical and psychological effects of dizziness and sometimes cannot understand that the patient may be severely disabled by the condition.

THERAPEUTIC INTERVENTION

Not all patients with dizziness have balance disorders. There appear to be three categories: those with dizziness, those with balance disorders, and those with balance disorders and dizziness. Each of these categories of older adults should be treated differently. The treatment program should be based on the functional deficits of the patient.

During the assessment of dizziness, it is important to determine if patients have fallen and if so, how often. Frequent falls (more than two within the past 6 months when no environmental hazards were present) are reason for significant concern. These individuals should be seen more frequently in the clinic and should be monitored closely at home by a family member. The patients who fall frequently might benefit from some type of alarm device to notify emergency personnel when a fall occurs.

Exercise

In an exercise program for a patient with vestibular dysfunction, the patient is asked to perform movements that increase symptoms. The objective is to let the patient feel dizzy in a safe environment. How quickly to advance a program is difficult to determine because if it progresses too rapidly, the patient might get worse, discontinue the exercises, and not return for future therapy. A combination of easier and more difficult exercises is often best so that the patient will be successful with at least a few of them. Keeping the number of exercises under five at each visit also helps with compliance.

When designing an exercise program, it is usually important to warn the patient that he or she will initially feel worse because of the exercises. If the patient remains severely dizzy as long as 45 minutes after the exercises have been completed, the exercises were too intense and must be modified in terms of intensity or number.

It is extremely important to get the patient to progress as quickly as possible while in a safe place so that confidence can be restored. Functional retraining, muscle strengthening, eye and head exercises, and having the patient attempt to perform difficult tasks are components of an individualized exercise program for a patient with vestibular dysfunction (Box 62–2).

Older adults most likely to benefit from a vestibular rehabilitation program include those with unilateral vestibular hypofunction (peripheral vestibular disorders) and those with bilateral peripheral vestibular disorders. Other patients that may be helped by physical therapy include those with head trauma, cerebellar atrophy or dysfunction, and multiple sclerosis. Patients who have been diagnosed with bilateral disorders may continue to improve with physical therapy up to a year after the insult, although the functional result may not be as successful as it is in patients with unilateral peripheral disorders. Patients with bilateral disorders often walk with a wide-based gait and may continue to require assistive devices after intervention. It is much more difficult to treat persons with central disorders, anxiety disorders, and combined central/peripheral vestibular disorders.

Older patients with dizziness can be helped by

Box 62–2

Exercises for the Patient with Dizziness

Exercises for the patient who experiences dizziness with transitional movements	• Head movements	Supine Sitting Standing Walking Walking and performing a functional activity
	• Functional activities	Pivots Circle and figure eight walking Ball toss Obstacle course
Balance exercises	• Consider the head, foot, and arm position plus whether the eyes are open or closed • Use the Clinical Test of Sensory Organization to help you plan your treatment • Hip and ankle strategies • Weight shifts • Single-leg stance • Stepping forward and back • Side stepping • Standing on foam • Kicking a ball • Walking backwards • Crossovers • Tandem walking • Romberg • Step-ups • Move objects to different surfaces • Trace the alphabet • Heel raises • Racquetball against the wall • Walk and carry an object • Walk in a dark room • Catch a ball while sitting on a gym ball • Stepping on a compliant surface • Jump rope • Ankle "proprioceptive" boards • Weight shift with a weight around the waist • T-Band weight shifts • Heel walking • Single-leg stance with kicking a ball on a string • Bus-step up • Stand on one leg and rotate the head • Functional movements for weight shift like golfing • Tilt boards • Toe walking	

Box continued on following page

Box 62–2 *Continued*

Exercises for the Patient with Dizziness

Eye movements (can be assessed with Frenzel glasses)	• Examples of eye exercises[a]	Head stable, eye tracking an object
		Object stable with the head moving
		Object and head both moving to track an object
	• Eye-head exercises	Focus on a card and move head to left and right
		Track a moving object up and down
		Focus on a card and move the head up and down
		Move head and card in the same direction at arm's length
		Look left and right quickly and focus on an object
		Look up and at eye level at two cards, head still
		Look up and at eye level at two cards, head moving
		Move head and card up and down
		Look right and left at the card while it is held in front of you
		Simon Says
		Mall walking
		Play ping pong
		Spin in a chair that rotates
		Laser tag
		Imaginary target exercise
		X2 viewing[a]
	• Otolith stimulation	Bounce on a ball
		Jump rope
	• Benign Paroxysmal Positional Vertigo (BPPV) Maneuvers[a]	Epley maneuver
		Semont's maneuver
		Brandt-Daroff exercises

[a] See Herdman S. *Vestibular Rehabilitation.* Philadelphia: F. A. Davis; 1994.

rehabilitation. At one time it was thought that they could not improve by means of a customized exercise program, but this has been shown to be a false assumption.

One of the most important components of the exercise program is getting patients to comply with the prescribed exercise routine on a regular basis. When compliance is an issue, it may be necessary to treat those patients more frequently. Older adults may be fearful of performing exercises alone at home even though a home exercise program always includes very specific instructions for performing the exercises safely.

The exercise usually recommended for older adults with dizziness is a walking program. Walking challenges the patients, especially outside the home, and exposes them to various amounts of visual stimuli. In some older individuals, initiating a walking program may not be possible because they live alone and may be afraid of falling.

CONCLUSION

Older adults present with many different causes of dizziness. They can be central, peripheral, psychiatric, or caused by other various systemic diseases, as noted in Box 62–1. Treatment is best initiated after a through medical workup to determine the medical diagnosis of the patient. Dizziness is an elusive symptom that can be difficult to diagnose. If the cause of the dizziness is vestibular, individually tailored exercise is of great benefit in the recovery of functional skills.

SUGGESTED READINGS

Connell B, Wolf S for the Atlanta FICSIT Group. Environmental and behavioral circumstances associated with falls at home among healthy elderly individuals. *Arch Phys Med Rehabil* 1997; 78:179.

Herdman S. *Vestibular Rehabilitation*. Philadelphia: F. A. Davis; 1994.

Herdman S. Advances in the treatment of vestibular disorders. *Phys Ther* 1997; 77:602.

Horak R, Henry S, Shumway-Cook A. Postural perturbations: new insights for treatment of balance disorders. *Phys Ther* 1997; 77:517.

Ludin-Olsson L, Nyberg L, Gustafson Y. "Stops talking when walking" as a predictor of falls in elderly people. *Lancet* 1997; 349:617.

Shumway-Cook A, Woollacott M, Kerns KA, Baldwin M. The effects of two types of cognitive tasks on postural stability in older adults with and without a history of falls. *J Gerontol A Biol Sci Med Sci* 1997; 52A:M232.

Whitney SL, Walsh MK. The home exercise routine for vestibular physical therapy. In: Kaufman IK, ed. *Dizziness and Balance Disorders*. New York: Kugler Publications; 1993: 721.

Chapter 63

Balance Testing and Training
Robert H. Whipple, M.A., P.T.

INTRODUCTION

Neurobiological vulnerability and diversity are important considerations when balance testing and training older adults. For the preponderance of independent older adults, deficits of balance are unlikely to be due to specific diagnoses but, rather, to ill-defined degenerative processes. These processes, in turn, may be caused by or influenced by an intricate web of factors such as genetic endowment, activity history, socioeconomic factors, personality, education, self-confidence, and undiagnosed disease. Not the least of these modifiers of balance is neurologi-

cal integrity. Longstreth,[1] for example, in a study of 3301 randomly selected ambulatory, community-dwelling elderly, found that 96% of the subjects had at least some degree of white matter degeneration, with the changes appearing moderate to severe in two thirds of the sample. However, even in the "super-healthy" old-old (subjects of age 90 and above, selected for having no trace of disease), there are dramatic losses in certain measures of balance, in spite of the presence of relatively normal MRIs and EEGs.[2, 3]

Disease aside, there may be both a variety as well as an inevitability to balance impairments in aging. As is so for most regions of the brain, there is a great degree of intercommunication and redundancy of information transfer among the various sites responsible for balance regulation. This could imply that all older adults with balance problems show a similar profile of deficits upon testing—for example, that it is likely that people with abnormally slow gaits are more likely to perform poorly on single-leg standing and turning.

There are people, however, with pathologically slow walks who nonetheless test out normally on an unstable surface with eyes closed, do a sit-to-stand in under a second, and show normal reactions to surface translation. An abundance of examples is possible. Their diversity is likely to reflect the multifocal and idiosyncratic distribution of lesions and sites of degeneration. Hence, the patchwork of neural losses may become manifested in a specific mix of balance deficits that can be brought to light only if the test battery is also sufficiently diverse and capable of revealing multiple components of balance.

RANGE OF ENVIRONMENTAL CHALLENGES TO BALANCE

In contrast to a patient's often distinctive and lesion-dependent profile of balance aptitudes is the vast array of potentially destabilizing conditions encountered in the course of daily function. Many of these challenges to balance have been found to be measurable and reproducible and have been effectively employed within currently used balance and functional assessment batteries.[4, 5]

Recently, a categorization scheme was proposed that attempted to account for a wide gamut of destabilizing circumstances that could be found during daily activities (excluding specialized movements, as in athletics).[6] Operationalizing balance functions in this manner was regarded as a first step toward helping to identify the components of an idealized balance intervention and test battery. Tables 63–1 and 63–2 and Figure 63–1 depict three

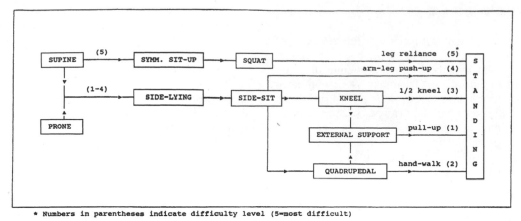

* Numbers in parentheses indicate difficulty level (5=most difficult)

Figure 63–1 Ground-level transfers to stand. Numbers in parentheses indicate difficulty level (1 = least difficult, 5 = most difficult). (Reprinted with permission from Whipple R. Improving balance in older adults: identifying the significant training stimuli. In: Masden JC, Sudarsky L, Wolfson L, eds. *Gait Disorders of Aging: Falls and Therapeutic Strategies*. Philadelphia: Lippincott-Raven Publishers, 1997: 358.)

balance challenge domains (BCDs) of destabilizing conditions along with examples of associated real-life activities. Table 63–1 presents volitionally based and predictable challenges to erect balance on a stable surface. Figure 63–1 presents ground-level activities and transfers between ground and standing. Table 63–2 presents unexpected external provocations to erect balance. Thus, there are eight volitional, including ground-level (seven from Table 63–1 and one from Figure 63–1), and five provocative categories (from Table 63–2) of challenges to balance.

Based on the categories, the following three groupings of balance tests are shown: predictable challenges in Table 63–3, unpredictable challenges in Table 63–4, and turning challenges in Table 63–5. Each balance assessment in Table 63–3 and Table 63–4 is displayed in terms of its balance challenge category, characteristic deficits observed, and balance training options. Turning is a BCD category in its own right and therefore has references only to deficits observed and training options. Following each table are expanded descriptions of items in the table, which should allow the reader to apply these techniques. Table 63–6 and its accompanying descriptions deal with indirect factors that are of importance in any balance evaluation.

BALANCE RETRAINING OPTIONS

For most community-dwelling older adults, the prospect of at least some improvement of balance through training is now a reality.[6–8] Considering the wide range of balance behaviors and environmental contexts to which we are routinely exposed, two possible therapeutic strategies present themselves.

The first involves training that contains many separate motor activities in which each corresponds to a specific performance as measured in a balance test. In its purest form, this strategy would dictate that the exercises chosen for treatment directly reflect the profile of deficits seen on balance testing. Hence, if gait were slowed and one-legged stance time decreased, treatment would focus on increasing gait speed and practicing single-leg standing.

Alternatively, systematic, integrated, or holistic approaches to balance restitution exist that may be of such potency that improvements can be seen in areas of balance performance that are seemingly unrelated to the kind of training undergone. For example, training in such areas as tai chi,[9] body awareness through movement such as Feldenkrais,[10] gaze stabilization,[11] or sensory organization,[12] may prevent falls and lead to increases in diverse areas of balance function (e.g., one-legged stance, limits of sway, and gait) without concentrated and specific training having been carried out in that function.

Only the future can fully resolve these issues. This chapter first presents, in table form, balance treatment guidelines for older adults based on the results of a selection of balance tests chosen by the author (Tables 63–3 through 63–5). The tests can be carried out within approximately 75 to 90 minutes and are representative of most of the BCD balance categories described above. Many traditional tests typically found in popularly used batteries[4, 7] are included, as well as tests involving the use of a perturbation force platform (EquiTest, NeuroCom International, Clackamas, Ore.)* A

---

*Although the Foam-and-Dome tests[14] are reasonably good substitutes for an unstable surface and for sensory organization assessment, measured surface translations and tilts can be reliably carried out only electromechanically.

Text continued on page 343

Table 63–1 Common Challenges to Erect Balance in the Absence of External Provocations or Tripping[a]

Destabilizing Conditions	Real-Life Activities
1. Decreased bipedal base	
Normal-width foot separation	
Symmetrical weight on heels	Leaning or reaching backward
Symmetrical weight on balls of feet	Leaning or reaching forward
Asymmetrical weight between feet	Leaning or reaching in oblique directions
Narrowed stance	
Feet close together (Romberg)	Narrowed floor space (or diminished ROM)
Tandem, semitandem	Narrowed floor space (or diminished ROM)
Feet crossed	Dictated by available floor space
2. One-legged stance	Put on pants; leaning to side
3. Limits of stability	
(Maintenance of center of force on perimeter of base of support)	Extreme reaching (e.g., painting, dusting)
4. Ambulatory conditions	
Normal walk	
Forward, usual speed > 1 m/sec	Conventional walking
Backward	Dancing, IADLs[a]
Maximum speed walk	Hurrying, exercising
Running or jogging	Hurrying, exercising
Side-stepping	Dancing; navigation at home, crowds
Stepping over	Obstacles in path
Narrowed (tandem) walk	
Forward (heel-to-toe-like)	Limited floor space; diminished abduction ROM
Backward (toe-to-heel-like)	Limited floor space; diminished abduction ROM
Slow-as-possible walk	In dark or on uncertain floor conditions
Using reduced area of foot	
Walk on toes	Hiking, dancing, uncertain floor conditions
Walk on heels	Backward loss of balance, dancing, pain under forefoot
5. Turning	Twists in daily activities
Segmental rotations (head, torso, pelvis)	
Pivots/spins of whole body	Fast turns without stepping
Step-pivots, > 180 degrees	Turns with steps, reverse direction of walk
6. Upper extremity movements	Unstressed daily activities
Casual movements	
Fast	Reactive or catching movements
With loads	Lift bags, place objects
7. Vertical body movements	
Nonstepping	
Transfers	Sit-to-stand
Jumps, hops	Emergency movements, exercise
Other	Stoop, squat, bend, pick up
While stepping	Stairs, curbs, stools

  [a] While weight-bearing on feet on a flat horizontal surface that is at least equal to the weight-bearing surface of the foot or feet.
  [b] IADL, instrumental activities of daily living; ROM, range of motion.
  From Whipple RH. Improving balance in older adults: identifying the significant training stimuli. In: Masden JC, Sudarsky L, Wolfson L, eds. *Gait Disorders of Aging: Falls and Therapeutic Strategies.* Philadelphia: Lippincott-Raven Publishers; 1997.

Table 63–2 Unexpected or Unusual External Challenges to Balance

Destabilizing Conditions	Real-Life Activities
1. Surface instabilities	
Horizontal plane	
Translations	Buses, trains, boats, escalators, moving walkways
Slippery or loose surfaces	Ice, loose rugs, gravel (stance-phase challenges)
Sagittal and frontal plane (tilts)	
Inclines (static)	Ramps, sloping terrain
Evoked sudden tilts	Vehicles, small boats, planes
Compliant (yielding) tilts	Foam, floor-rug transitions, sand
Sway-referenced tilts	Posturography platforms
Vertical dimension	
Surface movement under both feet	Boats, elevators, escalators, buses
Surface movement under one foot	Boat-dock, floor-elevator
Surface height differential	Potholes, rugged terrain, missteps
Compliant surfaces	Rugs, sand, foam, mud, sneakers, snow
2. Body perturbations	
Sudden pushes and pulls	Crowds, pets, team sports
Gradual onset	Pets
Sudden cessation	Object (pet) giving way while leaning against it
3. Reduced surface area	
Reduced anteroposterior dimension	Stand/walk on short object or terrain
Reduced mediolateral dimension	Stand/walk on narrow beam, plank, irregular terrain
4. Obstacle contact-ambulation	
Trips and stumbles	Edges of rug, cracks, cords, clutter
Anticipated resistances	
At lower extremity level	Walk in snow, water, leaves
At body level	Push-pull doors, pets, mowers, vacuum
5. Aberrant visual input	
Reduced or absent input	Moving in darkness
Distorted or confusing input	In moving vehicles, ships

From Whipple RH. Improving balance in older adults: identifying the significant training stimuli. In: Masden JC, Sudarsky L, Wolfson L, eds. *Gait Disorders of Aging: Falls and Therapeutic Strategies.* Philadelphia: Lippincott-Raven Publishers; 1997.

Table 63–3 Test and Training Scheme for Predictable Challenges to Balance in the Absence of External Provocations

Assessment	BCD Category	Deficits Observed	Training Options
1. *Narrowed stances* Romberg, half-tandem, full tandem	Decreased bipedal base	Fall, increased sway or need to use arms	Practice at level that presents difficulty (see below)
2. *Asymmetrical mediolateral weight-bearing* Left-right distribution at rest	Decreased bipedal base	≥ 20% more weight on one leg than other	Attention on pressure under feet, electronic scale feedback, standing on sloping surface, limits of stability training (see below)
3. *Asymmetrical anteroposterior (AP) weight-bearing* Forward-backward misdistribution at rest	Decreased bipedal base	≥ 3.5° anterior (@ ≥ 1.3° posterior) of neutral	Discriminate pressure under front vs. rear of feet; center of pressure electronic feedback; limits of stability training (see below)
4. *One-legged stance*	One-legged stance	Falling in ~ < 8 seconds, and having to abduct arms to assist	Practice task while holding on with two, then one hand, using minimal pressure (see below)
5. *Limits of stability* Maximal voluntary AP leaning	Limits of stability	Decreased amplitude of AP lean; inability to hold lean at limits of sway for more than a few seconds	Practice leaning to maximal limits of sway in all directions as well as AP while maintaining vertical torso
6. *Normal walk* Forward at usual speed	Ambulatory conditions	Velocity ~ < 9 M/sec; classical gait deviations (see below)	Classical gait-training techniques
7. *Turning (see Table 63–5)*			
8. *Sit-to-stand* 5× at maximal velocity	Vertical body movements (transfers)	Poor foot placement, lack of terminal extension control, decreased trunk acceleration, insufficient forward trunk displacement	Correction of listed deficits; increased trunk/hip flexor, hip extensor, knee extensor strength; improve head on torso control and gaze stability
9. *Pick up object* Timed pencil pickup from floor	Vertical body movements (other)	Loss or near loss of balance; nonfluid or slowed	As in sit-to-stand above
10. *Stepping up and down* (6-inch step)	Vertical body movements (stepping)	Requires manual assistance, loss of balance or near loss of balance	Practice on stairs; supplementary lower extremity resistance training

BCD, body challenge domain

Table continued on following page

Table 63–3 Test and Training Scheme for Predictable Challenges to Balance in the Absence of External Provocations *Continued*

Predictable and Volitionally Based Challenges to Erect Balance on a Stable Surface

1. Narrowed Stances: employing hand support as needed; if unable to do half-tandem, either practice Romberg at just-tolerable separation width, progressively decreasing width; or practice at quarter-tandem, increasing AP separation progressively. To practice tandem, begin with 2–3 inches wider separation, then progressively narrow as able. Alternatively, practice most difficult task while holding with two, then progressing to one hand, eventually with minimal finger pressure. Once tandem mastered, try with eyes closed.
   Deficits observed: falling to side, increased amplitude or frequency of sway necessitating use of arms
   Comment: ability to perform adequate single-leg stance need not be considered a substitute for tandem stance training, as skills may not be equivalent

2. Asymmetrical Mediolateral Weight-bearing: left or right misdistribution of weight-bearing at rest
   Deficits observed: $\sim \geq 20\%$ more weight on one leg than the other at rest (based on viewing forceplate or electronic bathroom scale outputs)
   Training options: correct directional bias by focusing attention on sensations of pressure under feet, giving forceplate or electronic scale feedback, standing on sloping surface (thereby forcing weight to other side), body awareness enhancing techniques (e.g., tai chi); increase difficulty level by closing eyes and/or standing on foam; see also Limits of Stability training below.

3. Asymmetrical Anteroposterior Weight-bearing: forward or backward misdistribution of weight at rest
   Deficits observed: $\sim \geq 3.5°$ forward angle of sway ($\sim \geq 1.3°$ backward angle of sway) from neutral (based on viewing forceplate output)
   Training options: develop discrimination between pressure under front vs. rear of feet while swaying (can be aided with forceplate feedback), or through Limits of Stability training (see below); develop toe flexion strength and control; body awareness enhancement (e.g., tai chi)

4. One-legged Stance: the ability to stand for at least 10 seconds on one leg with the arms crossed over the chest, without hopping or movement of the stance footpractice task while holding on with two, then one hand, using minimal pressure. Keep torso and head vertically aligned, and belt-line horizontal, using mirror whenever possible. Teach self-palpation of gluteus medius while hip-hiking. Home in on transition from "contact-only" with foot to be lifted to "lifting only 1 inch" off ground. Unlocking knee frequently enhances COG control.
   Deficits observed: limited stance time. Tendency to avoid commiting weight to stance-side leg, lack of vertical alignment of trunk, and bracing of one foot against calf of other. (Comment: the somatosensory afference (or perhaps input processing) controlling foot inversion/eversion deteriorates dramatically, even in normal aging. To compensate, emphasis must be shifted to hip control, more meticulous truncal alignment, and pelvic (center of gravity) awareness.)
   Training options: practice task while holding on with two, then one hand, using progressively less pressure as skill improves. Keep torso and head vertically aligned, and belt-line horizontal, using mirror whenever possible. Teach self-palpation of gluteus medius while hip-hiking. Home in on transition from "contact only" with foot to be lifted, to "lifting only 1 inch" off ground. Unlocking knee frequently enhances COG control.

5. Limits of Stability: the ability to shift and then hold the center of pressure maximally forward for 5–10 seconds (and then backward) over the feet.
   Deficits observed: poor holding ability at limits and reduced amplitude of lean. Hips and trunk tend to flex in attempting to shift weight forward, and extend when shifting backwards. (Comment: maintenance of vertical trunk control cannot be emphasized enough, and is frequently difficult to achieve. The natural tendency to flex when leaning forward is counterproductive because this synergy tends to create a forward shear force which *prevents* forward weight shift.)
   Training options: ask patient to imagine standing in the center of a large clockface drawn on the ground. Assuming forward is veiwed as 12 o'clock, then the center of pressure can be brought toward the perimeter of the base of support (feet) in all directions of the "clock" and held at this maximal sway threshold for 5–10 seconds. As in one-legged stance, maintenance of the head and torso perfectly vertical throughout is critical; e.g., when shifting weight forward the lumbar spine must extend, whereas backward shifting requires lumbar flattening. Patient attention is to be constantly directed to foot perception and when shifting forward, to vigorous toe flexion.

Table 63–3 Test and Training Scheme for Predictable Challenges to Balance in the Absence of External Provocations *Continued*

6. Normal Walk: forward, at usual speed over a 4-meter course.
Deficits observed: note conventional deviations, such as guardedness, lurching, weaving, waddling, asymmetrical or decreased step length, reduced swing clearance. If velocity is within normal limits, then assess also for presence of arm swing, arm-leg reciprocation, and trunk-pelvis counterrotation.
Training options: conscious correction for deviations and other conventional gait-training approaches. Attention to axial segment (head, chest, pelvis) motions and orientations in the horizontal plane, principles of vestibulo-oculomotor control, and techniques for enhancing body awareness are fruitful areas of focus (see also "Turning").

7. Turning: See Table 63–5

8. Sit-to-Stand Transfers: time to come to a complete stand five times without assistance at maximal velocity, from armless straight-backed chair.
Deficits observed: e.g., poor foot placement, lack of terminal extension control, decreased trunk acceleration, insufficient forward trunk displacement, backward loss of balance.
Training options: correction of listed deficits; increased trunk/hip flexor, hip extensor, knee extensor strength; improve head-on-torso control and gaze stability.

9. Pick Up Object from Ground: time to pick-up of pencil placed on ground immediately in front of patient.
Deficits observed: loss or near loss of balance; excessively slow ($> \sim 5$ secs), or discontinuous
Training options: as for sit-to-stand; if arthritic pain in knees (hips), shift emphasis (ROM) to hips (knees). If dizziness occurs, try longer AP (lunging) or wider (straddling) stance with head held more erect. Practice progressively faster and larger amplitude alternating trunk (hip) flexion-extension movements while standing. Practice standing (with close guarding) transversely on shortened block of wood (3–4 inches), thus activating hip synergy.

10. Stepping Up and Down: to and from a 6-inch box, without assistance.
Deficits observed: too slow, arms abducted, delayed restabilization after steps, loss or near loss of balance, multiple attempts, prolonged time to choose descending leg, manual assistance
Training options: practice on stairs with proper degree of support; supplementary lower extremity resistance training. If knee pain is excessive on up-step, teach how to substitute increased plantar flexion for decreased knee extension.

Table 63–4 Unpredictable or Unusual External Challenges to Balance

Assessment	BCD Category	Deficits Observed	Training Options
1. *Sagittal plane surface instability:* AP tilts in which surface "gives way"; with eyes open, closed, and with inaccurate visual input	Surface instabilities	Falls in ≥ 2 out of 3 trials of each condition	Perception of foot pressure cues while standing and slowly swaying; balancing while on unstable surface, with eyes open, closed, or inaccurate input (e.g., Foam-and-Dome EquiTest)
2. *Pulls to pelvis:* Sudden forces displacing the body backwards	Body perturbations	Backward falls or failure to employ flexor synergy in response to forces of 1.5 to 3.0% of body weight	Unexpected manual perturbations to torso or pelvis, varying in intensity and direction; sudden onset and sudden offset forces; eyes open and closed
3. *Absent or unreliable visual inputs:* Eyes closed or wearing "dome"	Aberrant visual input	Falls, dizziness, or excessive sway with eyes closed, or targets move with head	Emphasis on "dome" use during Foam-and-Dome training; EquiTest training on conditions SO3 and SO6; eliminate vision during assorted balance challenges

BCD, body challenge domain

Unpredictable and External Challenges to Balance

1. Sagittal Plane Surface Instability: classically performed on a surface that "gives" (compliant), like an EquiTest, or on foam. Upon shifting the center of gravity on an EquiTest, the surface yields in a special way called "sway referencing"—it tilts in proportion to the estimated degree of body sway. Three visual conditions are used: (a) eyes open on an unstable surface, equivalent to "Sensory Organization condition 4 (SO4)," (b) eyes closed on a tiltable surface (SO5), and (c) inaccurate visual input (visual surround moves proportional to angle of body sway) while on an unstable surface (SO6). Each trial lasts 20 seconds and is repeated three times in succession. Note however, that tests can be designed for compliant tilts in the mediolateral plane and for evoked (externally initiated) platform tilts or horizontal plane movements (translations).

Deficits observed: falls in 2 or 3 out of 3 trials in each SO condition, with no evidence of adaptation; use of upper extremities for counterbalancing should not be permitted.

Training options: initially, while on a stable surface, patient focuses attention on sensations of varying pressure under each portion of each foot while standing still or slowly swaying toward all points of the compass; increase difficulty level by closing eyes, wearing a "dome" (Japanese lantern affixed to head with midline target adhered to inner surface) and/or standing on a tiltable or foam surface; can be made harder yet by using more compliant foam or by increasing gain of EquiTest. Most of control should feel as if coming from legs ("ankle"), but hip countermovements must be permitted ("hip strategy") in proportion to the degree of give of the surface. Note: Training may also be additionally enriched through the use of externally evoked translations and tilts, if such equipment is available.

Comment: as age, frailty, and disease burden increase, it becomes unfeasible to clearly differentiate the effects of diminished sensation from poor central processing, faulty sensory reweighting of inputs, or deficiencies of efferents on poor test performance. For similar reasons, training to improve tolerance for an unstable surface may overlap with training for the resolution of sensory conflict (wearing a dome while standing on foam).

2. Pulls to Pelvis: sudden forces applied to pelvis, destabilizing body backwards. Known and reproducible forces can be created by attaching a pulley cable to back of spotting belt worn by patient, and then dropping weights (first 1.5%, then 3.0% of body weight) a vertical distance of 2 feet (Postural Stress Test).[16]

Deficits observed: falls with 1.5% or multiple backward steps without synergies, with 3.0% of body weight.

Training options: unexpected manual perturbations to torso or pelvis, varying in intensity and direction; sudden onset and sudden offset forces; difficulty increased by closing eyes and/or standing on foam.

Table 63–4 Unpredictable or Unusual External Challenges to Balance *Continued*

3. Absent or Unreliable Visual Input: standing with eyes closed; standing with "dome" or on EquiTest with sway-referenced movement of the visual surround (Sensory Organization condition 3).

Deficits observed: loss of balance, excessive sway or dizziness.

Training options: visual occlusion during whatever tasks are challenging to balance; conditions can include normal standing, with feet together, half-tandem, tandem, slow walk, leaning, stooping, head or torso rotation, etc. Unreliable visual inputs can be simulated with a "dome" (on solid, foam, inclined, or minitramp surfaces), or by training on EquiTest or similar equipment that provides false visual feedback (sway-referenced visual signals).

---

category of associated assessment items (such as lower extremity strength, dizziness, judgment, efforting, and fear) that impact on balance is also included in Table 63–6.

Additionally, given the complexity of turning and the prominent relationship between turning and falls in the elderly,[13] a brief format will be presented for the testing (see Table 63–5) and training (see Table 63–7 and Figure 63–2) of axial segmental movements (eyes, head, trunk) in the horizontal plane. It is likely that underlying deficits in left-right spatial orientation and rotatory control are strongly implicated in turn-related falls.

Body awareness techniques (e.g., tai chi, Alexander,[15] and Feldenkrais,[10] as well as exercises based on these principles) are examples of systematic, integrated, "holistic," and process-based procedures in which practice may generalize to improvements in diverse and nonpracticed areas of movement and posture. They share in common their great reliance on the cultivation of body awareness, imagery, and the fine control of segmental movements in the horizontal plane,[6] that is, the roots of turning. The scheme referred to above for the practice of segmental axial control of movement (see Table 63–7) is drawn from these techniques. Principles based on body awareness systems can be introduced during treatment and can then be reinforced by having the patient join an instructor-led group upon discharge. Socializing, memory consolidation, and confidence-building through the group can also lead to effective self-guided home practice.

DISCUSSION

Diversity and Specificity in Testing and Training

A recent review of 25 training studies[6] involving older adults showed that the regimens incorporating the greatest number of BCD categories were the most effective. Since even in the studies with more successful outcomes, an average of only two balance tests was used, the recorded improvements may represent a gross underestimation of many other categories of balance challenges in which gains may have occurred. The results of two recent studies[8, 18] suggest that at least for some measures of balance (single stance, limits of sway, unstable surface, and random surface tilts) improvements may indeed be training-specific, and that, therefore, a range of different balance tests ought to be made available in order to detect the potential for change in diverse areas of the balance spectrum.

Hence, although probably not true for all kinds of balance (see the following two paragraphs), the limited evidence suggests that we should consider introducing both diversity and specificity into our training and testing repertoires. In the scheme introduced in this chapter (Tables 63–3, 63–4, and 63–5), 10 of the 13 BCD categories (Table 63–1 plus Figure 63–1 and Table 63–2) are represented. For purposes of accuracy of quantification, many of the tests should be performed on a dynamic force platform, but this is not an absolute necessity. There is far from universal agreement on the validity of many of the force platform balance measures, and low-tech versions of these tests (e.g., use of foam for an unstable surface, manual perturbations, visual estimation of angle of limits of sway) may ultimately prove to be equally meaningful. Furthermore, regardless of limitations in test accuracy imposed by lack of instrumentation, the underlying balance functions can, in most cases, still be easily accessed through training.

Generalizable Training Effects Through Body Awareness (Holistic) Training

As indicated in Tables 63–3, 63–4, and 63–5, treatment techniques such as tai chi[9] and Feldenkrais[10] should also be considered when tackling some of

Table 63–5 Turning: Movement and Spatial Orientation in the Horizontal Plane

Assessment	Deficits Observed	Training Options
1. *Postural axial segmental asymmetries at rest* Deviations in horizontal and frontal planes	Excessive head, trunk, and hip side bend or forward bend	Lower body awareness threshold for detection of deviation through verbal and tactile feedback, mirror, and techniques such as Alexander, Feldenkrais, tai chi; see also horizontal plane exercises in Table 63–7
2. *360° Turns* Timed, maximal speed turns in place	Loss or near loss of balance, dizziness, left-right differences	See text
3. *Horizontal head rotation* Active left↔right rotation (yaw)	Loss or near loss of balance, body follows head, asymmetry, dizziness	See text
4. *Gaze stabilization* Visual fixation during rhythmical head rotations	Blurring of image, dizziness, loss or near loss of balance, markedly increased sway, rotational asymmetries	See text

a Asterisked items are not established measures

Turning: Movement and Spatial Orientation in the Horizontal Plane

1. Postural Axial Segmental Asymmetries at Rest: while standing facing a wall squarely, assess for deviations of head, trunk, and pelvis in the frontal, but particularly the horizontal planes (can use directions in which nose, sternum, and navel are points of reference).
Deficits observed: any combination of right or left deviations of segments from midline, assuming feet are pointing symmetrically forward; note exact combination (e.g., head rotated slightly to right, chest moderately to left, and pelvis markedly to left of midline).
Training options: lower body awareness threshold for detection of deviation through verbal, visual (mirror), and tactile feedback, and through techniques such as Alexander, Feldenkrais, tai chi.

2. 360° Turns: timed maximal velocity turns in place.
Deficits observed: loss or near loss of balance; too slow ($\sim$ >3 secs); too many steps ($\sim$ >8); marked differences in left versus right turns.
Training options: maintenance of vertical segmental alignment, widening steps, turning body by pivoting on toe of nonweight-bearing leg after a step, slowing down, repeated visual targeting, rotate from hips rather than twisting from trunk (moves head torso and pelvis in tandem), keep navel aligned with foot on side ipsilateral to turn before transferring weight to that foot; supplement with body awareness training techniques (e.g., tai chi); reduce directional bias by practicing turns in either direction, pointing out differences to patient; complement with segmental axial control exercises (see gaze control below and Table 63–7 and Figure 63–2).

3. Horizontal Head Rotation: rhythmical maximal amplitude left↔right head turning in response to metronome at .5 and .75 Hz (60 and 90 beats/min)
Deficits observed: loss or near loss of balance, increased sway, body follows head, dizziness, asymmetry in speed, amplitude or body-following in turning to left versus right
Training options: using mirror, note and correct: deviations from verticality, asymmetry in amplitude of rotation, failure to isolate movement to head; complement with segmental axial control exercises (Table 63–7).

4. Gaze Stabilization:[17] Visual fixation of midline target (3/4″ printed letter) at eye level 1 yard in front of standing subject; head is actively rotated rhythmically (can use metronome) left↔right over a 30°ROM ($\sim$15° to either side of midline) for a maximum of 2 minutes at a maximum frequency of 2 Hz (120 excursions/minute). Performance measure is rate at which patient can move without experiencing blurring or movement of target.
Deficits observed: blurring of target at under 2 Hz
Training options: perform one set rotating head from side to side (in horizontal plane) as fast as possible at a rate that is below threshold for blurring of image, for a maximum of 2 minutes nonstop; do total of 3× per day. Dizziness during performance is not a contraindication if patient is able to tolerate. However, blurring or moving of image should not be allowed. If blurring occurs keep lowering the rate of movement until the image becomes stable (i.e., just below threshold for blurring). If image blurs despite this, try in a seated position. More complex variations can be performed with head held in partial flexion or extension, and while walking forwards and backwards.

Table 63–6 Associated Considerations

Assessment	Deficits Observed	Training Options
1. *Lower extremity strength*	Specific weaknesses	Traditional strengthening techniques, using body weight resistance whenever feasible
2. *Dizziness*	Note circumstances, e.g., at rest, constant, during head movement, etc.	See text
3. *Efforting*	Excessive cocontraction, stiffness, breathholding, hyperresponsiveness	Techniques such as contract-relax "letting go" of hand tension, breathing awareness, verbal instructions (see text)
4. *Fear*	Hyperresponsiveness, breathholding, guardedness (see also "*Efforting*")	As for *efforting* above; reassurance of safety of test
5. *Judgment*	Hazardous behavior	Safety training

Associated Considerations

1. Lower Extremity Strength: muscle weakness can cause or contribute to balance problems
Deficits observed: assess for specific strength deficiencies; a few quick functional criteria for balance-related strength adequacy are: (1) ability to perform 15–20 brisk, one-legged heel rises with body weight, (2) walk on heels 100 ft nonstop taking small steps and holding onto wall while keeping forefeet well off ground, (3) 10–15 single-legged bridges, (4) 15–20 rapid sit-to-stands in succession without arm assistance.
Training options: strengthen target muscle groups; if many muscle groups are involved and it is not feasible to strengthen all simultaneously, prioritize as follows: (1) dorsiflexors, (2) plantarflexors, (3) hip flexors, (4) quadriceps, (5) hip abductors.

2. Dizziness: note if present.
Deficits observed: note circumstances—at rest, intermittent, upon head movement, postural hypotension, etc.
Training options: gaze stabilization exercises, habituation exercises; Semont or Epley maneuvers if indicated.[11]

3. Efforting: the psychoemotional predisposition or mental "set" to perform a potentially challenging motor task; if excessive, it may render some test results inaccurate or lead to misinterpretations of performance.
Deficits observed: over-efforting may be characterized by excessive cocontraction, stiffness, breathholding, fist-clenching, and other unnecessary tonic contractions or postural bracings that impede coordinated and efficient movement; it is a state of increased arousal and hyperresponsiveness that may be indistinguishable from fear (see below).
Training options: relaxation techniques, such as contract-relax, "letting go" of tension in hand, shoulders, jaw, frontalis, etc; breathing control and awareness techniques, such as in Hatha yoga.

4. Fear: as for efforting; excessive fear of testing or of falling may degrade test results and often leads to fatigue and premature termination of testing.
Deficits observed: as for efforting, but often more intense.
Training options: as for efforting; verbal reassurance.

5. Judgment: evidence of predisposition for risk-taking behavior.
Deficits observed: history of multiple falls or near-falls; haphazard approach to all movement tasks with violation of safety principles.
Training options: safety training, including assistive devices.

Table 63–7 Segmental Axial Rotation Training in the Horizontal Plane

Movement Type	Movement Description
1. Visual fixation with head rotation	Eyes fixate midline target while head rotates without accompanying trunk or scapular movement
2. Saccades	Maximal amplitude lateral eye movements without accompanying head movement
3. Visual tracking with head still	Move thumb slowly in large arcs from side to side while following with eyes; keep head and trunk still
4. Head tracking with eyes still	Head moves in tandem with side-to-side movement of thumb; eyes remain fixated on thumb but do not move
5. Head and eyes move in same direction	Head and eyes move simultaneously as far to the same side as possible
6. Head and eyes move in opposite directions	Head and eyes move simultaneously to the side as far as possible in opposite directions
7. Chest rotates on pelvis; head is still	Head is fixed in space at midline while upper trunk (chest) rotates as far as possible to either side
8. Chest and pelvis rotate together about both hips; head is still	Head is fixed in space at midline while both upper (chest) and lower (pelvis) trunk rotate as far as possible to a side about both hips
9. Chest, pelvis, and ipsilateral lower extremity rotate together about contralateral hip; head is still	Head is fixed in space at midline while chest, pelvis and lower extremity on side ipsilateral to rotation rotate as far as possible to a side about the contralateral hip (external rotation of pelvis on contralateral thigh), while pivoting about the ipsilateral heel
10. Head, chest, pelvis, and ipsilateral lower extremity rotate as a unit about contralateral hip	The entire body (head, chest, pelvis, ipsilateral lower extremity) rotates about the weight-bearing hip to the opposite side, pivoting about the heel on that side

See Figure 63–2 for clarification.

the more complex challenges to balance, such as those encountered during turning, single stance, gait, swaying to limits of stability, and visual deprivation. Rather than attempting to address each of many specific training tasks piecemeal, these techniques coalesce a multitude of balance challenges under a single conceptual umbrella that might be termed "holistic." These approaches emphasize imagistic, attentional, conscious, and "open-loop" processing, and it is unlikely that there is a single underlying therapeutic mechanism at work.

In the case of tai chi (Yang style) it appears that many balance tasks are simultaneously and systematically engaged. For example, the center of gravity (COG) is kept low (through flexed knees) and over a larger base of support, hip and thigh muscles are preferentially engaged, turning occurs exclusively at the hips, the head and torso are kept vertically aligned, the pelvis is held horizontally, respiration rate (slow) and quality (diaphragmatic breathing) are modified, and movement velocity is slow and unvarying. A multiplicity of specific acts related to balance control is thus being practiced, and the person's attention can be directed either to the individual elements or to the integrated whole (the Gestalt). An emphasis on awareness is the common thread that links these approaches.[10]

Turning

Evidence is accumulating that ostensibly simple acts such as performing a one-quarter turn in place or merely modestly changing direction while walking may be unusually challenging to the balance of older adults and may be a substantial contributor to many falls.[13] The seemingly innocuous and matter-of-fact nature of these movements may lead to

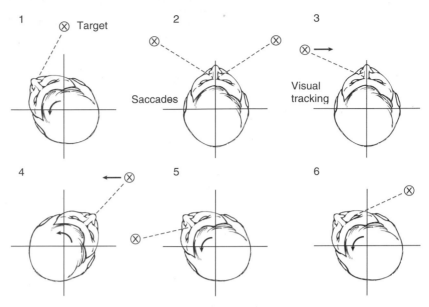

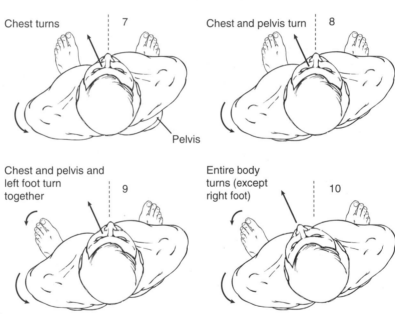

Figure 63-2 Overhead views of segmental axial rotation in the horizontal plane.

complacency and lack of vigilance, thereby increasing the risk for loss of balance. Features of turning likely to be particularly associated with neurobiological deficiencies of aging are deterioration in vestibular function, radical loss in one-legged stance capacity, marked deficiency in gaze stabilization function, and relatively greater declines in higher-order spatial-perceptual function.[2, 19] The complexities of intersegmental axial control in the horizontal and frontal planes as well as postural and arthritic decrements in neck, trunk, and hip range of motion (ROM) during a turn further aggravate the balance dysfunction.

Turning is a perfect context for the interaction of intersegmental axial control with certain holistic movement techniques.[9, 10] Experience with tai chi[9] or Feldenkrais[10] typically leads to a lowering of the threshold of awareness for segmental deviations from the true midline, vertical, and horizontal. Hence, practice of the segmental horizontal exercises (see Table 63 7) *while* focusing on subtle somatosensory body cues may, in a similar fashion, improve precision of segmental alignment and movement control while turning. In so doing, instead of "just turning," an individual may be able to successfully focus on where he or she is turning from (e.g., the hip); how far a segment has deviated off the vertical during weight transfer; if the head or eyes are lagging; and whether the center of gravity has arrived well within the base of support of the weight-bearing foot before the other foot is lifted.

Some FICSIT Evidence

Clinically and functionally speaking, there is currently no "right" theoretical framework within which to place the varieties of measurable balance dysfunction and their associated modes of retraining. Results, however, from the Farmington-FICSIT (Frailty and Injuries: Cooperative Studies of Intervention Techniques)[8] trial using elderly community dwellers of above-average health suggest that the type of balance improvement that is seen after training substantially mirrors the kind of training that is experienced. Three months of intensive (3×/week, 45–90 min/session) exposure to a balance-challenge package composed primarily of training in limits of stability, decreased bipedal base (tandem), one-legged stance, surface instabilities (foam), and aberrant visual input (eyes closed), led to measurable increases in maximal limits of stability, one-legged standing time, narrowed bipedal stance time, and decreased falling on an unstable surface (eyes open or closed). Thus, a training emphasis on five categories of the BCDs (see Tables 63–1 and 63–2) resulted in significant gains in the equivalent areas of performance. Categories in which there was no training such as fast walking and vertical body movements yielded no improvement on testing — that is, no increase in usual gait velocity or shortening of sit-to-stand time. Although the group undergoing lower extremity strength training alone improved significantly in strength, there was minimal carryover to any of the balance measures. It is possible, however, that in frailer and weaker individuals, some measures of balance might have increased from resistance training or from the indirect strengthening effects of a walking program.[20, 21]

As indicated earlier, tai chi encompasses a wide range of intermingled balance challenges. Studies in which tai chi has been used as a primary technique for balance enhancement in the elderly have yet to include multicomponent balance outcome measures in their test batteries. There are some early indications, however, that the effects of tai chi training may well generalize to multiple areas of balance performance. After the intense 3-month training period, the Farmington-FICSIT study used only low-intensity tai chi (once a week for 6 months) as a means of trying to maintain the balance and strength gains developed in the course of

prior high-intensity training (see above paragraph).[8] Nonetheless, after 6 months, this relatively low training dosage prevented the otherwise expected declines in one-legged stance time, unstable surface tolerance, and lower extremity strength[8] and significantly reduced the rate of falling in subjects who had received intensive 3-month balance or strength training prior to tai chi.[22] Interestingly, tai chi was unable to stem the loss of previous improvements in limits of stability. In retrospect, this finding could have been predicted, given that the variant of tai chi that was taught did not challenge subjects to lean to the maximal limits of stability.

Granted, these interventions took place outside the standard medical model which has its managed-care limits and its requisite reimbursement and regulatory issues. For example, Medicare limits on reimbursement, length, and duration of treatment ($1500 per calendar year, starting in 1999, for therapists in independent practice; no reimbursement for treatment longer than 1 hour; a frequency of fewer than three times weekly is not considered rehabilitative; and duration is usually shorter than 6 months) may not permit interventions identical to those described in the Farmington-FICSIT study. Nevertheless, data from these studies may be supportive of the practitioner's deciding to treat a patient for longer than 60 minutes or only once weekly. Furthermore, as noted above, instructor-led groups are valuable after discharge from medical therapeutic intervention.

CONCLUSION

It is now clear that good overall balance presumes competencies in a variety of balance categories. It is possible that some of these components can be responsive to training when specifically targeted (e.g., limits of stability, gait speed). Others may be more efficaciously influenced indirectly (e.g., the finding that one-legged stance time improved as a result of sensory organization training).[12] A third possibility is that techniques (e.g., tai chi, Feldenkrais, gaze control) that enhance the development of body or spatial awareness can integrate and "jump start" some of the intact, lower-order balance circuitries on the cortical level, leading to a generalized improvement in multiple balance components.

A related, more holistic prospect—again exemplified by tai chi—would be that multiple balance skills might be best learned through a systematized integration of a specific "package" of challenges to balance. The package could be held together (unified) by higher-order physiological "strings" such as body imagery, axial segmental control (principles of turning), slowness of movement, and the adoption of a pelvic spatial frame of reference.[23] Even if credible, such a scheme has its limitations. Despite its ability to reduce the incidence of falls, the Atlanta-FICSIT trial had no effect on resistance to perturbations,[18] and tai chi training in the Farmington-FICSIT study could not prevent the decay of previously acquired limits of stability skill.[8]

In the final analysis, all of these hypotheses are likely to be influenced by an individual's unique pattern of degenerative neural changes. At this time, prudence would dictate that we not limit our choice to *either* a diversified, multicomponent *or* a holistic, integrated strategy but, rather, that we choose a combination of *both* the diversified *and* the holistic approaches.

REFERENCES

1. Longstreth WT, Manolio TA, Arnold A, et al. Clinical correlates of white matter findings on cranial magnetic resonance imaging of 3301 elderly people. *Stroke* 1996; 27:1274–1282.
2. Kaye JA, Oken BS, Howieson J, Holm LA, Dennison, K. Neurologic evaluation of the optimally healthy oldest old. *Arch Neurol* 1994; 51:1205–1211.
3. Oken BS, Kaye, JA. Electrophysiologic function in the healthy, extremely old. *Neurology* 1992; 42:519–526.
4. Berg K, Wood-Dauphinee SL, Williams JI, Gayton D. Measuring balance in the elderly: preliminary development of an instrument. *Physioth Canada* 1989; 41:304–311.
5. Tinetti ME. Performance-oriented assessment of mobility problems in elderly patients. *J Am Geriatr Soc* 1986; 34:119–126.
6. Whipple RH. Improving balance in older adults: identifying the significant training stimuli. In: Masden JC, Sudarsky L, Wolfson L, eds. *Gait Disorders of Aging: Falls and Therapeutic Strategies.* Philadelphia: Lippincott-Raven; 1997: 355–379.
7. Tinetti ME, Baker DI, McAvay G, et al. A multifactorial intervention to reduce the risk of falling among elderly people living in the community. *N Engl J Med* 1994; 13:821–827.
8. Wolfson L, Whipple R, Derby C, et al. Balance and strength training in older adults: intervention gains and tai chi maintenance. *J Am Geriatr Soc* 1996; 44:498–506.
9. Kauz H. *Tai Chi Handbook: Exercise, Meditation and Self-defense.* New York: Doubleday; 1974.
10. Masters R, Houston J. Listening to the body: the psychophysical way to health and awareness. New York: Dell; 1978.
11. Herdman SJ. *Vestibular Rehabilitation.* Philadelphia: F.A. Davis; 1994.
12. Hu MH, Woollascott MH. Multisensory training of standing balance in older adults: 1. Postural stability and one-leg stance balance. *J Gerontol* 1994; M52–M61.
13. Topper AK, Maki, BE, Holliday PJ. Area actively-based assessments of balance and gait in the elderly predictive of risk of falling and/or type of fall? *J Am Geriatr Soc* 1993; 41:479-487.
14. Shumway-Cook A, Horak F. Assessing the influence of sensory interaction on balance. *Phys Ther* 1986; 66:1548–1550.
15. Alexander FM. The resurrection of the body: the essential writings of F. Matthias Alexander selected and introduced by Edward Maisel. New York: Dell Publishing; 1974.
16. Wolfson L, Whipple R, Amerman P, Kleinberg A. Stressing the postural response: a quantitative method for testing balance. *J Am Geriatr Soc* 1986; 34:845–850.
17. Denham T. Personal communication. Vestibular Unit, Rusk Institute of Rehabilitation Medicine, New York University, 1997.
18. Wolf SL, Barnhart HX, Kutner NG, McNeely E, Coogler C, Xu T. Reducing frailty and falls in older persons: an investigation of tai chi and computerized balance training. *J Am Geriatr Soc* 1996; 44:489–497.
19. Schaie KW. The course of adult intellectual development. *Am Psychol* 1994; 49:3–313.
20. Buchner DM, Larson EB, Wagner EH, Koepsell TD, DeLateur BJ. Evidence for a non-linear relationship between leg strength and gait speed. *Age Ageing* 1996;25: 386–391.
21. Buchner DM, Cress ME, DeLateur BJ, et al. A comparison of the effects of three types of endurance training on balance and other fall risk factors in older adults. *Aging-Clin & Exper Res* 1997;9:112–119.
22. Whipple RH. The effects of low intensity tai chi training on falls. Manuscript in preparation.
23. Mouchnino L, Aurenty R. Massion J, Pedotti A. Coordination between equilibrium and head-trunk orientation during leg movement: a new strategy built up by training. *J Neurophysiol* 1992; 67:1587–1598.

Chapter **64**

Fracture Considerations

Rosanne Lewis, M.S., P.T., G.C.S.
Timothy L. Kauffman, Ph.D., P.T.

INTRODUCTION

The fracture of a bone has a profound impact on any member of the the aging population, as the consequences may negatively impact on independence and can even lead to death. It is projected that by the year 2000 there will be 340,000 hip fractures per year in the United States. Vertebral compression fractures are more common but more difficult to diagnose because they are not always associated with trauma. Approximately one out of six vertebral fractures is found incidentally which suggests a gradual and possibly progressive onset with almost no symptoms.

A bone fractures when a force or stress is placed upon it that is greater than the bone can withstand. Bone has a tensile strength of approximately 140 MPa (mcgapascals; one MPa equals 145 pounds per square inch) in the second decade of life and it decreases to approximately 120 MPa by the eighth decade of life. The fracture threshold for the vertebrae and the femur is bone density of less than 1 gram per cubic centimeter.

NORMAL FRACTURE HEALING

Normal fracture healing can be divided into three overlapping phases. First, there is an immediate inflammatory phase in which there is bleeding resulting from the injury to the bone and surrounding soft tissue, and a hematoma forms (Fig. 64–1A). The bone cells at the fracture line die. The reparative, or proliferative, phase starts shortly after the injury, usually 24 to 48 hours if a good local blood supply to the fracture exists (Fig. 64–1B). Good reduction and immobilization of the fracture also help the bone during the reparative phase. Osteogenic cell proliferation lifts the fibrous layer of the periosteum from the bone and, somewhat more slowly, the osteogenic cells of the bone marrow cavity also proliferate (Fig. 64–1C). This proliferation gradually forms a collar, or callus, around the fracture line, which usually takes place in 2 to 4 weeks, but radiographic evidence of external callus formation may not appear until 3 to 6 weeks. A bone scan usually reveals increased metabolic activity shortly after the fracture and before the callus can be seen on an x-ray.

The remodeling phase starts during proliferation as the osteogenic cells begin to differentiate into osteoblasts, which start to form bony trabeculae that bridge the living and dead bone across the fracture line (Fig. 64–1D). Some of the osteogenic cells differentiate into chondrocytes and form cartilage in the fracture callus which eventually calcifies, becoming bone. Osteoclasts gradually remove the necrotic bone at the fracture site. The callus, consisting mostly of cancellous bone that has now formed across the fracture site, is fusiform. The cancellous bone is slowly remodeled into compact bone and finally, the original fracture line is no longer discernable.

FRACTURE REPAIR IN THE AGING PERSON

The rate of fracture repair in the aging patient should always be considered to be similar to that of a younger person—that is, early callous formation in 2 to 4 weeks and bony bridging over the fracture in 6 weeks, as shown on x-rays. However, a host of factors may impede this normal progression. First, osteoporotic bone may not heal as well as bone with normal tissue density. The inflammatory response to the injury and the blood supply may be inadequate. Failure to immobilize the fracture site also delays the healing process. The role of morphogenetic proteins and growth factors in fracture healing in aging patients is unclear, but adequate nutrition is crucial. Overall health or frailty as well as cognition can delay the healing process as well.

In the case of open reduction and internal fixation of a fracture, there is greater risk of further bone injury, called a stress riser, due to the orthopedic hardware. The use of screws and plates may weaken or pull out from bone that is already osteopenic.

SPECIAL FRACTURES IN THE ELDERLY

Not all fractures in the elderly are considered to be complete fractures. Stress fractures, also referred to as insufficiency fractures, occur in areas of repeated trauma when the bone remodeling is insufficient to repair the stresses of repetitive loading. This is particularly likely to occur in a patient who has been in a nonweight-bearing circumstance and in a person who has been fitted with a new orthotic device. The sedentary elderly are at risk when they start new, strenuous physical activities. Physically, these patients will present with pain, swelling, and warmth. Stress fractures or pseudofractures may arise in bone that has faulty mineralization which results in the subsequent inadequate repair of microtraumas.

Microfractures of the bony trabeculae have been demonstrated. The proclivity of these microfractures to cause pain is unclear. However, they may progress and lead to the silent fractures that are recognized on x-ray but may be old fractures. Despite the x-ray evidence of fracture, a patient can be unaware of having experienced any frank trauma; hence the term "silent fracture." This may be one of the causes of the lumbar kyphosis that is seen in some individuals who spend excessive amounts of time sitting.

Occult fractures, also referred to as insufficiency fractures, are best diagnosed with a bone scan or magnetic resonance imaging (MRI). This type of fracture is usually intramedullary and undisplaced and frequently occurs as a result of some minor or major trauma, but x-ray examination is negative. Typically, occult fractures occur in the proximal femur or humerus after a fall but they have also been reported in the sacrum, acetabulum, calcaneus, tibia, and spine. Quickly, these patients present with moderate to severe pain and tenderness. There is a concomitant reduction in range of motion and strength and, if in the femur, there is a marked antalgic gait. In nursing and rehabilitation, this type of fracture should be treated seriously even if it has not been confirmed on initial x-ray. If pushed too aggressively, complete disruption of bone may occur. Protected ambulation with a walker is requisite while the femoral or pelvic occult fracture heals.

A pathological fracture results from primary or metastatic malignant tumors in bone. These types

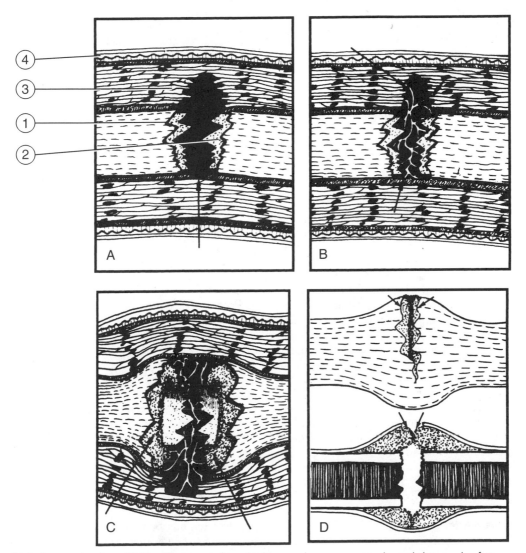

Figure 64–1 Fracture healing. (A) Bleeding occurs from the bone ends, marrow vessels, and damaged soft tissues, with the formation of a fracture hematoma that clots (closed fracture is illustrated). (1, periosteum; 2, haversian systems; 3, muscle; 4, skin) (B) The fracture hematoma is rapidly vascularized by the ingrowth of blood vessels from the surrounding tissues, and for some weeks there is rapid cellular activity. Fibrovascular tissue replaces the clot, collagen fibers are laid down, and mineral salts are deposited. (C) New woven bone is formed beneath the periosteum at the ends of the bone. The cells responsible are derived from the periosteum, which becomes stretched over these collars of new bone. If the blood supply is poor, or if it is disturbed by excessive mobility at the fracture site, cartilage may be formed instead and remain until a better blood supply is established. (D) If the periosteum is incompletely torn, and there is no significant loss of bony apposition, the primary callus response may result in establishing external continuity of the fracture ("bridging external callus"). Cells lying in the outer layer of the periosteum itself proliferate to reconstitute the periosteum. (Reprinted with permission from McRae R. *Practical Fracture Treatment*, 3rd ed. New York: Churchill Livingstone; 1994:19.

of fractures usually present as pain without any reported history of trauma; however, at times, metastatic bone disease is found in a patient who is being x-rayed because of trauma. Significantly, these patients complain of increased pain at night and of being awakened by the pain. The pain frequently increases with bedrest and the severity increases with time. Persons presenting with primary tumors of the breast, prostate, thyroid, kidney, or other organ should be suspected of having metastatic disease if pain complaints fit these descriptions. Standard x-rays are helpful for specific bony sites; however, a bone scan is important for a total skeletal evaluation.

FUTURE METHODS OF PROMOTING FRACTURE HEALING

As stated above, natural fracture repair in the elderly may not proceed in precisely the same pattern as repair proceeds in younger persons. However, several medical and physical methods for enhancing bone repair are being investigated. A number of growth factors have been found that influence fracture repair, including fibroblast growth factor, platelet-derived growth factor, transforming growth factor-β, and bone morphogenic protein. Insulin-like growth factor may stimulate fibroblast proliferation.

Ceramic composites of calcium phosphate have been used for bone grafts. Electrical stimulation and ultrasound at specific parameters are two physical modalities that are currently being used to promote fracture healing. Fracture treatment in the future is likely to involve active intervention to promote healing and thereby reduce morbidity.

THERAPEUTIC INTERVENTIONS

Osteoporosis-related Fractures

Osteoporosis is caused by increased action of cells that absorb bone or decreased action of cells that lay down bone. It affects cancellous (trabecular) bone more than cortical bone. The areas of the human skeleton that are likely to fracture as a result of osteoporosis are the neck of the femur, the vertebral bodies, and the wrist. Compression fracture of a vertebral body is a common occurrence in an individual with osteoporosis, and often it is the first indication that a person has osteoporosis. Estrogen is protective of bone and prevents osteoporosis, whereas long-term steroid use has the effect of weakening the bone and increasing osteoporosis. Weight-bearing exercise has been shown to be protective of bone strength, causing the cells that lay

down bone to be more active. Postmenopausal women in Western culture are at the highest risk. See Chapter 19, "Osteoporosis" and Chapter 61, "Estrogen Replacement Therapy" for further discussion of this subject.

Treatment of a person with an osteoporosis-related fracture consists of promoting healing, preventing deformity, and facilitating the person's return to full functioning. This type of fracture should not be viewed as an isolated event. It is usually the harbinger of future fractures. Thus, prevention of future fractures should be part of the treatment plan. In working with a patient with a compression fracture, the nurse or therapist should carefully screen for any signs of neurological compromise. By definition, compression fractures do not involve the posterior portion of the vertebral body and so do not involve a risk for protrusion of fractured bone into the spinal canal. If neurological signs are present, the client should be referred for studies to determine the presence of burst fracture or fracture dislocation.

Pharmacological Interventions to Promote Healing

An individual with a compression fracture may be given medications that seek to restore bone strength. A postmenopausal woman may be given hormone therapy. Alendronate is a medication that inhibits bone resorption and does not impair bone formation. The nurse or therapist treating a person who is taking Alendronate may assist by ensuring that the medication is being taken correctly. It must be taken on an empty stomach with 8 ounces of water. The individual should be upright after ingestion and should wait 30 minutes before eating. The side effects of gastrointestinal upset may be worsened if these guidelines are not followed. Another medication that inhibits bone resorption is salmon calcitonin which is either injected or used as a nasal spray. It can be given to those who cannot take either of the above medications.

Pain Management

An individual with a spinal compression fracture is likely to have pain with movement and might need instruction in log-rolling (moving with no trunk rotation while rolling). The use of a lumbosacral corset or Jewett brace may prevent extraneous motion and thus minimize pain. Clinical experience indicates that modalities such as heat, cold, and massage are effective in reducing pain, but its return is inevitable. It will, however, decrease with time and should be expected to resolve within a period ranging from 6 weeks to 6 months.

Prevention of Further Injury

Although the effects of a diet change on bone strength will take longer to be seen, the individual who has suffered a fracture may be amenable to changes in diet that will help to prevent future fractures. Referral to a registered dietitian is indicated. Further information about dietary calcium can be found in Chapter 19, "Osteoporosis."

All measures possible should be taken to prevent additional fractures and, above all, to avoid falling. The person's environment should be inspected for hazards that could cause a fall and they should be removed. A gradual resumption of mobility is necessary to prevent other medical complications such as pneumonia. Indeed, the person should be encouraged to slowly increase his or her participation in the activities of daily living. At that point, useful instruction would include a demonstration of how to perform activities without flexing the trunk. Sitting and forward flexion have been shown to increase intervertebral disk pressure, so these postures are to be avoided. As the individual begins to tolerate sitting, the use of a lumbar support will help to achieve some measure of lordosis in the lumbar spine. A person with a spinal compression fracture may be given a walker to assist in ambulation, but a four-legged, or pick-up, walker can place strain on the back because the individual must lean forward slightly to reach it, and then must lift it, which puts a great deal of pressure on the intervertebral disks and vertebral bodies. A walker with front wheels does not completely solve this problem, as the individual still has to lift the walker for turns and for backing up.

Clinical experience shows an individual with a history of compression fractures remains in a forward-flexed posture as a consequence of using a walker. The neurological system, particularly the vestibular system, learns that the "normal" walking posture involves a forward-flexed trunk. Skeletal muscle lengths may change, too, and contribute further to this new "normal" posture. The person never experiences a truly upright posture and loses control of posterior sway, becoming fearful of standing up straight. One means of preventing this problem is to have the individual work on exploring his or her limits of posterior stability while standing in a place perceived of as providing protection from a backwards fall. The most useful exercise is wall slides, in which the person stands with his or her back to a wall, hands lightly on the walker, and moves up and down and side to side. Progress can

be made toward requiring less and less support from the wall and from the walker.

Prevention of Further Deformity

During rehabilitation after a spinal compression fracture, it is vital to strengthen muscles that have become weak from disuse. Particular attention should be paid to exercises that encourage extension and upright posture. Of course, consideration must be given, during exercise programs, to restoring the length of tightened muscles and concurrently developing strength in them to provide the necessary stability. It is well documented that contracted muscles require strengthening exercises after they have been stretched, or weakness and instability will prevail in that area.

Water exercises can be done, as the buoyancy of water provides a comfortable, gravity-free environment, but the client must eventually transition to a land-based program in order to develop strength and polish the skills necessary to live in a gravitational environment.

Various studies that have investigated methods of improving bone mineral density (BMD) have shown that weight-bearing exercises improve BMD in the lower extremities and the spine, and weight-training exercises, which include upper and lower extremity resisted exercises, improve BMD in the upper extremities as well as in the spine and lower extremities.

Exercises should be instituted even with people who are not ambulatory because of the positive effects exercise has on bones. For individuals who are attempting to regain mobility after an episode of bedrest necessitated by an osteoporotic fracture, balance exercises that address the individual's specific impairments and unique needs are necessary. Some generic exercises are included in Box 64–1. They are helpful as general exercises for middle-aged and older persons, but it is important to remember the necessity of tailoring an exercise routine to the idiosyncrasies of the individual.

CONCLUSION

Fractures are major problems for aging persons, and in the great majority of cases, rehabilitation is a necessary follow-up. Understanding normal fracture healing and the possible factors that alter it will assist in the provision of optimal care. The special fractures such as the occult and insufficiency fractures and metastatic lesions are requisite considerations in geriatric rehabilitation. Proper therapeutic exercise, balance and gait training, pain control, and

Box 64–1

Exercises for Persons 55 Years Old and Older

These exercises are to be gradually increased. Work at your own pace and level of ability. Start with 5 or 10 repetitions and do fewer if you must or more if you can. Slowly increase by adding 2 to 4 or more repetitions every 5 to 10 days. Progress until you can do approximately 15 to 25 repetitions of each exercise. Do these exercises at least three times a week.

1. High Step
   Hold on to a chair for balance; stand up straight. Raise one foot off the floor so that your knee is as high as your hip. Reverse legs. Try not to lean on the chair too much. As you get stronger, you may be able to raise your leg higher, hold for a count of 5 (less if necessary), and decrease the amount of leaning on the chair.
   Purpose: To increase hip and leg strength and balance

2. Side Step
   Hold on to a chair for balance; stand up straight. Move one leg out to your side and hold it in the air. Don't bend at the waist. Hold leg up for 5 seconds, or less if necessary. Reverse legs. At first, you may be unable to hold your leg in the air. If so, simply move your foot out to the side.
   Purpose: To increase hip and leg strength and balance

3. Stand Up-Sit Down
   This is the key to being independent. Simply stand up, then sit down. To do this, you must get your feet under the front of the chair. Move your center of gravity forward and then up. If necessary, use the chair's arm rest. As you get stronger, decrease the amount of push that you need from your arms.
   Purpose: To improve strength, balance, coordination, and joint motion

4. Shoulder Shrug
   Sit up or stand up straight. Shrug your shoulders up high and release. Pull your shoulders back. You should feel your shoulder blades pull together.
   Purpose: To strengthen back, stretch chest muscles, and improve posture

5. Cervical Range of Motion
   Sit up or stand up, head erect but not forward. Turn your chin to your left shoulder, then reverse to the right. Lean your ear to your left shoulder, then reverse to the right. Lightly place your finger on your chin and push your chin back. *Do not* roll your head back as if looking up at the ceiling.
   Purpose: To improve posture, balance, and range of motion

6. Walk, Walk, Walk
   Walk at whatever level of ability you have. If you can walk only 50 feet, start at that level and try to increase the distance and improve your gait speed. Avoid stops and starts. If you are walking longer distances, such as a half mile or longer in 5 to 10 minutes, do a little stretching before starting. When finishing your walk, cool down by simply walking slowly, stretching, and doing a few of these exercises or your favorite ones.
   Purpose: To enhance overall health of muscles, bones, joints, circulation, heart, lungs, digestion, bowels, and mind
   If you need help getting started or if you have any concerns about your health, show these exercises to your physician.

prevention of further injury facilitate rehabilitation and enable the patient to attain as high a quality of life as is possible.

SUGGESTED READINGS

Buckwalter J, Glimcher M, Cooper R, Pritchard D. Bone Biology II: Formation, form, modeling, remodeling and regulation of cell function. In: Pritchard D, ed. *Instructional Course Lectures,* Vol. 45. Rosemont, IL: American Academy of Orthopaedic Surgeons; 1996:387–395.

Cornell C, Lane J. Newest factors in fracture healing. *Clin Orthop Rel Res* 1992; 277:297–311.

Feldman F, Staron R, Zwass A, Rubin S, Haramati N. MR imaging: Its role in detecting occult fractures. *Skeletal Radiol* 1994; 23:439–444.

Gerhart T. Fractures. In: Adams W, Beers M, Berkow R, Fletcher A, eds. *The Merck Manual of Geriatrics,* 2nd ed. Whitehouse Station, NJ: Merck Research Laboratories; 1995:79–98.

Hayes W, Myers E. Biomechanical considerations of hip and spine fractures in osteoporotic bone. In: Springfield DS, ed. *Instructional Course Lectures,* Vol. 46. Rosemont, IL: American Academy of Orthopedic Surgeons; 1997:431–438.

Koval K, Zuckerman J. Orthopedic challenges in the aging population: Trauma treatment and related clinical issues. In: Springfield, DS ed. *Instructional Course Lectures,* Vol. 46. Rosemont, IL: American Academy of Orthopaedic Surgeons: 1997:423–430.

Melton LJ, Kan S, Frye M, Whaner H, O'Fallon WM, Riggs BL. Epidemiology of vertebral fractures in women. *Am J Epidemiol* 1989; 129:1000–1011.

Chapter **65**

Stiffness

Lynn Phillippi, M.S., P.T.

INTRODUCTION

Stiffness, or loss of extensibility, is a common complaint of the elderly. Stiffness has the potential to limit numerous functional activities in the daily life of an elderly individual, by interfering with the initiation and completion of movement patterns.

In the elderly, the exudation of fibrinogen into the tissue spaces increases, so more fibrin, an elastic filamentous protein, tends to be deposited in the tissue spaces of older persons. If physical activity is not maintained, complete breakdown of fibrin may not occur, and increased amounts of sticky fibrin may accumulate in the tissue spaces, producing adhesions that restrict movement between adjacent structures. Fibrinous adhesions also form in a localized area following damage to the tissues.[1]

In many cases, restoration of normal physical activity is sufficient to cause the breakdown of fibrinous adhesions, but in some cases, when the

mass has become consolidated, it may be necessary for stretching to be applied using passive movements or even manipulation under anesthesia.

COMMON CAUSES OF STIFFNESS

Traditionally, the clinician has considered stiffness to be a natural part of the aging process, perhaps without examining the actual causes, some of which may be prevented. Four common causes of stiffness are:

- Biomechanical changes in connective tissue and related structures
- Hypokinesis
- Arthritis
- Trauma

Biomechanical Changes in Connective Tissue and Related Structures

Numerous characteristics of connective tissue and related structures cause stiffness in the elderly; a select few are highlighted here.

Myofibroblasts

Connective tissue cells that produce unusually large amounts of contractile protein are termed myofibroblasts.[1] When damage occurs to connective tissue there are two stages of response: cells multiply and cells increase secretion. If hyperplasia creates excessive production of actomyosin, the resulting contractile force may be significant enough to prevent normal range of motion in the affected area.

Collagen

Collagen is the main supportive protein in the skin, tendon, bone, cartilage, and connective tissue. A decrease in the elasticity of collagen and in ground substance is associated with the aging process. Also, cross-linking between collagen fibers increases with age, inactivity, and trauma, thereby restricting mobility of the connective tissue. The decrease in ground substance creates a loss of critical interfiber distance which restricts the ability of the fibers to move smoothly over each other. With intervertebral disk disease of the spine, decreased collagen mobility in the annulus and decreased water in the nucleus pulposus may compromise not only spinal mobility, but also spine length, which may impair breathing patterns.[2]

Contractures, frequently the result of tight joint capsules, fibrotic or short muscles, or other scar tissue are part fibrinous adhesions and part collagenous shortening. Newly developed contractures have a greater portion of fibrinous adhesion, whereas chronic contractures are more collagenous. Normal activity may break down fibrinous adhesions, but collagenous shortening often requires heat, prolonged stretching, and possibly surgical intervention (see Chapter 17).

Hyaluronic Acid

Hyaluronic acid is secreted from the hyaline cartilage which covers the surface of synovial joints. Compression of the joint enhances this secretion which entraps the synovial fluid among the hyaluronic acid molecules and lubricates the joint during movement. Secretion of hyaluronic acid decreases with age, thus causing a diminution in the effectiveness of joint lubrication.[1]

Cartilage

Cartilage, having no direct blood supply of its own, receives its nutrients from the blood flow in adjacent bones and the synovial fluid in the joint cavity. Chondroblasts secrete the glycoprotein chondroitin sulfate into the surrounding matrix and, through osmosis, attract water containing dissolved gases, inorganic salts, and other organic materials necessary for normal cartilage cell metabolism. Dehydration occurs with increasing age because the secretion of chondroitin sulfate decreases.[1]

Normal loading and unloading of cartilage is necessary for movement of materials in and out of chondrocytes. Without compression, metabolites remain in the matrix and oxygen content is lowered, which causes a reduction of glycoprotein secretion and an increase in the collagen precursor, procollagen. This process may convert hyaline cartilage to fibrocartilage. After degeneration of the cartilage occurs, it is not reversible. However, further changes can be avoided through regular activities that promote alternating compression and relaxation of the joint.

Hypokinesis

Too little or less than normal movement is termed hypokinesis. Any joint or muscle that is put in its lengthened or shortened state for a long period of time develops collagenous adhesions. To avoid these adhesions, physical activity several times during the day must be encouraged.

Arthritis

Osteoarthritis and systemic and rheumatic arthalgias are common causes of decreased flexibility, or stiffness, in the elderly individual; usually they are found in the knees, hips, and distal interphalangeal joints. These complaints may be attributed to acute synovitis, minute fragments of articular cartilage in the synovial fluid, inability of the joints to glide smoothly, muscle spasms, osteophytes at the joint margins, stretching of the periosteum, or muscle weakness secondary to disuse.

Polymyalgia rheumatica, a systemic arthritis, is a syndrome that occurs in older individuals. It is characterized by pain, weakness, and stiffness in proximal muscle groups, along with swelling, fever, malaise, weight loss, and a very rapid increase in the erythrocyte sedimentation rate. Most commonly affected are the neck, back, pelvis, and shoulder girdle. Corticosteroid therapy is effective in the acute phase. However, following this phase, soft-tissue mobilization along with strengthening exercises can be helpful.[2]

Trauma

Trauma caused by a significant external force, a repetitive internal or external microtrauma, or surgery can produce long-standing soft-tissue changes and scarring.[3]

It is important to focus on how a particular trauma has affected the functional abilities of an elderly person. For example, have the biomechanics of an individual gait pattern been altered by trauma to the pelvic girdle? Decreased mobility of the pelvic girdle may limit the ability of the individual to propel the lower extremity during gait, to shift weight equally, to perform effective arm swing, and to maintain head, neck, and trunk in alignment.

CONNECTIVE TISSUE AND STRETCHING TECHNIQUES

The unique qualities of deformation of connective tissues are referred to as viscoelastic ("viscous" refers to a permanent deformation characteristic and "elastic" to a temporary deformation characteristic). The explanation of Cantu and Grodin (1992) is as follows:

The elastic component of connective tissue represents the temporary change in length when subjected to stretch (spring portion of model). The elastic component has a poststretch recoil in which all the length or extensibility gained during stretch or mobilization is lost over a short period of time (Fig. 65–1). . . . The elastic component is not well understood but is believed to be the "slack" taken out of connective tissue fibers.

The viscous (or plastic) component represents the permanent deformation characteristic of connective tissue.

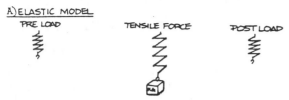

Figure 65–1 Schematic representation of the viscoelastic model of elongation—an elastic component in which no permanent elongation occurs after application of tensile force. (Reprinted with permission from Cantu RJ, Grodin AJ. Histology and biomechanics of myofascia. In: Grodin AJ, Cantu RJ, eds. *Myofascial Manipulation: Theory and Clinical Application.* Gaithersburg, Md.: Aspen Publishers; 1992:31.

After stretch or mobilization, part of the length or extensibility gained remains even after a period of time (hydraulic cylinder portion of the model). There is no postmobilization recoil or hysterasis in this component (Fig. 65–2).

If force is applied intermittently, as in progressive stretching, a progressive elongation may be achieved. In Figure 65–3A, strain or percent of elongation is plotted against time for the purposes of illustrating this phenomenon. . . . If the stress is reapplied to the tissue, the curve looks identical, but starts from a new length (Fig. 65–3B). . . . With each progressive stretch, the tissue has some gain in total length that is considered permanent.[4]

In the clinical setting, the above description of elastic versus viscous deformation is evidenced by range of motion that is measured before treatment, immediately after treatment, and 1 to 2 days later when the patient returns for subsequent treatment. Although the patient may demonstrate an increase in range of motion (the viscous portion) after treatment, part of that increased range may be lost from the elastic portion of the connective tissue by the time the patient returns for a subsequent treatment. Repeated treatments along with an effective home exercise program should result in overall increase in range of motion and improved function.

Connective tissue, like bone, responds to Wolff's law and adapts in the direction in which stress is applied. Since the half-life of collagen is 300 to 500 days (see Cantu and Grodin[4]), newly synthesized collagen will be laid down in the direction of the stress applied. Therefore, it is critical to focus on effective home exercise programs that enhance optimal postural and movement retraining.

An important factor to consider when stretching the connective tissue of the elderly is that the tissue responds optimally to slow and prolonged stretching. The elderly individual requires a longer time to loosen the connective tissue because of changes in biomechanical properties such as decreased ground substance and collagen flexibility. Heating modalities that produce tissue temperatures in the 42.5° to 45.0°C range in conjunction with prolonged stretching have been shown to produce a residual lengthening of tendon. Collagen fibers have to be heated to 42.5°C or above and have continuous force applied to them for at least 30 minutes. Ultrasound (at 1 MHz with an intensity of 1.0 watts/cm^2 for 10 minutes) may be used to raise temperature.[5]

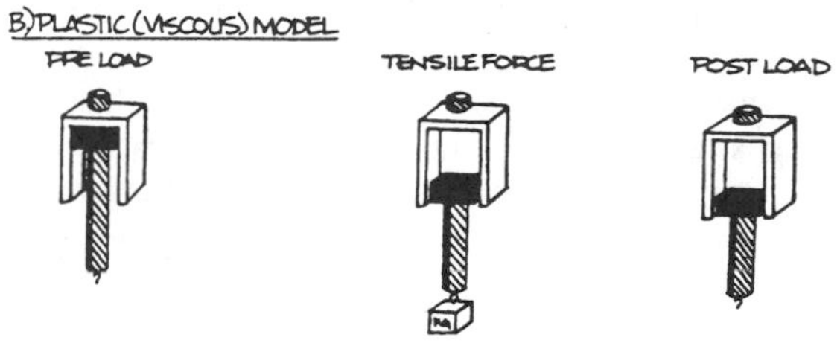

POSTURE, STIFFNESS, AND MOBILITY

A common and often preventable postural change in the elderly is the forward-flexed posture. This posture exhibits varying degrees of forward-thrust head and shoulders, decreased chest and rib cage mobility, increased kyphosis, elevation of the first rib, decreased flexibility of hips and knees, and a shift in the center of gravity. Functionally, the individual has greater difficulty in performing sit-to-stand motions, walking on uneven surfaces, turning, walking backwards, and performing abrupt starts and stops. As posture changes over time, collagenous adhesions increase, with resultant joint structural deformities. Table 65–1 highlights areas where the elderly commonly report stiffness and discomfort that limit functional activities and movements.

Pelvic Mobility

Pelvic anterior/posterior tilts and diagonal motions should be assessed with the patient side-lying, sitting, and standing. If restrictions exist, identify the tissues involved and perform soft-tissue mobilization and stretching techniques. Muscles commonly involved are the psoas major, the quadratus lumborum, and the paraspinals. At the same time the therapist is releasing the restriction, the patient can be performing an active movement such as the pelvic tilt, which may assist the release. As in all the following examples, it is important to educate the patient about how to improve movement pat-

Figure 65–2 Schematic representation of the viscoelastic model of elongation—a plastic component in which deformation remains after the application of tensile force. (Reprinted with permission from Cantu RJ, Grodin AJ. Histology and biomechanics of myofascia. In: Grodin AJ, Cantu RJ, eds. *Myofascial Manipulation: Theory and Clinical Application.* Gaithersburg, Md.: Aspen Publishers; 1992:32.

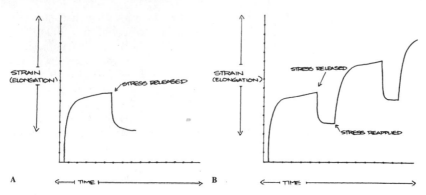

Figure 65–3 (A) Elongation of connective tissue (strain) plotted against time. (B) Repeated elongations of connective tissue (strain) plotted against time. (Reprinted with permission from Cantu RJ, Grodin AJ. Histology and biomechanics of myofascia. In: Grodin AJ, Cantu RJ, eds. *Myofascial Manipulation: Theory and Clinical Application.* Gaithersburg, Md.: Aspen Publishers; 1992:33.

terns and to formulate an individualized home exercise program.

Trunk Mobility

Assess the patient's trunk mobility in supine, sidelying, sitting, and standing positions. Identify any restrictions in the abdominal muscles, such as the rectus abdominis or the lumbar extensors, and combine various trunk motions performed actively by the patient with soft-tissue release to the areas.

Hip Mobility

Assess the patient in all of the above positions with the patient performing the hip motions actively as much as possible. Pay particular attention to restric-

tions in the gluteal muscles, the rectus portion of the quadriceps, the hip adductors, the tensor fasciae latae, and the iliotibial band.

Knee Mobility

Assess the knee in the positions described above, focusing on the quadriceps, hamstring, and gastrocnemius muscles, as well as the mobility and tracking of the patellae. The knee, hip, and ankle should be assessed in isolation as well as in combination, including the trunk and pelvis, because areas of stiffness may involve muscles and connective tissues that cross over two joints.

Ankle Mobility

In addition to assessing motions of the ankle, observe the position of the foot (pronation/supination) and restrictions in the talus/calcaneus and other bones of the foot, particularly in the standing position.

Shoulder Mobility

Assess the shoulder in all the described positions, noting restrictions in the pectoralis major and minor, the rotator cuff muscles, the long head of the triceps, and the latissimus dorsi. Scapular/humeral and scapular/thoracic motions should be evaluated along with motions in the rib cage, sternum, and clavicles.

Head and Neck Mobility

Assess all neck motions and identify restrictions in the scaleni, upper trapezii, levator scapulae, sternocleidomastoids, and paraspinals of the cervical area.

Table 65–1 Areas of Stiffness and Discomfort and the Muscles Involved

Area of Stiffness and Discomfort	Key Muscles Involved
Pelvic girdle and trunk	Psoas, iliacus, quadratus lumborum
Hips	Rectus/hamstrings, internal/external rotators
Knees	Quadriceps, hamstrings
Ankles	Dorsi and plantar flexors, gastrocnemius, soleus, tibialis anterior, plantar fascia
Shoulders	Pectoralis major, pectoralis minor
Rib cage	Intercostals
Neck	Suboccipitals, scaleni

Rib Cage

Identify restrictions in the intercostal muscles, diaphragm, and overall mobility of the rib cage.

Stiffness or loss of flexibility of the thorax in the aging person can be partially reversed through soft-tissue mobilization and stretching techniques, movement reeducation, and specifically designed home programs that focus on further resolving connective tissue restrictions. Great caution and individualized attention must be given to each patient because of the high risk for injury due to osteoarthritis, osteoporosis, and soft-tissue changes, especially skin atrophy. Improvement in posture facilitates other movements such as transfers, bed and mat mobility, ambulation, and other functional activities.

CONCLUSION

Stiffness, a frequent symptom in geriatric patients is caused by a variety of factors and may lead to functional declines in posture and mobility. Some of the factors that contribute to stiffness may be mitigated by proper assessment and appropriate heating modalities, therapeutic exercises, and manual techniques. The technique of slow and prolonged stretching is optimal to increase the length of connective tissues in aging persons.

REFERENCES

1. Pickles B. Biological aspects of aging. In: Jackson O, ed. *Physical Therapy of the Geriatric Patient*. New York: Churchill Livingstone; 1983.
2. Lewis CB. Clinical implications of musculoskeletal changes with age. In: Lewis CB, ed. *Aging: The Health Care Challenge*. Philadelphia: F.A. Davis; 1985.
3. Johnson GS. Soft-tissue mobilization. In: Donatelli RA, Wooden MJ. *Orthopaedic Physical Therapy*, 2nd ed. New York: Churchill Livingstone; 1994.
4. Cantu RI, Grodin AJ. Histology and biomechanics of myofascia. In: Cantu RI, Grodin AJ, eds. *Myofascial Manipulation: Theory and Clinical Application*. Gaithersburg, Md.: Aspen Publishers; 1992.
5. Lehmann JF, Masock AJ, Warren CG, Koblanski JN. Effect of therapeutic temperatures on tendon extensibility. *Arch Phys Med Rehabil* 1970; 51:481.

Chapter **66**

Pain
Ann K. Williams, Ph.D., P.T.

INTRODUCTION

Pain is a major complaint of many patients involved with the health-care system. In fact, people often wait until pain becomes severe or even intolerable before they go to a health-care professional. Pain may be a symptom or a sequela of injury, illness, or surgery. A definition of pain is the perception of an unpleasant sensory and emotional experience associated with actual or potential tissue damage.

The perception and experience of pain are affected by many factors, including the pain's source and the individual's cultural background, previous experiences, and emotions. Therefore, pain threshold and pain tolerance are quite variable among individuals and even within the same individual under varying circumstances. Pain is a common concern of elderly persons, who are more likely than younger people to have both acute and chronic conditions that result in pain. Surgical procedures are more frequently performed on older people. Also, elderly persons are more likely to have various long-term diagnoses that are associated with significant pain, such as osteoarthritis, osteoporosis with spinal fractures, diabetes with peripheral neuropathy, cancer, peripheral vascular disease, and postherpetic neuralgia.

CATEGORIZATION OF PAIN

Pain is categorized in various ways. Acute pain is considered to be pain of recent onset, usually, but not always, with a demonstrable cause. Acute pain may last from minutes to days. Pain lasting longer than 72 hours is sometimes categorized as subacute. Causes of acute pain include recent injury, illness, and surgery.

On the other hand, chronic pain can last for months or years. Definitions of chronic pain vary. A common timeline associated with chronic pain defines it as pain lasting longer than 3 months, though this limit is somewhat arbitrary. Other experts consider as chronic any pain that lasts longer than the expected resolution of the problem; with this definition, the time span of chronic pain is variable.

Pain can be referred to a site distant from its source. Referred pain is common with internal organ damage; for example, problems with the visceral organs such as the kidneys, colon, uterus, and rectum may refer pain to the low back. The anatomical basis for referred pain is thought to be that somatic and visceral tissues are innervated by afferent nerve fibers from the same spinal cord segments. Primary nociceptive pathways overlap and interconnect over several spinal cord segments so that the perception of pain may be in a location other than the site of the actual pathology. Nociceptive input may create hyperexcitability in nerve cells in the spinal cord that can refer pain to related tissues.

Pain can radiate from its source so that a large area may be painful. Some experts speculate that pain radiating over a large area indicates a particularly severe lesion and that the pain will become more localized as healing occurs.

PHYSIOLOGY OF PAIN

The perception of pain begins with the stimulation of primary nociceptors (pain receptors) in the skin or deeper tissues. The two types of nociceptors, A-delta and C fibers, can be stimulated by thermal stimuli, chemical means, or mechanical deformation. The number and type of pain receptors in tissues vary. For example, ligaments and bone periosteum are richly supplied with pain receptors, so injuries to these areas are quite painful. Normal articular cartilage has no pain receptors and can be severely damaged without the occurrence of pain. The visceral pleura also has no pain receptors and disease may be quite widespread in the abdomen while causing little pain. When tissue is damaged, various chemicals such as histamines, prostaglandins, and bradykinins are released; these chemicals not only cause the pain receptors to fire but also make them hypersensitive to further stimulation. Thus, once an injury or tissue damage has occurred, that area is particularly tender and irritable. Ischemia results in tissue damage and subsequently in pain primarily because of these chemical stimulants. Ischemia of nerve cells resulting from blood vessel damage is considered the cause of peripheral neuropathies such as those that occur in persons with diabetes.

The primary pain receptors enter the spinal cord at each nerve root and synapse with other neurons before the pain stimulus ascends to higher centers in the thalamus and midbrain. The strength of the pain stimulus can be modified at the spinal cord level and is the basis for such treatments as transcutaneous electrical nerve stimulation (TENS) and other sensory counterstimulation techniques. Centers in the thalamus, midbrain, and medulla can also modify the perception of pain through various descending inhibitory pathways. The brain and spinal cord also produce endogenous opioids such as enkephalins and endorphins that reduce the perception of pain.

Damage to nerve tissue, either peripheral or central, can result in neurogenic pain. Neurogenic pain is a poorly understood phenomenon; however, some studies indicate that pain in the elderly is more frequently neurogenic and may therefore have a greater perceived intensity.

Experimental studies indicate that in the absence of pathology, there are no age-related differences in pain threshold or pain tolerance. However, these studies should be interpreted cautiously, as experimentally induced pain may have little relationship to the clinical experience of acute and chronic pain. All of these studies were cross-sectional; the change in pain perception over the life span of individuals has not been studied. Also, these studies did not include the oldest old, those over the age of 85, a group that would be expected to have high levels of pathology and pain.

Some research indicates a decrease in the levels of endorphins and enkephalins in the elderly. Certain experts have hypothesized that reduced levels of these endogenous opioids and possible reduced levels of transmitters in pain-inhibitory pathways may result in an increased perception of pain in older persons. If endogenous opioid production is reduced in the elderly, treatments such as TENS would be expected to be less effective. However, clinical research has shown the opposite, and TENS may be effective in treatment of chronic pain problems in the elderly.

Despite the stereotype of the elderly as people who magnify their pain complaints, studies have repeatedly shown that older persons may be less likely to complain of pain, perhaps because they consider pain a normal part of aging. As is true of persons of all ages, complaints of pain may be intensified by depression, anxiety, and loneliness.

PSYCHOSOCIAL ASPECTS OF CHRONIC PAIN

Chronic pain has strong psychological, emotional, and sociological components. Many studies have demonstrated a strong relationship between chronic pain and depression and anxiety for persons of all ages. This relationship between chronic pain and depression is complex, interactive, and poorly understood. The long-term effects of pain on the physical, psychological, and social well-being of an individual are certain to make a person with chronic pain more prone to depression.

Conversely, depressed persons may take longer to recover and this may influence the pain experience. Other factors associated with pain and depression are high levels of physical disability and low levels of social support. Social support networks become stressed by the demands of caring for someone with long-term disability and pain, and depression can make the provision of this care even more difficult. Older persons tend to have smaller social support networks. Lack of key support persons is often the cause of increased use of costly formal support services and even of institutionalization. Most research indicates that age has no effect on the association between chronic pain and depression; however, a few studies show that stoicism and reluctance to acknowledge pain may be part of the chronic pain experience in older persons.

MEASUREMENT OF PAIN

Measurement of pain is critical for the assessment and control of pain. The various components of pain that can be measured include intensity, location, quality, and duration. One of the most common ways of measuring the intensity of pain is a verbal scale in which the patient is asked to indicate her or his level of pain on a scale of 0 to 10, with 0 indicating no pain and 10 indicating the worst possible pain. Visual analogue scales present the measurement of pain intensity on a graphic line on which the patient marks the level of pain. Body diagrams indicate the location of pain complaints, and lists of descriptive words such as those used in the McGill Pain Questionnaire provide an indication of the quality of pain (Fig. 66–1). All of these methods of pain measurement have been successfully utilized in clinical studies with elderly subjects; however, cognitive deficit such as that which occurs in persons with Alzheimer's disease may make the use of complex indices such as the McGill Pain Questionnaire difficult.

THERAPEUTIC INTERVENTION

Pain can be treated with both passive and active modalities. A commonly known passive mechanism for pain relief is medication. The pharmacological treatment of pain is convenient, prevalent, and generally effective with older persons, but care must be taken, as altered drug responses, drug interactions, and adverse drug reactions are well documented in the elderly. Thermal modalities such as heat or cold are other passive means that are often used for the treatment of pain. A warm whirlpool

bath promotes relaxation, increased circulation, and relief of muscle spasm and soreness. The use of cold or icepacks can be helpful with acute pain, especially when swelling is present. Cryotherapy reduces bloodflow to an area, decreases the secretion of pain-causing chemicals, and may serve as a counterirritant to the perception of pain. Research has demonstrated that treatments such as heat and cold are effective in pain reduction in older persons. However, whenever thermal means such as heat or cold are used, great care must be taken to be sure that the patient does not have decreased sensation or circulation; otherwise, tissue damage could occur. Contraindications such as decreased sensation or circulation are common with persons who have diabetes or neurological deficits, both of which increase in frequency in the elderly. Older persons with severe cognitive deficits such as Alzheimer's disease also may not be capable of alerting caregivers to a problem when thermal modalities are used.

As pain perception is heightened by anxiety and stress, any means of relaxation may help reduce pain. Massage is an ancient mechanism for relaxation and pain relief, especially of mild muscle soreness or spasm. Massage provides the benefits of therapeutic touch in addition to the mechanical effects of increased circulation, edema reduction, and loosening of tight tissue. Care should be taken, especially in the very old, to ensure that the skin can tolerate the stress of massage. Relaxation training and visual imagery are practices that also promote relaxation. Studies have indicated that health professionals are less likely to use modalities such as imagery and relaxation training with elderly persons, but there is no indication that these techniques would not be quite successful with older persons in pain.

Positioning or support to relieve stress on an area can help reduce pain. A common means of relieving stress on a painful joint in the lower extremity is with the use of assistive devices. These assistive devices may be a cane or walker or an orthosis such as a soft cervical collar or foot orthosis. Orthoses can also provide support to prevent additional injury. For example, an ankle/foot orthosis may be applied to the lower extremity of a stroke patient to prevent lateral ankle sprains.

More specialized modalities for pain relief such as ultrasound, TENS, electrical stimulation, or joint mobilization may be used by the physical therapist. Ultrasound is a form of mechanical and thermal energy that may promote tissue healing and reduce pain. TENS involves the application of electrical current through electrodes on the skin to inhibit the transmission of nociceptive input. Other forms of

McGill Pain Questionnaire

Patient's Name _____ Date _____ Time _____ am/pm

PRI: S _____ A _____ E _____ M _____ PRI(T) _____ PPI _____
       (1—10)   (11—15)   (16)   (17—20)   (1—20)

1 FLICKERING —
  QUIVERING —
  PULSING —
  THROBBING —
  BEATING —
  POUNDING —

2 JUMPING —
  FLASHING —
  SHOOTING —

3 PRICKING —
  BORING —
  DRILLING —
  STABBING —
  LANCINATING —

4 SHARP —
  CUTTING —
  LACERATING —

5 PINCHING —
  PRESSING —
  GNAWING —
  CRAMPING —
  CRUSHING —

6 TUGGING —
  PULLING —
  WRENCHING —

7 HOT —
  BURNING —
  SCALDING —
  SEARING —

8 TINGLING —
  ITCHY —
  SMARTING —
  STINGING —

9 DULL —
  SORE —
  HURTING —
  ACHING —
  HEAVY —

10 TENDER —
   TAUT —
   RASPING —
   SPLITTING —

11 TIRING —
   EXHAUSTING —

12 SICKENING —
   SUFFOCATING —

13 FEARFUL —
   FRIGHTFUL —
   TERRIFYING —

14 PUNISHING —
   GRUELING —
   CRUEL —
   VICIOUS —
   KILLING —

15 WRETCHED —
   BLINDING —

16 ANNOYING —
   TROUBLESOME —
   MISERABLE —
   INTENSE —
   UNBEARABLE —

17 SPREADING —
   RADIATING —
   PENETRATING —
   PIERCING —

18 TIGHT —
   NUMB —
   DRAWING —
   SQUEEZING —
   TEARING —

19 COOL —
   COLD —
   FREEZING —

20 NAGGING —
   NAUSEATING —
   AGONIZING —
   DREADFUL —
   TORTURING —

PPI
0 NO PAIN
1 MILD —
2 DISCOMFORTING —
3 DISTRESSING —
4 HORRIBLE —
5 EXCRUCIATING —

BRIEF —   RHYTHMIC —   CONTINUOUS —
MOMENTARY —   PERIODIC —   STEADY —
TRANSIENT —   INTERMITTENT —   CONSTANT —

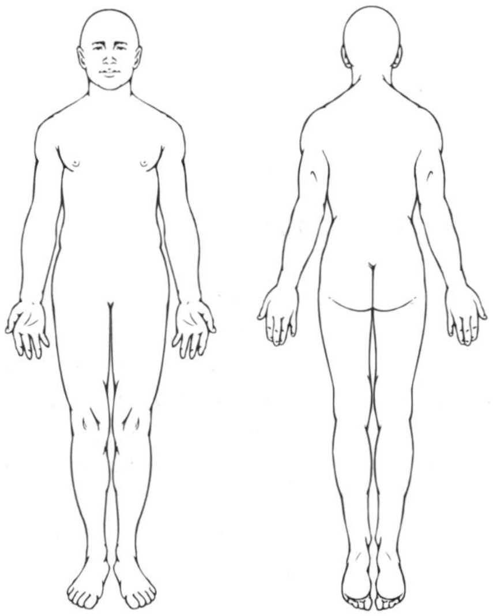

E = EXTERNAL
I = INTERNAL

COMMENTS:

Figure 66-1 McGill Pain Questionnaire. The descriptors fall into four major groups: sensory, 1–10; affective, 11–15; evaluative, 16; and miscellaneous, 17–20. The rank value for each descriptor is based on its position in the word set. The sum of the rank values is the pain rating index (PRI). The present pain intensity (PPI) is based on a scale of 0–5. (Redrawn from Wall PD, Melzack R. *Textbook of Pain*, 3rd ed. London: Churchill Livingstone; 1993:341. From Melzack R. The McGill Pain Questionnaire: Major Properties and Scoring Methods. *Pain* 1975; 1:277–299.)

electrical stimulation may promote relaxation of muscle spasm or act as a counterirritant. Active movement such as range-of-motion activities, gentle exercise, and joint mobilization can decrease stiffness, promote circulation, and relieve pain. Often, recovery from surgery or injury is a difficult balance between rest for healing and motion to prevent stiffness, debilitation, and pain. The healing process results in the deposition of additional collagen and this tissue must be mobilized to prevent loss of function and additional pain. For elderly persons, it is often the case that early but gentle activity is required following injury in order to prevent loss of function that is difficult if not impossible to regain later.

The extremes of pain associated with terminal illnesses such as cancer require special treatments such as large doses of opioid medications or surgical procedures such as neurectomies, cordotomies, or intraventricular morphine pumps. These have been shown to be equally effective in all age groups.

Another important aspect of pain control that is sometimes neglected when dealing with elderly persons is the educational component that results in cognitive understanding and reduction of anxiety. Studies have indicated that elderly persons are more likely than younger persons to perceive that they have received limited information about the causes and consequences of their painful conditions. When given instruction in coping techniques and informed of expected sensations and outcomes, elderly persons are able to reduce pain perceptions.

Special Precautions to Consider with Some Older Persons

While the pain complaints of many acute conditions do not change with age, some conditions, paradoxically, may present with fewer pain complaints in the elderly. For example, a myocardial infarct can be "silent" and occur without significant complaints of chest pain. In the frail elderly, confusion or fatigue can be the signal of illness rather than the more classic symptoms of pain or systemic symptoms.

Older persons with severe cognitive deficits present special problems when it comes to pain management. Studies have indicated that these persons can accurately describe their immediate experience of pain, but memory problems make it difficult to obtain information about the interactions of injury, illness, and pain. Long-term pain management is more complex for these persons.

Pain Management Programs for Elderly Persons

Some chronic painful conditions in elderly persons can create special challenges in pain management. Postherpetic and trigeminal neuralgia pain are difficult to control; TENS has been shown to be especially effective for these conditions. TENS can also be useful for the treatment of peripheral neuropathies in persons with diabetes, whereas methods such as heat are contraindicated because of the circulatory and sensory problems associated with diabetes. Pathological fractures from osteoporosis or cancer occur frequently in older persons. Active or active-assistive exercise despite pain is important for maintaining function and preventing debilitation. Orthotic support, use of assistive devices, and exercise in a hydrotherapy pool combined with pain medication are examples of methods to control pain and promote function for these persons. Spinal stenosis, or narrowing of the spinal canal, can cause severe lower extremity pain and usually occurs in older persons. Some cases require surgery to decompress the spinal structures, but many older persons may not be surgical candidates because of chronic diseases associated with aging. Pain for persons with spinal stenosis may be reduced through positioning to reduce pressure in the spinal canal as well as through the use of modalities to control symptoms. All patients, regardless of age, can present with unique circumstances that require customized plans of care and pain management. Additional special considerations are called for when treating elderly persons.

C O N C L U S I O N

Pain is a significant problem for members of the aging population, even though they may not express concern because they consider it a normal part of aging. Traditional treatments such as medication are effective, but caution is warranted because of changes in pharmacodynamics and pharmacokinetics in older people. Other forms of treatment that may be effective include thermal modalities such as heat and cold, TENS, relaxation and visual imagery, assistive devices, active treatments such as exercise and stretching to reduce stiffness and improve circulation, and education to improve cognitive understanding. Surveys have indicated that despite problems with pain, many elderly persons are able to maintain functional levels of activity.

SUGGESTED READINGS

Barr John O. Conservative pain management of the older patient. In: Guccione AA, ed. *Geriatric Physical Therapy*. St. Louis: C.V. Mosby; 1993: 283–306.

Ferrall BA. Pain management in elderly people. *J Am Geriatr Soc* 1991; 39: 64–73.

Gibson SJ, Katz B, Corran TM, Farrell MJ, Helme RD. Pain in older persons. *Disabil Rehabil* 1994; 16: 127–139.

Harkins SW, Kwentus J, Price DD. Pain and the elderly. In: Benedettic, ed. *Advances in Pain Research and Therapy*, Vol. 7. New York: Raven Press; 1984: 103–121.

Jessell TM, Kelly D. Pain and Analgesia. In: Kandel E, Schwartz JH, Jessell TM. *Principles of Neural Science*. Norwalk, Conn.: Appleton & Lange; 1991: 385–399.

UNIT V

SPECIAL PHYSICAL THERAPEUTIC
INTERVENTION TECHNIQUES

Chapter 67

Gait Training

Patricia Hageman, Ph.D., P.T.

INTRODUCTION

Gait training is one of the most frequently prescribed rehabilitation techniques because gait is the most common of all human movements and, as such, any pathology that affects it requires immediate attention. Rehabilitation therapists must be aware that a healthy geriatric gait includes a wide variety of "normal," yet disruptions in the sequence of actions are easily identified.

Treatments may vary among patients because of individual needs and pathologies, but general geriatric gait training should be directed toward (1) improving lower extremity muscle strength, particularly of ankle plantar- and dorsiflexors, quadriceps, and hip abductors and extensors at a moderate intensity of 70 to 80% of the one-repetition maximum (1-RM); (2) attempting a normal active postural alignment; (3) achieving improvement in weight-shifting and ankle push-off; (4) coordinating lower extremity movements with trunk and upper extremity movements; and (5) providing the most stable gait with the fewest restrictions possible—only those needed for safety and mobility by analysis of the need for assistive devices. Environmental conditions should be assessed and modified where possible, including routes and distances traveled, lighting, uneven or even surfaces, stairs, and safety hazards.

COMPONENTS OF GAIT

Gait training consists of any combination of (1) mobility and transfer activities, (2) pregait mat and standing activities, (3) static and dynamic balance activities, (4) interventions during gait, and (5) adaptation of assistive devices or environment.

Mobility and transfer activities include rising-to-standing and returning-to-sit. High-level activities include floor-to-standing activities.

Pregait exercises are designed primarily to improve trunk and extremity strength and control. Appropriate mat exercises include pelvic tilt movements, hip raising (bridging), trunk twisting, sitting push-ups (latissimus dorsi dips), and hands-and-knees activities including rocking and arm and leg reaching. Pregait standing activities include weight shifting, arm raising, push-ups, toe raising, hip hiking and leg swinging, and a progression of drills from 4-point to swing-to to swing-through. Advanced standing activities include sideways and backwards ambulation. These pregait standing activities may be progressed from using the parallel bars to using an assistive device to free-standing movement.

Static and dynamic balance activities for gait training may be performed in sitting and standing positions. Sitting activities include controlled reaching and leaning within the base of support, with movement side to side, forward, and backwards. Sitting postural control may be challenged by using external disturbances such as a gentle push. Standing balance may be enhanced with the use of weight shifting activities in which the patient is asked to move as far in all directions as he or she is comfortably able to without needing to bend at the hips or take a step. Controlled reaching, lifting, and weight shift activities assist in training for standing balance. The level of difficulty may be increased by performing reaching, lifting, and weight shift activities while standing on high-density foam. Sophisticated computerized force platform systems offer monitoring for various weight shifting and response activities, which in some cases might include responding to a moving floor. The type of shoe worn has been shown to influence balance, with the preferred shoe type being a laced-up hard-soled shoe.

Interventions during gait training include assessment for assistive devices (a cane, crutches, a walker, orthoses), feedback for movement control (manual, electrical stimulation, biofeedback, vi-

Table 67–1 Normal versus Pathological Gait in Elderly

Normal Aging Gait	Pathological Gait
Decreased free and fast velocity, although ability remains to voluntarily increase speed from free to achieve fast gait	Significant decrease in free velocity (<.85 or 1 m/s) with loss in ability to increase speed from frcc to fast gait
Smaller step and stride lengths but symmetrical	Significant decrease in step and stride length and/or nonsymmetrical steps
Mild decrease at push-off; flat foot heel-strike or decreased ankle movement	Significant decrease at push-off or foot slap at heel-strike
Step width 1–4″	Step width >4″
Pelvic rotation 8–12 degrees	Pelvic rotation <8–12 degrees
Small toe clearances	Large toe clearance or tripping or both

Table 67-2 Treatment Techniques for Common Gait Deviations

Observed Deviation	Activity
Difficulty rising-from-sitting	Scoot forward in chair
	Lean forward to rise
	Push from chair
	Adapt chair height/firmness
	Triceps/latissimus dorsi strengthening
	Forward rocking/weight shift in sitting
Leaning backwards in standing	Correct cervical spine position in sitting if patient has adapted to upper cervical extended position
	Visual feedback in standing
	Standing weight shift, one foot in front of the other
	Development of ankle strategy through weight shifting from the ankles
Asymmetrical weight distribution	Weight shift for equal distribution while standing with feet apart or together (forward, sideways, backwards)
	Provide feedback verbally, visually (mirror, computer system), biofeedback, etc.
Flexed standing posture	Reduction of contractures
	Strengthen hip, knee, and ankle extensors
	Feedback for normal posture with emphasis on head position
	If walker is needed, raise height of walker
Foot clearance issues	Parallel bar hip hiking and leg swinging exercises and other weight shift activities
	PNF gait facilitation techniques
	AFO set with dorsiflexion at neutral to 5 degrees
	Electrical stimulation of dorsiflexors
Difficulty with reciprocal swing of legs	Trunk rotation mat exercise
	Sitting and standing trunk twisting
	Parallel bar 4-point gait drills
	PNF facilitation during gait
	Trunk rotation on upper body ergometer (UBE)
	Feedback using footprints on floor
Decreased endurance	Adapt appropriate assistive device to gait pattern that requires less energy (e.g., convert 4-point gait to swing-to-gait pattern) or use wheeled walker vs. regular walker
	Progress tolerance by varying repetitions and distances
	Overall endurance training (UBE, cycling, etc.)
Asymmetrical step lengths	Parallel bar leg swinging
	PNF gait-swing facilitation
	Lower extremity strengthening
Decreased push-off	Plantarflexor strengthening including multiple repetitions of standing toe rising
Decreased balance	Decision making for appropriate assistive device
	Postural control training to include sitting and standing reach, awareness and training of standing limits-of-stability
	Assess footwear; hard-soled, well-fitted, lace-up shoes with thick, absorbant socks are preferred
	Environmental modifications for safety (lighting, clear paths, etc.)

sual), practice of dynamic balance, and progression from performing the standing activities listed above within the parallel bars to performing them outside of the bars. Treatment progression may advance from even surfaces to uneven surfaces, ramps, and stairs. Forward gait training may be progressed to sidestepping, turning, backward stepping, reaching, and carrying objects.

Environmental concerns include assessment of the distances and velocities that have to be covered,

Box 67–1

Components of the Gait Assessment Rating Score (GARS)

A. General Categories
  1. Variability—a measure of inconsistency and arrhythmicity of stepping and of arm movements
    0 = fluid and predictably paced limb movements
    1 = occasional interruptions (changes in velocity), approximately < 25% of time
    2 = unpredictability of rhythm approximately 25–75% of time
    3 = random timing of limb movements
  2. Guardedness—hesitancy, slowness, diminished propulsion, and lack of commitment in stepping and arm swing
    0 = good forward momentum and lack of apprehension in propulsion
    1 = center of gravity of head, arms, and trunk (HAT) projects only slightly in front of push-off, but still good arm-leg coordination
    2 = HAT held over anterior aspect of foot and some moderate loss of smooth reciprocation
    3 = HAT held over rear aspect of stance-phase foot, and great tentativeness in stepping
  3. Weaving—an irregular and wavering line of progression
    0 = straight line of progression on frontal viewing
    1 = a single deviation from straight (line of best fit) line of progression
    2 = two to three deviations from line of progression
    3 = four or more deviations from line of progression
  4. Waddling—a broad-based gait characterized by excessive truncal crossing of the midline and side-bending
    0 = narrow base of support and body held nearly vertical over feet
    1 = slight separation of medial aspects of feet and just perceptible lateral movement of head and trunk
    2 = 3–4" separation of feet and obvious bending of trunk to side so that cog of head lies well over ipsilateral stance foot
    3 = extreme pendular deviations of head and trunk (head passes lateral to ipsilateral stance foot) and further widening of base of support
  5. Staggering—sudden and unexpected laterally directed partial losses of balance
    0 = no losses of balance to side
    1 = a single lurch to side
    2 = two lurches to side
    3 = three or more lurches to side

B. Lower Extremity Categories
  1. % Time in swing—a loss in the percentage of the gait cycle constituting the swing phase
    0 = approximately 3:2 ratio of duration of stance to swing phase
    1 = a 1:1 or slightly less ratio of stance to swing
    2 = markedly prolonged stance phase, but with some obvious swing time remaining
    3 = barely perceptible portion of cycle spent in swing
  2. Foot Contact—the degree to which heel strikes the ground before the forefoot
    0 = very obvious angle of impact of heel on ground
    1 = barely visible contact of heel before forefoot
    2 = entire foot lands flat on ground
    3 = anterior aspect of foot strikes ground before heel
  3. Hip ROM—the degree of loss of hip range of motion seen during a gait cycle
    0 = obvious angulation of thigh backwards during double support (10°)
    1 = just barely visible angulation backwards from vertical
    2 = thigh in line with vertical projection from ground
    3 = thigh angled forward from vertical at maximum posterior excursion
  4. Knee Range of Motion—the degree of loss of knee range of motion seen during a gait cycle
    0 = knee moves from complete extension at heel-strike (and late-stance) to almost 90° (~70°) during swing phase
    1 = slight bend in knee seen at heel-strike, and late-stance and maximal flexion at midswing is closer to 45° than 90°
    2 = knee flexion at late stance more obvious than at heel-strike, very little clearance seen for toe during swing
    3 = toe appears to touch ground during swing, knee flexion appears constant during stance, and knee angle during stance and knee angle during swing appears to be 45° or less.

Box continued on following page

Box 67–1 *Continued*

Components of the Gait Assessment Rating Score (GARS)

C. Trunk, Head, and Upper Extremity Categories
   1. Elbow Extension—a measure of the decrease of elbow range of motion
      0 = large peak-to-peak excursion of forearm (approximately 20 degrees), with distinct maximal flexion at end of anterior trajectory
      1 = 25% decrement of extension during maximal posterior excursion of upper extremity
      2 = almost no change in elbow angle
      3 = no apparent change in elbow angle (held in flexion)
   2. Shoulder Extension—a measure of the decrease of shoulder range of motion
      0 = clearly seen movement of upper arm anterior (15 degrees) and posterior (20 degrees) to vertical axis of trunk
      1 = shoulder flexes slightly anterior to vertical axis
      2 = shoulder comes only to vertical axis, or slightly posterior to it during flexion
      3 = shoulder stays well behind vertical axis during entire excursion
   3. Shoulder Abduction—a measure of pathological increase in shoulder range of motion laterally
      0 = shoulders held almost parallel to trunk
      1 = shoulders held 5–10 degrees to side
      2 = shoulders held 10–20 degrees to side
      3 = shoulders held more than 20 degrees to side
   4. Arm-Heelstrike Synchrony—the extent to which the contralateral movements of an arm and leg are out of phase
      0 = good temporal conjunction of arm and contralateral leg at apex of shoulder and hip excursions all of the time
      1 = arm and leg slightly out of phase 25% of the time
      2 = arm and leg moderately out of phase 25–50% of the time
      3 = little or no temporal coherence of arm and leg
   5. Head Held Forward—a measure of the pathological forward projection of the head relative to the trunk
      0 = ear lobe vertically aligned with shoulder tip
      1 = ear lobe vertical projection falls 1″ anterior to shoulder tip
      2 = ear lobe vertical projection falls 2″ anterior to shoulder tip
      3 = ear lobe vertical projection falls 3″ or more anterior to shoulder tip
   6. Shoulders Held Elevated—the degree to which the scapular girdle is held higher than normal
      0 = tip of shoulder (acromion) markedly below level of chin (1–2″)
      1 = tip of shoulder slightly below level of chin
      2 = tip of shoulder at level of chin
      3 = tip of shoulder above level of chin
   7. Upper Trunk Flexed Forward—a measure of kyphotic involvement of the trunk
      0 = very gentle thoracic convexity, cervical spine flat, or almost flat
      1 = emerging cervical curve, more distant thoracic convexity
      2 = anterior concavity at midchest level apparent
      3 = anterior concavity at midchest level very obvious

Reprinted with permission. Wolfson L et al. Gait assessment in the elderly: a gait abnormality rating scale and its relation to falls. *J Gerontol* 1990; 45:M12–M19. © The Gerontological Society of America.

Box 67–2

Tinetti Assessment Tool

BALANCE TESTS

Initial Instructions: Subject is seated in hard, armless chair. The following maneuvers are tested.

1. Sitting balance

Leans or slides in chair	= 0
Steady, safe	= 1

2. Arising

Unable without help	= 0
Able, uses arms to help	= 1
Able without using arms	= 2

3. Attempts to arise

Unable without help	= 0
Able, requires >1 attempt	= 1
Able to arise, 1 attempt	= 2

4. Immediate standing balance (first 5 seconds)

Unsteady (swaggers, moves feet, trunk sways)	= 0
Steady but uses walker or other support	= 1
Steady without walker or other support	= 2

5. Standing balance

Unsteady	= 0
Steady but wide stance (medial heels > 4″ apart) and uses cane or other support	= 1
Narrow stance without support	= 2

6. Nudged (subject at maximum position with feet as close together as possible, examiner pushes lightly on subject's sternum with palm of hand 3 times)

Begins to fall	= 0
Staggers, grabs, catches self	= 1
Steady	= 2

7. Eyes closed (at maximum position of no. 6)

Unsteady	= 0
Steady	= 1

8. Turning 360 degrees

Discontinuous steps	= 0
Continuous	= 1
Unsteady (grabs, staggers)	= 0
Steady	= 1

9. Sitting down

Unsafe (misjudges distance, falls into chair)	= 0
Uses arms or not a smooth motion	= 1
Safe, smooth motion	= 2

Balance score: _____ /16

Box continued on following page

Box 67–2 *Continued*

Tinetti Assessment Tool

GAIT TESTS

Initial Instructions: Subject stands with examiner, walks down hallway or across room, first at usual pace, then back at "rapid, but safe" pace (using usual walking aids)

10. Initiation of gait (immediately after told to go)

Any hesitancy or multiple attempts to start	= 0	
No hesitancy	= 1	_____

11. Step length and height

a. Right swing foot

Does not pass left stance foot with step	= 0	_____
Passes left stance foot	= 1	
Right foot does not clear floor completely with step	= 0	
Right foot completely clears floor	= 1	_____

b. Left swing foot

Does not pass right stance foot with step	= 0	
Passes right stance foot	= 1	
Left foot does not clear floor completely with step	= 0	
Left foot completely clears floor	= 1	_____

12. Step symmetry

Right and left step lengths not equal (estimate)	= 0	
Right and left step lengths appear equal	= 1	_____

13. Step continuity

Stopping or discontinuity between steps	= 0	
Steps appear continuous	= 1	_____

14. Path (estimated in relation to floor tiles, 12" diameter; observe excursion of one foot over about 10' of the course)

Marked deviation	= 0	
Mild to moderate deviation or uses walking aid	= 1	
Straight without walking aid	= 2	_____

15. Trunk

Marked sway or uses walking aid	= 0	
No sway but flexion of knees or back or spread of arms while walking	= 1	
No sway, no flexion, no use of arms, and no use of walking aid	= 2	_____

16. Walking stance

Heels apart	= 0	
Heels almost touching while walking	= 1	_____

Gait score: _____ /12
Balance + gait score: _____ /28

Reprinted with permission. Tinetti ME. Performance-oriented assessment of mobility problems in elderly patients. *J Am Geriatr Soc* 1986; 34:119–126.

Box 67–3

Functional Ambulation Profile

Name: _____

Static Weight-bearing Capacity

Date							
Bilateral Time							
Left Unilateral Time							
Right Unilateral Time							

Dynamic (in place) Weight Transfer Rate

Date							
Time to complete 4 transfers (8 steps)							

Basic Ambulation Efficiency

Date								
Through // bars Holding on	time							
	steps							
Through // bars Not holding on	time							
	steps							
12 foot distance Outside // bars	time							
	steps							

Comments

_____
_____
_____
_____
_____
_____

Reprinted from *Physical Therapy* with the permission of the American Physical Therapy Association. Nelson AJ. Functional ambulation profile. *Phys Ther* 1974; 54:1059–1064.

Box 67–4

Get-up and Go

Instructions: The patient is instructed to perform the following tasks while a trained observer watches and evaluates. The observer then gives the patient a score based on the following criteria:

1 = normal
2 = very slightly normal
3 = mildly abnormal
4 = moderately abnormal
5 = severely abnormal

Tasks:

Patient is asked to sit comfortably in a chair.
Patient is then asked to rise.
Patient is asked to stand still.
Patient is asked to walk toward a wall.
Before reaching the wall, patient is asked to turn without touching the wall and return to the chair.
Patient is asked to turn around and sit down.

Data from Mathias S, Nayak USL, Isaacs B. Balance in elderly patients: the "Get-up and Go" test. *Arch Phys Med Rehabil* 1986; 67:387.

edition (ICD-9) recognizes the existence of gait abnormalities that have causes that cannot be determined but that produce symptoms that represent important problems in medical care. The ICD-9 codes include code 781.2 Abnormality of Gait, which describes ataxic, paralytic, spastic, or staggering gait patterns. This code may be appropriate to describe the gait conditions for which many elderly people require training.

Many assessment and outcome tools demonstrate high reliability and validity for use in documenting gait training in the elderly population, including the Gait Assessment Rating Scale (GARS), the Tinetti Gait Scale, the Functional Ambulation Profile (FAP), the Get-up-and-go test, and others (see Boxes 67–1 through 67–4).

CONCLUSION

Declining mobility is a common complaint among aging persons, and it is likely to lead to diminutions in the performance of daily living activities and the quality of life. Gait training involves several components of mobility, including transfer, mat, balance, and ambulation activities. Various pathologies may contribute to declining mobility and pathological gait in an elderly person, but significant improvements may be documented by using appropriate assessment tools and proper intervention.

the surfaces traveled, and the safety of paths and transfers at home.

Rehabilitation therapists may expect significant improvements for most geriatric individuals after gait training, although the expectations for rehabilitation should not exceed what would be expected in the normal geriatric population (see Table 67–1).

GAIT DEVIATIONS AND INTERVENTIONS

Many specific pathologies (orthopedic, neurological, biomechanical, cardiopulmonary), may contribute to gait deviations but the elderly client usually presents with multiple problems. Individual pathologies may result in a typical pattern of gait deviation, but many elderly adults have one or more common gait deviations. Some common gait deviations of the elderly and recommended treatment techniques are noted in Table 67–2.

The International Classification of Diseases, 9th

SUGGESTED READINGS

Basmajian JV. Crutch and cane exercises and use. In: Basmajian JV, Wolf SL, eds. *Therapeutic Exercise*. Baltimore: Williams & Wilkins; 1990:125.

Gowland C, Torresin W, VanHullenaar S, Best L. Therapeutic exercise for stroke patients. In: Basmajian JV, Wolf SL, eds. *Therapeutic Exercise*. Baltimore: Williams & Wilkins; 1990:207.

Hageman PA. Gait characteristics of healthy elderly: a literature review. *Issues Aging* 1995; 18:14–18.

Lewis CB, Bottomley JM. *Geriatric Physical Therapy: A Clinical Approach*. Norwalk, Conn.: Appleton & Lange; 1994.

Prince F, Corrieveau H, Hebert R, Winter DA. Gait in the elderly. *Gait Posture* 1997; 5:128–135.

Schmitz T. Preambulation and gait training. In: O'Sullivan SB, Schmitz TJ, eds. *Physical Rehabilitation: Assessment and Treatment*. Philadelphia: F.A. Davis; 1988.

Voss DE, Ionta MK, Myers BJ. *Proprioceptive Neuromuscular Facilitation: Patterns and Techniques,* 3rd ed. Philadelphia: Harper & Row; 1985:259–269.

Woollacott MH, Tang P-F. Balance control during walking in the older adult: research and its implications. *Phys Ther* 1997; 77:646–660.

Chapter 68

Heat and Cold Therapy

Wayne K. McKinley, P.T.

INTRODUCTION

The application of heat and cold modalities, including their use in treating the elderly, is certainly nothing new in rehabilitation medicine. Many have coined these modalities passive therapy. Whether the word "passive" refers to the modality itself, its application, or the patient's role is left up to individual interpretation. The use of heat and cold modalities is, in this author's opinion, not passive therapy; there is a definite use of energy involving changes in temperature and the release of energy. The physical therapy practitioner judiciously using these modalities is certainly using a component of medicine that provides benefits to patients.

HEAT

The use of heat for medical purpose may be traced back to the earliest time when people bathed in the warmth of the sun or lay in the warm sand. The use of hot springs may have coincided with sun

---

Box 68-1

Effects of Heat

1. Increases arteriolar dilatation
2. Increases capillary blood flow
3. Increases metabolism
4. Promotes analgesia
5. Promotes muscle relaxation
6. Enhances collagen extensibility
7. Encourages edema resulting from increased capillary pressure and cell permeability

Systemic Effects

(dependent on area exposed

and time applied)

8. Increases in cardiac output, pulmonary ventilation, body temperature, and pulse rate
9. Increases cerebral oxygen saturation and metabolism

Box 68-2

Benefits Derived from Heat

1. Reduces pain
2. Reduces stiffness
3. Alleviates spasms
4. Increases range of motion
5. Improves tissue healing by increasing blood flow
6. Improves electrical conductivity of skin

---

bathing or may have come later. With scientific inquiry came greater understanding of the effects, reasons for using, and contraindications to using heat, which are enumerated in Boxes 68–1, 68–2, and 68–3. As time has changed technology, so has it changed the ways in which heat can be applied, as is shown in Box 68–4 and described in the following sections.

Heat can be conveyed or transferred in four ways. The first is radiation—"a process by which energy is propagated through space or matter."[1] An example of radiation is the use of the infrared ray. The second is convection—"the transfer of heat by means of current in liquids or gases."[1] The most popular example of convection is the whirlpool. The third method is conduction "the exchange of thermal energy in which there is physical contact between the two surfaces."[1] The most commonly used example of conduction is the hydrocollator, or hot pack. The fourth is evaporation—"the form of heat transfer that dissipates heat from the body."[1] Evaporation occurs not only when the body perspires but also during exhalation, a significant factor that may contribute to dehydration in cold dry climates.

Methods of Applying Heat

Radiant Heat from Luminous and Nonluminous Infrared

Heat lamps and infrared units have been two of the most common ways of applying heat, but in recent years, they have been supplanted by new technology. The luminous, or near infrared, is a lamp that produces visible light within the wave-length range of 770 to 1,500 nanometers. Nonluminous, or far infrared, is a lamp that produces nonvisible radiation in the wave-length range of 1500 to 12,500 nanometers. Infrared can be directed only to an exposed area or surface that is facing the lamp. Output is determined by wattage and the distance from the lamp to the

---

Box 68–3

Contraindications for the Use of Heat

1. Acute inflammatory conditions

2. Existing fever

3. Malignancies (potential metastasis)

4. Active bleeding

5. Cardiac insufficiency (the additional stress on the heart may not be tolerated when generalized heat is used)

6. Treatment of geriatric patients (the frail elderly may have unreliable thermoregulatory systems and may easily develop a fever as a result of generalized heat treatment)

7. Peripheral vascular disease (decreased capacity to meet the increased metabolic demands of heated tissues)

8. Treatment of patients undergoing radiation treatment (their tissues are devitalized and should not be heated)

9. Existing edema (may be increased)

10. Treatment of patients who suffer from sensory loss (they are unreliable judges of heat levels; if use of heat is justifiable, close monitoring is required)

11. Treatment of confused patients (they are unreliable judges of heat levels; if treated with heat at all, extreme caution and close monitoring are required)

---

or some other hydrophilic substance are heated in thermostatically controlled cabinets to temperatures of 160° to 170°F (71.1° to 76.7°C). A pack is applied to the patient after being wrapped in a terry cloth towel, usually of 6 to 8 layers. Lying on top of a hot pack is not recommended, but if this position is best for the patient, extra toweling is needed. The sensation for the patient should be a mild to moderate, comfortable feeling of heat. In all cases, the patient should be checked frequently to guard against overheating or burning. Home-use heating pads that are electronically controlled or microwavable are also available. Length of treatment time is usually 15 to 30 minutes. The elderly patient may not be able to lie prone, so if the lumbar spine is the area to be treated, the patient may be more comfortable sitting in a chair with the heat source placed behind the back. Extra toweling and close monitoring are needed in these cases. Nylatex straps, although popular, present a problem. The extra pressure can cause hot spots, especially over bony prominences.

Patient comfort, not age, appears to be the more important factor in obtaining results from heating, so any comfortable position can be used during the heat application. Peak skin temperature from moist heat application in a clinical environment is reached in 7 to 11 minutes, regardless of the person's age. Significantly, skin temperature may remain elevated for up to 40 minutes or longer, after removal of the moist heat pack.[3]

Diathermy: Shortwave and Microwave

Shortwave diathermy produces heat by converting high frequency electromagnetic energy into heat

surface. The area perpendicular to the lamp is heated more than a surface at an angle.[1, 2]

The advantages of infrared lamps over hot packs are that there is no weight of an object on the patient and that the area being treated is visible during the treatment. But the geriatric patient commonly is bothered by bright lights; thus, the glare from the luminous infrared can be irritating to a patient's eyes. Protection with shaded glasses or goggles or by blocking the light from the face is recommended. A white towel over the area being treated decreases the intensity for the sensitive patient by reflecting back some of the radiation.

Hydrocollator Packs/Hot Packs

Hot packs are used to provide moist heat through the transfer of heat energy by conduction. Chemical packs filled with bentonite, a hydrophilic silicate,

---

Box 68–4

Methods of Heat Application

1. Radiant heat from luminous and nonluminous infrared

2. Hydrocollator packs/hot packs

3. Shortwave diathermy

4. Microwave diathermy

5. Whirlpool

6. Paraffin bath

7. Fluidotherapy

8. Ultrasound

9. Moist towels

---

energy in the patient's tissues. Frequencies vary among manufacturers but are controlled in the United States by the federal government. Available frequencies include 45, 27, and 13 MHz, or megahertz. (The wavelength is the reciprocal of the frequency. The product of frequency × wavelength is equal to a constant—the speed of light, or 300,000 km/sec: f × w = c).[4] The wavelengths are 11 and 22 meters in the United States; a wavelength of 7 meters is available in Europe.

A condenser field or an induction field is utilized by the shortwave diathermy to produce heat. Setting up the condenser field requires airspace, plates, and electrodes. The induction field requires a cable to form a coil around an extremity or flat helix. The drum electrode contains a coil in a plastic housing. Refer to each manufacturer's specifications for proper placement, spacing, and toweling to deliver the proper dosage. Depending on conditions, treatment time is 15 to 30 minutes.

Microwave diathermy is similar in concept to shortwave diathermy, but it uses a much shorter frequency.[4] The wavelength used to produce this heating effect is most commonly 12.2 cm and it has a frequency of 2,450 MHz. The microwave diathermy uses a magnetic oscillator to produce a high-frequency current. This is picked up by a co-axial cable and beamed to the patient by an antenna. This antenna is contained within a reflector. The

two together are called a director. The director is what is placed over the patient to direct the energy to the patient. Once again, each manufacturer's guidelines should be consulted for the proper placement, size of director, spacing, and toweling for proper treatment. The heating effect from the microwave is more concentrated than shortwave diathermy, but it must be remembered that absorption is dependent upon tissue density, with fat, muscle, connective tissue, blood, and bone being different from each other (see Fig. 68–1).

The most notable contraindication to the use of these diathermies is the presence in a patient of a pacemaker or metal implant.[5] The electromagnetic field interferes with the pacemaker's function. Implanted metal becomes hot and can damage surrounding tissue. Also, extreme caution is necessary when treating debilitated patients, as they cannot tolerate strong generalized heating.

Whirlpool

Hydrotherapy is one of the oldest methods of treating physical ailments—Nature provided hot springs for our ancestors. Today, whirlpools are available in many sizes and shapes. Immersion of the full body or just an extremity is possible. Temperatures from 94° to 104°F (36.5° to 40.5°C) are used for heating patients without circulatory problems.

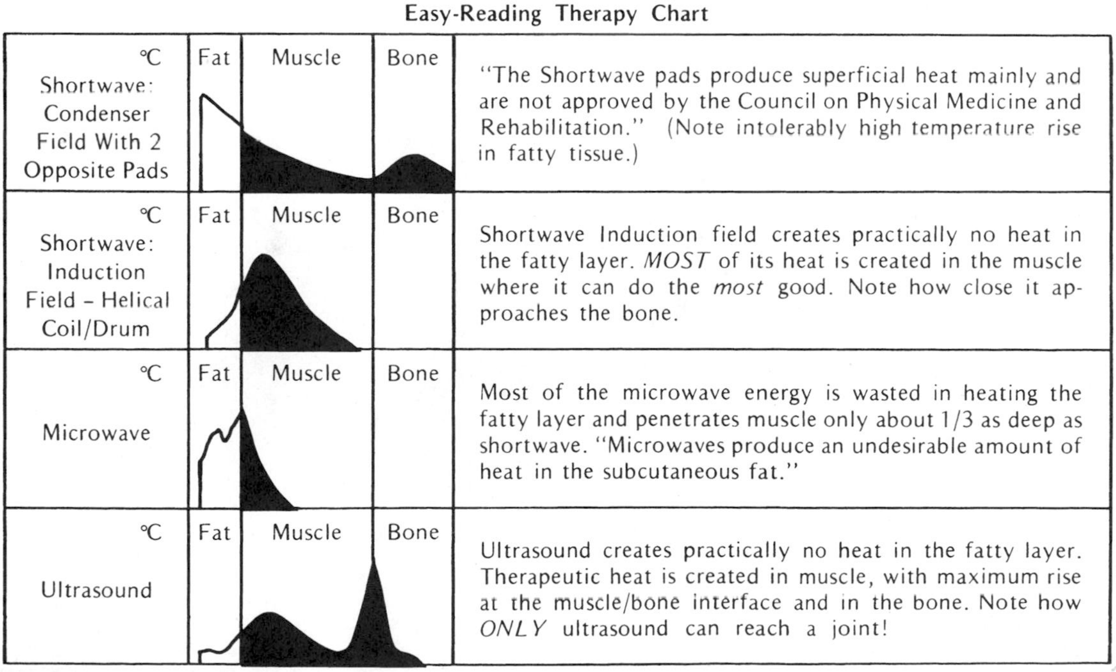

Easy-Reading Therapy Chart

Figure 68–1 Choosing the best heat therapy method. (From Paetzold J. Physical laws regarding the distribution of energy for various high-frequency methods applied in heat therapy. *Ultrasound Med Biol* 1956; 2:58, as modified by Kahn J. *Principles and Practice of Electrotherapy*, 3rd ed. New York: Churchill Livingstone; 1994:7.)

Length of time for immersion is usually 20 minutes. The geriatric patient can usually tolerate whirlpools to the extremities without complications. Greater caution must be exercised with full-body immersion, as faulty thermoregulatory control could easily lead to heat exhaustion or heat stroke.

Paraffin Bath

A paraffin bath is the application of a paraffin wax and mineral oil mix, which is used primarily for heat application to the hands and feet. The temperature of the mix is kept between 118° and 130°F (47.0° and 54.4°C).

Two methods of application exist:

(1) Dip and wrap. Dip the part to be heated 8 to 10 times into the paraffin wax and oil mix; then wrap the part in a plastic bag. Wrap a second time with a terry cloth towel to help retain the heat.

(2) Dip and reimmerse. Dip the part to be heated 8 to 10 times to create a solid coating, then reimmerse the part for the remainder of the treatment. The therapist must pay particular attention to the integrity of the skin when using this modality. The geriatric patient's skin is usually thin, and the temperatures of this modality may be too intense for this age group.

Fluidotherapy

This is a convection-type heating unit in which warm air is circulated through the unit to agitate the medium of fine cellulose particles. Units come in different sizes, from small ones for distal extremity treatment to larger ones that treat the trunk. Treatment and particle agitation can be controlled to vary the treatment approach. Temperatures usually range from 102° to 118°F (38.8° to 47.0°C). Particle agitation is used to help with desensitization of hypersensitive areas. If an open wound is present, the area can be protected with a plastic bag to prevent particles from coming into contact with the wound. As is the case with paraffin, the temperatures of this modality may be too high for the sensitive skin of the geriatric patient.

Ultrasound

Ultrasound is considered to provide the deepest penetration of all heat modalities. It is generally intended for heating deeper tissues, namely the deep ligaments or the capsular ligaments of joints (see Fig. 68–1). It makes use of acoustic energy and has been found to increase tissue temperature to depths of up to 5 cm. For ultrasound to be most effective in heating deeper tissues, the 1.0 MHz frequency

should be used at intensities of 1.0 to 2.0 W/cm² at continuous wave for 5 to 10 minutes, depending upon the size of the area being treated. The heating of superficial tissues is more effective with a 3.0 MHz frequency. The nonthermal effects of ultrasound cause the separation of collagen fibers, which increases the extensibility of connective tissues. A second effect is the increase of ionic exchange due to increased membrane permeability. Special caution must be used to avoid sonating over implanted joints because some plastics selectively absorb ultrasound waves which may cause the component to become unseated.

Moist Towels

Terry cloth towels soaked in warm water and then wrung out can be an effective heat treatment. The down side is that the heat dissipates quickly into the atmosphere, requiring multiple applications over the course of a 20- to 30-minute treatment session. Microwaving the wet towel can aid in the heating process, but caution must be used to avoid causing burns at the higher temperatures.

COLD

Cold is defined as the absence of heat or as heat at its lowest temperature.[3] Snow and ice were used long before there was artificially made ice. Cold spring water and snow water were used for stomach problems and other diseases.[2] Historically, cold wa-

---

Box 68–5

Effects of Cold

1. Decreases local metabolism
2. Vasoconstricts local blood vessels
3. Reduces inflammation
4. Reduces edema and hemorrhage
5. Slows nerve conduction velocity, which leads to pain relief
6. Decreases spasticity
7. Stimulates muscle contraction with quick or short application
8. Decreases pulse and respiratory rates, vasoconstricts systematically, decreases muscle tone, and provokes muscle shivering, depending upon area exposed and length of time applied

Box 68–6

Benefits Derived from Cold

1. Relieves pain
2. Reduces fever
3. Controls bleeding
4. Prevents or reduces edema
5. Decreases muscle guarding and spasms
6. Tempers diminished elasticity
7. Allows increased range of motion (through use of stretch after vapor coolants)
8. Facilitates muscle contraction[1]

ter has been recommended for gout, meningitis, ulcers, rheumatism, arthritis, and swollen joints.

Cold can be applied to reduce tissue temperature by convection (the movement of air over the skin), by evaporation (the spray of coolant such as fluoromethane), or by conduction (the application of solids, liquids, or gases that are lower in temperature than the skin).[2] The effects and benefits of and the contraindications for cold applications are shown in Boxes 68–5, 68–6, and 68–7, respectively.

When applying cold to living tissue, it is vital to be vigilant about possible injury. Acute red wheals are indicative of possible skin injury and may occur

Box 68–7

Contraindications for the Use of Cold

1. Cardiac or respiratory insufficiencies
2. Treatment of geriatric patients (the frail elderly have unreliable thermoregulatory systems)
3. Peripheral vascular disease and circulatory insufficiency
4. Sensory loss (treat with caution as when using heat)
5. Confusion (treat with caution as when using heat)
6. Hypersensitivity to cold (Raynaud's phenomenon)
7. Dislike of cold (especially geriatric patients)

at a temperature as high as 18°C (64.4°F). Temperatures below 10°C (50°F) may cause pain, weakness, loss of fine motor ability, and eventual numbness. Tissue damage ensues at 10°C. Human tissue freezes between −.53°C (31°F) and −.65°C (30.8°F). Duration, as well as temperature, is important to consider in preventing injury to skin with the application of cold. At 1.9°C (35.4°F), irreversible tissue damage will not occur if the cold is applied for 7 minutes or less. However, after 11½ minutes at the same temperature, hyperemia and tenderness result and last for several days. Repeated exposure can cause blistering of the skin.

Another factor to consider when applying cold, especially to geriatric patients, is the cold pressor response. This is a systemic response to placing the hand or any other body part into 4°C (39°F) water for 1 minute. Blood pressure in the opposite arm rises. Hypertensive patients show a large, or hyperreactive, response that may be interpreted to be characteristic of essential hypertension or of a predisposition to it. The cold pressor response is probably mediated by sensory reception of cold-induced pain and not by essential hypertension, however. There is a risk that the cold pressor response will occur at 15°C (59°F) or lower. The colder the modality, the greater the increase in blood pressure.[3]

Methods of Applying Cold

Cold Packs

Cold may be applied in a variety of methods, as shown in Box 68–8. One popular method is with the use of cold packs, which can range from the commercially made vinyl pack of silica gel or sand slurry mixture to the inexpensive bag of ice cubes or frozen peas. A mixture of 1 part rubbing alcohol

Box 68–8

Methods of Cold Application

1. Ice cubes/ice packs
2. Ice massage
3. Ice water-soaked towels
4. Cold baths
5. Vapor coolant sprays
6. Controlled cold compression units
7. Cold room, air conditioning

to 3 parts water also makes a reusable ice pack when placed in a zip-lock bag. The temperature of the cold pack should be $-5°C$ (21°F) prior to use. Moist towels facilitate energy transfer by eliminating the interference of air. Using warm water to wet the towel makes the initial contact with the cold more comfortable for the patient. Commercial cold packs hold their low temperatures for approximately 15 to 20 minutes. Chemical cold packs are also available and are usually a one-time use item for the emergency first-aid situation. Caution should be used when activating these packs so as not to break the packaging, as the packs usually contain chemicals of alkaline pH that can cause skin burns.

Ice Massage

For an ice massage, water is frozen in a paper or styrofoam cup. The cup is then peeled back to expose the ice but leaving the remainder of the cup to insulate the hand of the therapist. Ice "popsicles" can be made by placing a wooden tongue depressor in a cup of water. The therapist then holds the popsicle by the wooden handle and rubs the ice over the skin in small circular motions. A dry towel is used to dab off the excessive moisture every 30 to 40 seconds. An area of 10 × 15 centimeters is covered in an 8- to 10-minute period. The patient's sensation will be of intense cold, burning, aching, then analgesia, or numbness.

Ice-water–Soaked Towels

Terry cloth towels can be placed in ice water or a slushy ice mixture. Excessive water is wrung out. The cold towel is applied directly to the area being treated. Towels are changed every 4 to 5 minutes.

Cold Baths

Cold baths are used primarily for cooling the distal extremities; the body part to be chilled is immersed in cold water with or without ice cubes. Water temperatures may vary from 13° to 18°C (55° to 65°F).[4] The lower the temperature, the shorter the immersion time. Immersion in a cold bath of 13°C (55°F) is usually very uncomfortable. Temperatures this low are likely to be too intense for the geriatric patient.

Vapor Coolant Sprays

Fluoromethane vapor coolant spray is a noninflammable, nontoxic spray used for treatment of trigger points and tight, painful muscles. The area of treatment is placed into a passive stretch and then the coolant is sprayed directly over that area. Further stretching of the area is performed as tolerated. The spray is applied from a distance of approximately 45 centimeters from the skin at a 30-degree angle.[1] Spraying is done with unidirectional parallel sweeps along the muscle at the trigger points and into the area of referred pain. To treat the muscle to allow greater range of motion, the entire muscle should be sprayed, from origin to insertion. Spray two to three times over the entire area at a rate of 10 centimeters per second.[1] This type of spray is used to facilitate stretching, not to cool the body.

Controlled Cold Compression Units

Cold compression units direct water, at temperatures of 10° to 25°C (50° to 77°F), through special sleeves that fit over the extremities. The sleeve is controlled pneumatically to pump or to compress fluid from a swollen extremity.

Cold Rooms or Air Conditioning

Patients with certain diseases such as multiple sclerosis may perform better in cooler temperatures. Many of these patients find extreme heat increases fatigue levels. Air conditioning a room to temperatures of 18.3° to 20°C (65° to 68°F) can enhance performance and delay fatigue. Extreme caution must be exercised to prevent hypothermia resulting from lowering the geriatric patient's core temperature (see Chapter 11).

APPLICATION OF HEAT AND COLD IN GERIATRIC PATIENTS

The application of heat and cold modalities in the elderly requires more consideration than is necessary with younger patients. Conditions such as heart disease, arthritis, peripheral vascular disease, and diabetes are common in the elderly, especially after the seventh decade.[3] Changes in the body's physiology, especially in the circulatory and nervous systems, may seriously decrease the body's ability to respond to temperature changes. The therapist must assess each individual patient's ability to tolerate heat and cold.[6]

Checking the patient's history thoroughly for pertinent diseases and medications that could alter the patient's response to heat or cold is essential. The overall physical condition of the patient—cardiovascular fitness, muscle tone, and skin integrity—should be examined as well. Trial assessment of tolerance to heat and cold can be made by

Table 68–1 Modalities and Applications of Heat and Cold

Modality	Temperature (F)	Application	Time (minutes)	Considerations
Heat				
Hydrocollator pack/hot pack	140°	Localized Insulation necessary	20–30	Commercially available for home use May require assistance to apply Low to moderate cost
Paraffin wax	120°	Localized Dip and wrap in paper and toweling or dip and hold in wax	20–30	May require assistance for effective home use Low cost
Infrared lamp	500 + watt bulb	Localized Place several inches from exposed area	20–30	Convenient for home use Low cost
Electric heating pad/glove	100°–105°	Localized	20–30	Convenient for home use Low cost
Electric blanket	70°–80°	Generalized	20 min–several hours	Convenient for home use Moderate cost
Elastic joint supports/warmers, blankets, sleeping bags	Retain body heat	Localized or generalized	30 min–several hours	Convenient for home use Low cost
Ultrasound	$.5 \rightarrow 1.5$ w/cm^2	Localized Use coupling medium	5–15	PT-administered
Cold				
Hydrocollator pack/cold pack	50°	Localized Insulation necessary	20–30	Commercially available May require assistance to apply Low to moderate cost
Slush pack	35°–45°	Localized Fill doubled plastic zip-lock bags with 1 cup denatured alcohol and 2 cups water; freeze Insulation necessary	10–20	Convenient for home use Low cost
Home cold packs	35°–45°	Localized Apply slightly thawed bag of frozen vegetables or crushed ice Insulation may be necessary	10–20	Convenient for home use Low cost
Ice massage	35°–45°	Localized Rub large ice cube or ice "popsicle" over area	5–10	Convenient for home use

placing a hot pack or an ice pack on an uninvolved area and monitoring the patient's response.

Heat Versus Cold

The use of heat has many benefits. So does the use of cold. The decision to use one or the other should be based on the desired physiological effects (see Table 68–1 when deciding between heat and cold and determining treatment durations). Heat or cold—which should it be? What works well with one patient may not work with another. Patients' likes and dislikes will also enter into the decision. Patients who believe that cold is more beneficial will get better with the use of cold, and vice versa. Therefore, when a therapist has some leeway, it is best to use the modality the patient prefers, as a happier patient is likely to achieve better results.

The Future

The future of hot and cold packs is unclear. The United States Medicare system eliminated reimbursement for these modalities on the basis of budgetary constraints. The decision was rationalized by the suggestion that these treatment modalities are innocuous and do not require the skills of a healthcare provider for application. The information in this chapter indicates that there are reasons for concern when using heat and cold modalities, especially when caring for geriatric patients. (The Medicare decision applies only to hot and cold packs and not to the other deep-heating modalities.)

The concept that hot and cold packs are not sophisticated and have only minimal local effects may change in the future as a result of recent research that shows statistically significant changes in cerebral hemodynamics and cerebral metabolism with the application of standard hot packs and cold packs to the thighs of normal, healthy volunteers. Cerebral blood flow was measured in the middle cerebral artery with continuous transcranial Doppler sonography. Cytochrome aa_3 and cerebral oxygen saturation were measured by transcranial near-infrared spectroscopy. These investigators suggested that the rebound response of cerebral metabolism after cold stimulation may open new therapeutic possibilities in the treatment of central nervous system diseases by the use of thermal stimuli.[7]

CONCLUSION

Various modalities of heat and cold can be used in treating the geriatric patient. The methods of application, the desired effects, and the contraindications determine the therapist's choices of modality. The potential for misapplication and possible harm to the geriatric patient makes the use of thermal modalities a concern. Nonetheless, the indications and benefits of each modality for the individual geriatric patient should be the consideration, not the Medicare regulations or reimbursements.

REFERENCES

1. Michlovitz S. *Thermal Agents in Rehabilitation*, 2nd ed. Philadelphia: F.A. Davis; 1990.
2. Licht E. *Licht's: Therapeutic Heat and Cold*, 2nd ed. New Haven, Conn.: Elizabeth Licht; 1965.
3. Kauffman T. Thermoregulation and use of heat and cold. In: Jackson O, ed. *Therapeutic Considerations for the Elderly.* New York: Churchill Livingston; 1987.
4. Kahn J. *Principles and Practice of Electrotherapy.* New York: Churchill Livingston; 1994.
5. Hayes KW. *Manual for Physical Agents,* 3rd ed. Evanston, Ill.: Northwestern University Medical School; 1984.
6. Mathews D, Fox E. *The Physiological Basis of Physical Education and Athletics.* Philadelphia: W.B. Saunders; 1971: 104–124.
7. Doering Th, Brix J, Schneider B, Rimpler M. Cerebral hemodynamics and cerebral metabolism during cold and warm stress. *Am J Phys Med Rehabil* 1996; 75:408–415.

Chapter **69**

Electrotherapy
Joseph Kahn, Ph.D., P.T.

INTRODUCTION

A wide range of beneficial effects and some concerns should be considered when treating the geriatric patient with electrotherapy. The great variety of these modalities allows for specific selection based upon the desired effect. The purpose of this chapter is to describe briefly the different therapeutic choices and not to discuss in depth the physics of the various applications of electrotherapy. The reader is referred to Chapter 68 for more complete information on heat and cold therapy.

OVERVIEW OF ELECTROTHERAPY MODALITIES

Electrotherapy offers the geriatric patient a wide spectrum of therapeutic benefits. Among the modalities available are iontophoresis, transcutaneous electric nerve stimulation (TENS), other electric stimulation of various types, ultrasound, cold laser, pulsed magnetic fields therapy, and traditional diathermy.[1]

Iontophoresis involves the introduction of chemical substances into the tissues by means of direct current. Highly localized, this targets the treatment directly to the needy area. Which ion (chemical) is utilized depends upon the pathophysiology involved and the results desired (Box 69–1). Pharmaceutical precautions depend upon individual sensitivities, allergies, and prior experiences with each patient. Caution is advised regarding vasodilatation where vascular compromises are present.

TENS is designed specifically to alter the transmission of pain signals to the brain, minimizing or eliminating narcotic or other drug dependency for pain control. TENS is a particularly helpful modality to control pain caused by herpes zoster. Electrodes are placed at the offending nerve roots bilaterally, with parameters set for acute pain management, 150 Hz, 150 microseconds at minimal intensity for 1 hour, four times daily.

Ultrasound serves to reduce muscle spasm as it penetrates as deep as 4 to 6 centimeters into tissues. There are four basic physiological effects of ultrasound. First, chemical reactions are enhanced by

---

Box 69–1

Currently Utilized Ions: Properties and Sources

- **Hydrocortisone**: 1% ointment, various local sources, positive pole; anti-inflammatory; avoid ointments with "paraben" preservatives; used for arthritis, tendinitis, myositis, bursitis

- **Mecholyl**: mecholyl ointment, Gordon Labs, Upper Darby, PA; positive pole; vasodilator, analgesic; used for neuritis, neurovascular deficits, sprains, edema

- **Lidocaine**: Xylocaine 5%, Astra Pharmaceutical Co., Westboro, MA; positive pole; anesthetic analgesic; used for neuritis, bursitis, painful range of motion

- **Acetic acid**: 10% stock solution, cut to 2%; negative pole; used for calcific deposits, myositis ossificans, frozen joints

- **Iodine**: from Iodex (with methyl salicylate); negative pole; sclerolytic, antiseptic, analgesic; used for scar tissue, adhesions, fibrositis

- **Salicylate**: from Myoflex (Adria Labs, Columbus, OH) ointment, 10% salicylate preparation, or Iodex *with* methyl salicylate (Medtech Labs Inc., Cody, WY); negative pole; decongestant, analgesic; used for myalgias, rheumatoid arthritis

- **Magnesium**: from 2% solution of magnesium sulfate (Epsom salts); positive pole; antispasmodic, analgesic, vasodilator; used for osteoarthritis, myositis, neuritis

- **Copper**: 2% solution, copper sulfate; positive pole; caustic, antiseptic, antifungal; used for allergic rhinitis, dermatophytosis (athlete's foot)

- **Zinc**: from zinc oxide ointment 20%; positive pole; caustic, antiseptic; enhances healing; used for otitis, ulcerations, dermatitis, other open lesions

- **Calcium**: from calcium chloride, 2% solution; positive pole; stabilizer of irritability threshold; used for myospasm, frozen joints, trigger-fingers, mild tremors (non-Parkinsonian)

- **Chlorine**: from table salt (NaCl), 2% solution; negative pole; sclerolytic; used for scar tissue, adhesions

- **Lithium**: from lithium chloride or lithium carbonate, 2% solution; positive pole; specifically for gouty tophi

- **Hyaluronidase**: Wydase (Wyeth, Philadelphia, PA); solution to be mixed as directed on vials; positive pole; absorption agent for edema, sprains

---

From Kahn J. *Principles and Practice of Electrotherapy*, 3rd ed. New York: Churchill Livingstone; 1994. Used with permission.

the ultrasonic vibrations. Second, the permeability of membranes is increased by ultrasound. Third, mechanical responses may increase tendon extensibility but, if ultrasound is used to extreme power or duration, it may cause collapse of molecules and destruction of substances, which is a phenomenon called cavitation. The last physiological effect is the thermal effect.

Contraindications for the use of ultrasound in the geriatric population include the following:

1. Ultrasound should not be focused over bony prominences or used for ailments of the eye or of testicular tissue.
2. The presence of pacemakers may preclude the use of ultrasound.
3. Metallic implants and surgical fixation materials may be loosened by the use of ultrasound, and the metal/tissue interface may be a site for heat build-up and possible burning.
4. Healing fracture sites may not be appropriate locations for the use of ultrasound; however, some practitioners suggest that ultrasound may be a stimulant to bony growth.

Cold laser is an extremely valuable adjunct in the management of open wounds to enhance granulation rates.

Pulsed magnetic field therapy is a new addition to the physical therapist's arsenal and will be described later. It works by creating a magnetic field that aligns the polarities in the treated body area. Used commonly in Canada, South America, and elsewhere, it has yet to be fully utilized in the United States. It is particularly effective in the management of arthritic symptomatology.

"Old-fashioned," or traditional, diathermy is still a viable alternative to superficial heat, wherein the heat generated is at a much deeper level than can be achieved with heating pads, hot packs, or infrared lamps.

Last, but certainly not least, is electrical stimulation. There are several methods of stimulating neuromuscular tissues such as low-volt AC/DC, high-volt pulsed DC, interferential, and microampere techniques. Each has specific characteristics offering the clinician a complete array of procedures.

CONSIDERATIONS OF USE IN AGING PATIENTS

Pacemakers negate the use of any modality with a frequency of 500 Hz or more. This eliminates diathermy, microthermy, ultrasound, high-volt electrical stimulation, interferential therapy, Russian stimulation, and electrical stimulation in general. That leaves only cold laser and probably microam-

perage stimulation for the treatment of the pacemaker patient. Also, all geriatric patients should be checked for cardiopulmonary deficiencies before using any procedure. Sudden increases in circulation could be a problem.

With geriatric patients, however, some of the electrical stimulation parameters must be changed or adapted to the characteristics of the individual patient. Thin or dry skin, diminished circulation, less than optimal muscle strength, and commonly limited range of motion due to arthritis mandate changes in the parameters. Thin, dry skin offers higher resistance to current and requires higher voltages to obtain proper amperages (Ohm's law). Diminished circulation hinders optimal transmission of current, as the capillary flow is, in reality, a "second circuit" within the body. Muscle strength loss and limited ranges of motion provide practical limits for electrical stimulation. The astute physical therapist should be able to assess the individual patient's needs and to adjust the parameters accordingly.

There are no special rules concerning administration of electrical stimulation to geriatric patients other than to take extra care because of the factors mentioned above. General precautions and contraindications for electrical stimulation include active hemorrhage, phlebitis, demand-type pacemakers, and fresh fractures in order to avoid unwarranted bony movement.

ELECTRICAL STIMULATION CONSIDERATIONS

Electrodes should be thoroughly moistened, with no wrinkles or dry spots, or adequately covered with transmission gel. It is recommended that only electrical transmission-type gels be used, not ultrasonic preparations. Electrodes should be secured in position with light-weight sandbags, nonconductive tape, or Velcro straps. Tight, constrictive, or moist (and therefore conductive) strapping should be avoided. Self-adherent electrodes are convenient but expensive and may cause skin irritations that should be avoided or managed with common-sense skin care.

Hydrocollator packs should *not* be placed across two electrodes, as conduction will take place through the hot pack, affecting the voltage in the circuit. If simultaneous heating is desired, an insulating layer such as cellophane placed between the electrodes and the pack eliminates this problem without lessening the heat transfer. An alternative is an infrared lamp placed about 36 inches from the skin. Never allow the full weight of the body or a heavy limb to rest on an electrode. The weight will squeeze out the needed moisture in the electrodes, leaving dry spots that will inevitably cause burns. Many patients, especially members of the geriatric population, prefer to be treated in a sitting position as opposed to lying supine or prone. Proper positioning, with pillow supports for back, popliteal areas, and shoulders, is mandatory for a comfortable session.

Functional Electrical Stimulation

Weight-free exercise is one of the prime benefits of functional electrical stimulation and should be considered when positioning the body part to be treated. When circulatory problems are encountered, be aware of dependent positioning of the lower and upper extremities. Duty-factor limitations, that is, on/off times, with the older patient are usually in order because relatively easy or early fatigue may be a present caution. A cycle of 4 to 6 seconds on and 4 to 6 seconds off is suggested. Whereas the younger, athletic type may require 30 to 45 minutes of stimulation, the older patient would do better with only 10 to 15 minutes. This rule is subject to variations depending upon individual characteristics. Current intensities should be kept minimal to obtain the desired results rather than maximal. Following the tenets of the Arndt-Schulz law in physiology ("the less the better"), it has been noted that "visible contraction at patient tolerance" will serve the geriatric patient to a much greater extent than the full, often painful but impressive maximum contraction sought by and for athletes. (Although many senior patients are also athletic, it is recommended that age take precedence in treatment design.)

Low Volt

With traditional low-volt AC/DC stimulation, "visible contraction at patient tolerance" is the best guide for the AC circuitry. The chemical effects associated with DC make this a current with a "bite," and it should be administered in the presence of reaction of degeneration (RD). With neural damage, the ability to respond to AC is lost. Pulsed (interrupted) DC is indicated.

High Volt

High-volt pulsed DC is not usually favored for geriatric patients. The higher voltage necessary to produce this twin-spiked, pulsed DC presents a problem: the extremely short duration (in microseconds) of each pulse offers deeper penetration. This

shortened pulse, with the accompanying higher frequency (2500 Hz), may indeed bypass the superficial nerve endings, which is thought to make the treatment more comfortable. However, the higher frequency and shorter wave length requires the higher voltages which, in turn, may be uncomfortable to the less than athletic geriatric patient. Whether a particular patient of any age is frequency-sensitive or voltage-sensitive will determine the comfort levels of high-voltage pulsed DC units. Clinicians may administer both separately to test for acceptability and effectiveness (see Chapter 52 for a discussion of the use of high-voltage pulsed direct current for wound healing).

Interferential

Interferential currents combine the advantages of penetration by the two carrier medium frequencies (4000 to 4100 Hz) with the optimal therapeutic stimulating "beat" frequencies in the 1 to 100 Hz band. Usually, with minimal sensation, deep muscle contractions are felt by the patient with very little surface discomfort. In addition, the "sweep" mode of most interferential units offers a greater fiber recruitment pattern by involving a spectrum of individual frequencies, that is, they sweep across a band of beat frequencies during each session. Because there is a differential frequency response for each fiber, this is a distinct advantage. Interferential current is more comfortable but less dramatic and visible in most instances. As mentioned previously, increased fiber recruitment via the sweep mode, and precise localization with targeting, are two additional benefits of the modality.[2]

Microampere

Microampere stimulation (MENS; as no neural fibers are stimulated at these extremely low intensities, there should be no "N" in the name) is designed to enhance the flow of ions within the capillary circulation, bringing needed nutritional and therapeutic substances to traumatized or diseased tissues. Normally, these injured tissues are walled off by a strong electrical charge[3] that prevents the needed ions from entering and beginning the healing processes. The slight boost provided by microampere stimulation aids in bringing the required ions to the target site by helping to overcome the higher resistance of the injured tissues. This modality is ideally suited to the geriatric patient as there is no sensation and no muscle contraction and as neither motor nor sensory nerves are stimulated by parameters in the micro ranges. It is a useful method of increasing circulation gently without the systemic effects of a vasodilation drug. One of the better techniques with microamp stimulation is the manual approach. Here, the physical therapist places one electrode on his or her hand and the other on the patient. The therapist then proceeds to massage the area, simultaneously administering the microamp stimulation and adding the hands-on touch so necessary with all ages!

Microampere stimulation produces neither sensation nor muscle contractions, so it comes as a complete surprise to patients who have experienced traditional electrical stimulation treatments. However, the outcomes usually dispel any notion of "nonfunctioning equipment." Keeping the front of the unit in view is suggested because it allows patient and physical therapist to note the display indicating current flow; when one electrode or the hand of the manually treating clinician is removed, the current flow indicator is seen to disappear. The variations available among intensities, frequencies, and wave-forms for microampere stimulation make this modality clinician-oriented, requiring knowledge, training, and individual techniques, rather than the standardized and protocol-controlled procedures favored by managed care facilities and insurance carriers.

Magnetic Field

The latest modality to be considered is magnetic field therapy. Commonly utilized in Europe, South American, and Canada, this interesting procedure is slowly finding a place in our therapeutic arsenal. Whether as clinical models with special applicators or personal-sized units worn by the patient, these devices present a unique form of administration. There is no sensation felt by the patient, nor is there a need to disrobe. Magnetic fields penetrate across all tissues and materials. We are subjected daily to the Earth's own magnetic field. The physiological effects of exposure to concentrated natural magnetic fields are currently being studied, and they seem to include analgesia, increased circulation, enhanced healing, and improved membrane ionic exchange.[4] Favorable and enthusiastic reports from clinicians invite further study of this modality.

CONCLUSION

A wide variety of available electrotherapeutic techniques make up the arsenal of treatments that can be administered to the geriatric patient. The clinician's decisions regarding parameter variations adaptable to the geriatric population make the difference be-

tween routine care and expertise. Let's strive for expertise!

REFERENCES

1. Kahn J. *Principles and Practice of Electrotherapy*, 3rd ed. New York: Churchill Livingstone; 1994.
2. Stephenson R, Johnson M. The analgesic effects of interferential therapy on cold-induced pain in healthy subjects: a preliminary report. *Physiother Theory Pract* 1995; II:89–95.
3. Nordenstrom B. *Biologically Closed Electric Circuits*. No data given.
4. Magnetherapy, Inc. 760 US Highway One, Suite 101, North Palm Beach, FL 33408.

Chapter **70**

Orthotics
David Patrick, M.S., P.T.

INTRODUCTION

An orthosis is a mechanical device applied to the body in order to support a body segment, correct anatomical alignment, protect a body part, or assist motion to improve body function. In accomplishing these objectives, orthotic devices assist in promoting ambulation, reducing pain, preventing deformity, and allowing greater activity. Orthotic devices are often indicated as a component of the rehabilitation process for a variety of diseases and conditions that affect the geriatric population. Successful orthotic intervention when working with aging individuals demands a practical balance between the objectives that are ideally desired and what the elderly individual will reasonably tolerate.

Orthotic devices accomplish their objectives by applying forces to the involved body segments. As a rule, the more aggressive the orthotic intervention, the greater the force generated. In general, elderly individuals are less tolerant of the resultant discomfort of aggressive orthotic intervention, and their skin and subcutaneous tissue are less tolerant of the external forces generated. This frequently results in the need to compromise between an ideal and an acceptable orthotic outcome and to choose more "forgiving" orthoses in terms of comfort and tolerance—that is, less rigid orthotic devices. This discussion focuses on the lower extremity and spinal orthotic interventions, which are commonly associated with the geriatric population.

LOWER EXTREMITY ORTHOTIC SYSTEMS

Shoes

Proper distribution of forces in order to maintain the integrity of the skin of the foot is of primary importance. The shoe should fit properly and the volume of the shoe should appropriately accommodate the foot and any additions such as a foot orthotic or plastic ankle-foot-orthosis (AFO). Generally, a sneaker with a removable inlay or an extra-depth shoe with a removable inlay is recommended. The inlay can be removed to accommodate fluctuating edema or the addition of an orthosis. In unilateral involvement the inlay can remain in the shoe on the uninvolved side, maintaining the fit on that side and balancing the patient in terms of height. It is recommended that the shoe have a soft upper (the portion of the shoe covering the dorsum of the foot) to reduce pressure in the presence of minor foot deformities such as bunions or hammer toes. Severe foot deformities may require a custom shoe made from a cast of the individual's foot.

Foot Orthotics

In general, flexible accommodative orthotics for the purpose of distributing forces to protect the skin and promote comfort are indicated. The bones of the foot of the geriatric patient are often functionally adapted and the joints may be restricted in terms of range of motion. Thus, attempting biomechanical control may be inappropriate and may, thereby, contraindicate the use of rigid orthotic devices and necessitate careful consideration of the application of even semirigid devices.

Ankle-Foot-Orthotics (AFO)

AFOs are frequently utilized with the elderly to improve ambulation status and gait quality. AFOs are capable of controlling the foot and ankle directly and the knee indirectly, for example, by positioning the ankle in dorsiflexion to produce a knee flexion moment to control genu recurvatum or by positioning the ankle in plantarflexion to produce a knee extension moment to assist in stabilizing the knee. Neuromuscular conditions such as a hemiparesis due to a cerebral vascular accident as well as musculoskeletal pathologies such as arthritis commonly result in foot and ankle dysfunctions in the geriatric population which can be managed in part with AFOs.

A common challenge is deciding whether to use a plastic or a metal AFO system. The metal AFO has little skin contact except for the calf band and shoe which are the reaction points of the orthosis. This quality is a distinct advantage of the metal system for patients with fluctuating edema or poor skin integrity. In comparison, the total-contact nature of the plastic AFO results in a greater ability to control the foot and ankle. Additionally, the plastic AFO is lighter in weight, more cosmetically acceptable, and has the practical advantage of easy interchange among shoes. Plastic AFOs would appear to be the orthosis of choice for geriatric patients whenever possible. One strategy to determine whether a metal AFO system is indicated for a particular patient is to consider the sensory status and volume stability (i.e., presence or absence of fluctuating edema) of the patient and the reliability of the patient or support person, because the skin integrity of the involved lower extremity must be monitored. Negative findings in two of these categories would indicate consideration of a metal AFO instead of a plastic orthosis.

A soft AFO such as a neoprene ankle sleeve may be appropriate for controlling minor discomfort from arthritis or to encourage ankle stability when a more rigid system cannot be tolerated. Such orthoses accomplish their goals remarkably well in some cases by retaining heat and acting as a kinesthetic reminder.

Knee-Ankle-Foot Orthoses (KAFO)

Although AFOs are tolerated well by the geriatric population, the addition of a knee joint and thigh cuff to form a KAFO system results in a much less acceptable orthotic intervention because a larger brace is more difficult for the patient to tolerate wearing. A KAFO has the advantage of controlling the knee as well, because the foot and ankle directly and indirectly influence the hip joint. A KAFO is the orthosis of choice in the presence of severe genu recurvatum, or knee buckling, that cannot be managed with an AFO. Additionally, significant coronal plane instabilities at the knee (genu varum or valgum) are effectively managed by a KAFO. Less severe knee problems may be managed using a knee orthosis (KO), but the shortened lever arm (the shorter length of the orthosis) results in greater skin pressures, and the softer nature of the elderly patient's lower extremity (LE) musculature can create suspension problems as the KO tends to slide distally during use.

Hip-Knee-Ankle-Foot Orthoses (HKAFO)

The addition of a hip joint and pelvic band to a KAFO results in an orthosis that is difficult to don and doff, less comfortable than shorter ones, and more cumbersome to wear. For the geriatric population, the hip joint and pelvic band are most commonly added when rotation control of the LE is required.

Hip Orthoses

A hip orthosis is commonly used with the elderly to limit the extent of hip joint adduction and flexion following the dislocation of a hip arthroplasty (hip rotation is controlled to a lesser degree). Premanufactured systems are available that allow the limits of hip ROM to be adjusted as required to protect the hip adequately and simultaneously allow the patient to perform the activities of daily living.

Knee Orthoses

A postoperative knee orthosis is commonly used after a knee arthroplasty. The knee orthosis is usually designed to allow ROM adjustment in graduating increments, as desired. A soft knee orthosis is commonly used to address arthritis-related pain and promote knee stability through a greater kinesthetic awareness. A knee orthosis with wraparound closure design is recommended for the elderly patient to facilitate donning and doffing. Some orthopedists order knee immobilizers postoperatively for their patients who have had total hip replacements. The rationale is that by preventing knee flexion, the operative hip flexion will be reduced, thereby mitigating risk for dislocation. This technique should be considered for individual patients only in the early postoperative period as it does impede mobility and may cause knee stiffness and hip pain because of the long lever arm.

Fracture Orthoses

Fracture orthoses are utilized with the geriatric population to reduce the amount of time the joints surrounding a fracture have to be immobilized in a cast. This reduces the potential negative effects of immobilization such as contractures and phlebitis. Additionally, lower extremity fracture orthoses may reduce the period of recumbency, thereby minimizing the risk of potentially life-threatening complications such as pneumonia. Fracture orthoses are tightened circumferentially around the involved area and, using the hydraulic effect of soft tissues (the noncompressibility of fluids) and gravity, they transmit forces that realign and support the fracture site while allowing motion in the surrounding joints.

Fracture orthoses must be worn snugly; they are commonly used for the management of nondisplaced or minimally displaced fractures, especially those of the humerus, tibia, radius, and ulna.

SPINAL ORTHOTIC SYSTEMS

Spinal orthotic intervention is particularly challenging when dealing with the elderly population. Older patients commonly present with a variety of pathologies involving the spine and soft tissues of the trunk that could well be treated by the application of a spinal orthosis. Tolerance to wearing such a device, however, is limited, particularly in the cases of the more rigid systems and those that cover extensive body area.

Spinal orthoses accomplish their objectives through one or more of the following biomechanical principles:

1. Three-point pressure control,
2. Indirect transfer of load by increasing intra-abdominal pressure,
3. Correction of spinal alignment, or
4. Sensory feedback (kinesthetic reminder).

Three-point pressure control (the design of the orthosis) determines which spinal motions are limited. The magnitude of control (the degree of limitation) is directly related to the rigidity of the orthosis and the degree of tightness with which it is worn. A rigid orthosis is capable of applying greater forces to the body to restrict motion than is a more flexible system. However, the geriatric patient is less tolerant of the resulting discomfort and potential breathing restriction, and the skin of the older patient is less capable of withstanding the forces generated without its integrity being compromised. The decision to use a rigid rather than a more flexible system should therefore be based on the degree to which spinal motion restriction is required. For example, a geriatric patient with an unstable fracture of the spine requires a rigid orthotic system to restrict motion in the involved spinal segment, whereas management of a stable compression fracture offers greater latitude to use a more flexible device without compromising the patient's safety. It should be noted that a more rigid device is often preferred in terms of protecting the involved spinal segment, but the decision to use a more flexible system is based on the practical issue of orthotic tolerance and thus compliance with wearing the orthosis. The ideal orthosis serves no purpose at all if it is not worn and, particularly with the geriatic population, it it sometimes necessary to make practical decisions that involve relinquishing orthotic control to gain patient acceptance.

Soft and rigid spinal systems applied to the trunk typically incorporate a means of applying abdominal pressure, thereby increasing intra-abdominal pressure, which has been shown to reduce the load on the vertebrae and intervertebral disks. Some literature suggests that this may be the primary effect of the corsets and soft binders that are frequently used in geriatric applications.

The principle of correcting spinal alignment is seldom applied to the geriatric population because of restriction of spinal flexibility and poor tolerance of the required forces.

Flexible spinal orthoses serve to limit motion by acting as kinesthetic reminders to volitionally restrict movement as opposed to exerting three-point pressure control. Motion restriction accomplished through a flexible orthosis would obviously be better tolerated by the elderly.

Cervical Orthoses (CO)

Among cervical orthoses (COs), soft cervical collars are well tolerated and provide reasonable control of cervical flexion and extension. The Philadelphia collar offers greater control than the soft cervical collar and is also reasonably well tolerated.

Cervical-Thoracic Orthoses (CTO)

When more definitive control of the cervical spine and upper thoracic region are required, a cervical orthosis with a thoracic extension (a cervical thoracic orthosis, or CTO) is indicated. Rigid four-poster and sternal-occipital-mandibular immobilizer (SOMI) systems are poorly accepted by the elderly. The Minerva CTO tends to be better tolerated and does maintain appropriate spinal control.

Thoraco-Lumbo-Sacral Orthoses (TLSO)

Thoraco-lumbo-sacral orthoses (TLSOs) are utilized to address spinal pathologies from approximately the T6 to the L3–4 region. An over-shoulder overlap may allow control of the T4–5 levels, and a cervical extension addition to the TLSO is recommended for more definitive control above the T6 level. TLSOs most effectively control the T12–L1 region and offer diminishing control of spinal segments farther away from this region. Rigid immobilization is typically accomplished using a "body jacket" made of plastic with a soft foam interface (lining). Soft, high-density body jackets can incorporate high-density outer foam instead of plastic. Plastic stays (permanent or removable) or a plastic frame

can be incorporated into the foam for additional restriction of motion if desired. These systems, when custom-fabricated, offer excellent alternatives to the rigid body jacket. They tend to be much better tolerated by the elderly patient and offer moderately effective restriction of spinal motion.

The TLSO corset (semiflexible) is often used for patients whose acceptance of a more rigid spinal orthosis is questionable or for patients who require minimal restriction of spinal motion. Compression fractures are very common in the geriatric population and frequently an attempt is made to manage them with a corset. Rigid systems such as the Taylor and Knight-Taylor are less frequently used for the elderly because they are difficult to tolerate.

Lumbo-Sacral Orthoses (LSO)

Utilized to address spinal pathologies from approximately L1 to L4–5, the lumbo-sacral orthosis (LSO) most effectively controls the L3–4 spinal level. As with the TLSO, a rigid system is used in the presence of spinal instability, whereas more flexible systems are preferred and better tolerated by the geriatric population and should be used whenever possible. Corsets are commonly used to manage soft-tissue injuries that result in back pain. The custom-made, soft, high-density LSO is an excellent alternative to the rigid body jacket or corset, offering a balance between comfort and control. It should be noted that successful orthotic outcomes with the soft, high-density system appear to be more readily accomplished in patients with average to thin body types. Again, rigid LSO systems like the Chairback and Knight are poorly tolerated by geriatric patients.

CONCLUSION

The use of orthotics to support a body segment, correct anatomical alignment, protect a body area, or assist body movement is an important therapeutic consideration in geriatric rehabilitation. It is crucial to involve the patient in the choice of orthotic in order to attain a balance between objective ideals and patient adherence. Attention must be given to possible harmful effects of the orthotic device on the skin and the subcutaneous connective tissues of aged persons.

SUGGESTED READINGS

Bunch WH, Keagy R, et al. *Atlas of Orthotics: Biomechanical Principles and Application.* St. Louis: Mosby; 1985.

Edelstein JE. Orthoses. In: Myers RS, ed. *Saunders Manual of Physical Therapy Practice*. Philadelphia: W.B. Saunders; 1995: 1183–1227.

Nawoczenski DA, Epler ME, eds. *Orthotics in Functional Rehabilitation of the Lower Limb*. Philadelphia: W.B. Saunders; 1997.

Chapter **71**

Prosthetics
David Patrick, M.S., P.T.

INTRODUCTION

The elderly make up the largest group of patients requiring lower extremity (LE) amputations; peripheral vascular disease (PVD) and complications of diabetes are the leading causes. Progress in the fields of rehabilitation and prosthetics has resulted in a large number of geriatric amputees' being successfully fitted with prostheses and subsequently requiring rehabilitation.

EVALUATING THE PATIENT

The physical therapy program starts with a comprehensive evaluation of the patient. This is particularly important with the elderly amputee who commonly presents with a number of comorbid conditions that can impact on his or her functional outcome. A format for the evaluation of the LE amputee is provided in Figure 71–1. The following elements represent important considerations in the evaluation and treatment of the geriatric amputee.

Age   Consider overall wellness and conditioning, functional abilities, and motivation as being more important than chronological age.

Secondary Diagnosis   Investigate the presence of comorbid conditions. Elderly vascular amputees can demonstrate multiple secondary conditions in addition to the amputation. The presence of cardiac disease is common, as the same factors that increase the incidence of PVD in diabetics also increase the incidence of atherosclerotic coronary artery disease. This leads to an increased death rate (there is an estimated 25 to 50% 3-year survival for a diabetic with a major amputation) and an increase in the symptoms of angina, congestive heart failure (CHF), and arrhythmias.

Cognitive Status   Determine the patient's ability to understand and remember instructions. Pro-

vide instructions in writing that clearly state the wearing schedule of the shrinker, socks, and prosthesis. Review the instructions with the patient frequently. Direct the patient to maintain a written diary of sock-ply use and color-code the various sock plys to assist the patient in maintaining proper socket fit.

Wheelchair   Recommend availability of a lightweight, easily transportable wheelchair for long-distance transportation, limited ambulation endurance, discontinued prosthetic use (because of skin breakdown), and prosthetic breakdown. Bilateral LE geriatric amputees commonly depend on wheelchairs as opposed to walking with prostheses.

Transfers and Mobility   Train patients to change positions slowly to avoid episodes of syncope that could result in loss of balance. Reduced proprioceptive feedback through the prosthetic extremity and the predisposition of the elderly for postural hypotension increase the risk of balance loss when changing positions.

Ambulation   Prioritize the maintenance of skin integrity, the prevention of falls, and the control of energy expenditure.

Skin Integrity   The loss of elements of the connective tissue, the thinning of the dermis, and alterations in the content of elastin and collagen represent characteristic skin changes that occur with aging and predispose the amputee to skin breakdown during prosthetic use (see Chapter 54, "Skin Disorders"). Particularly with the transtibial (below-knee) amputee, use a conservative, methodical progression of weight-bearing and ambulation distance and continue to monitor the skin of the residual limb (in the past, it was referred to as the stump) on a frequent basis. Consider shear-force-absorbing socket interfaces and prosthetic componentry to reduce forces on the residual limb.

Fall Prevention   Conservative advancement of assistive devices is recommended, prioritizing safety over progression. The transfemoral (above-knee) geriatric amputee is less prone to skin breakdown than is the transtibial amputee, but the transfemoral amputee is at greater risk for falls.

Energy Expenditure   The geriatric amputee should not be encouraged to walk at a "normal" walking speed. Allowing the patient to self-select ambulation velocity results in a more normal rate of metabolic energy expenditure, decreasing perceived exertion and potential cardiac difficulties. A slower self-selected walking velocity should be expected at higher amputation levels.

Date therapy initiated _____

Name _____ Age _____ Room # _____

Diagnosis (Date/Cause of amputation) _____

_____

Secondary diagnosis _____

Precautions _____

Past medical history _____

_____

Social history _____

_____

Orientation and ability to follow directions _____

_____

Functional level
    1. Wheelchair _____
    2. Transfers _____
    3. Bed mobility _____
    4. Sitting balance _____
    5. Standing balance _____
    6. Ambulation—level surface without prosthesis _____
               —level surface with prosthesis _____
               —elevations without prosthesis _____
               —gait deviations _____

               _____
    7. Floor transfer _____
    8. Donning/doffing prosthesis _____
    9. Stump wrapping _____
  10. Endurance
Residual limb length: below knee—left or right
    a. _____ cm from MTP to end of bone
    b. _____ cm from MTP to end of flesh
Residual limb length: Above knee—left or right
    a. _____ cm from perineum to end of bone
    b. _____ cm from perineum to end of flesh

Girth measurements: Reference point

Date Proximal Distal					

	(R)—ROM—(L)	(R)—Muscle Stength—(L)
Hip flexion Hip extension Hip abduction Hip external rot Hip internal rot Knee flexion Knee extension Ankle P/F Ankle D/F		

Knee A-P Stability (L) _____ (R) _____

Knee M-L Stability (L) _____ (R) _____

Figure 71–1 Sample lower extremity amputee evaluation form

Illustration continued on following page

Residual limb condition:
Shape _____
Scar _____
Skin _____
Bones _____
Musculature _____
Sensation _____
Pulses _____
Phantom sensation/pain
Description of prosthetic appliance _____
_____

Condition of remaining LE:
Skin condition _____
Pulses _____
Sensation _____
Ulcerations _____
Upper extremities:
ROM (L) WNL except for _____
(R) WNL except for _____
Strength: (L) WNL except for _____
(R) WNL except for _____
Back _____
Abdominals _____
Additional comments: _____

Goals: Treatment plan:

Date   Therapist

Figure 71–1 *Continued*

Prosthetic Donning and Doffing Difficulty in donning and doffing the prosthetic may result from limitations in manual dexterity as well as visual dysfunction. Self-suspending systems, Velcro closures versus buckles, and oversized extensions on belts and socket inserts should be considered.

Range of Motion (ROM) Adequate ROM is required for successful prosthetic outcome. Degenerative joint disease predisposes elderly amputees to contractures. Common areas of LE contractures include:

- the partial foot level: plantar flexors (due primarily to muscle imbalance),
- the transtibial level: knee flexors and hip flexors, and
- the transfemoral level: hip flexors, hip abductors, hip external rotators.

Strength and Endurance Deconditioning is common with aging and may limit ability to participate in the rehabilitation program. Initiate a strengthening and endurance program as soon after surgery as possible.

Volume Containment Controlling the volume of the residual limb is an important aspect of preparing it for definitive prosthetic fitting, reducing pain in the limb that is related to edema, and facilitating healing after the amputation surgery. Comorbid con-

ditions such as renal failure and dialysis or CHF predispose the geriatric amputee to significant girth fluctuations. Shrinker socks are recommended instead of Ace wraps because of the relative ease of donning and the greater consistency of fit (they require less frequent reapplication and adjustment). A rigid dressing should be considered when protection of the residual limb is a priority. Regular girth measurements of the residual limb are recommended to monitor the effectiveness of the volume-containment program.

Sensation Sensory evaluation is important to accurate prediction of the amputee's ability to detect abnormal forces during prosthetic use and to detect soft-tissue trauma in the remaining limb. Vascular insufficiency and particularly diabetes may result in polyneuropathy involving the sensory nerve fibers and predisposing the elderly amputee to skin problems.

Condition of the Remaining LE It is essential to evaluate the remaining LE for evidence of vascular insufficiency or sensory deficits that could lead to further amputation. Unilateral amputees with diabetes have more than a 40% risk over 4 years of having an amputation of the remaining LE. Polyneuropathy associated with diabetes may involve sensory, motor, and autonomic nerve fibers. Motor deficits may cause atrophy of the foot intrinsics and muscle imbalances in the foot, resulting in foot deformity and skin injury caused by fitting problems with shoes. Sensory deficits result in the lack of an appropriate avoidance response to abnormal forces. Autonomic involvement may result in dry skin which creates greater susceptibility to breakdown and infection. The importance of this evaluation cannot be overemphasized, as peripheral neuropathy has been identified as the primary underlying cause of amputation in the elderly with diabetes. Patient education that emphasizes proper footwear and skin management is an essential component of the amputation prevention program.

PROSTHETIC PRESCRIPTION

Advances in the technology of prosthetic components have improved the possibility of successfully fitting the geriatric amputee with a prosthesis. Innovations in socket designs, lightweight components, improved suspensions, and stable knee design options all contribute to improved prosthetic tolerance and better functional outcomes for elderly amputees. The application of advanced prosthetic componentry also results in increased expense, so judgments must be made about the relative costs and benefits of these components to each patient. The Lower Limb Prosthetics Medical Review Policy (LLPMRP) developed by Medicare structures financial sponsorship of the various prosthetic ankle, foot, and knee components based on the patient's anticipated functional outcome (Box 71–1). The LLPMRP should be considered by the prosthetics team in the process of prescribing prostheses for the many geriatric amputees with Medicare coverage.

Preparatory vs. Definitive Prosthesis. A preparatory prosthesis that is functional although not fully finished or cosmetic is strongly recommended over a definitive prosthesis as the first prosthetic device for a geriatric amputee. The preparatory prosthesis allows earlier prosthetic fitting by avoiding the need to wait until shrinkage of the residual limb is complete. This may help to prevent secondary complications resulting from immobility that are potentially life-threatening to the elderly patient. The definitive prosthesis is the near-final or finished product, with all the appropriate modifications and cosmetic touches.

Endoskeletal vs. Exoskeletal Design

The exoskeletal design has a hard, laminated plastic shell that provides the weight-bearing support. The space between the ankle block and the bottom of the socket is hollow to reduce weight. In contrast, the endoskeletal design consists of a tubular structure that constitutes the internal support to which the foot, ankle, and knee assemblies are attached. The endoskeleton is covered with a pliable surface that is shaped and colored to match the opposite limb.

Endoskeletal prosthetic design is usually recommended for geriatric amputees because of the ease with which adjustments can be made and components interchanged, the reduced weight, and the cosmetic benefits in transfemoral applications. Weight restrictions have been identified by the manufacturers of some endoskeletal components.

Prosthetic Sockets

At the level of the transtibial amputation, the patellar tendon-bearing (PTB) socket with a soft insert is commonly utilized. A patient with fragile skin or sensitivity in the residual limb may benefit from soft insert materials such as silicone that are designed to dissipate shock and shear forces. A flexible inner socket supported in a rigid outer frame may result in greater comfort for the elderly amputee by providing relief to pressure-sensitive structures.

After a transfemoral amputation, a geriatric patient can be successfully fitted with either a quadrilateral or an ischial containment socket. A patient with a short residual limb, poor residual limb muscle tone, obesity, or a high activity level would be expected to achieve the greatest benefit from the ischial containment socket design. The elderly amputee may experience more comfort when sitting if he or she has chosen a flexible socket design that is capable of accommodating its shape to the supporting surface.

Prosthetic Suspensions

The following prosthetic suspensions are recommended for transtibial-level amputation:

- Supracondylar cuff with Velcro closure on strap;
- Supracondylar wedge self-suspension with tab extensions attached to medial and lateral insert wings;
- Sleeve suspension (determine if the patient has the hand dexterity to manage the sleeve);
- Silicone suction suspension (consider the patient's ability to manage the sleeve and the patient's skin's tolerance to silicone);
- Joint and corset (which may be necessary due to hypersensitivity, skin problems, or knee joint pathology that prohibits full weight-bearing through the residual limb).

Box 71–1

Medicare's Lower Limb Prosthetics Medical Review Policy (LLPMRP)*

A determination of the medical necessity for certain components/additions to the prosthesis is based on the patient's potential functional abilities. Potential functional ability is based on the reasonable expectations of the prosthetist and ordering physician, considering factors including, but not limited to:

a. the patient's past history (including prior prosthetic use, if applicable),

b. the patient's current condition, including the status of the residual limb and the nature of other medical problems, and

c. the patient's desire to ambulate.

Clinical assessments of patient rehabilitation potential should be based on the following classification levels:

Level 0: Does not have the ability or potential to ambulate or transfer safely with or without assistance and a prosthesis does not enhance patient's quality of life or mobility.

Level 1: Has the ability or potential to use a prosthesis for transfers or ambulation on level surfaces at fixed cadence. Typical of the limited and unlimited household ambulator.

Level 2: Has the ability or potential for ambulation with the ability to traverse low-level environmental barriers such as curbs, stairs, or uneven surfaces. Typical of the limited community ambulator.

Level 3: Has the ability or potential for ambulation with variable cadence. Typical of the community ambulator who has the ability to traverse most environmental barriers and may have vocational, therapeutic, or exercise activity that demands prosthetic utilization beyond simple locomotion.

Level 4: Has the ability or potential for prosthetic ambulation that exceeds basic ambulation skills, exhibiting high-impact stress or energy levels. Typical of the prosthetic demands of the child, active adult, or athlete.

In the following sections, the determination of coverage for selected prostheses and components with respect to potential functional levels represents the usual case. Exceptions will be considered in an individual case if additional documentation is included which justifies the medical necessity. Prostheses will be denied as not medically necessary if the patient's potential functional level is "0."

Feet:

A determination of the type of foot for the prosthesis will be made by the prescribing physician and/or the prosthetist based upon the functional needs of the patient. Basic lower extremity prostheses include a SACH foot. Prosthetic feet are considered for coverage based upon the functional classification.

External keel, SACH foot or single axis ankle/foot are covered for patients with a functional level 1 or above.

Flexible keel foot and multiaxial ankle/foot candidates are expected to demonstrate a functional level 2 or greater functional need.

Flex-foot system, energy-storing foot, multiaxial ankle/foot dynamic response, or flex-walk system or equal are covered for patients with a functional level 3 or above.

Knees:

Basic lower extremity prostheses include a single axis, constant-friction knee. Prosthetic knees are considered for coverage based upon functional classification.

Fluid and pneumatic knees are covered for patients with a functional level 3 or above.

Other knee-shin systems are covered for patients with a functional level 1 or above.

Ankles:

Axial rotation units are covered for patients with a functional level 2 or above.

Sockets:

No more than two of the same socket inserts are allowed per individual prosthesis at the same time.

Socket replacements are considered medically necessary if there is adequate documentation of functional and/or physiological need. There are situations where the explanation includes but is not limited to: changes in the residual limb; functional need changes; or irreparable damage or wear/tear due to excessive patient weight or prosthetic demands of very active amputees.

---

*From U.S. Department of Health and Human Services.

For transfemoral-level amputation, the following prosthetic suspensions are suggested:

- Neoprene belt with Velcro closure;
- Hip joint and pelvic band with Velcro closure (indicated when hip stability or rotational control is required);
- Silicone suction.

Prosthetic Feet

The weight of the foot and the function of the foot's keel in relationship to the patient's activity level are the two primary considerations for the geriatric amputee. The keel provides the inner rigidity of structure to control the function of the prosthetic foot.

SACH Feet The solid ankle, cushion heel (SACH) feet are low cost and dependable. Geriatric lightweight versions are available. The rigid keel can interfere with the ability of the amputee to roll over the forefoot during the terminal stance phase.

Single-axis Feet More readily plantar flex from heel strike to foot-flat during the early loading phase of gait, single-axis feet are recommended for the geriatric transfemoral amputee using an unlocked knee when greater knee stability during the early stance phase of gait is desired.

Multiple-axis Feet Accommodating to uneven surfaces, multiple-axis feet are recommended for geriatric patients with sensitive skin, who may benefit from the reduction in shear forces transmitted to the prosthetic socket-skin interface. Typically, this is a heavier prosthetic foot.

Elastic Keel Feet The flexible nature of the elastic keel foot facilitates ambulation by allowing easier rollover at the terminal stance phase of gait. Lightweight designs are available. This prosthesis is appropriate for the moderately active individual.

Dynamic Response Feet Typically more expensive, dynamic response feet are appropriate for an individual with a high activity level. They incorporate foot keels that bend in response to the patient's weight during rollover, then "spring back," providing propulsion during the push-off phase of the gait.

Prosthetic Knees

Insuring knee stability during stance is the highest priority for the geriatric transfemoral-level amputee.

Lightweight versions of the various designs of prosthetic knees are available and are recommended for examination by the elderly amputee.

Manual-locking Knees Maximum knee stability during gait is important, and manual-locking knees provide it, but the resulting gait is the least cosmetic gait because the knee remains in extension during the swing phase.

Weight-activated Friction Knees (Safety Knees) Frequently used with geriatric patients, weight-activated friction knees provide inherent knee stability during the stance phase by locking in response to the patient's weight-bearing, then unlocking allowing the knee to bend during the swing phase, which provides a more natural gait appearance.

Polycentric Knees Inherent alignment stability is provided by polycentric knees, but they are not commonly used by geriatric patients because of their greater weight and complexity.

Hydraulic or Pneumatic Swing-phase Controls A very active individual might consider hydraulic or pneumatic swing-phase controls.

CONCLUSION

Amputations occur with increasing incidence as age rises. The conditions that most commonly necessitate amputation are peripheral vascular disease and complications of diabetes. Because of the high frequency of comorbid conditions in the elderly patient, a comprehensive evaluation is requisite. A preparatory prosthesis is strongly recommended for the geriatric patient because it allows early fitting and thus discourages the secondary complications of immobility. The various types of prosthetic components should be studied, and then chosen to meet the individual patient's needs. The patient's date of birth is less important when considering a prosthesis than is overall wellness, fitness, functional ability and motivation.

SUGGESTED READINGS

Bowker JH, Michael JW. *Atlas of Limb Prosthetics: Surgical, Prosthetic, and Rehabilitation Principles.* St. Louis: Mosby–Year Book; 1992.
Edelstein JE. Lower limb prosthetics. *Top Geriatr Rehabil* 1992; 8:1.
Patrick DG. Prosthetics and geriatric patients. *Phys Ther Today* 1993; 16:4.
Patrick D. Prosthetics. In: Myers R, ed. *Saunders Manual of Physical Therapy Practice.* Philadelphia: W.B. Saunders; 1995: 1121–1182.

VI

PHYSIOLOGY/PATHOLOGY AND
ETHICS OF DEATH AND DYING

Chapter 72

Legal Considerations
Ron Scott, J.D., M.S. (P.T.), O.C.S.

INTRODUCTION

Rehabilitation professionals and support personnel who treat geriatric patients face potential malpractice liability exposure for their conduct, just as health-care professionals do in any other care-delivery setting. The majority of the reported physical therapy health-care malpractice cases published in the legal literature involve geriatric clientele as plaintiffs, or parties bringing legal action against their health-care providers.

The United States is a highly litigious society. In 1992, approximately 19 million new civil lawsuits between private parties were initiated nationwide. Although only a small proportion of these legal cases involved health-care malpractice, the risk of liability exposure in health-care practice generally, and in geriatric rehabilitation practice in particular, is significant. Geriatric rehabilitation professionals must strike a careful balance between providing optimal quality patient care (a prospect made more difficult in the current cost-containment-focused managed care environment) and minimizing their own health-care malpractice liability risk exposure incident to practice.

In geriatric rehabilitation, professional practice in compliance with legal standards also includes knowledge by care-givers of, and compliance with, the Patient Self-Determination Act and state statutory reporting requirements for suspected elder abuse, among a myriad of other relevant laws. Because nearly one third of the population over age 55 is employed, health-care professionals should also be cognizant of laws protective of the employment rights of their geriatric clients, including the Age Discrimination in Employment Act, the Americans with Disabilities Act, and the Family and Medical Leave Act.

HEALTH-CARE MALPRACTICE

Negligence

Health-care malpractice is defined as physical and/or mental injury incurred by a patient in the course of health-care examination or intervention, coupled with a legal basis for imposing civil liability on a health-care provider for the harm suffered by the patient. Traditionally, the only basis for imposing health-care malpractice liability was professional negligence, or substandard care.

In a professional negligence lawsuit brought by a patient against a health-care professional, the patient normally must prove four core elements by a preponderance, or greater weight, of evidence. These four elements are:

- That the defendant health-care professional owed a special duty of care to the plaintiff-patient;
- That, in the course of health-care delivery, the health-care professional breached, or violated, the duty owed, by failing to meet at least minimally acceptable care standards;
- That the breach of duty by the health-care provider caused injury to the patient; and
- That the patient sustained injuries of the type for which a judge or jury may legally order compensation in the form of a money damages judgment, designed to make the patient "whole" again.

In addition to being legally responsible for his or her own conduct, a health-care professional providing geriatric rehabilitation is also normally vicariously, or indirectly, responsible for the conduct of supportive personnel acting under the supervision of the licensed or certified professional. Health-care professionals must clearly communicate orders to support personnel to whom care tasks are delegated, and establish competency standards and actually assess the competency of supportive personnel on an ongoing basis.

Additional Legal Bases for Malpractice

Other legal bases for imposing health-care malpractice liability, in addition to professional negligence, include:

- Intentional misconduct, including battery (injurious or otherwise offensive physical contact with a patient) and sexual battery (physical contact intended to gratify a health-care provider's illicit sexual desires);
- Strict product liability, for patient injury by dangerously defective treatment-related equipment, such as durable medical equipment supplied to a geriatric client; and
- Breach of contract liability, for failure to fulfill a therapeutic promise made to a patient.

Geriatric rehabilitation professionals and clinic and agency managers are advised to develop, educate staff about, and enforce formal risk management policies and procedures designed to minimize health-care malpractice liability exposure of professional employees and organizations. Legal counsel should be consulted proactively for advice on developing and implementing such initiatives.

Consider the following hypothetical example:

A home-health physical therapist is charged by a geriatric patient with sexual battery. In this case involving myofascial release, there was, in fact, no therapist misconduct; the patient was simply confused about the nature of the therapeutic touch and honestly believed it to be improperly applied by the therapist to her torso. What risk management measures should the physical therapist and agency have undertaken to prevent this kind of allegation?

The agency and its professional and support staff should have developed and practiced under a professional-patient relations policy that requires:

1. Patient understanding of and informed consent for intensive hands-on therapy, such as myofascial release and massage;

2. Notification by the treating health-care provider to the patient of the right to have a same-gender chaperone present during treatment (SUCH A POLICY OBLIGATES THE EMPLOYER TO MAKE AVAILABLE A CHAPERONE UPON THE PATIENT'S REQUEST); and

3. Respect by providers for patient autonomy and modesty, including appropriate patient draping procedures prior to and during treatment.

In this scenario, the physical therapist faces primary liability exposure for his or her conduct, and the employing agency possible vicarious liability for the physical therapist-employee's conduct within the scope of employment.

PATIENT INFORMED CONSENT

In any health-care delivery setting, adult patients with full mental capacity have the right to give informed consent before evaluation or intervention. The duty to make relevant information disclosure and obtain patient informed consent to treatment is premised on respect for patient autonomy, or self-determination. Although the exact disclosure requirements for patient informed consent vary from state to state, the following elements are commonly included:

- Disclosure of the patient's diagnosis and relevant information about a proposed intervention;
- Disclosure of serious risks of possible harm or complication associated with a proposed

intervention that would be material to the patient's decision about whether to accept or refuse the intervention;
- Discussion about the expected benefits, or goals, associated with the proposed intervention; and
- Disclosure of reasonable alternatives to a proposed intervention, and their material risks and benefits.
- After the above disclosure elements are discussed with the patient, the provider is additionally obligated to solicit and satisfactorily answer the patient's questions and formally ask for patient consent to proceed before doing so.

It may not be necessary to individually document in patients' records each patient's informed consent for routine care. An agency, institution, or group may elect instead to memorialize an informed consent policy in a policy and procedures document; orient providers upon employment of their informed consent obligations; monitor informed consent processes on an ongoing basis; and reinforce the duty to obtain patients' informed consent with providers on a regularly recurring basis during in-service education.

Managed care "gag clause" employment provisions requiring providers to refrain from discussing with patients care options that are not offered by patients' insurance plans derogate from respect for patient autonomy and the informed consent requirement for disclosure of reasonable alternatives to proposed care options, and are therefore unethical and in many jurisdictions illegal.

REPORTING SUSPECTED ELDER ABUSE

Geriatric rehabilitation professionals have a legal duty to act reasonably to identify elder abuse in their clients and to take appropriate action to prevent further abuse. This may include reporting suspected elder abuse to social service departments or agencies or to law enforcement agencies, as appropriate.

Elder abuse may be less often recognized and reported by health-care professionals than domestic or child abuse. Most state laws on reporting abuse provide for qualified immunity from defamation or other bases of liability for persons making good-faith reports of suspected abuse.

Signs and symptoms of possible elder abuse may be present in a geriatric client and in the client's abuser, who may be present with the client during examination or treatment. Signs and symptoms in the geriatric client may include, among others, unexplained or untreated injuries; reticence; poor hygiene; malnutrition and dehydration; and dirty or inappropriate dress for conditions. Indices of elder abuse in abusers, who may be care-givers or family members, include, among others, aggression toward or verbal abuse of the geriatric patient; speaking for the client during an examination or treatment; and indifference to instructions or suggestions offered by the provider.

Consider the following case:

Mr. Doe is an 83-year-old patient who is status post-right cerebrovascular accident, with mild left upper limb hemiparesis. He has just been referred as an outpatient to ABC Rehab, Inc. His examining physical therapist notices the following about Mr. Doe:

1. He is accompanied by his 51-year old daughter, Sue, who does most of the talking for the patient;

2. He has scratches and petechiae on the dorsal forearms;

3. He is dressed in a Navy pea-coat, long-sleeved shirt, and wool trousers, despite its being June and 78°F.

How should the physical therapist proceed, based on the above information?

Based on the presentation above, Mr. Doe may be a victim of elder abuse. The physical therapist should annotate pertinent objective examination findings in Mr. Doe's health record and should consult with a supervisor or professional colleague about this patient. The therapist may also, as an exercise of professional judgment, report his or her suspicion to the facility's social service department for follow-up. Whether or not a report to social service is made at this time, the physical therapist should closely monitor Mr. Doe for any further indicators of possible abuse.

PATIENT SELF-DETERMINATION ACT

The Patient Self-Determination Act of 1990 (PSDA) is a federal statute that memorializes a patient's right to control routine and extraordinary treatment-related decisions. The PSDA, like the law of patient informed consent, is premised on respect for patient autonomy.

The PSDA does not create any new substantive patient rights; it simply requires health-care facilities—including hospitals and long-term care facilities—to ask patients about any advance directives that they might have in effect and to honor the provisions of those advance directives.

Advance directives are legal instruments that memorialize patients' desires regarding care options in the event of such patients' incapacitation. They are of two basic types: living wills, which spell out patients' wishes concerning the scope of permissible health-care interventions in the event of patient incapacity, and durable powers of attorney for health-care decisions, which empower third parties to act on behalf of incapacitated patients. Patient health records should include information about existing patient advance directives.

EMPLOYMENT PROTECTION FOR OLDER WORKERS

There are three federal statutes that serve primarily to protect the employment interests of older workers. These are the Age Discrimination in Employment Act, the Americans with Disabilities Act, and the Family and Medical Leave Act.

The Age Discrimination in Employment Act of 1967 (ADEA) prohibits employer discrimination against workers age 40 or older. The broad prohibition of discrimination against older workers encompasses nearly all aspects of the employment relationship, from recruitment and selection to training and promotion to employee benefits. Under case law developed after implementation of the ADEA, employers may discharge older workers from employment if such workers contractually waive their ADEA rights in exchange for monetary compensation.

The Americans with Disabilities Act of 1990 (ADA) offers significant protection from discrimination to older workers and patients. Under Title I of the ADA, business organizations having 15 or more workers are prohibited from discriminating against physically or mentally disabled employees, and must provide reasonable accommodation for employees' disabilities that affect their ability to carry out essential functions of their jobs. Title III of the ADA protects the rights of disabled consumers to equal access to public accommodations, including privately owned health-care facilities.

The Family and Medical Leave Act of 1993 (FLMA) requires employers having 50 or more full-time employees to allow employees to take up to 12 weeks per year of unpaid, job-protected leave for personal or familial illness or for adoption or childbirth. Unlike the ADEA and ADA, which are enforced by the federal Equal Employment Opportunity Commission, the FLMA is administered by the federal Department of Labor.

Consider the following scenario:

A 68-year-old rehabilitation client informs a physical therapist during the patient history interview of circumstances that might constitute employment discrimination (age-related discharge) related to the client's disability. What should the therapist do?

Even though the therapist is generally familiar with employment laws, the therapist should not attempt to advise the client about possible legal options. Instead, the therapist should inform the client of the right to seek legal advice with an attorney of choice or through the public service county bar association's legal referral service, which is available in every county and parish in the United States at no cost or for a low charge for initial legal advice.

CONCLUSION

Geriatric rehabilitation professionals must be cognizant of key laws and legal requirements affecting their practice and their clients' civil rights. Under managed care, the rehabilitation milieu has become extremely businesslike and impersonal, making malpractice avoidance more difficult. Clinicians and managers must simultaneously strive for optimal quality patient care and effective clinical risk management in order to survive and thrive.

Knowledge of laws respecting patient autonomy, including the Patient Self-Determination Act concerning patients' advance directives, and of employment protections benefiting elderly clients, enables geriatric rehabilitation professionals to better serve their clients. Legal advice, however, should be given to clients only by attorneys.

The information presented in this chapter is intended as legal information only and not as specific legal advice for any health professional. Individual legal advice can be given only by a person's personal or institutional attorney, based on the distinct laws of the particular jurisdiction (state or federal law, as applicable).

SUGGESTED READINGS

Hyman A, Schillinger D, Lo B. Laws mandating reporting of domestic violence. *JAMA* 1995; 273:1781–1787.
Scott RW. *Health Care Malpractice: A Primer on Legal Issues for Professionals,* 2nd ed. New York: McGraw-Hill; 1998.
Scott RW. *Professional Ethics: A Guide for Rehabilitation Professionals.* St. Louis: Mosby–Year Book; 1998.
Scott RW. *Promoting Legal Awareness in Physical and Occupational Therapy.* St. Louis: Mosby–Year Book; 1997.
Scott RW. *Legal Aspects of Documenting Patient Care.* Gaithersburg, Md.: Aspen Publishers; 1994.

Chapter **73**

Ethics
Mary Ann Wharton, M.S., P.T.

INTRODUCTION

Decisions regarding moral choices—what is right versus what is wrong—are difficult, and they frequently complicate treatment interventions and service delivery in geriatric rehabilitation. These moral decisions are often made more difficult by factors such as ageism, societal attitudes, and available reimbursement for health-care services. This is especially true in the current health-care delivery system, which intermingles patient care with technology, a reimbursement-driven environment, and a societal mandate to conserve health-care dollars. An understanding of ethical principles and theory can provide a framework for analyzing the values involved in moral decision-making in geriatrics.

ETHICS AND MORALITY

Morality is defined by Churchill as "behavior according to custom."[1] It is further defined by Purtilo as guidelines that are designed to preserve the fabric of society.[2] Ethics, on the other hand, can be viewed as "a systematic reflection on and analysis of morality."[2] As such, ethics is based on principles that provide a conceptual framework within which it is possible to place perceptions of ethical cases and problems. These principles allow the imposition of some sense of artificial order on a story, and they affect peoples' response to it. Ethical concepts are tied to society's customs, manners, traditions, and institutions. In essence, these concepts define how members of a society deal with the world.[3]

Professional ethics that arise in the context of health care provide guidelines that are ultimately no different from those that arise from religious, philosophical, cultural, and other societal sources.[2] Ethical situations in geriatrics are no different from the ethical situations in other aspects of health care. Similar reasoning processes should be observed to answer questions of morality when dealing with older individuals.

ETHICAL PRINCIPLES

Ethical principles serve as one tool for solving complex ethical problems. Ethical theories provide a sense of order. They can help to simplify a complicated case for initial problem-solving, and that simplification in itself can be useful in ordering and focusing a wide range of disparate intuitions.[3]

The foundational principles of biomedical ethics that govern geriatric rehabilitation professionals include the following ethical duties and rights:

- Beneficence—the duty to do the best possible,
- Nonmaleficence—the minimal duty to do no harm,
- Justice—the allocation of time and resources, and
- Autonomy—the ethical right of self-determination.

Autonomy

Respect for patient autonomy is an ethical principle that requires further understanding and definition. According to the ethical principle of autonomy, the patient has the right to actively negotiate his or her own health-care decisions. In geriatrics, issues of autonomy may revolve around questions of individual competency to make decisions. Health-care providers must recognize that questions of patient competency are determined legally and are not to be presumed by the professional or by family members or care-givers. One concern specific to the autonomy of the older patient may be the reliance of the professional on family members or care-givers to make decisions for that individual. In situations in which the older client is legally competent to make decisions, the moral appropriateness of consulting such individuals must be determined by the patient himself or herself. This is an especially difficult issue for care-givers when the patient is ill, recovering from surgery or pathological insult, or taking certain medications, all of which can negatively affect the patient's judgment.

One factor that may influence the ability of older individuals to make autonomous health care choices is their own beliefs or expectations regarding health care. Specific factors to consider might include whether they view health care as a right or a privilege. They must also analyze whether they believe that they are a passive recipient of health care versus the more current concept that stresses an individual's responsibility to actively participate in the rehabilitation process.

Informed consent, which provides the legal basis for autonomy, requires patient education according to the "reasonable man standard." Specifically, this standard obligates the health-care professional to provide information in terms understandable to a reasonable individual of like circumstances. Informed consent is recognized as one way to achieve patient adherence.

In the previous chapter, Scott notes that legal disclosure requirements vary from state to state but commonly include the following:

- The patient's diagnosis and pertinent evaluative findings,
- The nature of a proposed or ordered intervention,
- Any material risks for harm or complication associated with the proposed intervention,
- Reasonable alternatives, if any, to the proposed intervention, and
- The goals of the intervention.

Scott goes on to state that the goals of geriatric rehabilitation intervention must be jointly developed and implemented by the patient and the rehabilitation professional. Both parties to the rehabilitation "contract" then feel that they have a stake in achieving an optimal patient outcome (see Chapter 72, "Legal Considerations").

One additional factor to consider with respect to ethics and patient autonomy is the issue of paternalism. Paternalism may be defined as coercion, or interference with another person's freedom of action. It is justified by reasons related to the welfare and happiness of the individual being coerced. In ethics and health care, paternalism stems from the principle that the practitioner should act to bring about the maximum benefit for the patient, even at the expense of the patient's autonomy. It is rooted in the health-care provider's knowledge and professional understanding coupled with the duty of beneficence and the health-care provider's desire to bring about the best outcome. In its extreme, paternalism can result in a violation of autonomy, which is not considered acceptable in this society. On the other hand, contemporary health care may accept gentle paternalism, which combines with informed consent to achieve patient adherence. In geriatrics, questions of competency frequently complicate this issue.[4]

The issues of patient autonomy and paternalism may also be complicated by Medicare or other insurance regulations that require specified treatment times and frequencies. Thus, the ill or depressed patient may be coerced into going to rehabilitation in order to protect Medicare payment benefits, which may be suspended if the patient fails to attend the regulated number of daily hours or treatment days per week, depending upon the treatment setting—rehabilitation unit or skilled nursing facility, respectively. Some medical providers maintain the attitude that the patient may not refuse the required care, which is paternalistic.

FIDELITY, VERACITY, CONFIDENTIALITY

Secondary ethical duties inherent in health care include the following:

- The fidelity/fiduciary relationship, or faithfulness; it entails meeting a patient's reasonable expectations;
- Truth-telling, or veracity and honesty; it obligates a health-care provider not only to the patient but also to other sources such as the reimbursement source, and this is a frequent source of conflict;
- Confidentiality, or the patient's expectation that the health-care provider will honor personal information as private; legal basis for this exists in the concept of the right to privacy.

SOURCES OF CONFLICTS IN GERIATRIC REHABILITATION

Several broad sources of ethical conflicts in geriatric rehabilitation have been outlined in Guccione and Shefrin.[5] They can be listed as follows:

Personal vs. Professional Beliefs In dealing with older patients, a health-care professional must recognize that occasionally a conflict exists between personal feelings about a patient or situation and professional duties. The professional must know how to weigh personal values against professional obligations and responsibilities.

An Interdisciplinary Team's Perceptions and Conflicts Expectations of team members involved in the care of geriatric patients may differ or not be clearly understood. Conflicts may develop regarding the role and responsibility of each professional. It is important that each individual on the team clarify the promises implicit in the commitment to work on an interdisciplinary team.

Organizational and Societal Conflicts Current health care reflects rapid changes in delivery and service models, especially as managed care principles have come to predominate in organizations. Conflict often exists between the health-care professional's obligations to the patient and obligations to the organization. Our society expresses a wide variety of opinions about the attitude that should be taken toward elders. Recent dilemmas involve the allocation of health-care resources, especially the financing of care and the reimbursing for services. Therapists must look at each case on an individual basis and at the same time consider that case in the context of societal issues.

ETHICAL DECISION-MAKING

Purtilo has identified the following five-step process as a tool that can be used to address ethical problems[2]:

1. Gather relevant information,
2. Identify the type of ethical problem,
3. Determine the ethics approach to be used,
4. Explore the practical alternatives, and then
5. Complete the action.

SPECIAL TECHNIQUES TO PROMOTE ETHICAL DECISION-MAKING IN GERIATRIC CARE

A variety of techniques can be used to promote ethical decision-making in geriatric care. Included in these techniques are value histories, use of ethics committees and team conferences, and recognition of legal remedies, including guardianship and power of attorney.[1]

Value History A value history is a summary of a patient's values and beliefs. The information is obtained prior to the onset of a cognitive impairment that impedes the exercise of autonomous judgment. It can also be constructed with the help of family members or significant others. This tool helps to preserve respect for the individual patient and his or her autonomy.

Ethics Committees Groups of individuals in an institution may be identified as an ethics committee. Such committees have the authority to facilitate the resolution of ethical dilemmas in health care. They can develop policy and guidelines, provide consultation and case review, offer theological reflection, and educate others in the institution regarding matters of morality. Membership varies and often is determined by the purpose of the committee. Generally, membership includes attorneys, clergy, ethicists, medical practitioners, and community representatives. Specific limits of authority vary, depending on the policy developed by the institution. One model specifies optional consultation with the committee, leaving compliance with their recommendations to the discretion of the professionals involved in the case. Another model specifies mandatory review of certain decisions, for example, those regarding life support measures, but continues to allow professionals to retain their authority in the final decision. A third model dictates mandatory review by the ethics committee and mandatory compliance with its conclusions.

Team Conferences The interdisciplinary team may be used for additional input when ethical issues about patients must be addressed. In order to effectively consider issues of morality and value as they affect geriatric patient care, both patients and appropriate family members and care-givers should be included on the team.

Legal Remedies

1. Guardianship: a mechanism that allows a surrogate or surrogates to exercise rights for an older person who is no longer mentally competent.
2. Power of Attorney: a form of voluntary guardianship in which a competent individual freely appoints a surrogate decision-maker. The decision may be invalidated automatically in some states if the individual becomes incompetent, but some states recognize a durable power of attorney, which does not expire if an individual becomes mentally incompetent. The authority of a durable power of attorney can include the ability to make health-care decisions.

The Relationship of Ethical and Legal Obligations

Scott, in Chapter 72, summarized the relationship between ethical and legal obligations. He states that in geriatric rehabilitation, discipline-specific professional codes of ethics govern the official conduct of members of that discipline if they are members of the professional association that promulgates and enforces the ethics rules. Rule of law, on the other hand, governs the conduct of all members of society. Currently, in health care the ethical duties and law have become blended to the point where they are often interchangeable. For example, it is a violation of civil and criminal law and of health-professional ethical mandates to commit sexual battery upon a patient. Similar parallels exist in the commission of health-care fraud, professional practice without the requisite license or certification, and other activities of clinical practice.

SPECIAL AREAS OF ETHICAL CONCERN IN GERIATRIC REHABILITATION

Discharge Planning

Complex ethical concerns can be identified with respect to discharge planning in geriatric rehabilita-

tion. Typically, discharge involves transition from a hospital to a site of continuing care. It also can be viewed as a transition from illness to rehabilitation and health. Ethical conflicts can be identified in relation to patient autonomy and involvement in the decision-making process. Additionally, ethical concerns may be identified with respect to discharge plans as they impact on the interests of multiple parties, including the patient, the family, the health-care providers, the institution, the reimbursement sources, the referral sources, and society itself. Specific concerns arise in the context of the current health-care delivery system, which is based on prospective payment systems with defined lengths of stay and managed care principles designed to control the expenditure of health-care dollars.

One variable in discharge planning may be that the health-care providers' prescription for long-term care may not show sufficient respect for individual autonomy. Typically, an individual's ability to participate in any decision-making process is determined, at least in part, by performance on mental status examinations. These exams, although considered reliable in judging mental capacity, are of limited value in judging capacity to make complex decisions related to discharge. Of primary importance is that such exams fail to account for an elderly individual's ability to function in the community, based on social ability and the strength of support networks, in spite of the fact that both of these factors are strong predictors of success in community living. An ethical decision related to discharge that truly accounts for patient autonomy should include some prediction of the individual's ability to address the challenges of independent living.[6]

Another factor that complicates the ethics of discharge plans is that every decision affects the rights of many people and must account for competing obligations. It is widely recognized that the elderly individual has the moral and legal right to decide autonomously what is appropriate, but the impact of that decision on the rights, duties, and obligations of family members must also be considered. Specifically, the patient's goal must be accommodated to the family's ability and willingness to help, if such support is part of the proposed discharge plan. Conversely, the rights of family members must not have more influence on the discharge plan than the rights of the older patient. One temptation is to consult and address the needs of family members while virtually ignoring the decision-making right and ability of the older individual, even when that individual is capable of involvement in the process.

From an administrative standpoint, discharge involves balancing the good of the patient against other goods, including the needs of the hospital and of society. Conflicts may arise between the financial interests of the institutions and society and the welfare of the patients. These are especially evident when financial considerations are viewed in light of the mission of the institution and its administrative obligations to the staff and the community. The Code of Ethics of the American College of Hospital Administrators specifically addresses such conflicts of interest by stating that the welfare of the individual must prevail. The code, however, is silent on issues of conflicts in administrative obligations. Therefore, an underlying motivation in effecting discharge or transfer of a patient from an institution may be the administrative obligation to ensure that the institution remains viable. This obligation may be seen to supersede the obligations of the institution to the community, the medical staff, and even the patient. As a result, needs of individual patients may play a relatively minor role in ethical frameworks espoused by administrators. Rather, in this context, a patient's needs are balanced against the needs and interests of others. This may pose an ethical dilemma to those care-givers directly involved in effecting an appropriate discharge plan for an individual patient.[7]

Discharge plans that involve placement in long-term care are often among the most difficult. The health delivery system provides the older individual with little opportunity to choose either the site of care or its details. Such decisions are often made by discharge planners or social workers who have little opportunity to consult with the individual patient. Frequently, the discharge plan is determined without discussing the circumstances with the patient and is based on the physician's judgment that the older patient "needs 24-hour care." Additionally, the patient is rarely informed that the primary purpose of the discharge planner is to facilitate prompt discharge while automatically following rules for referral to postacute care settings. The older individual is expected to make a critical life decision with inadequate time and information and may be being advised by professionals who have not fully disclosed the constraints imposed on them by their jobs. Furthermore, little consideration is given to the individual's right to make an informed, autonomous decision to return home when that decision is considered risky or hazardous by the physician or health-care team. This is often the result not only of the health-care professionals' desire to do what they know is best for the patient, but also of the fear of litigation resulting from the adverse outcome of a risky discharge decision.[8]

Ethics and Long-Term Care

Long-term care, in current health services delivery, refers to a broad range of services that are available to assist an individual who has functional impairments. These services can include personal care, social support, and health-related services. Settings for the provision of long-term care include an individual's home as well as a variety of institutional settings. The same ethical issues described above arise in the care of any older person receiving long-term care.

As noted previously, a primary ethical concern in decisions about long-term care involves the admission process itself. Frequently, decisions are made with little respect for patient autonomy. An individual may be denied the right to choose what is perceived as a risk-laden choice (to remain at home), and that may be a violation of his or her autonomy. In order to preserve autonomy and allow a patient to return home, he or she must understand the risks and consequences and must also understand that the decision should not have an adverse impact on the rights of others.

Another consideration in long-term care is the issue of privacy and dignity. Providers of geriatric rehabilitation services must be cognizant of individual dignity when assisting with personal-care services such as bathing and toileting. In institutional settings, sensitivity to issues of privacy and dignity must be heightened, as the environment, by its nature, is not conducive to either. Examples of situations that may lead to violation of these rights include multiple-occupancy rooms, responsiveness to call buttons, and the use of first names without permission from the patient.

Rehabilitation in long-term care may evoke ethical dilemmas unique to that setting. By definition, rehabilitation implies fostering maximum patient independence in functional tasks. Geriatric patients seek long-term care precisely because they are dependent to some degree. An ethical challenge exists between respecting a patient's autonomy and complying with his or her request for help and encouraging independence. In a broader sense, a similar challenge may exist in decisions related to protecting a patient from risky situations such as falls or adverse health events. Health-care providers must determine when a person needing care should be allowed to consciously choose a course that professionals consider risky in order to maximize values versus allowing a patient to be unattended and potentially unsafe.

The lack of patient autonomy in long-term-care living environments may be the result of the care-givers' and administrators' roles, their job descriptions, the physical environment, and the regulations that govern these institutions. Administrators and staff may be trained to be task-oriented, which provides little opportunity to consider autonomy or even clients' involvement in daily decisions about their own care. The physical environment is often one of little space for storage of clothing and personal possessions, minimal security for personal items, and limited privacy. Care plans and routines dominate the timing and the content of daily activities. Regulations, although designed to protect the welfare and safety of residents, frequently discourage residents' participation in decision-making and often allow for little freedom of choice. Examples include restrictions on what residents can keep in their rooms, requirements about supervision and the charting of patient activity, and safety requirements. Conversely, some regulations may enhance patient autonomy, such as those that mandate the availability of consumer information, enforce privacy regulations, and place limits on the use of restraints.[8]

Restraints

The use of restraints in the care of the elderly poses several ethical and legal questions that must be addressed by health-care providers. A restraint is defined as any device that restricts freedom of movement. The rationale for restraint use with the elderly is frequently cited as prevention of injury to self or others, but many times the underlying motivation is fear of institutional liability.

When considering the use of restraints to control a patient for safety or because of behavior, the rehabilitation professional must be cognizant of the fact that the literature reports little scientific basis to support the efficacy of restraints in safeguarding patients from harm. In fact, adverse effects cited in relation to restraint use include such consequences as reduced functional capacity secondary to immobilization, as well as physiological changes including contractures, decreased muscle mass and strength, loss of bone integrity, decubitus ulcers, and adverse psychological response to stress. It should also be noted that, with respect to geriatric rehabilitation, the use of restraints is inconsistent with and frequently in conflict with the goals of rehabilitation.

Hieleman identifies several issues that must be addressed when weighing the option of using restraints:[9]

- informed consent,
- risk versus benefit analysis,
- determination of competency,
- the resident's rights and empowerment, and
- risk reduction.

It should be noted that the use of restraints without the patient's informed consent may be legally restricted. The Omnibus Budget Reconciliation Act of 1987 (OBRA) regulations strongly imply that nursing facilities must obtain informed consent for whatever approach is taken to effect resident safety. Also, the Fourteenth Amendment to the U.S. Constitution guarantees freedom from harm and unnecessary restraints.[10]

It may be ethically permissible to override the refusal of a competent patient to apply a mechanical restraint if that individual is jeopardizing the safety and welfare of others. In such cases, the ethical principle of preventing harm to others supersedes the patient's right to refuse, and the negative rights of an individual to be free of interference ends as the autonomy of others is violated. In this case, the professional must balance professional responsibility to an individual patient with societal and legal obligations to protect the public health.[10]

If restraints are used as a punitive measure, there is no ethical justification for their application. Such a practice would be defined as abusive.

When the use of restraints is consistent with treatment goals, their application may be ethically indicated. One example is when a restraint such as wrist cuffs is applied to prevent interference with a life-sustaining treatment such as a nasogastric tube. In such cases, it should be emphasized, the treatment goal is to restore the patient to health.[10]

Managed Care

Managed health care poses special challenges in geriatric rehabilitation and ethics. One consideration is the managed care organization, structure, and function itself. In the managed care structure, there are multiple actors with incompatible interests. For example, the rehab provider has a fiduciary responsibility to patients but may also be an employee of or contractor with the organization. The organization itself may have legal and financial obligations to shareholders to maintain low cost, yet an ethical obligation to patients to provide quality care.

Another current source of ethical conflict is the morality of market-driven health care, which has the potential to threaten professionalism. The introduction of market-driven practices into health care may divide professional loyalties between providing the best treatments in order to improve the patient's quality of life and keeping expenses to a minimum by limiting services, increasing efficiency, and lessening the amount of time spent with each patient. The result may be that the professional must chose between best interests of the patient and economic survival. Frequently, reimbursement drives the care.

The integrity of the patient/provider relationship may also be threatened in the current health-care delivery climate. Focus on the patient is the primary concern of health care. Managed care, however, may threaten this relationship through policies that deny access to care, restrict the professional's ability to perform tests, and withhold or limit treatment. Such policies create conflicting loyalties and undermine trust between provider and patient. The provider may be in the dual and potentially conflicting positions of being guardian of society's resources and being a primary advocate for the individual patient.[11–13] With respect to geriatric patients, it can be stated that ethically the profession may not be able to afford to rehabilitate someone who is about to die—in which case rehabilitation would not be effective anyway. On the other hand, it is imperative that the profession never withhold treatment just because a person is old. The difficulty is determining who is ready to die and who may benefit, and how much, from rehabilitation efforts.

Managed care may impact on the ethical principle of patient autonomy, and it potentially threatens the patient's freedom of choice. When health-care coverage is provided as an employee or retirement benefit, the employee's choice may be even more restricted. In order to take advantage of health-care coverage as a benefit, the employee or retiree is often forced to accept a plan that limits service access and doesn't meet health-care needs. A person has the responsibility of understanding the terms of his or her own health-care plan.[13, 14]

Finally, one more factor related to patient autonomy is the perceived right to have all treatment choices funded. It is paramount to acknowledge that autonomy does not guarantee funding. Rather, some balance must be achieved between conserving society's health-care dollars and paying for individual health-care needs. Providers and elderly patients must recognize that autonomy also entails responsibility. It obligates individuals to use resources wisely, to assist in conserving resources, and to live a healthy lifestyle.

Elder Abuse

Abuse of the elderly may take many forms, from causing actual physical harm or mental anguish to denial of needed medical and social services to financial exploitation. Abusive behavior toward the elderly may come from family members, care-givers, or health-care providers themselves. Often, the abuse may not be overt or intentional, but may stem from personal and professional values, including the desire to protect the elderly patient at the expense of his or her right to make autonomous choices.

One ethical consideration that must be acknowl-edged when health-care providers become aware of actual abuse is the need to maintain a balance between sensitivity to patient trust and the need to abide by regulatory statutes that mandate reporting. This is especially important if knowledge of the abusive situation was gained through confidential disclosure of information.[5]

As recognized previously, components of elder abuse must be acknowledged in discharge planning, use of restraints, and denial of services enforced through regulations and managed care.

CONCLUSION

Ethical concerns and sources of conflict abound in regard to the rehabilitation of the geriatric patient. It is imperative that the health-care practitioner who works with elders be sensitive to these issues, understand the underlying ethical principles, acknowledge the legal basis of these principles, and incorporate moral values into the decision-making process.

REFERENCES

1. Henderson ML, McConnell ES. Ethical considerations. In: Matteson MA, McConnell ES. *Gerontological Nursing Concepts and Practice*. Philadelphia: W.B. Saunders; 1988.
2. Purtilo R. *Ethical Dimensions in the Health Professions*, 2nd ed. Philadelphia: W. B. Saunders; 1993.
3. Elliott C. Where ethics comes from and what to do about it. *Hastings Cent Rep* 1992; 22:28–35.
4. Weiss GB. Paternalism modernized. *J Med Ethics* 1985; 11:184–187.
5. Guccione AA, Shefrin DH. Ethical and legal issues in geriatric physical therapy. In: Guccione AA, ed. *Geriatric Physical Therapy*. St. Louis: Mosby–Year Book; 1993.
6. Dubler NN. Improving the discharge planning process: distinguishing between coercion and choice. *Gerontologist* 1988; 28 [suppl]:76–81.
7. Spielman BJ. Financially motivated transfers and discharges: administrators' ethics and public expectations. *J Med Humanities Bioeth* 1988; 9:32–43.
8. Kane RA. Ethics and long-term care. *Clin Geriatr Med* 1994; 10:489–499.
9. Hieleman F. Restraint reduction in nursing facilities: the issues involved in decision-making. *Geri-topics* 1991; 14:26–27.
10. Moss RJ, La Puma J. The Ethics of Mechanical Restraints. *Hastings Cent Rep* 1991; 21:22–25.
11. Kassirer JP. Managed care and the morality of the marketplace. *N Engl J Med* 1995; 33:50–52 [editorial].
12. Rodwin MA. Conflicts in managed care. *N Engl J Med* 1995; 332:604–607.
13. Council on Ethical and Judicial Affairs, American Medical Association. Ethical issues in managed care. *JAMA* 1995; 273:338–339 [comment].
14. Emanuel EJ, Dubler NN. Preserving the physician-patient relationship in the era of managed care. *JAMA* 1995; 273:338–339 [comment].

Chapter **74**

Physical Therapy and the Generational Conflict

Timothy L. Kauffman, Ph.D., P.T.

INTRODUCTION

The conflict between the older generation and the younger generation is an age-old problem. The issue is particularly poignant in societies and nations that do not venerate their seniors. Physical therapy care in an aging world population was the subject of an editorial 10 years ago in which T.F. Williams, former Director of the National Institute of Aging, was quoted as saying, "Of all human beings who have ever lived on the earth and have reached age 65 years, the majority are alive today."[1] "This statement holds significant implications for the society in general and especially for health-care providers and their aged patients."[2] By now, everyone has heard the demographic litany about the increasingly aging population and the rising costs of caring for the elderly. The problem that we, as a civilization, face is how to handle this growing dilemma, both fiscally and ethically.

PARTISAN POLITICS

A member of the U.S. House of Representatives addressed a group of physical therapists at the 1996 Combined Sections Meeting of the American Physical Therapy Association. He presented a scenario in which a family had a choice between health-care for a terminally ill mother or more money for the discretionary use of the younger family members through tax savings derived from reduced health-care benefits for Medicare patients and pensioners. The Congressman insisted that we must cut the health-care benefits, even though it is cold-hearted, because we must offer hope and a future (which is being "warm-hearted") to our children and grandchildren. This simplistic either/or verbiage is the source of an increasingly intense generational conflict that pits one generation against another.

Dollars, ecus, yen, and the other monetary units drive this conflict, aided by partisan politics, abuse of elders by the media,[3] and sensationalism. Political concerns about health-care costs are heard around the world, especially in countries with aging populations. The Social Democratic Party (SPD) in

Adapted and reprinted with permission from Physiotherapy Theory and Practice 1996; 12:193–196.

Germany is campaigning for true health-care reform, and a member of the German Bundestag was recently describing the same generational conflict between young and old. The year 1993 was declared the European Year of Older People and Solidarity between Generations in order to highlight the challenges and focus on finding solutions to this phenomenon of aging.[4]

DEMOGRAPHICS

The need to grapple with these demographic and financial issues is very real, for estimates indicate that approximately 25% of the population of Europe has reached pension age and it is thought that this increase in the percentage of aging persons will continue.[5] Within the European Union, the country with the highest percentage of aging persons is France; Belgium, Germany, and Italy have a greater number of old (60 years plus) persons than young (under 19 years old). Across the European Union, 80% of social protection expenditures are for old-age pensioners.[6]

In the United Kingdom, between 1983 and 1993, the total population had increased by 3%. But the number of persons 65 years old and older had increased by 8%, the number in the 75 to 84 age group had increased by 13%, and in the group that included people 85 and over, the increase was 50%. Expenditures (1993–1994) for those over 65 years of age, who are only 1 of 7 in the population, accounted for 45.5% of U.K. Department of Social Services expenditures and 40.5% of U.K. Department of Health expenditures.[7]

A similar trend is occurring in the United States, where the over-85 age group is growing the fastest.[8] Adding to the Medicare problem is the looming postwar baby-boom cohort, which reaches retirement age beginning in 2010. Compounding the problem further is the fact that the U.S. birth rate reached unprecedented lows in the mid-1970s,[9] which means the taxpaying workforce will be smaller when the mandated social costs are likely to be the highest ever. Projected Medicare costs, using 1987 dollars, will nearly double by the year 2020.[8]

POLITICAL STALEMATE IN THE UNITED STATES

The zenith of the generational conflict in the United States occurred in November of 1995, when the American people suffered through the debacle of the closing down of the U.S. government because it was announced by some that Medicare, the American old-age health-care system, would be bankrupt by the year 2000 or shortly thereafter. The impasse occurred because of partisan political maneuvering by a Congress that wanted to cut costs and to eliminate the U.S. federal debt in order to save something for future generations. Blocking this move was President Clinton, who wanted to protect the health-care benefits for the elderly.

It is a profound truth that democratic governments built on consensus and compromise must painfully allocate limited resources to numerous mandated, needy, and exigent programs and projects.

Former Soviet Bloc

The difficulty of developing workable and ethical solutions to problems of health-care and aging may be greater in the countries of the former Soviet bloc. The paternalistic system of government provided many social supports for retirees, including free health-care and medications. In the present period of transition, the rehabilitation possibilities in Hungary, for example, are limited by few resources and few health-care specialists, which may account for the extensive use of medication there.[10]

PARADIGM SHIFT

The drawing here, by the German artist B. Stolz, illustrates the problem by depicting the weight (or burden) of the young and the old resting upon the shoulders of healthy young working adults. The question to be answered is, Must the generational difference be viewed as an either/or situation? The answer is no. What if the headlines of the newspapers reported that nearly 100% of education costs go to persons under the age of 19 years? Should pensioners in the United Kingdom stop paying community charges and other taxes that benefit younger persons? Public education in the United States is funded largely by real estate taxes on property owners. Some fixed-income Medicare retirees must sell their homes because they can no longer afford their real estate taxes.

Harbingers of doom aside, not all the information is catastrophic. First, although the population of the world is aging, there is some indication that the rate of increase of aging is starting to decline. Second, the morbidity of the aging population is being compressed into a shorter time period.[11] Of persons in the United States over the age of 85, 80% are *not* living in nursing homes, and half of the over-85 patients in nursing homes are there because of chronic conditions that have definable and modifiable antecedent risk factors.[11] This means

that people are living longer and healthier lives. This, it is hoped, will reduce the per capita cost. That is, adding years to life does not automatically mean adding excessive cost to the system.

Lubitz and associates[12] took a sample of actual 1990 Medicare costs and simulated lifetime costs for persons who became Medicare beneficiaries in 1990 and for people who will enter the system in 2020. These writers suggested that the effect of increased longevity on Medicare cost per individual may be minimal, (even though the overall costs will, of course, increase because of the greater number of enrollees). Physical therapy, both rehabilitative and preventive, is integral to the compression of morbidity and, thus, to the control of costs.

The trend toward home health-care,[5] which clearly should involve rehabilitation care, may help to reduce costs to the system and possibly to preserve individual dignity and family integrity,[13] but the trend is not without problems. It shifts the costs to families, which already provide the majority of care for the elderly,[14] and it may increase stress on the care-givers. Recognizing these increased bur-

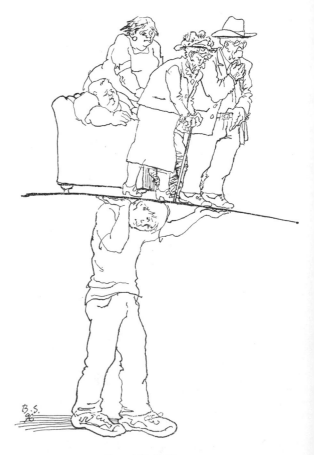

Bernd Stolz 96

dens on families, a plan was designed in Germany to help families offset these additional costs, but the demand exceeded what the system could manage.[15] Also, family structures are changing as more women enter the workforce, and social and international mobility are increasing.[16] Better screening of individuals through the use of a geriatric intermediate-care facility may help to predict those who are likely to be discharged to home and, thus, to prevent institutionalization. However, this study conducted in Japan did not deal with the changing structure of the family and workforce.[17]

The Role of Health-care Providers

Health-care providers are very much involved in the entire process. We are involved as care-givers with our patients and our families. We are involved as researchers hoping to find better ways of providing the best possible care within the social structures and financial constraints of each country, and we share that information through this text and many others. We are involved as citizens, hoping that our governments will listen to our needs and the needs of our patients. We are seeking the wisdom and the ability to amalgamate our personal interests with our professional interests and the interests of our societies. However, Robert Binstock, past president of the Gerontological Society of America, reminds us of an enduring and universal truth: "Politics, not research, will resolve value conflicts regarding the nature and extent of hardship and what actions, if any, governments should undertake to alleviate hardships."[18] Maybe we need to remind our politicians that "When, due to financial restrictions, resources are allocated in a hard and pitiless manner, society's response to its vulnerable old and ill members becomes an even greater sign of its humaneness."[13]

No Easy Answers

The determination to remain independent despite the travails of age-related pathology and the fear of becoming a burden on family and society, is an attitude that correlates with the compression of morbidity. This phenomenon of aging has forced society to consider issues like advance directives or living wills and do-not-resuscitate orders. Hesse[19] reported that in persons 85 years old and older, during terminal hospitalizations, there have been significant declines in high-intensity medical interventions such as cardiopulmonary resuscitation, invasive tests, and minor surgery. Requiring consent-to-treatment may reduce undesired and costly medical and surgical interventions. Palliative care *must* be maintained out of human decency and this requires physical therapy for comfort and for pain control. At this time, there is very little support for the highly emotional subjects of euthanasia, deliberate acts that lead directly to death, or assisted suicide, the provision to a knowing patient of medical means to cause self-death. Civilization must continue to wrestle with these issues, especially as we enter this Age of Aging.

CONCLUSION

The issues of generational conflict are not new and they need not be magnified. The biblical story of Abraham and Isaac serves as a concluding comment. Abraham, a centenarian, was tempted by God to sacrifice his only son, Isaac, who was then only a lad. Abraham instructed his servants to wait for him and Isaac and stated, "We will return." Seeing the wood, fire, and knife, Isaac asked, "Where is the lamb?" Abraham answered, "God will provide himself a lamb" (Genesis 22:1–13, Authorized [King James] Version). The important message is that Abraham never lost sight of what he needed to do, and a desirable solution to his dilemma was reached. As this world ages, the solution will be found by young people and old people working together for the common good. We, as health-care providers, must be participants in that solution.

REFERENCES

1. Williams TF. The future of aging. *Arch Phys Med Rehabil* 1987; 68:335–338.
2. Kauffman T. Physiotherapy as the world ages. *Physiother Pract* 1988; 4:61–62.
3. Cohen GD. Journalistic elder abuse: it's time to get rid of fictions, get down to facts. *Gerontologist* 1994; 34:399–401.
4. Jamieson A. The role of the European Union in promoting healthy ageing. *Soc Sci Med* 1994; 39:1497–1499.
5. Dall JLC. The greying of Europe. *Br Med J* 1994; 309:1282–1285.
6. Watson R. Making the most of ageing populations. *Br Med J* 1995; 310:554.
7. Impallomeni M, Starr J. The UK Community Care Act (1990) and the elderly. *Lancet* 1994; 344:1230.
8. Schneider EL, Guralnik JM. The aging of America *JAMA* 1990; 263:2335–2340.
9. Ycas MA. The challenge of the 21st century: innovating and adapting social security systems to economic, social, and demographic changes in the English-speaking Americas. *Soc Secur Bull* 1994; 57:3–9.
10. Blasszauer B. Institutional care of the elderly. *Hastings Cent Rep* 1994; 24:14–17.
11. Fries, JF. The sunny side of aging. *JAMA* 1990; 263:2354–2355.
12. Lubitz J, Beebe J, Baker C. Longevity and Medicare expenditures. *N Engl J Med* 1995; 332:999–1003.

13. Allert G, Sponholz G, Baitsch H. Chronic disease and the meaning of old age. *Hastings Cent Rep* 1994; 24:11–13.
14. Topinková E. Care for elders with chronic disease and disability. *Hastings Cent Rep* 1994; 24:18–20.
15. Karcher H. Germany's home care scheme faces problems. *Br Med J* 1995; 310:1025.
16. McCormick WC, Rubenstein LZ. International common denominators in geriatric rehabilitation and long-term care. *J Am Geriatr Soc* 1995; 43:714–715.
17. Ishizaki T, et al. Factors influencing users' return home on discharge from a geriatric intermediate care facility in Japan. *J Am Geriatr Soc* 1995; 43:623–626.
18. Binstock R. Perspectives on measuring hardship: concepts, dimensions, and implications. *Gerontologist* 1986; 26:60.
19. Hesse, KA. Changes in the way we die. *Arch Intern Med* 1995; 155:1513–1518.

Chapter **75**

Medicare

Timothy L. Kauffman, Ph.D., P.T.

INTRODUCTION

In the United States, the rehabilitation of geriatric patients takes place largely within the Medicare and Medicaid systems. As the population ages, the systems have become an increasingly partisan political battleground with a moderate to high level of distrust, frustration, and confusion among the various players on the field, including the beneficiaries and their advocates, lobbyists, and families; the care providers, both individuals and institutions; the insurance companies; and the politicians and regulatory bureaucrats.

There is some justification for this sociopolitical quagmire because the Medicare and Medicaid systems are large, changing, and expensive. Over 38 million people, or approximately one out of seven Americans, are covered by the Medicare system, and Medicaid covers over 32 million beneficiaries, of whom over half are children. Medicare accounts for about one third of all payments to hospitals and one fifth of payments to physicians. In 1996, over $200 billion were spent by the Medicare system; that accounts for approximately 2.3% of the gross domestic product. The alarm about Medicare costs and expenditures has been ringing for over a decade because of the looming demographic shift of the initial wave of postwar baby boomers reaching Medicare age in the year 2011. The good news is that the average rise in Medicare costs has been on the decline since its inception. In its first 10 years, the average increase in Medicare costs was approximately 17%. This decreased to 16% from the middle 1970s to the middle 1980s, and it is projected to be 8% from the middle 1990s to the year 2005.

HISTORY

The bill that initiated the Medicare program was signed into law by President Lyndon Johnson on 30 July 1965. Symbolically, he signed the bill at the Truman Library in Independence, Missouri, because President Harry Truman had publicly endorsed and fought for government health insurance in the 1940s and 1950s. Interestingly, at that time, then-Senator Lyndon Johnson was only one of several southern Democratic senators who supported President Truman's legislative effort. Truman's ideas were not new, as they were based on European hospital insurance models that were shaped at the turn of the century. Truman's proposals were defeated by Congress in 1951, but the tenets were debated and reworked during the Eisenhower administrations, which offered scaled-down alternatives under the name "medicare."

As President, John Kennedy determined that hospital health-care for the aged was "must" legislation. Introduced by Representative Cecil King (D, CA) and Senator Clinton Anderson (D, NM), the bill was blocked by opponents, including Senator Wilbur Mills (D, AR). Kennedy's death and Johnson's landslide victory in 1964 led to a new make-up of Congress. By then, Mills not only supported the Anderson-King Bill (hospital insurance, now known as Medicare Part A), he also expanded it to outpatient services (now known as Medicare Part B). Thus, Title XVIII of the Social Security Act became the law of the land and the Medicare system went into effect 11 months later on 1 July 1966.

The Medicaid legislation was also enacted in 1965 as Title XIX to provide for a combined federal and state program for poor families. Medicaid covers children and some long-term care service, but it varies with the state.

THE KEY PLAYERS

The American government is based on a system of checks and balances, so it should be no surprise that this comes into play within the Medicare system, too. The key players are in all three branches of the government, as shown in Figure 75–1. First of all, Congress enacted the legislation that authorized the Medicare system. Congress can and does alter the system by passing new laws; indeed, the Balanced Budget Act of 1997 is likely to have a strong impact on geriatric rehabilitation.

A second and equal player is the Chief Execu-

The Medicare System

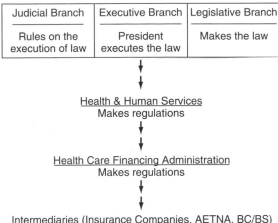

Judicial Branch	Executive Branch	Legislative Branch
Rules on the execution of law	President executes the law	Makes the law

↓
↓

Health & Human Services
Makes regulations

↓
↓

Health Care Financing Administration
Makes regulations

↓
↓

Intermediaries (Insurance Companies, AETNA, BC/BS)
Interpret and enforce regulations

Figure 75–1 The key players in the Medicare System are in all three branches of the federal government.

tive, or President, who signs the legislative bills into laws. The President is responsible for executing the law. This is done by asking the appropriate executive branch department to implement the wishes of Congress. In 1965 it was the Secretary of Health, Education and Welfare, John Gardner, who was responsible for promulgating the regulations to implement the grand idea of providing health-care to elderly Americans. In 1980, during the Jimmy Carter administration, the Department of Health, Education and Welfare was dismantled and the new Health and Human Services Department emerged. Thus, the law comes from the Congress and the regulations come from the Department of Health and Human Services. Most changes in the Medicare system now take place through the regulatory process.

Shortly after the inception of the Medicare system, the Department of Health, Education and Welfare recognized that it did not have expertise in administering the financial aspect of federally mandated health-care programs. Thus, the Health Care Financing Administration (HCFA) became a new federal agency, and it now oversees all of the financial aspects of the Medicare and Medicaid systems and the regulatory process. In today's health-care arena it does appear at times that HCFA's purpose is to control costs, not to assist in the delivery of care.

HCFA is not designed as an insurance company, so it contracts with private insurance companies to administer the Medicare regulations and to handle the reimbursement and health-care delivery processes. These fiscal intermediaries, or insurance companies, also reinterpret and implement the Medicare regulations that come from the Department of Health and Human Services and from HCFA. The intermediaries will, at times, release guidelines for implementing the regulations.

There is no single fiscal intermediary for the entire Medicare system. Thus, the interpretation of the regulations is not uniform. This causes some confusion among care providers and patients, especially as they move from one location to another in the United States. Further confounding the situation is the tendency toward larger and larger business organizations for health-care delivery; thus, one may be providing rehabilitation services in Massachusetts when the Medicare intermediary is located in Tennessee. Also, the health-care provider companies may further refine and make declarations in writing concerning what is coverable or allowable according to their interpretations of the intermediary guidelines or HCFA regulations.

Several other government agencies are involved in overseeing the implementation of the Medicare system, too. They are the United States General Accounting Office (GAO) which is occasionally funded to review the system to determine its appropriateness. For example, the GAO released a report (GAO/HRD—87–91) in July of 1987 that has had a profound effect upon geriatric rehabilitation; it said that rehabilitation services were being paid for by the Medicare system without receipt of adequate information. This was the major justification for the tightening of requirements for documentation. Another very important report (GAO/PEMD—93–97) was released by the GAO in August of 1993; it found that the methods being used by four Medicare carriers to pay claims under the supplemental medical insurance program, or Medicare Part B, were not effective in determining whether the medical care was appropriate or not. Thus, since this report, greater emphasis has been placed on establishing medical necessity.

Also, the Office of the Inspector General of the Department of Health and Human Services is at times called upon to review the implementation of the Medicare system. Additionally, the Office of Management and Budget and the Congressional Budget Office are involved in auditing the Medicare programs and forecasting future expenses.

A third equal player in the Medicare system is the judiciary branch, as lawsuits are brought by Medicare beneficiaries or plaintiffs against the Medicare system. A major case was the Fox v. Bowen decision in 1986 which had a profound impact upon outpatient geriatric rehabilitation by implementing screens or edits which delimited the length and number of treatments allowable according to diagnosis.

SOCIAL SECURITY TRUST FUNDS

As mentioned above, during the historic debate over the Medicare legislation, the initial thrust was to provide hospital insurance, with acute-care benefits in mind. This is administered under the Hospital Insurance Trust Fund (HI) and is best recognized as Medicare Part A. Currently, Medicare beneficiaries are required to pay $764.00 as a deductible for the first day in the hospital. After 61 days, a copayment is implemented at $191.00 until day 90, after which the copayment increases to $382.00. HI, or Medicare Part A, also pays for "inpatient" care and services provided in a patient's home if there is reasonable rehabilitation potential and the patient is currently homebound. This will be discussed in further detail later.

As mentioned above in its historic context, the Medicare Part B system, or Supplemental Medical Insurance (SMI), was added to the legislative effort late in the process. It provided for outpatient services. In addition to these two social security trust funds, there are the Old Age and Survivors Insurance (OASI) and Disability Insurance. The most well-recognized social security payment system falls under the OASI program. This is the program to which employers and employees contribute and, upon retirement, or if the worker dies, payment is made to the employee or to his or her survivors, respectively. At the present time, one can retire at age 65 and receive full social security benefits; the age will rise to age 67 by the year 2027. The OASI, or social security fund, currently brings in more money through payroll deduction taxes than it spends. This payroll deduction tax is 6.2% which is deducted from employees' wages, plus an additional 6.2%, which is contributed by employers. This amounts to a payroll deduction tax of 12.4% to support the OASI. Further, the Medicare Hospital Insurance Trust Fund is supported by an additional payroll deduction tax amounting to 2.9%, which is split evenly between the employee and the employer, coming to a contribution of 1.45% from each. At this time the Hospital Insurance Trust Fund for Medicare Part A is also solvent but is the focus of major political and public discussion.

The Medicare Part B system, or SMI trust fund, is supported by the payment of premiums by beneficiaries. Typically, when an individual turns 65 years of age he or she is able to receive retirement benefits under the OASI system. At that time the Medicare retiree receives the Hospital Insurance Part A protection without any further financial outlay. However, the Medicare Part B system is financed by a deduction from the social security retirement amount as a premium payment for the SMI or Part B insurance. In 1966 this SMI premium amounted to $3.00 per month, and by 1996 this premium amount had increased to $42.50. In 1997–1998 the amount rose to $43.80 and is now projected to grow to $74.00 by 2003. The increased monthly Part B premiums are projected to bring improved outpatient care, especially for mammograms, pap smears, prostate and colorectal cancer screening, some bone mass measurements, and diabetes self-management. There is a great deal of discussion about this changing amount and possibly attaching it to a means test or allowing people to opt out of the system. At the present time, Medicare Part B pays for 80% of allowable expenses and carries a $100 annual deductible.

CRITERIA FOR MEDICARE REIMBURSEMENT

Geriatric rehabilitation services are covered by the Medicare system when there is an expectation of restoring the patient's level of function if it has been compromised by an injury or illness. Repetitive care to maintain a level of function is not eligible for reimbursement. It is crucial to have an appropriate diagnosis, with specific treatment goals, both short-term and long-term. The frequency of treatment should be enumerated, and for Part A there is a minimum of 5 days per week. In most rehabilitation units, it takes place twice daily for a minimum of 4 hours at least 5 days a week, sometimes 7 days a week. For Medicare Part B, rehabilitation services are supposed to take place at least 3 times per week. Obviously, both of these guidelines may have to be modified in order to meet the individual patient's illnesses, schedules, and other confounding factors in the delivery of health-care. These confounding situations should be recorded in the patient's chart.

MEDICARE PARTS A AND B: THE CONFUSION

As stated above, Medicare Part A is a hospital insurance; however, services under the HI trust fund may be rendered in a hospital, rehabilitation unit, hospice system, skilled nursing facility, or home health care situation. In contrast, coverage under Medicare Part B may take place in an outpatient setting in the hospital, a patient's home, an extended-care facility, rehabilitation agency, Comprehensive Outpatient Rehabilitation Facility (CORF), or other outpatient treatment center. Additionally, it may be rendered to an individual who is living in a skilled nursing facility in a long-term care setting. Thus, the strict nomenclature of inpatient versus outpatient care is not fully appropriate. This continuum of health care under the Medicare system is shown in Figure 75–2. From the rehabilitation prospective there should be no difference in the sophistication of the level of care rendered to a patient, whether it falls under Part A or Part B. The differentiation arises only from the sociomedical factors that necessitate inpatient rather than outpatient care.

HOME HEALTH SERVICES

Geriatric rehabilitation taking place in the home is largely a result of legislative and regulatory decisions made in the 1980s. At that time the Prospective Payment System (PPS) with Diagnosis-Related Groups (DRGs) was enacted which encouraged hospitals to discharge persons as quickly as possible. The concept behind this prospective payment system was that the efficient hospitals would benefit and the inefficient hospitals would suffer financial demise. However, as the late Senator John Heinz reported, the DRG system encouraged patients to leave hospitals "sicker and quicker."

As a result, the home health-care industry grew so rapidly that by the late 1990s it has become a major concern for budget watchers because of the increase in home health-care costs. Home health services are usually covered under Medicare Part A, provided certain criteria are met. As stated above, the patient must have an appropriate diagnosis and there should be a reasonable expectation

that the patient will recover from the condition. Obviously, in the geriatric setting the functional declines are not always clearly attributable to an acute episode, and this creates some ambiguity about medical necessity.

A person who requires skilled rehabilitative services must be determined to be confined to home in order to receive home health-care. Also, the physician must certify that the patient is confined to home. If the patient is able to leave home, it should be achievable only with considerable and taxing effort. The patient may leave home for short durations to obtain medical care such as outpatient dialysis, chemotherapy, radiation, or for an occasional trip to a barber or a walk or drive around the block.

Further, the patient is considered homebound if he or she has a condition or illness that restricts the ability to leave home except with assistance from another person or requires special transportation, or leaving home is contraindicated. Any condition such as a stroke that may cause the loss of the use of the upper extremities so that the patient is unable to open doors or use handrails will fit the criteria of being homebound. Posthospital care with resultant asthenia or weakness, pain, or other medical conditions that restrict activities also qualify the patient for home health-care. For example, a person with atherosclerotic cardiovascular disease may have cardiac risk with physical activity and should not be

CONTINUUM OF HEALTH-CARE SETTINGS FOR THE GERIATRIC PATIENT

Figure 75–2 The delineation between Part A and Part B of Medicare should not be based on the skilled nature of the services, but should be based on sociomedical decisions that determine place of care. (SNF, skilled nursing facility; LTC, long-term care; ICF, intermediate care facility.)

Living Independently		Institutional Care		
PART B		PART A	PART A	PART B
Outpatient care ➝ ➝ ➝ ➝ ➝ ➝ ➝		Hospitalization ➝ ➝	LTC ➝ ➝ ➝ ➝ ➝ ➝ ➝	LTC
		Acute care	SNF	SNF
Hospitals		SNF	Rehab unit	ICF
Private Homes		Rehab unit		
Nursing Homes				
Therapy Offices				
Rehabilitation Agencies				
CORFs				
Dependent Living at Home				
Hospice (Part A)				
Home Health Agency (PartA)				

leaving home. Additionally, a psychiatric problem in which a patient refuses to leave home or a circumstance in which it is unsafe to leave a person unattended may qualify the person as homebound.

The patient is not confined to home if he or she has the ability to obtain health-care in an outpatient setting. The aged person who does not often travel from home because of feebleness and insecurity brought on by advanced age would not be considered homebound for purposes of receiving home health services unless he or she meets one of the above conditions.

THE MEDICAID SYSTEM

The Medicaid system is a federally mandated program under Title XIX which is administered by the individual states, so there is discrepancy concerning who and what is covered by the program. Basically, Medicaid is a safety net for poor families with dependent children, disabled and blind adults, and the elderly. In 1996 the poverty guide was $7,740.00 for a single person and $10,300.00 for a couple.

In 1993 over 32 million Americans were covered by the Medicaid system, accounting for nearly $113 billion dollars of expenditures of which 64% were federal. The Medicaid federal budget is expected to grow to $179 billion dollars by the year 2002. Significantly, Medicaid, unlike Medicare, pays for long-term care, which amounted to over $40 billion dollars in 1995.

THE OLDER AMERICANS ACT

Like the Medicare and Medicaid legislation, the Older Americans Act (OAA) was passed in 1965. It established the Administration on Aging which organizes and directs the delivery of community-based services at the state level and represents a federal grant program. The OAA supports education, research, and training. It has been the impetus for states to establish local agencies concerned with aging. These programs are often involved in establishing social services, nutritional services, and senior center programs.

THE FUTURE

The Balanced Budget Act passed in 1997 has promoted many radical changes within the health deliv-

ery system. Many of these changes will be phased in over the next several years and are likely to alter the present delivery of rehabilitation services to aging patients, although during that time they will be subject to changes in regulations and to new legislation that may refine some of the original components of the 1997 Balanced Budget Act. Among the various changes are the application of a prospective payment system for outpatient care beginning in 1999 in acute-care hospitals. Similarly, a prospective payment system has been mandated for rehabilitation hospitals beginning in the year 2000. Skilled nursing facilities and home health agencies will also have phased-in prospective payment systems.

On the outpatient side, there will be alterations in annual payments per beneficiary to rehabilitation agencies, comprehensive outpatient rehabilitation facilities, physical and occupational therapists in independent practice, and Part B skilled nursing facilities. At the present time there is a $900 limit for each patient for rehabilitation services rendered in an independent practice, and this will increase to $1500 in 1999.

CONCLUSION

From its inception, Medicare has been surrounded with controversy over costs, paperwork fraud, and types of services rendered. The great achievement of this mammoth system is that many, many patients have received quality health-care services that may not have been available to them in the past. The changing demographics of the aging population, including the increasing wealth of a large percentage of Medicare recipients, are likely to be considerations in determining the services to be rendered to the postwar baby boomers when they reach retirement and Medicare age.

SUGGESTED READINGS

Medicare Home Health Manual. HCFA Pub. 11-T273, Baltimore, MD, 1998.
Moon M. *Medicare Now and in the Future.* Washington, D.C.: Urban Institute Press, 1995.
National Academy on Aging, 1275 K. St., N.W. Suite 350, Washington, D.C. 20005:
Medicare: Hospital Insurance and Supplementary Medical Insurance, 1995
Medicare and Medicaid Dual Eligibles, 1997
The Older Americans Act, 1995
Social Security: The Old Age and Survivors Trust Fund, 1997
Poen MM. Harry S. Truman versus the Medical Lobby: The Genesis of Medicare. Columbia, Mo.: University of Missouri Press; 1996.

Chapter **76**

The End of Life
Timothy L. Kauffman, Ph.D., P.T.

Death and Dying

Death is a finite moment
  known only to God
Dying is a process that
  Everyone does differently and uniquely.
Death is a victory
  A gift from Jesus on the cross
Dying is a plethora of emotions
  frustration
  inconsistent days
    some joyful
    some angry
    some, maybe many, in pain
    or some days when you just sense
    an overall loss of wellness
Death is the final goodbye to life on earth
  as we know it
Dying is the goodbyes to people, events, yes, even things close to you.
The hardest and most overwhelming goodbye to me is leaving my children
  Their careers I'll not see develop & flourish
  Their weddings I'll never participate in
  The grandchildren I'll never hold or spoil and of course other immediate family, friends, colleagues, places
  I've traveled, forests, waterfalls, lakes, flowers, mountains, rustic roads, parks, oceans, my cats, Tabitha and
  Magnum, my stuffed animals, and more and more.
Death is our greatest victory
  propelling us to a peace beyond our own understanding.
Dying is the vehicle that transports us, not always a smooth and tranquil ride but at journey's end remains the
  promise of a safe arrival.

LYNN PHILLIPPI

Written at Linen & Lace B&B
June 26, 1997

INTRODUCTION

These words were composed by Lynn Phillippi who wrote Chapter 65 as she struggled with her own medical problems, shortly before her own death. As Lynn noted, death is but a finite moment and each person's death is different and unique. As health-care providers to geriatric patients we are faced with the reality of patients dying, but the process and timing of that moment are not always simple or clearly delineated. Therein lies a difficult and ethical problem, especially with the acute-care model dictated by the U.S. Medicare system. That is, when should rehabilitation services be stopped? This question does not concern medical or nursing services because Medicare requirements are not the same, as rehabilitation, which is ". . . performed with the expectation of restoring the patient's level of function which has been lost or reduced by injury or illness." But the dying process is often protracted, filled with repetitive losses and rebounds as the progressive decline and downward spiral transpire, so rehabilitation should be refined to meet the changing needs of increasingly frail and debilitated patients. In these commonly occurring cases the purposes of rehabilitation are to assist the patient and other care-givers with quality-of-life issues such as pain control, positioning, mobility, handling, and toileting and to provide dignity to a human being and his or her family.

THE END OF LIFE

When does the end of life start—after the second stroke or when a terminal illness is diagnosed or when a person is admitted to an extended-care facility or when a doctor says so . . .? In an abstract way, the end of life may start at the time of birth and luck, choice, and genetics determine how long the involution will be. Most health-care providers in the field of geriatrics recognize it when a patient is approaching the end of life; but most also realize that some patients will "hang on" for days, months, or even years. Therefore, to withdraw rehabilitation services too early or to deny those services may approach neglect or abuse, especially if rehabilitation specialists are not consulted.

Admittedly, constraints such as patient potential exist, but the decision should be arrived at by the family, care-providers, physicians, and rehabilitation specialists with due consideration given to pathology, family and patient desires, availability of services, and financial realities. Included among the family's and patient's desires are sociological differences, for the end of life is surrounded with a variety of habits, beliefs, customs, and values. Culture and religion are crucial considerations that influence the provision of health care to persons as they approach death.

Palliative Care

When a patient has little or no potential or refuses rehabilitative care, then respect, dignity, and physical as well as emotional comfort must be given freely by all ethical people who come into contact with this human being. At such a time, rehabilitation for the purpose of restoring or recovering function is obviously not appropriate; however, palliative care is. Palliation simply means to moderate the intensity of pain or to offer care or services that will allow for a better quality of life at the time when life is ending. Often, care is directed toward the dying patient's family as much as it is given to the patient. For example, the family might need help in accepting the harsh and sad reality of the impending expiration. Appropriate services from a physical or occupational therapist may be to help with proper mobility in bed, with sitting, and with assisting to toilet. Speech therapy may be helpful for teaching swallowing, mouth care, and communication modifications. Perhaps at this stage of life, the end, the ability to communicate at any level is a most crucial need, especially for the sake of family and intimate friends.

Palliative care is not something that is done only at the end of life. Efforts to moderate the intensity of pain and minimize functional limitations and impairment would have been made prior to clinical recognition that the patient has poor rehabilitative potential and is approaching the end of life. So

rehabilitative and palliative care are not mutually exclusive but are on a continuum, with the emphasis on curative recovery of function lost lying at one end of the spectrum and on comfort and moderating the intensity of pain lying at the other, when restoration is unlikely or impossible.

This concept fits well within the parameters of the *Guide to Physical Therapist Practice*. The interventions of coordination and communication are particularly pertinent, as they can be used to coordinate care of the patient with family, significant others, care-givers, and other professionals. This involves instruction in proper procedures and techniques but holds quality-of-life issues and palliation as the focus.

The Role of Rehabilitation

Because each individual patient and family approaches the dying process with a different set of medical, spiritual, and physical needs, the role of rehabilitation must be varied. In the early stages, mobility is an important treatment consideration and thus typical gait, balance, and therapeutic strengthening exercises may be appropriate. The use of assistive devices for balance, safety, pain reduction, and joint protection may enable the patient to maintain a sense of independence and involvement in life's activities. Joint protection with the use of an orthotic or splint may enhance functional capacity, and as a patient becomes more confined to bed, it may be used to prevent painful and disfiguring contractures, swelling, or pressure areas.

Therapeutic exercise to maintain breathing capacity and exercise tolerance is useful. The inability to breathe is frightening and can usually be controlled until the very last days or hours of life. Exercise tolerance should be aimed at sitting up on the bedside or in an easy chair or wheelchair. The world looks better from an upright posture and the patient may be able to eat or at least sit at a meal with family. Breathing and eating may be easier in the upright position.

Adaptive equipment for eating, dressing, and bathing may help to maintain independence and a sense of self-worth. A wheelchair is most useful for transport and to conserve energy; however, it can cause injury or at least pain and fatigue if it is ill-fitted. Pressure areas can occur and edema may result in dependent extremities. A poorly fitted wheelchair or prolonged sitting encourages kyphosis of the spine which can cause back pain, reduce chest expansion for breathing, and compress the abdomen, making eating more difficult.

Pain management for the terminally ill patient usually involves medication, especially narcotics.

Some patients and their families choose not to use these types of medications because of their beliefs or because of the lightheadedness or drowsiness that results. The physical modalities of the various heat or cold applications and electrical stimulation are beneficial, although realistic expectations are requisite. The effects of the portable and easily used transcutaneous electrical nerve stimulator (TENS) are less potent and not identical to the effects of a dose of morphine but they are of value. The physical modalities are described in detail in Chapters 68 and 69.

Range-of-motion exercises help to control pain and to prevent contractures, stiffness, and pressure areas. Often these can be taught to family members; that way, they have an opportunity to participate in the care of their loved one rather than being just bystanders. Further, these exercises require physical contact, which is an important human need that may be lost to the dying patient because of medical interventions or simply because family members don't know whether or not handling will cause harm. Gentle massage is therapeutic too, both physically and emotionally.

Emotions

When providing medical care, be it curative or palliative, it is vital to remember that patients and their families have real emotions that must be considered. Bereavement is a process that starts before death and continues after it. The family and intimate friends are facing a loss, sometimes one that they are not ready to accept, and denial is a common coping mechanism. Denial may be used by the patient, too, and that can impede the more important acts of completing one's life work, settling one's affairs, and saying goodbyes. When working with a patient and family members at a time when all of them may be in various stages of denial, it is necessary to be honest, but not brutally so. Empathy and honesty help, especially when they come from all members of the health-care team and from clergy.

Anger and frustration are also commonly encountered in a dying patient and may be directed at family members, at God, or at some or all of the medical-care providers. Fear and guilt may also be present, for death is an unknown. Several of the world's major religions have taught the concept of sin, and the dying person may have a sense of guilt about the commissions or omissions of life, and may regret the inability to do something about them in the last remaining days. Again, empathy, honesty, and dignity are important. At the end of life, a person should feel that he or she is okay and is valued by the medical providers as a human being until death and then as a memory.

Many patients and families are most appreciative of anything that can be done to provide additional comfort, dignity, and worth. Therein lies the inner strength to continue to work with patients and their families as life completes its journey.

Hospice

The concept of hospice developed in the 1960s in Great Britain; in the United States it is now a Medicare Part A program which usually starts when a patient is determined by a physician to have fewer than 6 months of life left to live. A wide variety of physical capabilities and needs are found among hospice patients. In the early stages of hospice care, rehabilitation services may indeed be curative and in the end, only palliative. The blending of one phase into the other is usually gradual, but the consultation and care provided by rehabilitation specialists as members of the hospice team will maintain the quality of life at its optimal level.

Impending Death

Certain signs indicate that death will occur soon. In the final days, the patient may become increasingly somnolent and diaphoretic, and intake of fluids and food may nearly cease. The toes and fingers as well as the nose and ears may become cyanotic as the circulation and oxygen perfusion decline. The death rattle, a frequent cause of distress for family members, results from bronchial congestion or palatal relaxation. If desired, clergy should be consulted, and the family can be present and hold hands or touch or rub the loved one to say final goodbyes. Peace, dignity, and respect must prevail.

CONCLUSION

As Lynn Phillippi wrote, "Death is the final goodbye to life on earth." It is an individual experience inherent in life. Knowing what stops life allows a better understanding of what life is. Health-care providers to aging and dying patients participate in this universal college frequently. Rehabilitative services, curative and palliative, enhance the quality of life for the dying patient and for the patient's family.

The following words were written as I sat at the funeral of a patient I had treated, off and on, for 8 years, both curatively and palliatively.

The Meaning of Life

What is the meaning of life?
The answer is unclear;
And it is not the same for all.
Part of the answer is in death
When it is not.
Death begets life
For it is the aging, the passage
  of time that nourishes the young;
Without someone before us,
  there can be none behind us.

Life is not easy.
It is filled with problems,
  heartaches, sadness, Yet
  there is joy abundant.
Sometimes it is hard to find.
Accept the bad, for it is life, too.
But search and focus on the good,
  the beauty.
It passes every day.

Those who precede us and those
  who pass through life with us
  are ALWAYS present.
They live with us forever
  in our thoughts,
  our actions,
  our lives.

In life, there is no absolute beginning
  and no absolute ending;
  there is only conception and there is death
  which mark these times.
  But what preceded and followed these events,
  both conception and death?

Are the lives of loved ones
  both giving and receiving love;
  sharing learning and living.
We are our parents, our spouses,
  our children, our grandparents, and
  grandchildren,
  and others who enter our lives
  sharing, learning, living, loving.

The meaning of life is the here and now,
  which are built upon what preceded
  and provide for what follows;
The meaning of life is to experience it,
  the good and the bad,
But most important is to focus
  on the beauty of its experiences.

SUGGESTED READINGS

Faulkner A. *Working with Bereaved People.* London: Churchill Livingstone; 1995.

Gillham L. Palliative care. In: Pickels B, Compton A, Cott C, et al., eds. *Physiotherapy with Older People.* Philadelphia: WB Saunders; 1995: 305–322.

Guide to Physical Therapist Practice. *Physical Therapy* 1997; 77(11).

Reuss R, Last S. Care of the terminally ill: Hospice, home, and extended care facilities. In: McGarvey C, ed. *Physical Therapy for the Cancer Patient.* New York: Churchill Livingstone; 1990: 163–171.

Squires A, Wardle P. To rehabilitate or not? In: Helm C. *Rehabilitation of the Older Patient.* London, 1988: 102–122.

Wood E. Quality of life: Physical therapy in hospice. *PT Magazine* 1988;6:39–45.

THE REHABILITATION TEAM

Chapter 77

Interdisciplinary Geriatric Assessment

David C. Martin, M.D.
Margaret Basiliadis, D.O.

INTRODUCTION

Many approaches to the care of the geriatric patient have been lumped under the rubric of "geriatric assessment." Indeed, in terms of process and outcome, geriatric assessment is one of the most widely studied aspects of geriatric health care. By 1996 there were more than 150 published reports on geriatric assessment and numerous meta-analyses had been performed or were under way.

The goal of this chapter is to examine the philosophical underpinnings of the interdisciplinary approach to geriatric medicine, to examine some of the models of how geriatric assessment has been operationalized, and to point out some of the weaknesses and future directions of research for this model of health care.

PHILOSOPHICAL UNDERPINNINGS OF GERIATRIC ASSESSMENT

Secondary Aging Must Be Distinguished from Primary Aging

Physiologists often divide the problems of aging into two categories—primary aging and secondary aging. Primary aging includes those physiological changes that can be ascribed solely to the passage of time. Several theories have been set forth to explain the changes caused only by aging. These include denaturation of proteins through crosslinking, cumulative damage from free radicals, and an internal biological clock that is genetically determined. This last theory gained credibility from cross-species studies that related longevity to the number of cell doublings that could occur in cell culture. The number of cell doublings proved to be species-specific and varied directly with the longevity of the species.

An exciting recent finding could further elucidate the exact nature of this biological clock. This finding is the discovery that repeating base pairs at the ends of strands of DNA, called telomeres, prevent unraveling of the DNA strands and preserve the genetic integrity through their repeated replication. The telomeres "harden" the DNA strand in a fashion similar to the way the plastic caps on the ends of shoelaces prevent the shoestring's unraveling. The length and stability of telomeres could be the physiological basis of the biological clock.

Secondary aging involves those decrements in function which can be ascribed to disease processes. Primary and secondary aging are sometimes difficult to distinguish from each other. For example, it was once thought that there was a substantive decline in cardiac output that was age-related and due to primary aging. When these data were reexamined excluding subjects with subclinical coronary artery disease, it was learned that the cardiac output is actually well preserved into advanced age. The effects were not due to primary aging at all but rather to secondary aging in the form of arteriosclerotic disease.

Likewise, in the era before autopsy studies had been done upon persons with dementia, it was believed that dementia was simply a primary process of the senium rather than secondary aging. Autopsy series later disclosed that cognitive losses could be explained by specific pathologies such as multiple strokes or the senile plaques and neurofibrillary tangles of Alzheimer's disease. It is now known that even though speed of effortful mental processing slows with aging, in the absence of disease, cognition remains well preserved.

How do these principles relate to geriatric assessment? It is the role of geriatric assessment to tease out the effects of secondary aging and to reverse them through specific treatments, to ameliorate them through interventions that may improve though not cure the underlying condition, or to assist the patient to function better by marshalling support services or altering the patient's environment to make that environment more conducive to the patient's needs.

Coexistence of Multiple Diseases and the Cascade of Illness

When clinicians are first trained in medicine, they are commonly taught to think in terms of the "chief complaint." This approach proves to be much too restrictive in the practice of geriatric medicine. Here, the most common scenario is one of multiple, coexisting pathologies that are all conspiring to harm the patient's functional ability. Many patients presenting for geriatric assessment may have more than four significant medical problems that need to be addressed.

An example of the cascade effect of multiple problems might be the patient who presents with delirium. Such a change in mental status is a final common pathway for many medical and psychiatric conditions. In this example, the pathology might be traced back as follows: the patient has some moderate renal insufficiency and prostatic hypertrophy. The prostatic hypertrophy leads to urinary retention which further worsens renal function which leads to azotemia and anorexia which leads to reduced fluid and nutritional intake which leads to even further worsening of renal function and a relentless downward spiral. This interrelationship of organ system function causes a cascade of illness that affects many organs.

A challenge of geriatric assessment is to trace the cascade of events back to find key points in each patient's unique pathophysiology where treatment may halt or reverse the downward spiral. Because of the complexity of this process, an interdisciplinary approach is often most successful. Also, there is no substitute for seasoned and experienced clinicians making expert diagnoses. The challenges of treating the frail elderly led Franklin Williams, a recent director of the National Institutes on Aging, to coin the phrase "the fruition of the clinician" in respect to the practice of geriatric medicine.

As Any Cohort Ages, Variability Increases

As noted earlier, it is often impossible to predict the specific decline of any particular organ system on the basis of aging alone. Likewise, it is impossible to predict the physiological function of any individual based on age alone. One may speak of chronological age versus physiological age. To speak of a young 80-year-old or an old 65-year-old does not sound like an oxymoron to the geriatric practitioner.

What can be predicted is that as people age, they become less and less like each other. (Anyone who has attended a 25-year class reunion has probably experienced this first-hand.) No two persons age identically. Some encounter diseases, others suffer traumatic injuries, and others cope with both. Lifetime habits, choices, and fortune add to the genetic variability of aging individuals.

The increasing diversity that comes with age has a direct effect on geriatric assessment. For geriatric assessment to work well, it is crucial that both diagnostic and therapeutic approaches be individualized for each patient. Attempting a "cookbook" approach to the solution of clinical problems in such a diverse group could easily lead to iatrogenic harm. The recent trend toward the creation and application of clinical pathways or clinical guidelines in the treatment of specific conditions must proceed carefully and contain greater flexibility when dealing with issues in geriatric medicine.

Again, the interdisciplinary approach, because of its greater clinical diversity, can better account for the pluralism of this unique population.

Diminished Homeostatic Reserve Blocks Recovery

Perhaps the best definition of aging is "increasing susceptibility to the forces of mortality due to decreased homeostatic reserve." Homeostasis concerns the body's ability to maintain itself in a steady state and to get itself back on track whenever there is perturbation from that steady state. Ability to maintain a constant temperature, constant blood pressure, and constant blood glucose level are all examples of homeostasis.

When homeostatic reserves are constrained, there is diminished likelihood of survival with any extreme stress. A key principle in geriatric assessment is to recognize that homeostatic reserves are diminished and that patients are more sensitive both to the disease processes and to the iatrogenic effects of intervention. This should lead to a more conservative and individualized approach in the application of therapeutic maneuvers and drug therapies.

These issues are especially important in geriatric rehabilitation. A common scenario is the elderly patient who has suffered a hip fracture and requires surgical repair. With postoperative pain and analgesia, the patient often suffers such setbacks as postoperative delirium, fever, anemia from blood loss, atelectasis, and hypoxemia. Thus, the rehabilitation measures may be delayed for several days by intercurrent illness. While at bedrest, the patient may be losing on the order of 4 to 5% of muscle strength and 1 to 2% of aerobic capacity daily. Whereas younger people may surmount these losses, in the geriatric patient who is already marginally compensated, these losses become highly significant and make rehabilitation and recovery all the more difficult.

In this setting the patient might not physically or psychologically cope well with the arduous exercise demands of rehabilitation. The twice-daily treatments of up to 4 hours imposed by government regulations may be too rigorous for some of these more frail individuals. Sometimes rehabilitation must occur at a more gradual pace and in the long-term-care setting.

Diseases Present in an Atypical Fashion

Among geriatric patients, the common presentations of illness are often replaced by the less specific and more global findings of increased confusion, weakness, anorexia, and tendency to fall. One sees such phenomena as "silent myocardial infarction," "afebrile pneumonia," and "depression without sadness." The first manifestation of urosepsis might be falling, or the presenting symptom of a myocardial infarction might be increased agitation. In geriatric assessment, the clinician must cast a wider net in attempting to make diagnoses.

Other diseases typically present only in the elderly or much more frequently in the elderly, and the index of suspicion for these problems must remain higher. These disorders include such entities as polymyalgia rheumatica, Parkinson's disease, and hypothyroidism.

Diseases are Underreported

Geriatric patients commonly underreport their problems. Sometimes cognitive impairment gets in the way of an accurate relating of historical information. At other times the patient is embarrassed to bring up certain problems. This may account for the fact that incontinence is so underreported. At other times depression may lead to a sense of hopelessness about the possibility of getting help; or patients may have acquired some of the ageist bias from the society in which they live and may feel that their problems are to be expected at their time of life and they should not complain.

The process of geriatric assessment strives for accurate and reliable historical information by collecting data through collateral interviews with caregivers and loved ones as well as with the patient himself or herself. The patient is also typically interviewed by several professionals. A patient might relate something to a nurse or social worker that would not have been mentioned to a doctor.

Self-report questionnaires and structured assessment tools to measure cognition, affect, and morale can yield quite useful information if they are administered carefully and in a nonthreatening manner. These tools add additional important information to the historical database.

THE PROCESS OF GERIATRIC ASSESSMENT

The process of geriatric assessment typically involves an interdisciplinary approach. The most consistent team members to have formed the traditional core of this assessment process have included the geriatrician or geriatric nurse practitioner, nurse, and social worker. Ancillary team members have included the occupational therapist, physical therapist, psychiatrist, nutritionist, speech therapist, exercise physiologist, recreational therapist, and respira-

tory therapist. One of the very first outpatient assessment programs even employed an architect because of the frequency with which changes in the patient's home environment were being recommended.

An example of the geriatric team in action may help to illustrate many of the principles of geriatric assessment:

Mrs. A was an 85-year-old widowed woman who was living with and being cared for by her 54-year-old daughter. She was referred by her daughter for outpatient geriatric assessment. The patient had been suffering from gradual and progressive memory loss for the preceding 3 years. Three weeks previously she had become more apathetic and withdrawn and had ceased to be able to climb the stairs because of arthritic complaints. On intake she was being treated with amitriptyline 25 mg at night for depression.

On further questioning, it was learned that the patient was becoming delusional, believing that people on the television screen were real. Her functional status a month earlier had been much better and her incontinence was new. She complained of a feeling of profound weakness. The social worker learned that the daughter was extremely resentful that the care-giving burden had fallen to her and was not being shared by her two siblings. She felt guilty about her resentment and this made her care-giving even more difficult.

Medical workup disclosed moderate degenerative joint changes, moderate hearing loss, and dysphoric mood. The patient made seven depressive responses on the Geriatric Depression Scale and scored 20/30 on the Folstein Mini-Mental Examination. She remembered zero out of three objects on early recall. Mobility testing showed profound weakness, with difficulty arising from the exam chair and broadening of the support base. Screening laboratory tests showed a mild anemia with a hemoglobin of 11.3 g/dL and an MCV of 81. The serum cobalamin level was low normal at 200 pg/mL. The sedimentation rate was markedly elevated at 110 mm/h. Other blood parameters were normal. An MRI scan showed periventricular hyperintensity and multiple lacunae. Soon after the initial assessment, the patient was begun on 15 mg daily of prednisone for a presumptive diagnosis of polymyalgia rheumatica. In addition, she was begun on cobalamin injections. The amitriptyline was discontinued. When the patient was returned to the clinic for a family conference, her mobility had improved dramatically, as had her pain symptoms. The incontinence had resolved because the patient was now mobile enough to get to the bathroom. The delusions had also disappeared but the patient remained dysphoric. The family was educated and counseled about the spectrum of the patient's problems. It was pointed out that her cognitive loss might not be due to Alzheimer's disease, as she had been previously told, and that the prognosis was uncertain. It was decided to continue to monitor the patient's mood for another month and to consider treating her with one of the newer selective serotonin uptake inhibitors if her mood remained depressed. The patient was referred to an adult day-care program. She began to attend 3 days per week.

Six months later, the patient was being maintained on 5 mg daily of prednisone. Her mobility remained good and the sedimentation rate was 26 mm/h. The patient had been started on sertraline 50 mg daily and her mood had improved. The hemoglobin had risen to 13.0 g/dL. She was still occasionally delusional and the score on the Mini-Mental exam had not improved. The patient's daughter, however, was feeling greatly relieved, and she perceived her mother to be functioning at a much higher level of cognition, even though this could not be objectively demonstrated. The daughter was planning to have her mother enter a 1-week respite program while the family went on a week-long vacation.

This case illustrates several key principles of geriatric assessment. This patient was suffering primarily from an illness (polymyalgia rheumatica) that is found exclusively in the elderly population. In the absence of any symptoms suggesting cranial arteritis, many clinicians would institute an empiric trial of corticosteroid therapy without doing a temporal artery biopsy and gauge the response to therapy. A dramatic response as was seen in this case helps confirm the diagnosis.

The next most important problems, those of the cognitive impairment and dysphoria, reveal how multiple coexisting pathologies can conspire to create dysfunction. The suddenness of the onset of the patient's delusions and cognitive decline suggested either a vascular process or a reaction to the anticholinergic effects of the amitriptyline. The low cobalamin level is also not an uncommon finding and could also be contributing to the cognitive loss. The use of oral rather than parenteral replacement therapy for a low cobalamin level is debatable but the decision was made to institute parenteral replacement just in case the patient could not adequately absorb the vitamin.

In many instances of geriatric assessment, the care-giver becomes as much a client as the patient. Predictable respite is one effective means of reduc-ing care-giver stress, and referral to an adult day-care program is an ideal way to provide predictable respite. When alleviated of some of the care-giving burden, the daughter could once again enjoy her relationship with her mother.

The perception on the part of family members that the patient was functioning much better cognitively even though objective improvement could not be measured represents another phenomenon deserving of mention. Significant disparity between "perceived" and "measured" improvement often exists.

In order to coordinate and implement the various recommendations of the separate professionals involved in the interdisciplinary approach, a team conference is typically held after the assessment. The care plan is crafted with input from the various team members. Often a family conference is held with the patient and all involved family members and care-givers. The purpose of this conference is to educate the patient and care-givers, to make official recommendations, and to answer questions. It also provides yet another opportunity to assess for care-giver burden and to move to alleviate it if it is clinically significant.

The interdisciplinary model of geriatric assessment has been applied to a variety of settings. The most common have been adult medical-surgical hospital wards, outpatient clinics, inpatient geropsychiatry units, nursing homes, rehabilitation hospitals, patient homes, and hospital-based consulting services. There are also more complex models that involve many team members and that are found in the inpatient and consultation models.

From many outcome studies that have been performed on the various manifestations of geriatric assessment, one can make several generalizations. First, and perhaps most important, is that assessment without implementation is of almost no value. The programs with the most robust outcomes have been those with direct links to rehabilitation services and those in which the geriatric team had direct responsibility for the implementation of care plans. Second, not all geriatric patients can be expected to benefit from geriatric assessment. Patients who have relatively high function and those who are hopelessly ill are less likely to derive benefit, so many programs attempt to target those who would be most likely to benefit. On the other hand, one would also not wish to be too quick to judge a patient as hopelessly ill, because geriatric assessment has scored some of its greatest successes in patients who had been previously written off by the traditional health-care system.

In terms of traditionally measured outcomes (such as mortality, functional status, frequencies of hospitalization, and nursing home placement), research study results are mixed. Because of the mixed models of geriatric assessment and differing sites of practice, meta-analyses and generalizations about the value of geriatric assessment are difficult. Nevertheless, some reviewers have felt that the data are convincing in terms of reduction of mortality, lowered rates of nursing home placement, and lowered levels of care-giver burden.

DIRECTIONS FOR FUTURE RESEARCH

The technology of geriatric assessment has been under attack because it is viewed as labor-intensive and inadequately reimbursed. Were the data of research studies more conclusive in regard to outcomes, it would be easier to advocate for the widespread application of interdisciplinary geriatric assessment. The main challenge in the light of what has been learned seems to be selective application of this interdisciplinary approach, targeting those subjects and contexts in which geriatric assessment is determined to be cost-effective.

Other areas of active research in this field include investigation into the optimal place to perform geriatric assessment. Some intriguing studies suggest that the optimal site may be in the patient's own home. Other important questions also have to be answered. Do data that have been collected largely through interview reflect what the patient is actually able to perform? Do data on functional status, which are often garnered by physical therapy and occupational therapy in a laboratory setting, correlate well with what the patient can do in his or her own home?

The development of critical pathways, or clinical algorithms, is a process that is being repeated at virtually every acute-care hospital in an effort to standardize care and reduce costs. As health-care systems become globalized to include the entire continuum, these pathways must become more extended. They will cease to be disease-specific or organ-specific and, rather, will evolve into a "syndromic" approach. To work effectively, these pathways must take into account the various principles of geriatric assessment that have been under discussion. The effects of application of such pathways on outcome remain to be seen.

Many other important questions about the approach to treating the geriatric patient must be addressed. Some of these are the following: What is the value of treating dysphoric mood that falls short of full-blown depression? Some data suggest that patients with dysphoria may be inappropriately high utilizers of health-care resources. How stable are people's advance directives? Do they change when patients are more immediately confronted with life-threatening situations and the issues are more immediate and less abstract than when the directive was originally formulated? How valuable are exercise prescriptions in late life? What are some of the long-term effects of nutrition on health? Higher folate intakes may have an antiatherogenic effect mediated through homocysteine levels. Are there ways to ameliorate the effects of bedrest deconditioning and the development of delirium that so often add to the morbidity of hospitalization of geriatric patients? Is there a role for anticipatory conditioning prior to elective hospitalizations or procedures (so-called prehabilitation)?

CONCLUSION

It remains for the upcoming generation of researchers and practitioners to improve the knowledge base and give good health and meaning to the latter stages of peoples' lives. Not enough students are entering this important field, yet it can be among the most rewarding and challenging of endeavors.

To recapitulate the previous clinical scenario of the 85-year-old woman with both physical and cognitive impairments, recall that the patient's subjective improvement vastly surpassed what could be objectively measured. When a patient is marginally compensated and just barely able to get by, then slight improvements in condition are often perceived as dramatic, even when the degree of improvement can scarcely be measured by our crude assessment tools. This magnified effect of intervention on the patient's and family's perceptions of health and well-being can be one of the most gratifying aspects of serving a frail geriatric population.

SUGGESTED READINGS

Applegate WB, Miller ST, et al. A randomized, controlled trial of a geriatric assessment unit in a community rehabilitation hospital. *N Engl J Med* 1990; 322:1572–1578.

Bortz W. Disuse and aging. *JAMA* 1992; 248:1203–1208.

Buchner DM, Wagner EH. Preventing frail health. *Health Promo Dis Prev* 1992; 8:1–17.

Creditor MC. Hazards of hospitalization of the elderly. *Ann Intern Med* 1993; 118:219–223.

Fiatarone MA, Marks EC, et al. High-intensity strength training in nonagenarians: effects on skeletal muscle. *JAMA* 1990; 263:3029–3034.

Folstein MF, Folstein SE, McHugh PR. Mini-Mental State: a practical method for grading the cognitive state of patients for the clinician. *J Psychiatr Res* 1975; 12:189–198.

Fretwell MD, Raymond, et al. The Senior Care Study: a controlled trial of consultative/unit-based geriatric assessment program in acute care. *J Am Geriatr Soc* 1990; 38:1073–1081.

Hirsch CH, Sommers L, et al. The natural history of functional morbidity in hospitalized older patients. *J Am Geriatr Soc* 1990; 38:1296–1303.

Hoenig HM, Rubenstein LZ. Hospital-associated deconditioning and dysfunction. *J Am Geriatr Soc* 1991; 39:220–222.

Landefeld CS, Palmer RM, et al. A randomized trial of care in a hospital medical unit especially designed to improve the functional outcomes of acutely ill older patients. *N Engl J Med* 1995; 332:1338–1344.

Reuben DB, Siu AL. An objective measure of physical function of elderly outpatients: the physical performance test. *J Am Geriatr Soc* 1990; 38:1105–1112.

Rubenstein LA, Josephson KR, et al. Effectiveness of geriatric evaluation unit. A randomized clinical trial. *N Engl J Med* 1984; 311:1664–1670.

Thomas DR, Brahan R, et al. Inpatient community-based geriatric assessment reduces subsequent mortality. *J Am Geriatr Soc* 1993; 41:101–104.

Tinetti ME, Inouye SK, et al. Shared risk factors for falls, incontinence, and functional dependence. *JAMA* 1995; 273:1348–1353.

Yesavage J. Depression in the elderly. *Post Grad Med* 91; 1992.

Chapter 78

Gerontological and Geriatric Nursing

Melen R. McBride, Ph.D., R.N.

INTRODUCTION

The nursing profession has a long history of providing health care to sick older people. Initially, geriatric nursing focused on physical care, comfort measures, and palliation. The care was often given almost entirely by nurses and their assistants in nursing homes or in people's own homes. As knowledge, technology, public policy, and societal expectations changed, the scope, types of geriatric services, and quality of nursing care also changed. The establishment of the first formal standards for nursing care for older adults, adapted in 1970 by the American Nurses Association (ANA), was a landmark initiative for nurses in geriatrics. It provided a link to nursing science, which is defined by the ANA as the deliberate problem-solving process, grounded in the biopsychosocial sciences, of diagnosing and treating actual or potential health problems.

As these practice standards were reviewed and modified over time, patient-centered care, family participation, and nursing services related to the prevention of disease and disability and the promotion of good health for older adults were articulated more explicitly as major components of geriatric nursing practice. This paved the way for the use of the term "gerontological nursing" to refer to a domain in the continuum of the science and practice of nursing that is devoted to the complex care of older people and their families and to balancing the effects of normal aging and pathology. Today, the term "geriatric nursing" indicates specialized clinical care for the medical problems of the sick and chronically ill elderly in various interdisciplinary patient-care settings. Nurses with advanced training who practice in this area are known as geriatric nurse practitioners or geriatric clinical specialists.

An overall goal for gerontological and geriatric nursing is to provide humanistic health care to older adults and their families by paying careful attention to individual circumstances, needs, and goals. Preventing impairment, restoring functions, and maintaining an enduring state of health and well-being are embedded in these goals. A key strategy that is used to meet these goals is the application of the nursing process that consists of assessment, planning, intervention, and evaluation within the context of health-care issues presented by the elder and the family.

As a discipline, nursing has agreed to a social contract to make its services available 24 hours a day. Thus, gerontological and the geriatric nurses have critical roles in the collaboration of the health-care team, as they must be involved in planning, implementing, and evaluating patient care. The nurses' roles and functions include nursing treatments and other therapeutic activities for direct patient care, case management, patient and family health education and counseling, administration, advocacy, public policy development, and education and research.

DIRECT PATIENT CARE

To ensure seamless care, continuous leadership and accountability are requisite. Professional nurses act on these responsibilities in acute-care units, ambulatory care clinics, long-term care facilities, home-care agencies, and other sites where the need for geriatric care can be fulfilled.

At least three different types of nursing expertise, using different levels of critical thinking and clinical decision-making skills, are available to older patients to assist them in meeting their health-care needs:

(1) Staff nurses have clinical, technical, and humanistic skills in one-to-one interaction so they can strengthen and support the biopsychosocial processes of recovery, rehabilitation, healing, preventing disease and disability, and dying with dignity. Nurses functioning in this role practice in acute-care settings, skilled nursing facilities, home health settings, and hospices, and a smaller number practice in ambulatory care clinics or doctors' offices.

(2) Geriatric clinical nurse specialists have expertise in working with complex nursing-care problems and draw from their advanced skills in hands-on clinical care, critical analysis and decision-making, teaching, counseling, and coordination and follow-up of interdisciplinary care plans. They practice in acute and long-term care settings and may be consultants to community clinics and home-based geriatric care programs.

(3) Geriatric nurse practitioners have expertise in performing comprehensive physical assessments, interpreting symptoms and physiological abnormalities, and developing treatment, management, and follow-up plans for medically induced problems, in partnership with the primary care physician and other team members. Their practice is closely linked with primary care services in ambulatory clinics, although a growing number of these nurses are providing services to elderly patients in long-term care facilities, adult day health programs, and physicians' offices.

The Four Steps of Nursing

The four-step nursing process guides the nurse to individualize, contextualize, and prioritize problem areas. The steps consist of assessment, planning, intervention, and evaluation.

Step 1, Assessment Biopsychosocial data about geriatric patients is collected by means of interviews, record reviews, direct observations, and other approaches, as time allows, to build a composite picture of the multiple and often competing needs of the geriatric patient and the informal caregiver. For example, the federally mandated multidisciplinary assessment called the Minimum Data Set (see Burke and Walsh, page 610) is used in nursing homes by long-term care nurses to record assessment data as part of the team approach to care planning and treatment.

Data from nursing assessments are necessary to identify problems in the order of clinical significance at a specific time and according to the urgent need for nursing interventions. The information may include general and specific data on the presenting problems as defined by the patient and the care-giver, medical diagnoses, prescribed medical treatments, status of physical and mental functions, alternate health-care resources, patient goals and expectations, safety risks, self-care abilities for recovery, including the ability to perform the activities of daily living, and other information that a nurse considers clinically relevant to the case or situation. Identifying nursing diagnoses and prioritizing these problem areas are the major intended

process outcomes. Since 1973, the North American Nursing Diagnosis Association (NANDA) has continued to develop a taxonomy of nursing diagnoses, and currently there are approximately 130 approved classifications of patient care problems in nine categories.

It is important for members of health-care teams to be aware that some problem areas that demand priority nursing interventions may not always be parallel to or target directly the "curing" goals of a medical plan.

Step 2, Planning The nursing care plan incorporates specific nursing interventions and nursing activities to treat specific nursing diagnoses or deal with problem areas such as changes in food intake, impaired capacity for personal care, risk for accidental injuries due to general weakness and mild dementia, grief unrelated to the health problem, and other needs of the geriatric patient and the caregiver. Included in the plan are nursing actions to ensure the continuity of all prescribed medical treatments and other intervention modalities for the geriatric patient. Clinical judgment is an important nursing skill in this process because it enables an accurate identification of the nursing diagnosis.

Step 3, Implementation The process of implementation unleashes the collective efforts of members of the nursing staff, including auxiliary nursing personnel, and directs them so that the nursing care plan can be carried out. Safe and compassionate approaches that are clinically and technically appropriate are used to achieve the desired clinical outcomes. Nursing actions include checking vital signs, changing the position of an immobilized elderly patient, orienting an elder with a memory deficit to time, place, and activity, interviewing a family caregiver prior to home care, consulting other health-care professionals, advocating for an elder to obtain a local community resource, and other actions aimed at resolving a nursing problem or reducing the impact of a nursing diagnosis.

Step 4, Evaluation A patient's physical, verbal, and behavioral responses, informal care-givers' reports, and observations by health-care providers from other disciplines are important aspects of the feedback mechanism that helps the nursing staff to maintain a dynamic, flexible care plan. Critical analysis of information obtained while nursing interventions are in progress may be used to modify nursing interventions, redirect patient and family participation in the overall treatment and management plan, reexamine the health-care team's understanding of the clinical problem, determine cost benefits, realign leadership, and support the standards of quality patient care.

CASE MANAGEMENT

The nurse case manager looks after a group of elderly patients and informal care-givers. As a rule, frailty, multiple chronic illnesses, unstable functional status, complex psychosocial and financial situations, and other multilayered clinical issues trigger the need for this type of professional nurse. Advanced skills in clinical decision-making, communication, resource identification, referral, management, systems analysis, and cost analysis are essential for effective case management. The role of nurse case manager involves consulting with health-care providers; meeting with patients, family members, and other support systems; advocating for need-specific health and social services; planning for discharge; ensuring safe termination of services; facilitating shared decision-making; and recording appropriate documentation. As health-care delivery systems change, the number of nurse case managers for older people is expected to increase, particularly in community-based programs such as home-based services, adult day health programs, and respite and hospice services. For example, in the home health arena, the nurse is the ideal team leader; in that role, the nurse can coordinate the case and facilitate the completion of required documentation by interdisciplinary care-providers, institutions, physicians in group or private practice, and payors. With the growing trend toward managed care, the nurse in such a role might be called a case manager. Other administrative functions may also be a part of the geriatric nurse case manager's responsibility in the practice sites mentioned earlier.

HEALTH EDUCATION AND COUNSELING FOR PATIENTS AND FAMILIES

A major focus of the teaching and counseling done by gerontological and geriatric nurses relates to the implementation of treatment and management prescribed by health-care providers in acute care, home care, or community care. Teaching patients before they are discharged to home or another site of care helps to prepare the patient and the family. Education in ways of preventing disease, disability, and complications of existing chronic health conditions becomes increasingly necessary as the shift to community care expands. Teaching and counseling by these nurses take place across the continuum of care of the elderly. This function may be combined with direct patient care and case management functions.

ADMINISTRATION

Professional roles for administrative nurses include director of nursing services in a skilled-nursing facility and administrator in a variety of settings, such as home care, adult day health, respite care, hospice, and other community care programs for older adults. Some nurse entrepeneurs take on the challenge of administering small board-and-care homes. The legislative mandates of Medicare and Medicaid, the regulations, and the standards of care, to name a few, are complex bodies of information that the geriatric nurse administrator is able to translate into practice in order to support quality standards of care and ensure fiscal responsibility.

ADVOCACY AND PUBLIC POLICY DEVELOPMENT

Although nurse activism is found among all types of practitioners of nursing, some nurses in gerontology and geriatrics build careers in advocacy dedicated to shaping and changing public policy. Their expertise in the legislative process and their analyses of public policies may be applied to issues related to health-care access for the aging population and other relevant concerns. They find employment in governmental agencies, in the offices of public officials, with advocacy organizations, or with other entities oriented toward public policy issues and aging.

EDUCATION AND RESEARCH

With the increasing number of education programs in gerontological and geriatric nursing being taught in colleges and universities, the need for faculty members with doctorals and masters degrees in gerontology and geriatrics will continue to grow. Clinical specialists, nurse practitioners, and nursing administrators predominate in the faculties of many nursing schools across the country. Gerontological and geriatric nurses with doctoral degrees have teaching and research responsibilities. They are prepared to function as principal investigators in research projects and clinical trials and to establish research programs in gerontological and geriatric nursing science. Generating evidence-based nursing practice is an important commitment of these nurse researchers. Some of the domains of nursing research are sleep disturbances, agitation, pet therapy, family care-giving, falling behavior, sensory disabilities, and self-care deficits. The body of knowledge produced by their studies contributes to improving health-care for older people and to advancing the science of aging. In addition, these researchers create opportunities for other nurses to experience the research process as assistants, graduate students, or participants in the study.

CONCLUSION

Gerontological and geriatric nurses have a variety of roles and functions. With the trend toward downsizing and the shift to managed care programs, these roles and functions are being fused and structured in different ways. New personnel who deliver direct bedside care but have limited formal education and training are being introduced into the clinical arena. The challenge to nursing, in particular to nurses in gerontology and geriatrics, is to maintain the standards of health-care for older adults, especially those who are disempowered by chronic disability, socioeconomic status, racial or cultural factors, environmental situations, or technological illiteracy. Also, the aging of the baby boomers, a social and historical phenomenon, is already shifting the focus of health care from the cure model to the prevention model. It is clear that new expertise and more advance-practice nurses will be needed in this specialty.

SUGGESTED READINGS

For information on practice models in gerontological and geriatric nursing, contact the American Nurses Association at 600 Maryland Avenue, S.W., Suite 100 West, Washington, D.C. 20024-2571, and the Sigma Theta Tau International Honor Society at 550 West North Street, Indianapolis, IN 46202.

American Nurses Association. *Scope and Standards of Gerontological Nursing Practice.* Pub. #GE-14. Washington, D.C.: American Nurses Association Publishing; 1995.

American Nurses Association. *Nursing Social Policy Statement.* Pub. #NP-107. Washington, D.C.: American Nurses Association Publishing; 1995.

Burke M, Walsh M., eds. *Gerontologic Nursing: Wholistic Care of the Older Adult.* St. Louis: Mosby–Year Book; 1997.

Chenitz WC, Takano Stone J, Salisbury J, eds. *Clinical Gerontological Nursing: A Guide to Advance Practice.* Philadelphia: W.B. Saunders; 1991.

Dash K, Zarle N, O'Donnell L, Vince-Whitman C. *Discharge Planning for the Elderly: A Guide for Nurses.* New York: Springer Publishing; 1996.

Eliopoulos C. *Gerontological Nursing,* 4th ed. Philadelphia: J.B. Lippincott-Raven; 1997.

Matteson MA, McConnell E, Dill Linton A, eds. *Gerontological Nursing: Concepts and Practice,* 2nd ed. Philadelphia: W.B. Saunders; 1997. Co.

Mezey MD, Rauckhorst LH, Stokes SA. *Health Assessment of the Older Individual: Springer Series on Geriatric Nursing.* New York: Springer Publishing; 1993.

NANDA. *Nursing Diagnosis: Definitions and Classifications: 1997–98.* Philadelphia: North American Nursing Diagnosis Association; 1997.

Needham JF. *Gerontological Nursing: A Restorative Approach.* Albany, N.Y.: Delmar Publishers; 1993.

Staab AS, Fennell Lyles M, eds. *Manual of Geriatric Nursing.* London: Scott, Foresman; 1990.

Chapter **79**

Geriatric Occupational Therapy
Joe Cipriani, Ed.D., OTR/L

INTRODUCTION

Occupational therapy (OT) involves the therapeutic use of self-care, work, and leisure activities to increase independent function, enhance development, and prevent disability. The focus of the profession is on functional performance in daily activities.[1] Ultimately, the goal of occupational therapy is to affect functional performance in such a way as to improve quality of life. The occupational therapist, therefore, plays a vital role on the interdisciplinary rehabilitation team of the geriatric client.

Occupational therapists can be found performing a wide variety of roles in geriatric settings. These roles include direct service provision, administration, education, consultation, and research. Common practice settings include acute-care hospitals, rehabilitation centers, psychiatric centers, adult day care, extended-care facilities, and home health.

OCCUPATIONAL THERAPY ASSESSMENT

Assessment in occupational therapy is designed to provide the therapist, client, and rehabilitation team with critical information on the ability of the client to perform various daily activities. For example, assessment can provide direct information on the level of independence the client has while performing such activities. Typically, a standardized or nonstandardized global assessment is used initially, with more specific assessment employed as needed. An example of a global assessment tool is the Functional Independence Measure (FIM)[2] (Fig. 79–1).

One classification system for activities refers to the self-maintaining activities of daily living (ADLs) and the instrumental activities of daily living (IADLs).[3] The term "ADL" is often used to describe basic self-care activities such as bathing,

FIM™ instrument

Functional Independence Measure

L E V E L S	7 Complete Independence (Timely, Safely) 6 Modified Independence (Device)	**NO HELPER**
	Modified Dependence 5 Supervision (Subject = 100%+) 4 Minimal Assist (Subject = 75%+) 3 Moderate Assist (Subject = 50%+) **Complete Dependence** 2 Maximal Assist (Subject =25%+) 1 Total Assist (Subject = less than 25%)	**HELPER**

	ADMISSION	**DISCHARGE**	**FOLLOW-UP**
Self-Care A. Eating B Grooming C. Bathing D. Dressing - Upper Body E. Dressing - Lower Body F. Toileting			
Sphincter Control G. Bladder Management H. Bowel Management			
Transfers I. Bed, Chair, Wheelchair J. Toilet K. Tub, Shower			
Locomotion L. Walk/Wheelchair M. Stairs	W Walk C Wheelchair B Both	W Walk C Wheelchair B Both	W Walk C Wheelchair B Both
Motor Subtotal Score			
Communication N. Comprehension O. Expression	A Auditory V Visual B Both V Vocal N Nonvocal B Both	A Auditory V Visual B Both V Vocal N Nonvocal B Both	A Auditory V Visual B Both V Vocal N Nonvocal B Both
Social Cognition P. Social Interaction Q. Problem Solving R. Memory			
Cognitive Subtotal Score			
TOTAL FIM Score			

NOTE: Leave no blanks; enter 1 if patient not testable due to risk

Copyright © 1993 Uniform Data System for Medical Rehabilitation, a division of U B Foundation Activities, Inc.

Figure 79–1 Functional Independence Measure (FIM). Functional Independence Measure, Copyright © 1996 Uniform Data System for Medical Rehabilitation (UDSMR℠). All rights reserved. Reprinted with permission of UDSMR, University of Buffalo, 232 Carter Hall, 3435 Main Street, Buffalo, NY 14214.

dressing, and toileting. The term "IADL" is used to describe more complex tasks such as meal preparation and medical management. Other assessments used by occupational therapists can provide information on sensory and perceptual functioning, neuromusculoskeletal and motor skills, cognitive skills, play and leisure skills, and social role performance.

OCCUPATIONAL THERAPY INTERVENTION

An intervention plan is developed from information gathered during the assessment process. Ideally, the process of data collection is highly collaborative, with the rehabilitation team, client, family, significant others, and therapist all contributing valid information. In particular, the central role of the client in the development of long- and short-term occupational therapy goals is critical. As there is an ex-

traordinary diversity of needs among different geriatric clients, and a variety of settings in which occupational therapy is provided, a "typical" geriatric rehabilitation plan for occupational therapy cannot be described.

One method of describing occupational therapy service delivery is by service programs. Box 79–1 illustrates five basic service programs—prevention, development, remediation, environmental adjustment, and supportive/health maintenance.[4]

Although one program can be the main basis of intervention, often multiple programs are used to meet client needs. The following example illustrates how service programs are delivered to a client in geriatric rehabilitation:

M.C. is an 89-year-old female who lives alone in a high-rise apartment complex designed for older

---

Box 79–1

Programs

A. Prevention
1. Entering level: the individual is currently functioning in the normal community environment to his or her relative satisfaction.
2. Objectives:
a. To prevent developmental, physical, and psychosocial regression, such as in a pediatric program in a general hospital
b. To prevent biogenic disorders, such as in a program for older adults with arthritis to prevent deformity and injury to their hands
c. To prevent psychogenic disorders, such as in a program for older adults to prevent isolation and depression
d. To prevent sociogenic disorders, such as in a program to prevent elder abuse
3. Skills fostered and techniques used in program implementation:
a. Scheduling and performing the activities of daily living
b. Instruction in efficient home management
c. Recommendation for change of work situation or job change
d. Instruction in the application of behavior modification
e. Instruction in the development and use of adapted equipment to prevent deformity or injury
f. Participating in programmed activities designed to prevent loss of sensorimotor functions, such as range of motion, coordination, muscle strength, physical tolerance, sensory perception, and integration
g. Instruction in work simplification and energy conservation
h. Instruction in the elimination of architectural barriers and hazardous furniture and equipment
i. Participating in planned activities to make constructive use of leisure time
4. Objectives are accomplished through:
a. Individual or group lecture, discussion, and demonstration
b. Development of illustrated booklets, tapes, films, and computer-assisted instruction
c. Consultation with community organizations concerned with the health and general welfare of its citizens
5. Working assumption: loss of functional ability skill (disability) can be prevented or mitigated by active intervention of therapists to inform citizens of potential dangers to health.
6. Certified Occupational Therapy Assistant (COTA)/OTR relationship: the COTA may collaborate and consult with the OTR or may be supervised by the OTR when providing prevention programs.

Box continued on following page

Box 79-1 *Continued*

Programs

B. Development
1. Entering level: the individual has not learned or developed skills or abilities appropriate to age level or life task; the program includes individuals throughout the life cycle.
2. Objectives:
a. To increase sensorimotor functions to appropriate age level or life task
b. To increase cognitive skills to appropriate age level or life task
c. To increase psychosocial (behavioral) skills to appropriate age level or life task
d. To increase ability to perform self-maintenance activities
e. To increase ability to perform life tasks, productive or leisure
3. Skills and techniques:
a. Instruction in and opportunity to perform skills and activities on the individual's developmental level
b. Instruction in performing activities of daily living (ADLs) and instrumental activities of daily living (IADLs)
c. Participation in programmed activities designed to develop the concept of self, interpersonal relationships, group interaction skills
4. Objectives accomplished through:
a. Explanation and demonstration
b. Normal developmental sequencing
c. Repeated practice
d. Behavior modification
e. Simulation, role playing
f. Task analysis
5. Working assumption: developmental disability can be understood in terms of a deviation from normal performance in a profile of skills by measuring the level of current functioning against the level normally expected for the person's age and lifestyle.
6. COTA/OTR relationship: the COTA assists the OTR in the assessment phase and must be directly supervised by the OTR during the implementation/management phase of the developmental program.
C. Remediation
1. Entering level: the individual has lost skills and ability due to illness or trauma but can be expected to regain at least some skills and relearn some activities, often adaptive, through specialized treatment and training.
2. Objectives:
a. To increase independence in performing ADLs and IADLs
b. To increase sensorimotor functions
c. To improve home management skills
d. To improve work proficiency and task performance
e. To improve cognitive functions
f. To improve job-related skills
g. To improve psychosocial performance
h. To prevent deformity
i. To prevent the extension of disease or trauma pathology
3. Skills and techniques:
a. Increase sensorimotor functioning in such areas as range of motion, muscle strengthening, coordination, physical tolerance, sensory discrimination, and cognitive function through planned activities
b. Instruction in performing ADLs and IADLs
c. Instruction in selected aspects of home management
d. Instruction in specific work-related skills
e. Instruction in the development of leisure activities
f. Instruction in psychosocial skills
4. Objectives accomplished through:
a. Individual or group—specific, planned activities
b. Environmental control—structured or nonstructured
c. Development of home program
5. Working assumption: disability can be understood as an inability or partial loss of ability to perform tasks; for example, donning a shirt can be difficult for an older adult after a cerebrovascular accident (CVA), and the occupational therapist can facilitate the increased independence of the client in performing this task by instructing the client in adapted techniques for upper extremity dressing.
6. COTA/OTR relationship: the COTA must be directly supervised by the OTR during all phases of the remedial program.

Box 79–1 *Continued*

Programs

D. Environmental Adjustment
1. Entering level: individual change and recovery have achieved a level of function that can be expected to continue through the immediate future or a longer period. Further improvement in function can be expected if the external environment is changed to reduce barriers to performance.
2. Objectives:
a. To further improve sensorimotor functions
b. To further improve psychosocial functions
c. To further increase ability to perform ADLs
d. To further increase ability to perform work and leisure activities
3. Skills and techniques:
a. Modification of and instruction in use of adapted equipment
b. Construction of and instruction in use of splints
c. Elimination of architectural barriers
d. Reconstruction of physical surroundings
e. Instruction in use of prosthetic devices
4. Objectives accomplished by:
a. Task analysis
b. Explanation and demonstration
c. Repeated practice
d. Consultation
5. Working assumption: devices and environments can be developed and applied that will extend, enlarge, and facilitate the desired behavior (physical and mental) of the older adult.
6. COTA/OTR relationship: the COTA may collaborate and consult with the OTR or may be supervised by the OTR in providing an environmental adjustment program.
E. Supportive/health maintenance
1. Entering level: the individual is living in a semiprotected environment, such as a residential home or other institution. A program is usually adopted for a group of persons and is frequently called an activity program.
2. Objectives:
a. To maintain general sensorimotor functions in the members of the group
b. To maintain or increase the psychosocial skills of the group
c. To maintain or increase the ability to perform life tasks, including ADLs and IADLs
d. To maintain the cognitive functions of the group
3. Skills and techniques:
a. Instruction in activities designed to encourage individual interaction with others and with the nonhuman environment
b. Programmed activities designed to maintain physical and sensory functions within the individual's current level of functioning
c. Selection of and instruction in activities within the individual's ability that enable the person to make constructive use of available time
4. Objectives accomplished through:
a. Group and individual explanation, discussion, and demonstration
b. Task analysis of group and individual abilities and task requirements
c. Consultation with staff personnel
5. Working assumption: disability in terms of increased loss of function can be slowed or avoided by active intervention.
6. COTA/OTR relationship: the COTA may collaborate or consult with an OTR or may be supervised by an OTR in providing a supportive/health maintenance program.

Reed KL, Sanderson SN. *Concepts of Occupational Therapy*, 3rd ed. Baltimore: Williams & Wilkins; 1992.

adults. Her level of functioning in ADLs can best be described as independent except for tub transfer. Prior to her hospital stay, she was being visited by a home health aide three times weekly for assistance with bathing. Her primary diagnosis was severe osteoarthritis of her left hip, with a secondary diagnosis of rheumatoid arthritis affecting primarily her upper extremities, especially her hands. She had a successful elective left total hip replacement 1 week ago. She has now been admitted to the rehabilitation unit of the acute-care hospital for a 2-week stay. The discharge plan is to return home with support services as needed. She has no immediate family in the area.

The occupational therapist performed a series of assessments with M.C. Through consultation with the rehabilitation team and M.C., three short-term goals were prioritized for her stay. The first goal was to increase her level of independence for dressing, using adaptive devices, so that M.C. could perform the tasks safely, maintaining her weight-bearing and hip surgery precautions. Increasing the level of independence for bathing was not a priority. M.C. was satisfied with the services of the home health aide.

The second goal was to increase her level of independence for functional ambulation. For example, her occupational therapist instructed her on the safe use of the walker during meal preparation in the clinic kitchen, as M.C. prepared light meals by herself. The third goal was to increase the level of independence for toilet transfer, using adaptive equipment such as a commode chair minus bucket placed over a regular toilet. This adaptation provided a secure base to transfer to and from the toilet while maintaining hip precautions. The occupational therapist also instructed M.C. on techniques of joint protection for her upper extremities and adapted an embroidery stand so M.C. could pursue her favorite hobby with less pain, making embroidered items for the holidays for her nieces. Finally, a home evaluation was performed to assess M.C.'s performance of daily activities and safety within her familiar environment. Recommendations such as removing throw rugs, arrangement of small appliances to table height, and proper lighting in the bathroom at night were made. In M.C.'s case, the combined use of the service programs of prevention, remediation, and environmental adjustment provided the most effective delivery of occupational therapy.

CONCLUSION

The occupational therapist is a key member of the geriatric rehabilitation team. The components of occupational therapy programs address the issues of prevention, skill or ability development, remediation, environmental adjustment, and supportive/health maintenance. Like all members of the geriatric rehabilitation team, occupational therapists and assistants work in a wide variety of settings to meet the needs of patients.

REFERENCES

1. Hasselkus Risteen B. Introduction to adult and older adult populations. In: Neistadt ME, Crepeau EB, eds. *Willard and Spackman's Occupational Therapy,* 9th ed. Philadelphia: J.B. Lippincott; 1997.
2. *Uniform Data System for Medical Rehabilitation: Guide for the Uniform Data Set for Medical Rehabilitation (Adult FIM).* Buffalo, N.Y.: UB Foundation Activities; 1993.
3. Law M. Evaluating activities of daily living: directions for the future. *Am J Occup Ther* 1993: 47:233.
4. Reed KL, Sanderson SN. *Concepts of Occupational Therapy,* 3rd ed. Baltimore: Williams & Wilkins; 1992.

SUGGESTED READINGS

American Occupational Therapy Association. Entry-level role delineation for registered occupational therapists (OTRs) and certified occupational therapy assistants (COTAs). In: *American Occupational Therapy Association: Reference Manual of the Official Documents of the American Occupational Therapy Association,* 6th ed. Washington, D.C.: American Occupational Therapy Association; 1995.

Crabtree J, Lawson O, Pedretti L, Stevens-Ratchford RG. *The Role of Occupational Therapy with the Elderly (ROTE): Revision.* Washington, D.C.: American Occupational Therapy Association; 1996.

Kiernat JM. *Occupational Therapy and the Older Adult.* Gaithersburg, Md.: Aspen Publishers; 1991.

Rogers JC. Geriatric psychiatry. In: Hopkins HL, Smith HD, eds. *Willard and Spackman's Occupational Therapy,* 8th ed. Philadelphia: J.B. Lippincott; 1993.

Chapter 80

Geriatric Physical Therapy
Jill Johnson, M.S., P.T.

INTRODUCTION

Physical therapy care is an important component of quality geriatric rehabilitation. An understanding of the referral mechanism and the potential assessments and interventions will enable other members of the geriatric rehabilitation team to use effectively the services of the physical therapy profession.

Physical therapists (PTs) are professionals who are involved in the examination, evaluation, treatment, and prevention of neuromuscular, musculoskeletal, cardiovascular, and pulmonary disorders that produce movement impairments, disabilities, and functional limitations.[1] A PT holds an undergraduate or graduate degree in physical therapy from a college or university program accredited by the American Physical Therapy Association (APTA) and is licensed by the state to practice after passing an examination. A physical therapist assistant (PTA) holds an associate degree in physical therapy from a college program accredited by the APTA and is licensed in many but not all states through examination. PTAs are educated to carry out many PT treatment activities, they cannot evaluate, reevaluate, or determine a plan of care. In some states, the PTA may not treat patients unless the PT is available to supervise and is physically on the premises where the treatment is rendered. In other states, the PTA may treat the patient without the PT's being present, but regularly scheduled supervisory visits and phone consultations are required.

Geriatric physical therapy has been identified as a physical therapy specialization in order to acknowledge the advanced-level skills of physical therapists who seek to address the unique medical and functional problems of older persons.[2] The first therapists were board-certified in geriatric physical therapy in 1992. Geriatric physical therapists can be found in multiple settings, including acute-care hospitals, rehabilitation centers, skilled nursing facilities, outpatient clinics, home health agencies, and hospice settings.

REFERRALS TO PHYSICAL THERAPY

How do health-care practitioners who work with the geriatric population know when it is appropriate to refer patients to physical therapy? Box 80–1 is a useful guide to referral to PT. These key indicators can be assessed by reading the patient's history, observing the patient's mobility, performing a functional evaluation, or interviewing the patient or care-giver.

Referral patterns to physical therapy during and after hospitalization have been studied in elderly patients hospitalized for general medical illness.[3] In this study patients were functioning at an independent level prior to hospitalization, with 95% independent in walking and 94% independent in transfers from a bed to a chair. At discharge, a high percentage of study patients were found to require assistance in walking (51%) and transfers (21%). Almost half of those patients who were dependent in either walking or transfer ability at discharge did not receive PT during hospitalization. Interestingly, those patients who participated in PT in the hospital

---

Box 80–1

Possible Indications for

Physical Therapy Referral

- The patient has had a recent fall or has a history of falls.
- The patient has strength or range-of-motion deficits.
- The patient needs a new assistive device for ambulation.
- The patient has musculoskeletal pain.
- The patient has difficulties with transfers and/or requires assistance.
- The patient has orthotic or prosthetic needs.
- The patient has poor balance.
- The patient ambulates very slowly.
- The patient is bedbound.
- The patient needs adaptive equipment to enhance safety in the home.

---

were significantly ($p < .05$) more likely to receive postdischarge PT. These results are important for several reasons:

1. It is possible that elderly medical patients are developing functional disabilities that are not being recognized by hospital staff.

2. Since the implementation of the Medicare Prospective Payment System, older Medicare patients are being discharged from the hospital quickly, which increases the likelihood that patients will not be referred to physical therapy.

3. The use of PT in the hospital served as a marker for the need for additional services after discharge.

Although this study did not analyze patient outcomes, it does point out that hospital staff should be more aware of the risk of functional decline faced by elderly patients and of the potential benefits of PT evaluation. It was suggested that on entry to the hospital, PT referrals be considered for patients who report a history of falls, mobility and transfer disabilities, or the need for an assistive device for walking prior to admission. In addition, during hospitalization, as part of routine hospital practice, all patients should be observed by the nursing staff for their ability to get out of bed and walk down a hallway. This approach to functional assessment could be accomplished with little effort or expense and would provide the information on which to base decisions to order PT during and after hospitalization.

ASSESSMENT OF THE GERIATRIC PATIENT

Once referred to PT, what are the unique services the patient will receive from the physical therapist? The assessment of a patient with impairments, functional limitations, disabilities, or other health-related conditions by a physical therapist includes but is not limited to obtaining the patient's history and performing a systems review and various tests and measurements. In some settings, physical therapists work as members of a geriatric assessment team and may be involved in routine screening of patients.

The following case study presents the details of a PT exam:

Mrs. W., a 96-year-old female, was referred to a home care agency for physical therapy following hospitalization for a fall in which she sustained a contusion of the right shoulder. A shoulder fracture was ruled out by x-rays, but Mrs. W. was complaining of pain and problems with shoulder movement, and she was having difficulty with self-care. She had a history of falls, was hard of hearing, and was legally blind. The patient's only medications were calcium tablets and Tylenol. She was discharged to the home of her 71-year-old daughter who had rheumatoid arthritis.

The geriatric physical therapist should look at function and not focus on impairment and range-of-motion measurements: What is the patient having difficulty doing that she could previously do? By using the systems approach (the systems are the cardiopulmonary, neural, integumentary, endocrine, musculoskeletal, and neuromuscular systems) the geriatric physical therapist will attempt to determine, whenever possible, which problem is age-related, which is pathology, and which is caused by disuse. In geriatrics, a one-system approach is rarely possible; comorbidity is the norm. Mrs. W.'s pre-hospitalization functional status had been fairly independent, as she had lived alone in a subsidized apartment complex for the elderly where meals were provided. Therefore, her potential for rehabilitation was good. Although she was legally blind, she had lived in her apartment for 18 years and was familiar enough with her environment that she could function quite well.

Multiple exams are utilized by physical therapists (Box 80–2), and choosing the appropriate

exam for the patient's condition is an important skill of a geriatric physical therapist. In this case, gait and balance, posture, joint integrity and mobility, range of motion, environment, cognition, self-care, and home management (including ADLs and IADLs) were assessed during the first few visits.

GOAL-SETTING AND INTERVENTIONS

Functional goals that are established with the patient and family are essential in developing the treatment intervention. Mrs. W.'s long-term goal was to return to her apartment. To meet this goal, several short-term goals were set:

- The patient will be able to transfer independently to a toilet or bedside commode and will be able to toilet herself independently.
- The patient will be able to have enough shoulder range of motion to dress herself, feed herself, and reach her dishes in the cupboard.
- The patient will have enough upper-body strength to lift a quart of milk, pour water from a tea kettle, make her bed, and do her laundry.
- The patient will be able to ambulate independently, using a wheeled walker, to the dining room in her apartment complex (a distance of 350 feet) with a target heart rate of between 102 and 110 beats per minute.

The target heart rate was based on the Karvonen formula[4] which in this case calculated the intensity of exercise between 60% and 79% of Mrs. W.'s target heart rate range or functional capacity. See Box 42–2 for the same formula for a 70-year-old person. The following formula was used:

Maximum heart rate (MHR) =	220
Age =	−96
	124
Subtract resting heart rate (RHR)	−70
	54
Multiply by intensity	
54 × 75% =	40
or	
54 × 60% =	32
Add back RHR 40	32
+70	+70
Target heart rate at 75% = 110 at 65% = 102	

To meet the functional goals, the intervention was focused on improving Mrs. W.'s impairments (decreased range of motion, strength, and balance, and unstable gait) in order to expand function. The program was tailored to the individual's needs and

Box 80–2

Examinations Provided by

Physical Therapists[a]

- Aerobic capacity or endurance
- Anthropometric characteristics
- Arousal, mentation, and cognition
- Assistive, adaptive, supportive, and protective devices
- Community or work reintegration (including instrumental activities of daily living)
- Cranial nerve integrity
- Environmental, home, or work barriers
- Ergonomics or body mechanics
- Gait and balance
- Integumentary integrity
- Joint integrity and mobility
- Motor function and coordination
- Muscle performance (including strength, power, and endurance)
- Neuromotor development and sensory integration
- Orthotic requirements
- Pain
- Posture
- Prosthetics
- Range of motion (including muscle length and flexibility)
- Reflex integrity
- Self-care and home management (including activities of daily living and instrumental activities of daily living)
- Sensory integrity (including proprioception and kinesthesia)
- Ventilation, respiration, and circulation

[a]From Guide to physical therapist practice. *Phys Ther* 1997; 77:1177–1466.

Table 80–1 Case Study Evaluation Findings and Interventions

Evaluation Findings	Interventions
Tinetti balance score = 16/26 (unable to reach or bend without losing balance, unable to turn without walker)	Instruction in balance exercises with support of the kitchen sink
Inability to perform toilet transfer independently	Order an elevated toilet seat with rails Instruct in a strengthening and coordination program Provide transfer training
Inability to walk unassisted because of decreased balance and decreased orientation to new apartment	Order wheeled walker Provide gait training Remove clutter and throw rugs
Decreased range of motion and strength of right shoulder, inability to dress independently, prepare meals, or do household tasks	Progress from passive range of motion to active/assisted to active exercises with added resistance

In addition to the above interventions, the physical therapist identified the need for other services. Referrals were obtained so that an occupational therapist could arrange for Mrs. W. to have adaptive equipment and ADL training and for the social work department to set up the services that would be necessary for Mrs. W. to return to her apartment. Instructions were given to the daughter to monitor the home exercise program and to communicate with other team members on a regular basis. Community services such as the Services for the Blind were also consulted.

Geriatric patients, in particular, benefit from a team approach. Because they are so commonly affected by a variety of interacting problems, input from several disciplines is essential. Team meetings can be an efficient way to discuss the many problems of an elderly client and to develop goals for that client based on each member's input. In the case of Mrs. W., her goal of returning to her own home required interventions by an RN, a PT, an OT, a social worker, and other family members.

tolerance. Table 80–1 contains some of the findings from Mrs. W.'s physical therapy assessment and shows how these findings were addressed in her treatment plan, based on the established goals.

CONCLUSION

The geriatric population is unique in its wide variation from individual to individual in the effects of both aging and disease processes. Some of the concerns that can affect older adults, such as dietary deficiencies, psychosocial problems, and limited finances may fall outside the realm of physical therapy, but they still affect the treatment provided by the therapist. Therefore, the team approach is most beneficial. Without support and conferencing with other team members, attainment of the goals of physical therapy may be hampered or the duration of rehabilitation lengthened.

In geriatric physical therapy, the therapist encounters a wide spectrum of individuals, ranging from those who require maximum assistance to those who function independently but require outpatient or group treatment. Geriatric rehabilitation offers a challenge to the talent and creativity of everyone involved.

REFERENCES

1. Guide to physical therapist practice, part I: a description of patient management: part II: preferred practice patterns. *Phys Ther* 1997; 77:1175–1650.
2. Geriatric Specialty Council, ed. *Geriatric Physical Therapy Specialty Competencies.* Alexandria, VA: 1990. [approved by the American Board of Physical Therapy Specialties, June 1990].
3. Johnson JH, Sager MA, Hirn G, Dunham NC. Referral patterns to physical therapy in elderly hospitalized for acute medical illness. *Phys Occup Ther Geriatr* 1994; 12:1–12.
4. Rimmer JH. *Fitness and Rehabilitation Programs for Special Populations.* Dubuque, IA: Wm. C. Brown Communications; 1994.

Chapter 81*

Geriatric Speech Pathologist

Colleen Reynolds, Director,
Speech/Dysphagia Department
Shelley Slott, Senior Speech Pathologist

INTRODUCTION

Speech language pathologists are highly skilled professionals who provide evaluation and treatment of adult and pediatric speech, language, and cognitive disorders across the continuum of care. The speech pathologist functions as an integral part of the rehabilitation team and facilitates the delivery of services that maximize the patient's functional inde-

pendence. The speech language pathologist's role is a crucial one that has major quality-of-life implications. Restoring the ability to think and to communicate can mean the difference between isolation and a return to meaningful life. Strokes, which occur with increasing frequency after middle age, are a common cause of communication disorders.

COMMUNICATION DISORDERS

The basic types of communication disorders include the following:

Left hemispheric damage often results in the loss of receptive language (understanding what is heard or read) or the loss of expressive language (the ability to convey thoughts, needs, and wants through speech, writing, gestures, or body language), or both. This is referred to as aphasia. The specific problem is determined by the location and severity of the brain damage. Language deficits can lead to frustration. In addition, the potential motor disruption resulting in right hemiplegia can significantly decrease the patient's mobility and independence.

Right hemispheric damage often results in reduced speech intelligibility due to muscle weakness and incoordination (dysarthria), impulsivity, flattened emotional affect, lability, visual and perceptual disorders, and pragmatic deficits. Receptive language deficits can be characterized by auditory processing problems and difficulty understanding high-level abstract language. Expressive language deficits may include verbosity and tangentiality, reflecting decreased content of structurally correct utterances. However, one must recognize that verbal communication deficits may be found in persons with hearing impairments.

Apraxia is a motor planning deficit characterized by the inability to purposely move parts of the body. There are many kinds of apraxia; however, the speech language pathologist typically deals with apraxia of the oral-motor structures, which include the following:

- oral apraxia, in which the patient cannot volitionally move his or her mouth in various ways, such as whistling, blowing, or moving the lips or tongue, and
- verbal apraxia, in which the tongue and lips and the vocal cords are unable to work together to form sounds or parts of words on command.

Dysarthria is a motor speech disorder that results from weakness, paralysis, or incoordination and causes problems that affect breathing and respiration, the ability to combine sounds to form audible and understandable words, and the pitch of the voice. There are many different types of dysarthria; it can result from neurological causes such as stroke and from progressive degenerative diseases, such as Parkinson's disease, amyotrophic lateral sclerosis, and multiple sclerosis. A speech pathologist can make an accurate diagnosis and provide specific management techniques such as teaching the patient exercises to strengthen weak muscles and providing alternative means of communicating such as a blackboard so that the patient is able to express needs and wants.

COGNITIVE DISORDERS

The speech/language pathologist also works to improve each patient's cognitive function. A patient with cognitive dysfunction can have difficulty thinking, reasoning, learning, and remembering. Deficits may range from mild to severe and may include interference with one or more of the following abilities:

Attention deficit results in the inability to focus on and be aware of stimuli; the patient has difficulty establishing, shifting, and maintaining focus; it can be accompanied by the inability to focus in the presence of relatively minor distractions.

Perception deficit results in the inability to recognize or identify meaningful symbols or to use the visual and auditory senses to process information about the environment. Deficits in the various areas of perception may make it difficult for the patient to recognize where he or she is, or to know how to get around, or to understand what is being said.

Memory deficit results in the inability to store and to recall information. Memory is divided into immediate, short-term, and long-term. A person with immediate memory deficits may not be able to repeat a series of numbers or words just presented; a person with short-term deficits may be unable to recall happenings from day to day or to recall information presented earlier the same day; and a patient with long-term memory deficits is unable to recall information from the past such as biographic information.

Problem-solving, organizing, and sequencing deficits result in the inability to isolate causes and effects, to determine consequences of actions, and to develop potential solutions. Problem-solving deficits become apparent as the patient attempts to become independent.

Reasoning, judging, and safety-awareness deficits result in the inability to plan, organize, or solve problems. The patient is unaware of the deficit and is prone to impulsivity and misinterpretations that result in decreased safety awareness and the inability to make appropriate decisions. This is one of the most difficult cognitive areas to remediate because problem-solving, reasoning, and making judgments are dependent on a combination of previously habituated learning strategies and skills. A person with these deficits may find it difficult to live independently and may require some level of supervision.

CONCLUSION

The speech/language pathologist's role, as a member of the rehabilitation team, is multifaceted. Diagnosis and treatment for a wide variety of communicative and cognitive disorders are highly individualized. The focus of rehabilitation is on improving intellectual, emotional, and behavioral capacities while assisting the patient and the family with any adjustments that may be required as a result of the patient's impaired language abilities and cognition.

SUGGESTED READINGS

American Speech and Hearing Association Committee on Communication Problems of the Aging. The roles of speech-language pathologists and audiologists working with older persons. *ASHA* 1988a; 30:80–84.

Kazandjian M. Communication impairments associated with traumatic brain injury in the older adult. In: Clark LW, ed. *Communication Disorders of the Older Adult; A Practical Handbook for Health Care Professionals.* New York: Hunter/Mount Sinai Geriatric Center; 1993.

Ripich D, ed. *Handbook of Geriatric Communication Disorders.* Austin, Tex.: PRO-ED; 1991.

Wheeler D. Communication and swallowing problems in the frail older person. *Top Geriatr Rehabil* 1995; 11:11–23.

Chapter **82**

Geriatric Social Worker
Patrick McDonald, M.S.W.

INTRODUCTION

Older adults are faced with a long series of losses and accommodations during the process of aging. This fact is brought home forcefully to the geriatric rehabilitation patient.

Apart from the physical damage caused by stroke, trauma, and other disabling conditions, the adjustment to loss, psychologically and practically, may be the most difficult problem the patient and family must face.

The social worker helps aging persons deal with this process in two ways: by counseling them and by planning and coordinating in-home services with them.

THE PATIENT AND THE FAMILY

The patient should be encouraged, but not forced, to deal with his or her depression, fears, denial, and all the other emotions attendant on significant change. The patient must be helped to see that rehabilitation is a process that includes therapy, counseling, and planning for the future.

The initial interview should focus on the patient's goal of returning home and on plans for that return (see Fig. 82–1).

Follow-up visits will begin to put the pieces of this plan together. Interviews with the patient and family will assure everyone of the practicality of

the plan and will ensure accurate communication among all involved.

The social worker's visits to the gym will provide first-hand knowledge of the patient's progress and abilities. A private interview with the patient's family or other care-givers will allow them to express their own emotional reactions to this experience. Oftentimes, their goals and expectations differ from those of the patient.

An elderly spouse may question his or her ability to provide adequate care for the patient at home. An employed spouse or child may be faced with very difficult choices upon the patient's return to the home.

Regular contact between the social worker and the patient and family prepares them for the rehabilitation experience, allows for ongoing assessment of the patient's progress, and reassures them that the discharge plan is workable. There may be occasions when the family does not desire the patient's return

---

SOCIAL WORK ASSESSMENT FORM

Room #: _____ Admission date: _____

Name: _____ Age: _____ D.O.B. _____

Address: _____ Hospital admitted from: _____

_____ Insurance info: _____

_____

Phone: _____ Physician: _____

Rehab DX: _____ Other DX: _____

Employment status: _____ Employer: _____

Income source (s): _____ Work phone: _____

FAMILY/CARE-GIVER

Marital status: M S D W Sep.   Spouse name: _____

Others in household: Name: _____ Age: _____ Emp. _____

Other contact: Name: _____ Phone: _____

Address: _____

Name: _____ Phone: _____

HOME/ENVIRONMENT

Type of home: Own: _____ Rent: _____ No. of Floors: _____ No. of Steps: _____

Primary entry: _____ No. of Steps: _____ Handrails: _____

Bedroom location: _____ Bath location: _____ Handrails: _____

Mental status and emotional reaction: _____

Alert? _____ Oriented? _____ Depressed? _____

Equipment at home: _____ Anticipated equipment needs: _____

Home health agency? _____ Other community services? _____

Patient family goals: _____

Plan: _____ Comments: _____

_____   _____

_____   _____

Social worker: _____ Date: _____

Figure 82–1

home; then contact with the social worker helps to prepare the family for the patient's discharge and perhaps helps to encourage them. The information gleaned by the social worker is essential for the rehabilitation team so it can prepare and evaluate the individual's treatment plan.

The Home

A home visit by members of the rehabilitation team allows family members to be interviewed in a familiar, nonthreatening setting. It allows the therapists to evaluate for barriers and adaptations that may be needed.

Occasionally, a home may be dangerous or inappropriate for a patient's return. Extreme clutter, filth, lack of utilities, or disrepair may require community intervention. The social worker will have to refer these rare situations to the Protective Service Unit of the Area Agency on Aging, or some other appropriate agency.

A first-hand view of the home environment helps the worker prepare the family for the patient's return and also helps to coordinate community services for the patient's return home.

Durable Medical Equipment

Most rehabilitation patients require the use of assistive devices, if only for a short time. Ordering durable medical equipment (DME) in a managed care climate requires knowledge of preferred provider relations and limits of coverage. Patients and families rely on social workers for this knowledge.

Basic items such as canes, walkers, and wheelchairs are covered by most insurance carriers for appropriate patients. Larger items such as lifts, passive-motion units, and even hospital beds are less readily available and may not be covered at all. Items like lift chairs or so-called stair glides are rarely, if ever, covered by insurance. Some DME suppliers have used lift chairs and stair glides as well as other items available at reduced cost.

Some patients injured under workers' compensation or automobile plans may be covered for special items such as lifts. Each individual has to be reviewed separately.

Some rehabilitation facilities or agencies for the handicapped may employ an equipment adaptor. This professional person modifies and customizes medical equipment to individual needs. This can be a very helpful service for the geriatric patient.

HOME HEALTH

Medicare and most major insurance plans cover rehabilitative and nursing services in the home after the patient has been discharged. If a skilled service (a PT or an RN) is ordered for home, a nurse's aide may be covered for personal care such as bathing. As with DME, many carriers are now requiring the use of preferred providers for home health services.

It should be noted that rural areas are often underserved by home health rehabilitative services. This can delay the initiation of care in the home.

Many people are under the impression that Medicare or other insurance companies provide for private nurses or aides in a patient's home. Medicare has never covered this service and most other plans have long since discontinued such benefits. There are many agencies that offer this help for a fee.

Community Services

The following are useful community services that have traditionally helped older people to remain at home; however, as public funds for these programs have dwindled, agencies have initiated fee-for-service arrangements. This has resulted in shorter waiting lists and faster start-up for services. Of course, it has also resulted in increased costs to the older consumer.

Area Agency on Aging   An Area Agency on Aging (AAA) is a local, public agency funded by federal and state monies; the agencies were created to provide support for older people in their homes. Some of the services offered include homemakers, personal care aides, friendly visitors, Meals on Wheels, and so forth. A means test determines eligibility, and the services are generally limited to 1 or 2 hours a week. Some AAA offer personal attendant care or Title XX (LAMP II or Options) programs designed to help the most physically challenged individuals stay at home. Agencies on Aging are generally run by county governments. Phone numbers and addresses can be found in the blue pages of the telephone book.

Chore   Chore services may be available through AAA or another public agency. This useful program can help to build ramps, attach handrails, or provide other minor adaptations. All materials are purchased by the individual receiving the service. Contact the Area Agency on Aging for more information.

Meals on Wheels   Perhaps the best known service, Meals on Wheels (MOW), provides a full meal for the homebound individual 5 days a week or more. There is generally a fee charged for this service. This agency is also listed in the blue pages of the telephone book.

Transportation   Adequate transportation services are the most common need of the elderly, especially for the geriatric rehabilitation patient. Most communities offer some type of subsidized transportation for eligible individuals. These programs function as a cross between a bus and a taxi. The vehicles, usually modified vans, travel specified routes but require advance notification of appointments.

Vans equipped with wheelchair lifts are available, but extra notice may have to be given. Ambulance transport for routine medical appointments is rarely covered by insurance and is very expensive. Many ambulance providers offer wheelchair van services at more reasonable rates.

PLACEMENT

Despite the best efforts of the professionals and the fervent hopes of all, the goal of returning home may not be possible for all patients. Inadequate progress in therapy or insufficient support at home may make nursing home placement the only appropriate course of action.

The social worker has to be sensitive to feelings of guilt, abandonment, and hopelessness as he or she guides the patient and family through the application process. Furthermore, if the realities of modern health care make the patient's first choice of a facility unachievable, the social worker must be frank and straightforward in dealing with placement issues. At all times, lines of communication must be kept open to make the patient's transition as smooth as possible.

CONCLUSION

The social worker's counseling skills help patients and their families to deal with their emotional reactions to infirmity, aging, and rehabilitation. The social worker's knowledge of community resources aids patients and their families in practical preparation for their future. These are the contributions of the social worker to the rehabilitation team as it helps the older patient reach the goals of maximum function and independence.

SUGGESTED READING

Gallo JJ, Reichel W, Andersen LM. *Handbook of Geriatric Assessment,* 2nd ed. Gaithersburg, Md.: Aspen Publishers; 1995.

INDEX

Page numbers in *italics* refer to figures;
page numbers followed by b refer to text in boxes;
page numbers followed by t refer to tables.

A

I